CW00938143

Medical Acupuncture

For Churchill Livingstone:

Commissioning editor: Inta Ozols
Project manager: Valerie Burgess
Project development editor: Valerie Bain
Design direction: Judith Wright
Project controller: Derek Robertson
Copy editor: Christine Wyard
Indexer: Elizabeth Ball
Promotions manager: Hilary Brown

Medical Acupuncture

A Western scientific approach

Edited by

Jacqueline Filshie MBBS FRCA
Consultant Anaesthetist, The Royal Marsden NHS Trust, Sutton, Surrey, UK
Honorary Senior Lecturer, Institute of Cancer Research, Sutton, Surrey, UK

Adrian White MA BM BCh LicAc
Research Fellow, Department of Complementary Medicine, University of Exeter, Exeter, UK

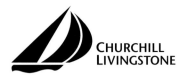
CHURCHILL
LIVINGSTONE

EDINBURGH LONDON NEW YORK PHILADELPHIA SAN FRANCISCO SYDNEY TORONTO 1998

CHURCHILL LIVINGSTONE
An imprint of Harcourt Publishers Limited

© Harcourt Brace and Company Limited 1998
© A new system of acupuncture – Felix Mann

 is a registered trademark of Harcourt Publishers Limited

All rights reserved. No part of this publication may be
reproduced, stored in a retrieval system, or transmitted in
any form or by any means, electronic, mechanical,
photocopying, recording or otherwise, without either the
prior permission of the publishers (Harcourt Publishers
Limited, Robert Stevenson House, 1-3 Baxter's Place,
Leith Walk, Edinburgh EH1 3AF), or a licence permitting
restricted copying in the United Kingdom issued by the
Copyright Licensing Agency Ltd, 90 Tottenham Court Road,
London W1P 0LP.

First edition 1998
 Reprinted 1998
 Reprinted 2001

ISBN 0 443 04976 9

British Library Cataloguing in Publication Data
A catalogue record for this book is available from the British
Library

Library of Congress Cataloging in Publication Data
A catalog record for this book is available from the Library of
Congress

Note
Medical knowledge is constantly changing. As new
information becomes available, changes in treatment,
procedures, equipment and the use of drugs become
necessary. The editors / authors / contributors and the
publishers have, as far as it is possible, taken care to ensure
that the information given in this text is accurate and up to
date. However, readers are strongly advised to confirm that
information, especially with regard to drug usage, complies
with the latest legislation and standards of practice.

Neither the publishers nor the author will be liable for any
loss or damage of any nature occasioned to or suffered by any
person acting or refraining from acting as a result of reliance
on the material contained in this publication.

The
publisher's
policy is to use
**paper manufactured
from sustainable forests**

Printed in China by RDC Group Limited
N/03

Contents

Contributors

Peter Baldry MBi FRCP
Emeritus Consultant Physician,
Ashford Hospital, London, UK

Robert Bekkering MD
Lecturer and former President of NAAV
(Dutch Medical Acupuncture Society),
Almere, The Netherlands

François Beyens MD
Medical Acupuncturist, Brussels, Belgium,
General Secretary of the International Council
of Medical Acupuncture and Related
Techniques

David Bowsher MA MD PhD FRCPEd FRCPath
Director of Research, Pain Research Institute,
Walton Hospital, Liverpool, UK

Robert van Bussel MD
Lecturer and former President of NAAV
(Dutch Medical Acupuncture Society),
Amsterdam, The Netherlands

A. Virginia Camp BSc MB ChB FRCP
Consultant in Rheumatology and
Rehabilitation Medicine,
St Mary's Hospital, Kettering, UK

Anthony Campbell MRCP (UK)
Consultant Physician, Royal London
Homoeopathic Hospital, London, UK

Jacqueline Filshie MBBS FRCA
Consultant Anaesthetist, The Royal Marsden
NHS Trust, Sutton, Surrey; Honorary Senior
Lecturer, Institute of Cancer Research, Sutton,
Surrey, UK

C. Chan Gunn MD FAAC FICAE
Director, Gunn Pain Clinic, and President of the
Institute for the Study and Treatment of Pain,
Vancouver, Canada; Honorary Fellow,
Peterhouse, Cambridge University, Cambridge,
UK; Clinical Professor, Multidisciplinary Pain
Center, University of Washington, Seattle, USA

Simon Hayhoe
Anaesthetist, Colchester District
General Hospital, Essex, UK

Joan Hester MBBS FRCA
Consultant in Pain Management and
Anaesthesia, Eastbourne NHS Trust,
Eastbourne, UK

George T. Lewith DM MRCP MRCGP
Honorary Visiting Clinical Senior Lecturer,
Southampton University and Partner, Centre for
the Study of Complementary Medicine,
Southampton, UK

Alexander J. R. Macdonald MB BS DLO
General Practitioner, Bristol, UK

Christine McMillan MMedSc BSc MCSP
Senior Physiotherapist, Department of
Rehabilitation Medicine, Royal Victoria
Hospital, Belfast, UK

Felix Mann MB BChir(Camb) LMCC
Private Practitioner/Lecturer in Acupuncture,
London, UK

Paul Marcus MD DipMedAc FFPM
Consulting Medical Acupuncture Practitioner,
Whitley, Cheshire, UK

Hagan Rampes BSc MB ChB MRCPsych LicAc
Senior Registrar, South Kensington and Chelsea
Mental Health Centre, Chelsea and Westminster
Hospital, London, UK

John W Thompson MB BS PhD FRCP
Honorary Physician and Honorary Consultant
in Medical Studies, St Oswald's Hospice,
Newcastle; Emeritus Professor of Pharmacology,
University of Newcastle; Emeritus Consultant
Clinical Pharmacologist, Newcastle Health
Authority, Newcastle upon Tyne, UK

Charles Vincent MPhil PhD
Senior Lecturer in Psychology,
University College London,
London, UK

Adrian White MA BM BCh LicAc
Research Fellow, Department of
Complementary Medicine, University of Exeter,
Exeter, UK

Acknowledgements

The editors are very grateful to each of the authors, who have contributed so generously with their time, their effort and their expertise. We are particularly indebted to Simon Hayhoe, our consulting editor, for his considerable expert help and advice throughout the preparation and realization of this book. We should also like to acknowledge our deep debt of gratitude to Julia Jeffery for her outstanding, long-suffering and dedicated secretarial support. Also to Barry Jenkins for his considerable contribution.

'We should let a hundred flowers blossom
and a hundred schools of thought contend,
but in a scientific manner'

Wong L P 1988 Successful treatment of paralysis of the lower extremity with acupuncture.
American Journal of Acupuncture 16:329–344

Introduction

SECTION CONTENTS

1

Introduction

Jacqueline Filshie
Adrian White

Our intention in putting this book together was to provide a scientifically based view of the place of acupuncture within modern medicine at the end of the twentieth-century. Experts were invited to contribute chapters on their own particular areas of interest using as much objective detail as possible. Much of the clinical material here is still based on experience rather than hard evidence, but we have purposely chosen authors who approach acupuncture scientifically, using their knowledge of neurophysiology but still respecting its traditional Chinese medical origins.

Acupuncture originated in China in prehistory and the theories of meridians and energy flow evolved by painstaking observation against a background of Chinese philosophy. Traditional theory and philosophical concepts are immensely charming and attractive. In addition to this instinctive appeal, we owe a considerable debt to all keen observers in the history of acupuncture for the valuable empirical knowledge that has been passed down the generations.

However, it seems that even experienced traditional practitioners find conflicting results when using traditional methods such as pulse (Vincent 1992) and tongue diagnosis. The traditional explanations of acupuncture are no longer the only available option: for many practitioners, both in the West and in China, there is every reason to believe that mechanisms of acupuncture will eventually be explained by science.

Acupuncture owes much of its respectability to the discovery that it releases opioid peptides

(Clement-Jones et al 1979, 1980). This may be regarded as the beginning of the 'Age of Enlightenment' of the ancient art. Current neurophysiological and neuroanatomical evidence is considered in detail in Chapter 6, but it is worth remembering that our knowledge is still likely to be incomplete.

Many diseases appear to be multifactorial, the end result of several harmful influences on a patient who may have a genetic predisposition to that condition. One of the common insults is psychological stress in one form or another. It seems possible that acupuncture can work in a variety of ways by reducing stress, by altering autonomic tone, by psychoneuroimmunomodulation, by influencing the hypothalamus, and by releasing neuropeptides with functions that we are still only beginning to understand. This multiplicity of mechanisms is one likely reason why it has proved so difficult to unravel simple and clear-cut explanations for acupuncture.

THE NEED FOR CLINICAL EVIDENCE

Ellis et al (1995) found that many orthodox treatments used today in the West are based on evidence from randomized controlled trials (RCTs). Evidence for the possible mechanisms of acupuncture is encouraging but does not guarantee that acupuncture works in patients. Most enthusiasts for acupuncture, whether practising in the traditional Chinese manner or in the modern Western way, accept that convincing proof of acupuncture's effectiveness is urgently required.

It seems probable that acupuncture has powerful non-specific (i.e. placebo) effects (Ernst 1994): to the patients it is a therapy that is unique and easily identified, it has the aura of Eastern mystique, it is often performed in a ritualistic manner, and it may be associated with long consultations that are in themselves likely to be therapeutic.

Placebo responses can be as high as 70–80% in appropriate circumstances (Benson & McCallie 1979, Richardson 1990, Wall 1994). Therefore it is essential to demonstrate that acupuncture has specific effects above and beyond its placebo effects. The 'gold standard' for clinical effectiveness is the RCT and it is somewhat embarrassing that the number of rigorous placebo-controlled RCTs in acupuncture is less than a hundred. We urgently need more evidence if acupuncture is to be adopted as part of orthodox medicine. The decision to provide a particular treatment must be based on the strength of evidence according to the following hierarchy (after Sackett 1989):

1. systematic review of randomized controlled trials
2. randomized controlled trials
3. non-randomized studies
4. case series, no controls
5. consensus of clinicians based on experience
6. clinical impressions.

There was an explosion of publications about acupuncture in the 1970s (Fig. 1.1). Many of these originated in America and China, but research has also been prominent in Russia (where acupuncture is often referred to as 'reflexotherapy') and there has been much research of good quality in Scandinavia. Acupuncture is one of the most researched of all complementary therapies. However, Figure 1.1 shows that the proportion of controlled trials is very small in comparison to subjective reviews, tutorials, case series and individual case reports. Much of this literature therefore contributes little to the evidence for acupuncture because it is not rigorous.

PROBLEMS IN ACUPUNCTURE RESEARCH

The problems in conducting research into acupuncture should not be underestimated and start with the identification of relevant previous studies. Searches of databases reveal large numbers of acupuncture references with promising titles but often the papers' contents are disappointing. These articles are often published in minor journals and there is considerable expense in retrieving them. It is tempting to rely on the authors' abstracts but these often draw over-optimistic conclusions from weak data. We hope

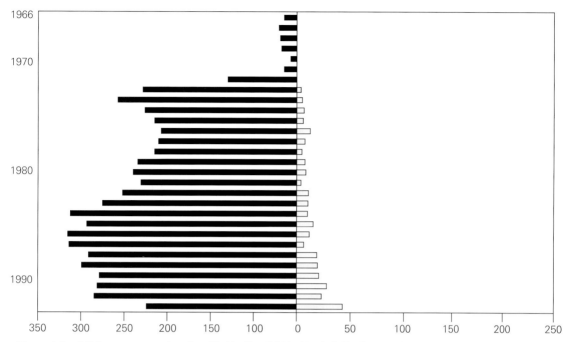

Figure 1.1 Articles on acupuncture listed in Medline (1966–1994): (left) all types of article; (right) clinical trials. (Data provided by J Barnes and reproduced with permission.)

that this book may help readers identify which articles are worth studying in the original.

Another problem in acupuncture research is the multiplicity of hypotheses and techniques included under the name 'acupuncture', some of which are listed in Figure 1.2.

In addition to the treatment variables detailed here, the individual's response must be taken into account. Some drugs more or less invariably bring about their desired effect (e.g. anaesthetic induction agents) whereas others have a less uniform effect that is dependent upon individual variation (e.g. anti-inflammatory agents). A similar variation is seen in the response to acupuncture (Fig. 1.3). It would be interesting to study the population responses to acupuncture for both painful and non-painful conditions.

Unfortunately many of the acupuncture studies that have been performed have not been reported in a way that makes them reproducible by other workers, which is a basic necessity for valid research. Reports frequently leave out technical details of the treatment given and so it is impossible to judge whether the acupuncture

was adequate. Another problem is the confusion caused by using different systems of nomenclature, for example in the different numbering systems for auricular acupuncture in France, Germany and China. This book uses the international nomenclature agreed by the World Health Organization (WHO) in 1989 (Jenkins 1990).

Acupuncturists who use Traditional Chinese Medicine (TCM) methods argue that these are so different from Western medicine that they cannot be tested by RCTs. It is true that TCM does make special demands on trial design, but there is no fundamental reason why these cannot be overcome and rigorous research done. For example, it has been argued that it is not appropriate to select patients according to Western diagnoses; however, it is perfectly possible to recruit patients according to the TCM diagnosis, for example all persons with 'Heart-Qi Deficiency'. Similarly, it has been argued that individualization of diagnosis and treatment is the essence of TCM, and cannot be incorporated into controlled studies. This is

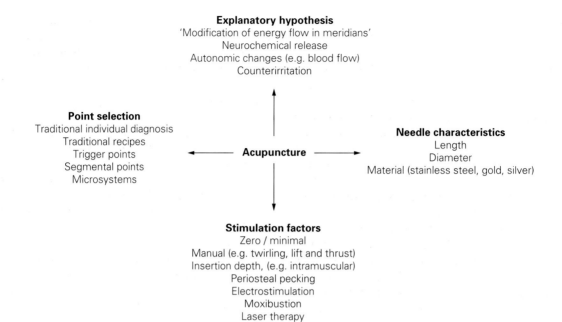

Explanatory hypothesis
'Modification of energy flow in meridians'
Neurochemical release
Autonomic changes (e.g. blood flow)
Counterirritation

Point selection
Traditional individual diagnosis
Traditional recipes
Trigger points
Segmental points
Microsystems

Acupuncture

Needle characteristics
Length
Diameter
Material (stainless steel, gold, silver)

Stimulation factors
Zero / minimal
Manual (e.g. twirling, lift and thrust)
Insertion depth, (e.g. intramuscular)
Periosteal pecking
Electrostimulation
Moxibustion
Laser therapy

Figure 1.2   Variables in acupuncture treatment.

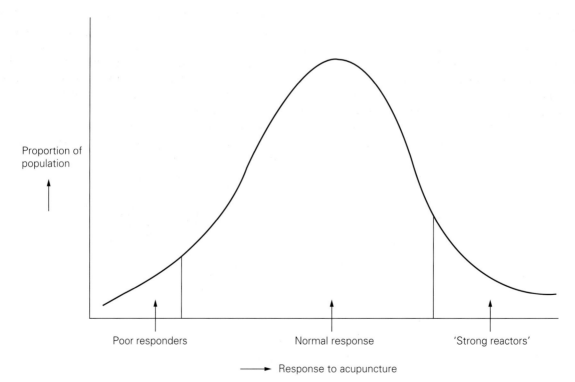

Proportion of
population

Poor responders   Normal response   'Strong reactors'

Response to acupuncture

Figure 1.3   Variation in the response to acupuncture treatment.

untrue; for example, Jobst et al (1986) used individualized treatments in a study of disabling breathlessness.

Rigorous trials should include blinding of the therapist in order to prevent therapist bias, but this is difficult in the case of an acupuncturist. One attempt to get round this problem is to train a novice to needle certain areas, not knowing which are active and which are inactive (Lagrue et al 1977). Another technique is to blind the acupuncturist to the real diagnosis (Godfrey & Morgan 1978). It is generally accepted that the problem of double blinding has not been solved; however, practitioner bias should be minimized by the method of 'standardized or minimal interaction' described by Hansen & Hansen (1983). This and the associated problem of designing a suitable sham procedure for the control group are discussed further in Chapter 13.

Another problem in acupuncture research has been that many outcome measures have been developed to measure symptoms, but few can assess the rather generalized beneficial effects that patients often report after they have been given acupuncture. However, there are now some reliable methods of measuring the quality of life, e.g. the Short Form-36 (Brazier et al 1992), and the Nottingham Health Profile (Hunt et al 1981). The recently introduced Measure Your Own Medical Outcome Profile (MYMOP) method (Paterson 1996) is a promising addition in which the patients nominate their own two worst symptoms. This measure may prove a useful single end point when a variety of conditions are treated by acupuncture.

ASSESSING THE EVIDENCE

An unbiased appraisal of the available clinical research into acupuncture would conclude that there are promising studies in many areas, but these are still mainly indecisive. However, the balance of evidence is convincingly in favour of acupuncture for one indication: antiemesis (Vickers 1996).

Research has concentrated, naturally enough, on the effect of needling. Yet this is only one component of the therapeutic interaction, whether acupuncture is being applied in a Western, TCM, or any other context.

The therapeutic relationship

Some of the variables that may influence the outcome of a consultation are given in Figure 1.4. There is considerable current debate about the precise definition of the 'placebo' and the percentage of patients who respond to each definition of it (Benson, 1996; Ernst & Resch, 1995; Roberts et al 1993).

What has become clear is that, in any consultation concerning illness, we must consider three components to any given therapy: the

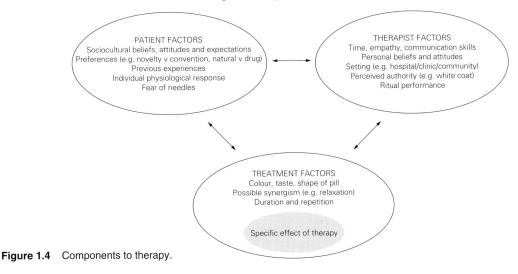

Figure 1.4   Components to therapy.

patient, the therapist and the treatment. Each may have its own cultural context (Fig. 1.4, adapted from Claridge 1970 & Helman 1994)

The shaded area in the third section represents the specific effect of the treatment itself (e.g. a new drug). In this book it is the specific effect of acupuncture that is to be examined.

Besides effectiveness, safety and cost-effectiveness are the other two crucial aspects of any treatment care. Safety is considered in Chapter 19, but currently there is insufficient information to warrant a chapter on the cost-effectiveness of acupuncture.

SUMMARY

Acupuncturists still face the exciting challenge of convincing the sceptics that the unlikely process of inserting needles into the body can help a medical condition. Too much of what our authors have contributed here has had to be based on clinical impressions and close observation instead of rigorous evidence. We can only emphasize the axiom: 'Lack of evidence of an effect, does not equal evidence of the lack of an effect'.

Our emphasis on research is not intended to undermine the value of clinical skills; we believe that careful observation is crucial to identifying possible effects, and clinical judgement will always be vital in applying evidence-based medicine sensitively and appropriately in our patients' best interests.

In reality, this book has proved somewhat harder to write than anticipated because of the lack of hard facts. We have attempted to cover nearly all aspects of modern acupuncture. Sadly, we have been unable to include a chapter on auricular acupuncture. Despite two valiant attempts by well-known experts, there simply are not enough scientific data to give sufficient substance to the text. We sincerely hope that this omission stimulates research in this area so that we can include a chapter on auricular acupuncture in a subsequent edition.

The editors would be glad to hear about any relevant information that has not been included in this edition; we apologise for any shortcomings, which are entirely the responsibility of the editors, and we shall try to make amends in further editions. We admit that most of the literature reviewed has been from journals in the English language and this will have resulted in a number of relevant omissions.

There is inevitably some overlap between authors but we have tried to keep this to a minimum. Not all the authors hold precisely the same views and we hope that readers will find this varied approach stimulating! It may be more accurate to regard this book as a collection of 'monographs' than a traditional text.

We would not expect our readers to devour this book from cover to cover at bedtime! It is more likely to act as a reference work in which current concepts about acupuncture are described by respected experts and backed by as many facts as possible. It is hoped that this textbook celebrates the emergence of acupuncture from its mystical, alternative roots and hastens its complete integration into conventional medicine over the next decade.

REFERENCES

Benson H 1996 Timeless healing. The power and biology of belief. Simon & Schuster, London

Benson H, McCallie D P 1979 Angina pectoris and the placebo effect. New England Journal of Medicine 300(25):1424–1429

Brazier J E, Harper R, Jones N M B et al 1992 Validating the SF-36 health survey questionnaire: new outcome measure for primary care. British Medical Journal 305:160–164

Claridge G 1970 Drugs and human behaviour. Allen Lane, London

Clement-Jones V, McLoughlin L, Lowry P J, Besser G M, Rees L H, Wen H L 1979 Acupuncture in heroin addicts: changes in met-enkephalin and beta-endorphin in blood and cerebrospinal fluid. The Lancet 2:380–383

Clement-Jones V, McLoughlin L, Tomlin S, Besser G M, Rees L H, Wen H L 1980 Increased beta-endorphin but not met-enkephalin levels in human cerebrospinal fluid after acupuncture for recurrent pain. The Lancet 2:946–949

Ellis J, Mulligan I, Rowe J, Sackett D L 1995 Inpatient general medicine is evidence based. Lancet 346:407–410

Ernst E 1994 Acupuncture research: where are the problems? Acupuncture in Medicine 12(2):93–97

Ernst E, Resch K-L 1995 Concept of true and perceived placebo effects. British Medical Journal 311:551–553

Godfrey C M, Morgan P 1978 A controlled trial of the theory of acupuncture in musculoskeletal pain. Journal of Rheumatology 5(2):121–124

Hansen P E, Hansen J H 1983 Acupuncture treatment of chronic facial pain—a controlled crossover trial. Headache 23(2):66–69

Helman C G 1994 Culture and pharmacology. In: Culture health and illness, 3rd edn. Butterworth Heinemann, Oxford, pp 194–223

Hunt S M, McKenna S P, McEwen J, Williams J, Papp E 1981 The Nottingham Health Profile: subjective health status and medical consultations. Social Science in Medicine 15a: 221–229

Jenkins M 1990 A new standard international acupuncture nomenclature. Acupuncture in Medicine 7:21–23

Jobst K, Chen J H, McPherson K et al 1986 Controlled trial of acupuncture for disabling breathlessness. Lancet 2:1416–1418

Lagrue G, Poupy J L, Grillot A, Ansquer J C 1977 Acupuncture anti-tabagique. La Nouvelle Presse Medicale 9:966

Paterson C 1996 Measuring outcomes in primary care: a patient-generated measure, MYMOP, compared with the SF-36 health survey. British Medical Journal 312:1016–1020

Richardson P H 1990 Pain and the placebo effect. Frontiers of Pain II, (4)

Roberts A H D G, Kewman L, Mercier M, Hael M 1993 The power of non-specific effects in healing: implications for psychosocial and biological treatments. Clinical Psychology Review 13:375–391

Sackett D L 1989 Rules of evidence and clinical recommendations on the use of antithrombotic agents. Chest 95(2)Suppl:25–45

Vickers A J 1996 Can acupuncture have specific effects on health? A systematic review of acupuncture antiemesis trials. Journal of the Royal Society of Medicine 89:303–311

Vincent C A 1992 Acupuncture research: why do it? Complementary Medical Research 6(1):21–24

Wall P D 1994 The placebo and the placebo response. In: Wall P D, Melzack R (eds) Textbook of pain, 3rd edn. Churchill Livingstone, New York, pp 1297–1308

2

Acupuncture in context

C. Chan Gunn

WHY 'SCIENTIFIC' ACUPUNCTURE?

In Europe, between 12 and 19% of the population report using acupuncture, according to consumer surveys (Fisher & Ward 1994). The Food and Drug Administration (FDA) of America estimates that 9 to 12 million acupuncture treatments are performed annually by non-medical acupuncturists and, in 1990, Americans made an estimated 425 million visits to providers of unconventional therapy, including practitioners of Traditional Chinese Medicine (TCM). Most sought these therapies for chronic rather than life-threatening medical conditions (Eisenberg et al 1993). Many jurisdictions have sanctioned non-medical acupuncturists (an issue that concerns the medical profession (Ulett 1992)), and the US National Institute of Health (1993) has recently established an Office of Alternative Medicine to offer exploratory grants for evaluating unconventional medical practice. Similar situations exist in many other Western countries; with increasing numbers of people, dissatisfied with the drug and surgery-orientated approach of Western medicine, turning to 'complementary' or 'alternative' medicine.

ANACHRONISTIC CONCEPTS OF CLASSICAL ACUPUNCTURE

The term 'acupuncture' is poorly defined, and has been used indiscriminately in the literature to refer to a number of related physical therapy techniques. 'Acupuncture' may refer to at least four distinct therapies with different rationales and efficacies (Chapman & Gunn 1990, Han & Terenius 1982):

1. classical acupuncture
2. scientific acupuncture
3. acupuncture as a form of trigger point therapy
4. acupuncture with electrical stimulation.

The aim of a physical therapy is to stimulate the nervous system, and acupuncture is by far the most effective therapy available for this (Ulett 1992). Needles of different types are invariably used, but the delivery of the stimulus may vary, and may be mechanical (by manipulation of the needle), thermal (moxibustion to the needle), or electrical (a pulsed, electrical stimulation to the needle). To avoid confusion the term 'acupuncture' should be used only when a needle penetrates the skin.

Practitioners of TCM use *classical acupuncture*, an old therapeutic modality that is based on the historical Chinese philosophical ideas of 'Yin-Yang' and 'Five Elements'. These were spontaneous, naive, materialist theories that also contain elementary dialectic ideas, and, combined with practical therapeutic experience, formed the fundamental theory of Chinese medicine. They were used to explain the physiological functioning of the human body and the occurrence and development of medical disorders, and to guide clinical diagnosis and treatment. Not only did they serve an active function in the historical development of medicine, but they are still used in Chinese clinical practice (Sivin 1987).

There are also Western physicians who practise a form of classical acupuncture, but many have undertaken a very rudimentary training in the metaphysical theories of TCM, and their acupuncture is based on a 'cookbook' approach in which routine sets of meridian points are used with minimal deliberation or variation for commonly encountered problems (Kao 1973). Sometimes as few as eight favourite points are employed (Lee & Liao 1990).

This ingenuous application of acupuncture is rejected by those medical acupuncturists who believe the theory of TCM to be in conflict with modern medical science. They promote *scientific acupuncture*, a Westernized version of acupuncture in which needle stimulation is given according to the observed principles of neurophysiology and anatomy. They emphasize that a contemporary physical examination and medical diagnosis are an essential preliminary to treatment, and that points to be needled in therapy are generally close to neural structures such as motor points and Golgi tendon organs (Gunn 1977, Gunn & Milbrandt 1976, Liu, Varela & Oswald 1975), and often in the same neurological segment as the injury (Wall 1974).

Probably the most compelling reason for medical acupuncturists to repudiate traditional Chinese philosophy is its intricate and inscrutable system of 'Yin and Yang', 'pulse palpation', 'Five Elements', and circulation of 'Qi' and 'Blood'. Such notions seem antiquated and even irrational to Western practitioners who lack the necessary background and inclination to understand the intricacy of TCM (Capra 1984, Holbrook 1981, Porkert 1983).

Health and disease are perceived differently by Western medicine and TCM. Western medicine has a narrow and specific definition of 'disease' as a 'definite morbid process, often with a characteristic train of symptoms': therefore, there are innumerable 'diseases'. Traditional Chinese philosophy has, on the other hand, a holistic concept of health. It regards good health as the ideal state in which there is total harmony and equilibrium within the body, and of the body within its environment. 'When Yin and Yang are in balance the vitalities and spirits will be in a well-ordered state (Gunn 1977). This concept of health agrees with the view held by modern epidemiologists that illness is caused by the loss of equilibrium in the simultaneous interaction of host, agent and environment (Itoh & Lee 1971). It also meets with the World Health Organization's definition of health as 'a state of complete physical, mental and social well-being and not merely the absence of disease and infirmity', (World Health Organization 1964).

In illness, TCM seeks to restore equilibrium in the body and rebalance the 'Yin and Yang'. Yin and Yang represent opposing forces or opposite ends of a scale or range of values. Rebalancing the Yin and Yang could mean, in a modern sense, re-establishment of normal biological values. When equilibrium is upset by an over-powering agent (e.g. a bacterial infection) TCM is ineffective and inferior to modern methods of intervention, such as antibiotics. But when disequilibrium is the result of a lowering of the host's power of resistance, or a dysfunction in the host, TCM stimulates the homeostatic powers or 'wisdom' of the body (Cannon 1963) to regain normal balance.

However, most TCM ideas are anachronistic and not compatible with contemporary science. Since Sir William Harvey, we have had a physiological version of the cardiovascular sys-tem and circulation of blood, but in TCM the cardiac system is responsible for mental, con-scious and higher nervous activity, and sweat is the dispersed fluid associated with the cardiac system. TCM's 'pulse diagnosis' is completely different in concept from Western pulse taking today. TCM physicians regard pulse diagnosis as the pinnacle of their examination and conduct it with great deliberation, almost as a ritual. A TCM physician is expected to be able to diag-nose any systemic disease solely by pulse diagnosis, but there are numerous systems of pulse diagnosis, all of which are extremely complicated. The conclusions reached on the supposed relationship between the pulse and internal organs can differ widely according to the system used; more often than not, no two interpretations are alike and indeed it has been recommended that 'the lore of the pulse be relegated to the domain of medical history' (Wong & Wu 1932). There seems no useful application for pulse diagnosis in scientific acupuncture.

TCM terminology remains popular with prac-titioners of classical acupuncture, but it is difficult to justify its use in scientific acupuncture because its anatomical and physiological termin-ology are vastly different from those in current Western medicine. For example, 'Lung' in TCM does not relate to diseases of the respiratory system, but to skin diseases; 'Kidney' is not concerned with the urinary tract, but with the genital system; and 'Spleen' regulates the diges-

tive functions. There is even an Organ, 'the Triple Energizer', which does not exist in modern anatomy (Liao 1973, Lu & Needham 1980).

Physiologists, electromyographers and physical therapists are aware that the peripheral nervous system is best stimulated at certain sites in the body where nerve fibres are most easily accessible (see Ch 9). Classical *acupuncture points* represent a selection of these sites. They are usually shown in acupuncture charts as situated on the skin (Chapman & Gunn 1990, Sivin 1987).

Meridians are lines that are created when strategic sequences of classical points are linked and named according to the internal organ with which they are supposedly associated. Although meridians may appear to be anatomically hap-hazard, they are useful surface anatomy charts of muscle motor points and musculotendinous junctions (Kao 1973, Sivin 1987). Meridians may be likened to contour lines on topographical maps, and they are useful clinical guides to important myotomal signs of peripheral neuro-pathy, such as increased muscle tone, tenderness over motor points (Gunn & Milbrandt 1976, Pomeranz & Stux 1989) and palpable muscle bands. For example, it is common knowledge that sciatic leg pain originates from the low back, and the back is always examined. How-ever, it is not well known that most musculo-skeletal pain conditions involve the spine; thus, when pain presents in a location supplied by the anterior primary ramus (e.g. in the elbow or shoulder), examination of the posterior ramus (i.e. the neck) is often neglected.

Meridians also indicate the source of pain when it is caused by the mechanical pull of a shortened muscle (Gunn 1990). For example, in chondromalacia patellae, crepitus and pain may present under the patella, but the strain is generated by shortening in the quadriceps femoris muscles. Finding concurrent spasm in the paraspinal muscles at L2–L4 confirms the diagnosis and reveals the segmental levels of radiculopathy (Gunn & Milbrandt 1978) (see Ch 9). Appropriate therapy would be to needle and release spasm in the quadriceps and paraspinal muscles (Gunn 1989). Because meridians are named according to their supposed association with internal organs, they are constant reminders that the peripheral nervous system is neurologically linked to internal organs through the autonomic system, and stimulation of the musculoskeletal system can reach and modify autonomic activity (Lee & Ernst 1983).

Classical acupuncture has placed great emphasis on the 'Qi' or 'flow of energy' in the body. It is an early concept similar to the Greek 'life force'. Vital life force is thought to flow through the meridians, and Excesses or Deficiencies in the flow of energy are said to cause pain, discomfort, hypo- or hyperfunction and, with time, trophic changes. By inserting the needles strategically along individual meridians or at their junctures, the acupuncturist is able to balance the flow of energy throughout the body. The concept of Qi is central to the theory of acupuncture. Functional disturbances in the nervous system can result from 'hypofunction' (e.g. deficits in nerve impulse conduction, neuromuscular transmission or muscle contraction) and also from 'hyperfunction' (e.g. paresthesia, neuralgias and involuntary muscle activity) (Culp & Ochoa 1982).

ACUPUNCTURE AND PAIN

With recent advances in the neurosciences, several scientific theories (Akil, Richardson & Hughes 1978, Mayer, Price & Rafii 1977, Pormeranz & Chiu 1976, Pomeranz & Stux 1989) have been advanced to explain the mechanism of acupuncture (Ch 6), but none has fully satisfied the scientific community (Vincent & Richardson 1986) and we are not at the 'threshold of a precise scientific explanation' (Peng & Greenfield 1990).

Western interest in acupuncture began in the mid 1970s following reports of its use for analgesia in surgery, so research has tended to focus on acupuncture's effects on acute and chronic pain. This preoccupation with pain, and to a lesser extent with behavioural events such as chemical dependency (Wen & Cheung 1973), depression and psychosomatic disorders (Li 1985), has led to a perspective of acupuncture that is too narrow to account for its application

in a wide variety of conditions. Any explanation for acupuncture must be able to account for its action in non-painful as well as in painful conditions.

Most acupuncture studies have concentrated on analgesia and the blocking of nociception (the immediate signalling of tissue threat or injury via Aδ or C fibres). Supporters of acupuncture theorized that endogenous opioids must be the mechanism for acupuncture pain control, and regarded acupuncture as a neuromodulating input into the CNS that can activate multiple analgesia systems in the spinal cord and brain, stimulating the endogenous pain suppression system to release neurotransmitters such as endogenous opioids (Ng et al 1992) (see Ch 7). Animal investigators have reported that 'acupuncture analgesia' (Bosset, Page & Stromberg 1984, Klide 1984, Wright & McGrath 1981) has been able to reduce experimental pain in animals. However, acupuncture analgesia alone cannot be depended upon to block the perception of noxious input and it is not a popular choice for surgery. Also, it is worth noting that the neurotransmitters, opioid and non-opioid, probably have wider physiological roles than analgesia alone.

Wall has described pain as a reaction pattern of three sequential behavioural phases: immediate (nociception), acute (inflammatory) and chronic (Wall 1979). Acupuncture is somewhat less effective in nociception or in inflammatory pain than in the chronic category.

Chronic pain may result from ongoing signals of tissue damage (nociception or inflammation) conveyed to the central nervous system (CNS) via a healthy nervous system; or it can be associated with psychological factors such as a somatization disorder, depression or operant learning processes. Pain can also arise when there is abnormal or altered function in the nervous system, e.g. hyperactivity at some level in the pain sensory system. Such functional disturbances generally occur in the peripheral nervous system when there is peripheral neuropathy (Thomas 1984). Peripheral neuropathy and denervation supersensitivity are responsible for a category of chronic neuropathic pain that can be managed very convincingly by acupuncture (see Ch 9).

Neuropathic pain is caused by abnormal physiology in the peripheral nervous system in the absence of tissue damage. Therapy in neuropathic pain is not to provide analgesia but to restore supersensitive structures to their norm.

Since neuropathic pain is associated with a lack of incoming impulses to the effector organ, a substitute excitatory input must be provided. Of all the physical therapies that can furnish this by reflex stimulation, acupuncture is the most effective.

REFERENCES

Akil H, Richardson D E, Hughes J 1978 Enkephalin-like material elevated in ventricular CSF of pain patients after analgesic focal stimulation. Science 201:463–465

Bossut D F, Page E H, Stromberg M W 1984 Production of cutaneous analgesia by electroacupuncture in horses: variations dependent on sex of subject and locus of stimulation. American Journal of Veterinary Research 45:620–625

Cannon W B 1963 The wisdom of the body. W W Norton and Company, New York

Capra F 1984 The tao of physics. Bantam New Age Books, Toronto

Chapman C R, Gunn C Chan 1990 Acupuncture. In: Bonica J J (ed) The management of pain, vol 2. Lea & Febiger, Philadelphia, pp 1805–1821

Culp W J, Ochoa J 1982 Abnormal nerves and muscles as impulse generators. Oxford University Press, New York

Eisenberg D M, Kesseler R C, Foster C, Norlock F E, Calkins D R, Delbanco T L 1993 Unconventional medicine in the United States: prevalence, costs and patterns of use. New England Journal of Medicine 328(4):246–252

Fisher P, Ward A 1994 Complementary medicine in Europe. British Medical Journal 309:107–111

Gunn C C 1977 Type IV Acupuncture points. American Journal of Acupuncture 5(1):51–52

Gunn C C 1989 Treating myofascial pain—intramuscular stimulation (IMS) for myofascial syndromes of neuropathic origin. HSCER, University of Washington, Seattle

Gunn C C 1990 Mechanical manifestations of neuropathic pain. Annals of Sports Medicine 5(3):138–141

Gunn C C, Milbrandt W E 1976 Tenderness at motor points—a diagnostic and prognostic aid for low back injury. Journal of Bone and Joint Surgery 58(6):815–825.

Gunn C C, Milbrandt W E 1978 Early and subtle signs in low back sprain. Spine 3(3):267–281

Gunn C C, Ditchburn F G, King M H, Renwick G J 1976 Acupuncture loci: a proposal for their classification according to their relationship to known neural structures. American Journal of Chinese Medicine 4(2):183–195

Han J S, Terenius L 1982 Neurochemical basis of acupuncture analgesia. Annual Review of Pharmacology and Toxicology 22:193–220

Holbrook B 1981 The stone monkey, an alternative Chinese–scientific, reality. William Morrow, New York

Itoh M, Lee M H M 1971 The epidemiology of disability as related to rehabilitation medicine. In: Kottke F J, Lehmann J F (eds) Krusen's Handbook of physical medicine and rehabilitation. W B Saunders, Philadelphia

Kao F F 1973 Acupuncture therapeutics: an introductory text. Triple Oak, Garden City, NY

Klide A M 1984 Acupuncture for treatment of chronic back pain in the horse. Acupuncture and Electro-therapeutics Research 9:57–70

Lee M H M, Ernst M 1983 The sympatholytic effect of acupuncture as evidenced by thermography. Orthopaedic Review 12:67–72

Lee M H, Liao S J 1990 Acupuncture in physiatry. In: Kottke F J, Lehmann F (eds) Krusen's handbook of physical medicine and rehabilitation, 4th edn. W B Saunders, Philadelphia, ch 16, pp 402–432

Li X R 1985 Acupuncture for psychiatric disorders—the past and the present. International Journal of Chinese Medicine 2(2) 17–20

Liao S J 1973 Acupuncture—an appraisal. Conn. Medicine 37:506–510

Liu Y K, Varela M, Oswald R 1975 The correspondence between some motor points and acupuncture loci. American Journal of Chinese Medicine 3:347–358

Lu G D, Needham J 1980 Celestial lancets, a history and rationale of acupuncture and moxa. Cambridge University Press, Cambridge

Mayer D, Price D, Rafii A 1977 Antagonism of acupuncture analgesia in man by the narcotic antagonist naloxone. Brain Research 121:368–372

National Institute of Health 1993 Exploratory grants for alternative medicine, National Institute of Health guide 22 (12), March 26

Ng L K Y, Katims J J, Lee M H M 1992 Acupuncture, a neuromodulation technique for pain control. In: Aronoff G M (ed) Evaluation and treatment of chronic pain, 2nd edn. Williams & Wilkins, Baltimore

Peng A T C, Greenfield W 1990 A precise scientific explanation of acupuncture mechanisms: are we on the threshold? Editorial review. Acupuncture: Scientific International Journal 1:28–29

Pomeranz B, Chiu D 1976 Naloxone blockage of acupuncture analgesia: endorphin implicated. Life Sciences 19:1757–1762

Pomeranz B, Stux G 1989 Scientific bases of acupuncture. Springer-Verlag, Berlin

Porkert M 1983 The essentials of Chinese diagnostics. Acta Medicinae Sinensis, Chinese Medical Publications, Zurich

Sivin N 1987 Traditional medicine in contemporary China. Science, Medicine, and Technology in East Asia Center for Chinese Studies, University of Michigan

Thomas P K 1984 Symptomatology and differential diagnosis of peripheral neuropathy: clinical and differential diagnosis. In: Dyck P J, Thomas P K, Lambert E H, Bunge R (eds) Peripheral neuropathy, 2nd edn. W B Saunders, Philadelphia, pp 1169–1190

Ulett G P 1992 3000 years of acupuncture: from metaphysics to neurophysiology. Integrative Psychiatry 8(2):91–104

Vincent C, Richardson P H 1986 The evaluation of therapeutic acupuncture: concepts and methods. Pain 24:1–13

Wall P D 1974 Floor discussion on acupuncture for pain therapy. In: Bonica J J (ed) 1974 International Symposium on Pain. Raven Press, New York

Wall P D 1979 On the relation of injury to pain. The John J Bonica lecture. Pain 6:253–264

Wen H L, Cheung S Y C 1973 Treatment of drug addiction by acupuncture and electrical stimulation. Asian Journal of Medicine 9:138–141

Wong K C, Wu L T 1932 History of Chinese medicine. Tientsin Press, Shanghai

World Health Organization 1964 Constitution of the World Health Organization, Geneva

Wright M, McGrath C J 1981 Physiologic and analgesic effects of acupuncture in the dog. Journal of the American Veterinary Medical Association 178:502–507

Practical aspects

SECTION CONTENTS

3

Methods of acupuncture

Anthony Campbell

The word 'acupuncture' is from the Latin and refers simply to 'piercing with a sharp instrument'. It is sometimes taken to refer exclusively to the traditional Chinese method of treatment, but in the present context it should be taken to mean the therapeutic use of needles, without any presupposition of an underlying theory structure. By common usage it is often extended to cover certain other forms of therapy, such as manual pressure (so-called 'acupressure'), transcutaneous electrical nerve stimulation TENS and, more recently and controversially, laser therapy. The traditional system makes use of local heating (moxa) and in recent years the Chinese and others have tried injecting various substances at acupuncture points. Although it will be necessary to glance at some of these methods briefly, most of the discussion will focus on the use of 'dry' needles.

ACUPUNCTURE WITH DRY NEEDLES

TYPES OF NEEDLE

The traditional acupuncture needle consists of a pointed shaft, made usually of steel but sometimes of gold or silver (according to some sources, these metals have special therapeutic properties). The upper part of the shaft may be wound round with fine steel or silver wire, terminating in a small loop; this winding forms a handle that allows the acupuncturist to manipulate the needle more easily. The length of the shaft varies considerably; the commonest size is 25–30 mm, but 15 mm and 50 mm needles are frequently used and longer needles still are sometimes chosen, especially by traditionalists. The thickness of the needles is generally 0.3 to 0.5 mm at least in the case of the Chinese needles; much thinner needles are used by some practitioners, especially the Japanese, but these require special techniques of insertion.

Formerly needles were reused many times. They were cleaned and sterilized and sometimes they were resharpened on a stone to get rid of the small hooks that tended to form at the tips. With increasing awareness of the risk of transmitting hepatitis and HIV, however, most practitioners have abandoned reusable needles and employ disposable needles exclusively. As a consequence of this change in practice, disposable needles have become widely available and better in quality than they used to be. It is now possible to buy sterilized disposable needles that are exactly the same as those used previously; that is, they have a steel shaft and a wire-wound handle. However, it is also possible to obtain needles with plastic handles; these are equally satisfactory unless the practitioner wants to use electrical stimulation or apply moxa to the needle.

In addition to the commonly used types of needle just described other kinds are available for special circumstances. Stud needles are used for ear acupuncture. These may be either very short fine needles with a small ball at the top or else needles made of fine wire and shaped like a small drawing pin. Needles of this kind are intended to be left in place for varying lengths of time. Practitioners of TCM sometimes use a 'plum blossom hammer'; this is a hammer with short needles set in its face, which allows scarification of the skin over an area. This can create serious sterilization problems.

Doctors often ask whether ordinary injection needles can be used for acupuncture. They can, but have certain disadvantages. Theoretically, the fact that they are hollow might mean that they are more likely to cause infection. A more serious drawback is that they have a cutting edge, whereas a traditional acupuncture needle lacks this edge and is therefore less likely to cause

bleeding or to damage internal structures. Finally, it seems to be more difficult to elicit the subjective and objective features known collectively as 'De Qi' (p 27) with injection needles. These needles can, therefore, be used if nothing else is available but authentic acupuncture needles are preferable.

DIFFERENT WAYS OF USING NEEDLES

Needling can be done in a variety of ways. The number of needles used on a single occasion may range from one to 20 or more. The depth of needling also varies; the tip of the needle may be inserted just through the skin, or the tissues may be penetrated to a depth of several centimetres. The needles may be left in for 20 or 30 minutes, sometimes even longer, or they may be withdrawn almost immediately, within 1 or 2 seconds. The needles may be left alone when they are in place, they may be manipulated manually in various ways, or they may be stimulated electrically. Last, but by no means least, there is the question of where the needles are to be inserted; this in turn depends in part on the kind of acupuncture being practised (traditional, modern, 'neoclassical', or whatever).

Choosing the sites to needle

There are many different ways to practise acupuncture (Fig. 3.1) and to a large extent the method a practitioner chooses will depend on his theoretical assumptions. The main possibilities are as follows.

Traditional

The needles are inserted in accordance with the traditional theoretical framework of TCM: Yin–Yang polarity, Qi, channels ('meridians'), points and so on. In the full-blown system the symptoms are diagnosed according to the traditional categories, using the pulses and the appearance of the tongue. In this version of acupuncture the location of the points is considered to be important and much attention is paid to locating them precisely.

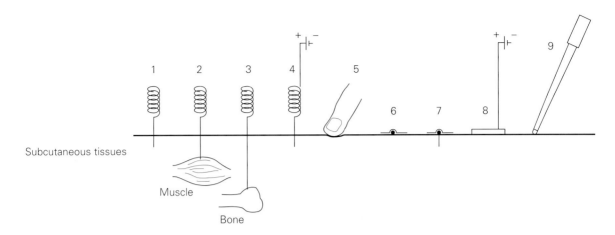

1 Superficial needling of subcutaneous tissue
2 Intramuscular stimulation
3 Periosteal stimulation
4 Electroacupuncture
5 Acupressure
6 Acupressure balls
7 Press-needles
8 TENS
9 Laser therapy

Figure 3.1   Types of acupuncture stimulation.

Neoclassical

This refers to a variety of methods that have arisen over the last few decades and bear some relation to the traditional system though they are not identical with it. Examples are ear acupuncture (auriculotherapy) and Ryodoraku. These systems are difficult to categorize but most tend to use concepts of 'energy balancing' and they may use electrically based diagnostic methods. Some of these methods are discussed further below.

'Cookbook' acupuncture

There exist numerous books containing lists of points to try in various disorders. These 'cookbooks', as they are often rather disparagingly called, are generally based on the traditional system. Their advantage is that they may give confidence to beginners; their main disadvantages are that they do not afford any insight into the principles of practice and may tend to encourage a mechanical approach to acupuncture.

Trigger point acupuncture

Practitioners who favour this approach base the choice of sites to needle on examining the patient and identifying the trigger points (TPs) by local tenderness and other criteria, such as the radiation of pain from the site, the 'jump sign' (flinching when the trigger point is pressed), muscle twitching on pressure, and changes in the overlying skin. Taut bands in muscles are also characteristic. This method, though modern, is not wholly incompatible with the traditional system. Traditional acupuncture has always recognized the existence of 'Ah Shi' points, which are not classic acupuncture points but become tender when there is pathology. Moreover, traditional acupuncture points and trigger points, though not identical, overlap considerably.

The term 'trigger point acupuncture' is somewhat elastic and covers a number of treatment variants. Some practitioners believe that it is desirable to needle the trigger point as accurately as possible. They use whatever length of needle is required to reach the trigger point and if they fail to strike it at the first attempt they partially withdraw the needle, alter the angle of insertion, and try again. Others prefer to use quite superficial needling over the trigger point and find that this is equally effective as well as less painful. At present there are no published trials that would enable one to choose the most effective method, so it is really a matter of personal choice which of the alternatives the practitioner adopts.

Periosteal acupuncture

As the term implies, this consists in needling the periosteum. It produces a peculiar, rather unpleasant type of pain that differs from that produced by needling other tissues. The main use is to treat painful disorders of individual joints. For example, pain in the knee might be treated by needling the medial surface of the tibia, and osteoarthritis of the big toe might be treated by needling the first metatarsal and first phalanx. Some practitioners also use periosteal acupuncture to produce remote or more generalized effects.

It does not seem to be very important to localize sites of periosteal needling precisely; any conveniently accessible site around the joint will usually work. Periosteal needling could therefore be thought of as a strong form of regional acupuncture, within a particular sclerotome.

Single-point acupuncture

Some research studies have been carried out using a single point to treat every patient. For example, PC-6 has been used as an antiemetic treatment. It is, however, unusual to use just one point in everyday clinical practice.

Minimalist acupuncture

As already mentioned, there are wide variations of opinion about the desirable duration and depth of needling. One school of thought favours the use of very superficial acupuncture, the needle being inserted just through the skin and left in for a very short time with little or no manual stimulation. This technique is less likely to cause aggravations, though they certainly can still occur. Surprisingly, it is not the case that minimalist acupuncture necessarily has a weaker effect than more forceful or prolonged needling; indeed, for some people it has a stronger effect.

Eclectic approach—the 'acupuncture treatment area'

Some practitioners use a non-traditional approach that borrows elements from many types of acupuncture without necessarily accepting the presuppositions of any of them completely. For example, an acupuncturist might use trigger point needling for perhaps 80% of the time but also needle traditional points on the ear on occasion. Some acupuncturists who are sceptical about the existence of acupuncture points in the full sense of the term nevertheless accept that there is probably a valid base of observation underlying the idea. From this viewpoint it is unnecessary to try to localize acupuncture points precisely. There are some people—'strong reactors'—in whom it hardly matters where a needle is inserted; a therapeutic effect is produced almost regardless of the site of stimulation. In other patients, needling has to be done within a broad general region—perhaps anywhere in the leg might do. In yet others the site of needling has to be more or less precise. According to this view it would be more accurate to speak of 'acupuncture zones' than 'acupuncture points' (see Ch 5).

Often these zones are selected on the grounds that they are tender when pressed—that is, they are trigger points. But certain sites, especially those on the distal parts of the limbs (LR-3, LI-4) are not usually tender; they may be thought of as areas in which it is particularly easy to produce a profound general effect on the system. They can therefore be useful in generalized disorders such as chronic urticaria as well as in disturbances of function such as migraine or asthma.

One way of denoting the site of needling, for practitioners who favour this eclectic approach, is to use a theory-neutral expression such as 'acupuncture treatment area' (ATA). An ATA may be described simply as an area of the body of variable size in which it is possible to produce a therapeutic effect by needling. Thus, classic acupuncture points, trigger points and regions of periosteum around joints would all be ATAs. There are special ATAs, such as the auricle (see below) that are said to contain other, smaller, ATAs within them. Ah Shi points are also ATAs and there is even a sense in which the body as a whole could be considered as an ATA in view of the phenomenon of diffuse noxious inhibitory control. One advantage of using the ATA terminology is that it emphasizes the variability in size of needling sites; another is that it avoids the misleading implication that a needling site must always be tender to pressure.

USING THE NEEDLES

Insertion

The technique of inserting the needles is simple but requires practice if it is to be done skilfully and relatively painlessly. Acquiring good needle technique is an important part of achieving success in acupuncture.

The exact method of inserting the needles will vary according to the site being needled and also, to some extent, the preference of the individual acupuncturist. If an introducer (see below) is not used, the commonest method is to stretch the skin with the left hand (assuming a right-handed practitioner) and to hold the needle with the tip just above, or just touching, the skin. Then the needle is thrust quickly and smoothly through the skin, to a depth of at least a couple of millimetres, sometimes more. Some practitioners like to spin the needle a little as it is inserted since this seems to give a smoother insertion, but it is by no means essential to do this. (The modern disposable needles, being generally

sharper than the older kind, are easier to insert and less painful for the patient.)

It is possible to decrease the pain of insertion somewhat in the following way. If the tip of the needle is rested for a moment against the skin there may be a sensation of slight pain; the needle is then moved away 1 or 2 mm to a less tender spot before being inserted. This procedure has the disadvantage that it tends to increase any apprehension the patient may feel and is therefore better avoided as a rule; however, it may be worth imparting to patients who are being taught to treat themselves with acupuncture (p 28).

The basic method of needling just described may need to be varied in certain circumstances. If the subcutaneous tissues are thin a fold of skin may be pinched with the left hand and the needle passed into this. When a long needle (50 mm) is used it is generally necessary to steady the shaft with the tip of a finger and to flex the shaft slightly at the same time to make it more rigid. Alternatively the longer needle may be held between finger and thumb just proximal to the tip, but the flexion method is probably preferable.

The angle of insertion is usually normal to the skin (90°). If the underlying tissues are thin, however, a more acute angle of insertion may be required.

The depth of insertion depends on the particular approach the acupuncturist has chosen. Some practitioners use superficial (2–3 mm) needling almost exclusively. Others prefer deeper needling; if the aim is to reach muscle trigger points then deep needling will certainly be required quite frequently, and the same applies to periosteal acupuncture. In the traditional system the acupuncture points are held to lie at various depths and the depth of needling is prescribed at the different points. Even if superficial needling is preferred the needle should pass through the skin into the subcutaneous tissues, since intradermal acupuncture is unduly painful and relatively ineffective.

Introducers

A number of practitioners like to use introducers.

These are plastic tubes surrounding the needles; the mouth of the tube is placed against the skin and the projecting top of the needle handle is tapped to drive the point a couple of millimetres through the skin. The needle can then be advanced farther manually. It is possible to buy sterilized needles already fitted with introducers. Needles of this kind are certainly easier for beginners to insert, but many experienced acupuncturists find them unnecessary and prefer not to use them, although patients like them, as pressure on the skin by the introducer makes needle insertion virtually painless.

To swab or not to swab?

In the past it was customary to wipe the skin with an alcohol-impregnated swab before taking a blood sample or giving an injection. The evidence that this really achieves much is unconvincing unless the procedure is performed a good deal more elaborately than is usually the case, and it seems to be done less frequently now than formerly. Most acupuncturists do not swab the skin, and although there is no harm in doing so it is probably unnecessary.

Needlestick injuries

Provided that disposable needles are used there is no risk of transmitting infection to the patient. Not so, however, as regards the acupuncturist; needlestick injuries are a constant occupational hazard. Most health workers today have been immunized against hepatitis B but this does not guarantee protection, and there is of course no immunization at present against HIV. It is therefore essential to do everything possible to avoid injuring oneself with used needles. Unfortunately such injury is more likely to occur now than formerly, owing to the increased sharpness of most of the disposable needles.

Some practitioners like to use the same needle at multiple sites in the same patient. This is satisfactory so far as the patient is concerned but it carries a risk for the acupuncturist, who may prick himself with a contaminated needle, and it

is therefore safer to use each needle once only. If this is done then needlestick injuries are likely to occur with clean needles only.

The commonest way to stab oneself is to prick the (left) hand which is stretching or steadying the patient's skin. If the method just described is followed this is not a serious matter. It is also possible to prick the left hand as the needle is withdrawn. To avoid this, withdraw the needle with one hand only, keeping the other hand well away from the needle point.

Attempting to resheathe a used needle in an introducer is an unsafe practice and should be avoided. Another hazardous moment can occur as the needle is disposed of. The tip of the needle can catch on the edge of the disposal bin and fly up. To prevent this, the needle should be held horizontally above the opening of the bin and allowed to drop inside; it should not be thrust into the bin point first.

It might seem to be advisable to wear surgical gloves to practise acupuncture. However, these do not provide any real protection against needlestick injuries and they make manipulation of the needles difficult.

Stimulation

In many cases, although not invariably, the acupuncturist will choose to stimulate the needle after it has been inserted. This stimulation can be done in various ways, including electrically (see below). Manual stimulation is most frequently done by rotating the needle a few degrees in both directions, the action being similar to that of winding a watch. In the traditional system it is also said to be possible to 'sedate' the points, for example by altering the direction in which the needle is twisted.

Other methods of manual stimulation include lifting and lowering the needle point within the tissues ('pecking') and rubbing one's thumb nail along the handle of a wire-wound needle to transmit the vibrations to the tissues. 'Pecking' is the usual method of applying acupuncture to the periosteum.

All these procedures may be carried out with various degrees of intensity. Twisting the needles, for example, may be done by rotating it 15 or 20° in both directions; this would be medium-strength stimulation. Gentler stimulation might involve only one or two small twists of the needle. Stronger stimulation would consist in twisting the needle through a bigger arc and for a longer time. If really strong stimulation is required it can be obtained by winding the needle continuously in one direction so that the fibres wrap themselves round the shaft; this is generally painful.

The decision about how much stimulation, if any, to apply is a very individual matter and acupuncturists vary considerably in their attitudes to the question. At one extreme some hardly use stimulation at all; at the other some use strong stimulation frequently. In spite of this variability, getting the amount of stimulation right is important, and this is one of the main things the would-be acupuncturist must learn. Overstimulation is a bigger danger than understimulation; indeed, for many patients it is almost impossible to perform acupuncture too lightly but very easy to perform it too vigorously. If it is too vigorous the patient is likely to suffer an aggravation of symptoms (see p 28) and at the same time will probably have a poor therapeutic response or even none at all.

The number of needles inserted and the duration of needling are other factors affecting the intensity of treatment. In general, the more needles that are inserted the bigger the effect on the patient, although there is not a direct relation between number of needles and intensity of treatment.

The duration of needling varies widely from doctor to doctor. Some withdraw the needle after half a minute or even less, while others, especially those who favour the traditional system, leave them in place much longer. There is little objective evidence to favour either of these methods over the other, although on theoretical grounds there is some reason to think that the nervous system adapts so quickly to a new stimulus that most of the effect is produced within a very short time after the needle is inserted.

Withdrawal

Withdrawing the needle is generally simple. Traditionalists advocate massaging the puncture site to seal it against the 'leakage of Qi.' For reasons discussed earlier this is probably undesirable and indeed it is best to keep the (left) hand away from the needle as it is withdrawn.

It may happen that withdrawal of the needle is followed by a small amount of bleeding. This can be stopped by simple pressure with a tissue or cottonwool swab; if the bleeding site is on a limb the part may be elevated for a few minutes. Another possibility is the appearance of a small 'bump' under the skin as the needle is withdrawn. This is due to the formation of a small haematoma; it should be pressed for a few minutes to flatten it and stop the bleeding. Patients should be routinely warned about the possibility of a bruise appearing after acupuncture, since if they are not expecting it they may become anxious at the sight of the discoloured area.

Sometimes, especially if the needle has been inserted accurately into a muscle trigger point, it may be gripped so firmly by the tissues that it cannot be withdrawn. Attempts to overcome the resistance by hard pulling cause the patient much pain. The remedy is to wait for a few minutes until the resistance has worn off. It is sometimes said that another needle should be inserted a short distance away to produce relaxation, but in practice this is seldom necessary.

Needles may bend during acupuncture. This can occur through clumsy insertion, or it may be caused by muscular movement on the part of the patient after insertion. It is not generally a problem although theoretically there is a risk that a needle will break. The most likely site for breakage is where the shaft joins the handle; needles should therefore not be advanced 'right up to the hilt'.

Acquiring good needle technique

Although some doctors regard the actual performance of needle insertion and manipulation as a mechanical matter that can satisfactorily be left to someone else to perform, others think that how the acupuncture is carried out is very important and contributes largely to the outcome. If this idea is right it follows that doctors studying acupuncture need to spend a good deal of time learning how to use the needles. To a certain extent this can be practised on oranges, but these do not really give the same sensation as needling patients. The best solution is therefore to practise on a fellow student or on oneself. Practising on oneself has two advantages: one learns exactly what the patient is going to experience and one has an incentive to avoid overstimulation!

THE PATIENT

Introducing acupuncture to new patients

It is important to take some care in introducing the idea of acupuncture to new patients. The first, essential, consideration is the medicolegal one: informed consent. Has the patient clearly understood what the acupuncturist intends to do? If acupuncture is carried out on a patient who has not consented to it the practitioner could be open to a charge of assault. The patient may ask about possible complications of acupuncture; such questions should be answered frankly and a note should be made of the questions asked and the answers given.

Another reason for taking care over introducing the idea of acupuncture is to allay any hidden anxieties that the patient may have; remember that fear of acupuncture often inhibits a good clinical response. Patients often ask 'Does it hurt?' This question, like others, should be answered honestly. The amount of pain will vary according to the type of acupuncture being used, the site of needling and other factors, so different patients will need different answers.

The patient may already have had acupuncture from someone else. It is important to find out about this: who did it, how did they do it, what was the result? Perhaps the previous occasion was a disaster, or perhaps it gave good results but was done by a different method from that to be used at present. These things need to be taken

into account and the patient should receive an explanation of the reasons for any differences.

It is essential to avoid overpersuading patients to have acupuncture. If they appear at all reluctant they should be told to go away and think about it. (The result of saying this is often to make the patient decide there and then to have acupuncture!)

Positioning the patient

Choice of the best position in which to place the patient obviously depends on which sites are to be needled. Many sites are accessible with the patient sitting, but the possibility of fainting must be kept in mind and if this is thought to be a risk the patient should, if feasible, be treated lying down. However, it is difficult to needle the neck and shoulders in a lying patient; one way out of this dilemma is to seat him sideways on the couch and facing away from you. If a faint then develops you can manoeuvre the patient into a lying position without much difficulty.

For treating the back it might seem logical to make the patient lie prone. However, this tends to squash the vertebral spines together unless a pillow is placed under the abdomen, and it may therefore be preferable to place the patient in the left or right lateral position. The back can also be treated with the patient sitting rather than lying. A convenient way of doing this is to use two chairs; the patient sits on one and leans forward on the other.

PHENOMENA EXPERIENCED DURING ACUPUNCTURE

These can be divided into sensations experienced by the patient and those experienced by the acupuncturist.

Sensations experienced by the patient

Local sensations

There is often a momentary pain when the needle is inserted. This comes from the skin and should pass off quickly. If it persists or is severe the needle should be withdrawn. There may then ensue a variety of other sensations, for most of which there are no adequate descriptive terms in English; the Chinese expressions have been rendered as 'fullness', 'heaviness' and 'sourness' (a kind of deep muscular aching). These sensations can radiate around the needle site for a variable distance. Together with the sensations felt by the acupuncturist, they make up the phenomena called 'De Qi' (see below).

General sensations

The patient may experience a degree of relaxation; this is quite common and sometimes it goes on to become drowsiness or euphoria. Patients may say they feel as if they have taken alcohol or other drugs. If pronounced, these sensations suggest that the patient is a 'strong reactor' (see below, also Ch 5). The explanation for these effects is unknown. They have been ascribed to endogenous opioid release, but against this is the fact that they can develop very rapidly—within a few seconds of the needle's being inserted. An interesting variation on this theme is the occasional occurrence of prolonged laughter or crying. These emotional abreactions can occur un-expectedly, sometimes after a number of treatments; they do not usually recur subsequently although some patients experience them every time they are treated.

Strong reactors

Patients who show some or all of these effects to a marked extent are likely to be strong reactors to acupuncture. (The existence of this patient category was first pointed out by Dr Felix Mann; see Ch 5.) Such people are particularly likely to do well with acupuncture but they are also easily made worse by it. They must be treated lightly, with briefer and more gentle needling than usual. They can sometimes be identified in advance of treatment; they tend to have a lively, alert appearance and are said to be likely to possess an artistic temperament. They show sensitivity to environmental influences and may give a

history of reacting adversely to many conventional drugs and to alcohol. But although these features may raise the suspicion that a patient is a strong reactor, some patients who do not fit the description may nevertheless prove to be strong reactors, so all new patients should be treated gently as a precaution. Children should always be regarded as strong reactors.

Strong reactors are likely to become drowsy or euphoric after treatment. They may also experience radiation of acupuncture sensations to various parts of the body, which may be remote from the site of needling. These effects are usually immediate, often occurring within seconds of needle insertion, but they may also be delayed. For this reason, patients should generally not drive immediately after treatment, especially after the first treatment. On one occasion a patient of mine drove the wrong way round a roundabout after acupuncture.

True strong reactors continue to get the same effect from acupuncture each time they are treated, sometimes for months or even years. Moreover they get it even if they treat themselves. In contrast, there are some patients who appear to have a strong reaction the first time they are treated but react much less strongly the second time and hardly at all thereafter.

Non-responders

The converse of the strong reactor is the patient who does not show any therapeutic response to acupuncture. According to many surveys 20–30% of the population are likely to be non-responders. However, the fact that a particular patient shows no immediate local or general response to treatment does not necessarily indicate that he or she is a non-responder; this can only be assessed later, once the effect of treatment on the symptoms has become apparent.

Sensations experienced by the practitioner

The acupuncturist may feel a resistance to manipulation of the needle, and the needle may be gripped by the tissues so that it is difficult to withdraw.

Other phenomena

The needle may appear to be drawn inwards so that there is a dimple round it. The needle site may be surrounded by an area of erythema.

De Qi As mentioned above, the subjective and objective local phenomena are together referred to by traditionalists as 'De Qi'; they regard these phenomena as indicating that the needle has tapped into the flow of Qi circulating in the meridians (see Ch 20). Non-traditional acupuncturists also use this term, although in a purely descriptive sense. According to some sources it is essential to obtain De Qi if there is to be a therapeutic response but this is by no means a universal opinion; however, it is likely that the occurrence of De Qi makes a good response more probable.

POSSIBLE COURSES OF EVENTS AFTER ACUPUNCTURE

The course of events after an initial acupuncture session is always unpredictable. There may be no change at all in the patient's symptoms, or there may be an improvement ranging from slight to complete relief, while the effect may be anything from transient to permanent. There may also be an aggravation—that is, a (temporary) worsening of symptoms.

A common sequence of events is that after the initial treatment there is a fairly transient improvement, lasting perhaps 2 or 3 days. Subsequent treatments tend to give longer remissions, which may also be more nearly complete. Ideally the patient will become symptom free after perhaps three to six treatments and can then be discharged. Quite often, especially in chronic disease, relief is incomplete but still worth while, or the symptoms remit but keep returning after a number of weeks or months. Many patients therefore require repeated treatment at intervals.

It is also common for patients to experience an aggravation. Such worsening of existing symptoms seldom lasts more than 2 or 3 days, although occasionally it may last longer. Aggravations are never permanent but in some disorders (asthma, for example) they are potentially dangerous. They may indicate that treatment was too vigorous, in which case a more gentle approach, with fewer needles and little or no stimulation, may prevent the aggravation; but some patients have this reaction every time they are treated no matter what is done. As a rule the occurrence of an aggravation suggests that there will be a therapeutic response later, but exceptions do occur.

Like aggravations, improvement in symptoms may take a few hours or days to appear. This again tends to be constant for any individual patient. Because the duration of improvement after the initial treatment is sometimes quite brief, it is important to question the patient specifically about even short-term relief, otherwise the acupuncturist may get the misleading impression that the treatment failed to work at all.

When to give up

In most cases there should be at least some degree of improvement within two or three sessions of treatment; if there has been no response at all at that stage it is seldom worth continuing. Certainly there can be no justification for continuing treatment indefinitely in the hope that a response will ultimately occur. The two- to three-session rule is not inflexible and some exceptions do occur, but it is a fairly safe guide for beginners. If a patient shows an aggravation to treatment, that should be construed as a response, albeit a negative one, and it suggests that improvement may be obtained by repeating the treatment more gently. There are undoubtedly some patients who will respond favourably only to acupuncture carried out with the utmost delicacy and lightness of touch.

Patients who show only brief response

These patients present some of the most difficult

therapeutic dilemmas. Some patients have good relief of their symptoms for only 2 or 3 weeks after each treatment. In such cases a search should be made for factors that are continually precipitating the symptoms, such as sitting in an uncomfortable position at work or living in an unhappy domestic situation. It may or may not be possible to modify these circumstances. In other cases it may be advisable to try TENS (see Ch 11) or self-acupuncture (see below)

Short-lived relief of symptoms also occurs in patients in whom acupuncture is being used to treat the pain of malignant disease. The duration of relief tends to decrease in these cases as the disease progresses, and acupuncture can thus be used as an indication of the patient's state of health.

Self-acupuncture

Some patients respond for relatively short periods to acupuncture, but during that time get excellent relief. Some of these can be helped if they are taught to carry out their own acupuncture. There seems no reason why patients should not do this; after all, many diabetics routinely inject themselves twice daily with insulin, so why should people not insert a plain needle after adequate instruction? Naturally it is necessary to select both the site of needling and the patient who is to learn the technique with care. Sites that generally prove easy for patients to use are LR-3 and the superficial tissues of the lower abdomen (except in very thin people). Sometimes it is preferable to teach a relative to give the treatment.

The acupuncturist should put in one needle as a demonstration and then have the patient put in another on the opposite side. The patient is then given a supply of needles (usually short—15 mm—ones) and some alcohol swabs if these are to be used. It is also a good idea to give the patient a printed list of instructions as a reminder, and to tell him to telephone at any time if there are any problems; in practice there almost never are. Patients are instructed to keep to the same site or sites of needling and not to increase the frequency of needling without discussing it with the doctor first. The frequency is usually once

every 2 or 3 weeks, rarely more often. The results of self-acupuncture practised in this way are generally excellent.

OTHER KINDS OF ACUPUNCTURE

ACUPRESSURE

This is an unfortunate term, meaning literally 'pressure with needles'. However, it has been increasingly widely used in recent years to refer to manual pressing of acupuncture points. TPs in muscles and elsewhere can often be inactivated, at least temporarily, by firm pressure or massage with the fingers. This can be painful but it has the advantage that patients can do it for themselves. It is generally less effective than acupuncture and needs to be repeated frequently.

The disappearance of TPs with pressure can be a problem for the therapist. It often happens that a TP is initially identified by palpation, but the mere process of examination is enough to abolish the TP temporarily so that subsequent needling is made more difficult.

EAR ACUPUNCTURE (AURICULOTHERAPY)

This technique has already been mentioned several times in passing. The modern use of the external ear to treat disease derives from the work of Dr Paul Nogier in France (1972, 1981), although it has been claimed that the method was known in China for many centuries. The basic idea is that there exists a representation of the body in the ear, with the head at the bottom in the lobe of the ear, the legs and feet at the top, and the spine running along the outer part of the ear. This recalls the motor and sensory homunculi in the cortex of the brain. Maps of the ear showing the acupuncture points on it exist; some derive from Nogier, others come from China.

The simplest method of locating the points on the ear is just to probe for areas of tenderness. More sophisticated methods, using electrical apparatus of various kinds, also exist, and Nogier has pioneered the use of what he calls the 'auriculocardiac reflex': coloured filters are brought up to the ear and the acupuncturist looks for changes in the quality of the radial pulse.

Needling the ear is carried out with fine short needles. These should be inserted carefully, without piercing the cartilage of the ear. The ear is generally chosen to needle when acupuncture is used to treat smoking or other addictions; indwelling press studs are often inserted in such cases and left in for a week or longer. There is a risk of infection if this is done and there have been cases in the last few years of bacterial endocarditis caused in this way. This technique should therefore be used cautiously if at all.

OTHER SOMATIC REPRESENTATIONS

Ear acupuncture is the best-known instance of a claimed somatic representation in a small area but it is not the only one. In scalp acupuncture, needles are inserted in the scalp overlying the motor cortex to try to restore function after a stroke, for example. Reflexology is a method of treatment in which zones in the soles of the feet, which are held to correspond to various body areas, are pressed and massaged. Still another site of representation is said to be along the course of the first metacarpal bone. Numerous other types of representation ('microacupuncture') are said to exist.

MOXA

This is an ancient Chinese practice allied to acupuncture. It consists in applying a thermal stimulus to various sites; many moxa sites are the same as acupuncture sites but there are also special moxa sites. Moxa is dried fibre obtained from plants of the *Artemisia* genus. It may be wrapped round the handle of the needle, which then conducts the warmth into the tissues, or it may be laid on a slice of garlic or ginger. Another method, used for moxa at the umbilicus, is to fill the umbilicus with salt and place the moxa on this. Moxa is little used in the West except by adherents of the traditional system.

INJECTION TECHNIQUES

There is a fine line between acupuncture and the injection of various substances into TPs or classic acupuncture points. A number of reports have appeared in the West in recent years, describing treatments based on injecting local anaesthetic, saline, and even sterile water to treat musculoskeletal disorders. It is likely that these techniques work in the same way as acupuncture although for some reason the experimenters seem not to have taken the logical next step of simply inserting a needle without injecting anything. The Chinese have also tried injecting various substances into acupuncture points, including vitamins and amniotic fluid. In France the technique of 'mesotherapy' uses the hypodermic or intradermal injection of a very wide range of substances to treat musculoskeletal and other disorders.

ELECTRICAL ACUPUNCTURE AND ALLIED METHODS

The use of electricity in acupuncture was another Chinese innovation, although it has been taken up widely in the West. Electricity has been used in two main ways: for point detection and for treatment (see also Ch 10).

Point detection

Numerous machines for detecting acupuncture points have appeared. Most depend on measuring the electrical resistance of the skin, the assumption being that this is lower over the acupuncture points. Most of the available machines tend to yield points wherever the experimenter expects to find them, but some, such as the Ryodoraku machine (see below), give more accurate results. Opinions differ on the value of using machines for this purpose, even among those practitioners who believe in the existence of traditional acupuncture points. Probably most seasoned acupuncturists would prefer to rely on their hands and their experience in deciding where to insert the needles, but some find the machines helpful and accurate.

Treatment

The Chinese first developed the use of electricity to stimulate acupuncture points. To do this, a needle is inserted into the point to be treated and one terminal is attached to the handle, usually via a crocodile clip. The other terminal is connected either to a second needle or to a neutral electrode (such as an electrocardiogram (ECG) electrode). Several needles are often connected to multiple outlets in this way. Choosing the right kind of current is important; direct current is unsuitable because electrochemical forces will corrode and weaken the needles, so a square-wave interrupted current is used. This may be relatively slow (2–10 Hz) or fast (80–150 Hz). More sophisticated stimulation patterns, designed to delay the rate at which the nervous system adapts to the stimulus, have been developed.

There have been very few studies to compare the effectiveness of electrical and manual stimulation. The choice of which to use therefore comes down largely to personal preference and practical convenience. Doctors who wish to give prolonged stimulation at several sites simultaneously may well find electrical stimulation useful but those who use minimal or brief insertion of the needles will not have any opportunity or need to stimulate them electrically.

Ryodoraku

Ryodoraku is a Japanese form of acupuncture that uses a special electrical machine for both diagnosis and treatment. The electrical resistance of the skin is measured with the machine at three points on each wrist and ankle, giving a total of 12 readings; these are then compared with the expected readings at these sites and a diagnosis is made accordingly. The machine is then used to stimulate various points on the body via inserted needles; the stimulation is typically brief. The Ryodoraku machine can also be used to search for acupuncture points on the body or the ear, without reference to the full Ryodoraku therapeutic system. Used in this way, the machine seems to detect certain sites of reduced electrical resistance in quite a convincing

and reproducible manner, without producing artefacts, although how far these are identical with acupuncture points, and how useful it is to find them, are still undecided questions.

TENS

TENS (see also Ch 11) is a form of treatment that has something in common with acupuncture and is another form of stimulation-induced analgesia. A small battery-powered machine is used to generate an interrupted current, which is applied to the skin via electrodes. These may be placed on either side of the painful area, over a major nerve supplying the area, or over the spine at a level one or two segments above that of the pain. It is worth trying in patients who respond only briefly to acupuncture and also in those who would be expected to respond to acupuncture but who fail to do so. The optimum frequency is usually about 80 Hz. It is important to make sure that the patient clearly understands how to use the machine and realizes that the pain may well return soon after the machine is switched off. (This is not, however, invariably the case; in some fortunate people relief of pain may last up to 10 hours.)

Although generally thought of as a treatment for pain, TENS can also be useful in some non-painful disorders. It can, for example, relieve the spasticity in some patients with multiple sclerosis if it is placed over the femoral or sciatic nerve. Professor B Kaada (1986) has described the use of low-frequency (2 Hz) TENS to treat non-healing ulcers and other circulatory disorders, and it has on occasion proved helpful in patients with Raynaud's disease.

Laser therapy

There has been a considerable vogue in recent years for using low-power lasers to stimulate acupuncture points (see also Ch 12). There are obvious attractions in doing this: there is no risk of infection and the treatment is pain free so it seems suitable for children and for adults who are apprehensive about acupuncture. However, the equipment is expensive and clinical trials of the efficacy of laser therapy have given mixed results. To date, it is not clear that the effect of these lasers is different from that produced by machines producing intense non-laser light. There are also certain legal restrictions on the therapeutic use of lasers.

and no one way that is indisputably 'right'. In time, research will doubtless give better guidance to choosing the best methods to use, but at present dogmatism would be out of place.

CONCLUSION

As this chapter will have made clear, there are many possible ways of practising acupuncture

FURTHER READING

Anon 1973 An outline of Chinese acupuncture. Academy of Traditional Chinese Medicine, Beijing

Kaada B 1986 Treatment of peripheral ischaemia and chronic ulceration by transcutaneous nerve stimulation (TNS). Acupuncture in medicine 3:30

Kaptchuk T J 1983 Chinese medicine: the web that has no weaver. Hutchison, London

Macdonald A 1984 Acupuncture: from ancient art to modern medicine. George Allen & Unwin, London

Needham J, Gwei-Djen L 1980 Celestial lancets: a history and rationale of acupuncture and moxa. Cambridge University Press, Cambridge

Nguyen Duc Hiepm 1987 The dictionary of acupuncture and moxibustion. Thorsons, Wellingborough

Nogier PFM 1972 Treatise of auricular therapy. Maisonneuve, Paris

Nogier PFM (trans. Kenyon J N) 1981 Introduction to auricular therapy. Maisonneuve, Paris

Mann F 1980 The treatment of disease by acupuncture, 3rd edn. Heinemann, London

Mann F 1993 Reinventing acupuncture: a new concept of ancient medicine. Butterworth Heinemann, London

Baldry P E 1993 Acupuncture, trigger points, and musculoskeletal pain, 2nd edn. Churchill Livingstone, New York

Travell J G, Simons D G 1983 Myofascial pain and dysfunction: the trigger point manual, vol. 1 Williams & Wilkins, Baltimore/London.

Travell J G, Simons D G 1992 Myofascial pain and dysfunction: the trigger point manual, vol 2. Williams & Wilkins, Baltimore

Melzack R, Wall P 1992 The challenge of pain, revised edn. Penguin, Harmondsworth

Wall P D, Melzack R (eds) 1984 A textbook of pain. Churchill Livingstone, New York

4

Trigger point acupuncture

Peter Baldry

INTRODUCTION

One of the most important indications for acupuncture, so far as pain relief is concerned, is in the alleviation of pain emanating from trigger points, in what currently is called the myofascial pain syndrome (MPS).

Terminology

MPS is a disorder in which muscle pain, localized to one particular region of the body, develops in the presence of a normal erythrocyte sedimentation rate and in the absence of any specific histological, biochemical or serological abnormalities. It is important to distinguish this syndrome from the somewhat similar but generalized muscle pain disorder currently known as fibromyalgia.

It should be noted that all other terms for these two disorders, such as muscular rheumatism, non-articular rheumatism, psychogenic rheumatism, fibrositis, myalgia and myositis, together with many others, are now outmoded.

Some early observations

It was John Kellgren, later to become Professor of Rheumatology at Manchester University, who in 1938, when working as a young research assistant under Sir Thomas Lewis at University College Hospital, London, was one of the first to conclude that the pain in myalgia, or what is currently called MPS, emanates from small, circumscribed, exquisitely tender points in muscle. He came to this conclusion by observing that he could reproduce the spontaneously occurring pain by applying sustained pressure to these points and that he could alleviate it by injecting Novocain (procaine hydrochloride) into them. He also observed that this pain is not generally felt at the tender point site itself, but is referred to an area of the body some distance from it (Kellgren 1938). It was largely these observations that prompted the American physician, Janet Travell, to study patients with musculoskeletal pain. She soon decided that, as it is neural hyperactivity at what Kellgren called tender points in muscle and its surrounding fascia that triggers off this referred pain, it would be more apt to call such points 'trigger points'. She also introduced the terms 'myofascial pain' and 'zones of pain referral', in addition to calling the disorder itself MPS (Travell & Rinzler 1952).

AETIOLOGY OF MPS

Trauma is the main aetiological factor. The muscle or muscles affected may suffer a direct injury or alternatively become acutely, chronically or recurrently overloaded. In addition, they may be subjected to repeated microtrauma such as may occur occupationally in patients with what has come to be known as 'repetitive strain injury'.

Trigger point nociceptors

MPS develops as a result of the activation and sensitization of nociceptors at trigger point sites in muscle.

Nociceptors are of two types. In the skin there are high-threshold Aδ mechanothermal nociceptors and C polymodal nociceptors. In muscle the nociceptors corresponding to these are termed group III and group IV respectively. Activation of cutaneous Aδ nociceptors gives rise to a transient, so-called 'first' pain and activation of cutaneous C nociceptors gives rise to a persistent, dull, aching, so-called 'second' pain. It might be thought that the effect of

trauma on muscle is similarly to activate Aδ (group III) and C (group IV) nociceptors. Raja, Meyer & Meyer (1988), however, have pointed out that 'the differential role, if any, of the myelinated and unmyelinated muscle nociceptors is unclear at the present time'. Also, Mense (personal communication, 1993) is of the opinion that 'first and second pain corresponding to the activation of group III and group IV fibres respectively, does not seem to exist in muscle'. David Bowsher (personal communication 1993) has gone so far as to state that 'nobody knows what is felt when human muscle group III (Aδ) afferents are stimulated'. The situation therefore is far from clear.

However, as the persistent, dull, aching type of pain present in MPS is similar in every respect to that which arises when C afferent, cutaneous nociceptors are activated, it would seem reasonable to conclude that the pain in MPS develops as a result of the activation of C afferent (group IV) nociceptors at trigger point sites in muscle. In support of this view is the observation that the pain in this disorder may be abolished by means of stimulating cutaneous and subcutaneous Aδ nerve fibres with dry needles (i.e. acupuncture), for it is known that this procedure blocks the C afferent input to the spinal cord, both from skin and from muscle, by activating enkephalinergic inhibitory interneurons situated at the boundary between lamina I and II of the dorsal horn (Bowsher 1990).

Myofascial trigger point group IV nociceptor activation

Myofascial trigger point, group IV, nociceptors situated at unmyelinated, C afferent nerve fibre terminals are initially activated as a result of the muscle being subjected to high-intensity, mechanically induced trauma. Trauma of this severity also damages surrounding tissue cells with, as a result of this and an associated inflammatory response, the liberation of various chemical substances such as bradykinin, prostaglandins, histamine and potassium ions. These chemicals are high-intensity, noxious stimulators and thus augment the already physically induced nociceptor activation (Rang, Bevan & Dray 1991).

Sensitization of activated myofascial trigger point group IV nociceptors

The noxious chemicals above also sensitize the nociceptors, lowering their threshold so that they then respond to low-intensity as well as high-intensity stimuli with, as a consequence, pain and tenderness from stretching or firm pressure—a phenomenon known as primary hyperalgesia (Woolf 1991). It is because of this chemically induced sensitization of nociceptors at a trigger point site that the tissues in its immediate vicinity are tender, and the tissues directly overlying it are exquisitely tender when firmly pressed.

Myofascial trigger point pain referral patterns

During the past 50 years Travell has made a special study of myofascial trigger point pain referral patterns and in recent years she and her colleague, David Simons, have published an authoritative textbook in two volumes in which these patterns are described and clearly depicted in well-executed drawings (Travell & Simons 1983, 1992). Travell and Simons state that each muscle in the body has its own specific pattern of trigger point pain referral. With some muscles this pain referral is to a distant site (Fig. 4.1); with some, the referral is to a site in the vicinity of the trigger point (Fig. 4.2); and with some the referral is both local and distant (Fig. 4.3). It has been possible for me to recognize most of these patterns in my own patients (Baldry 1993); it is necessary to stress, however, that this has not been so in all cases and in view of this it would seem reasonable to suggest that in the years to come the collective experience of clinicians working in this field may lead to the recognition of a number of variants.

THE DETECTION OF TRIGGER POINTS

It is essential when searching for trigger points for the examination to be carried out in a systematic manner. Guidance as to which muscles are likely to be affected by trigger point activity is obtained by paying careful attention to descriptions of referred pain patterns and by observing which movements of the body are restricted. Each muscle under suspicion should then be placed slightly on the stretch and systematically searched for trigger points by drawing the fingers firmly across the muscle in a manner similar to that employed when kneading dough. The necessity for firm palpation has to be emphasized because trigger points are liable to be overlooked if the pressure exerted is too gentle. Firm pressure over normal muscles causes no discomfort, but in the vicinity of a trigger point it is slightly uncomfortable, and over a trigger point itself, because it is a site where the nerve endings have become sensitized, the discomfort is such as to cause the patient involuntarily to jerk (the jump sign—Kraft, Johnson & La Ban 1968) and to utter an expletive such as 'ouch', or in Chinese, 'Ah Shi' (oh yes)! The clinical detection of a trigger point, which by definition is a point of maximum tenderness, is primarily dependent on the elicitation of these reactions.

In view of a trigger point's excessive tenderness, it is possible to determine its presence objectively by measuring the pressure threshold over it and comparing it with that over a corresponding contralateral non-tender point (Fischer 1988). There is nothing to be gained, however, from the use of a pressure threshold meter in everyday clinical practice. Such an instrument is of value only for clinical trials and in compensation claims where postaccident myofascial trigger point pain is involved.

Myofascial trigger point sites

Myofascial trigger points are found at muscle insertion sites, in the free borders of muscles, and also sometimes in their bellies, particularly in the region of their motor points. They may be present in areas of muscle that otherwise feel entirely normal. Additionally, they may be found in palpable, taut bands and fibrositic nodules.

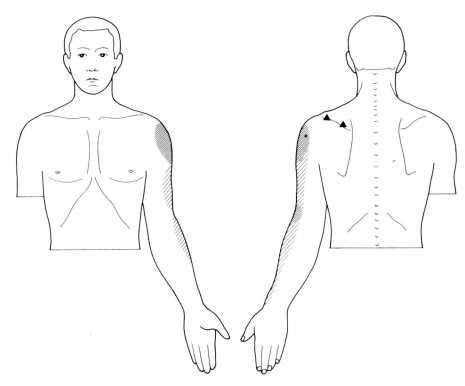

Figure 4.1 The pattern of pain referral from a trigger point or points (▲) in the supraspinatus muscle.

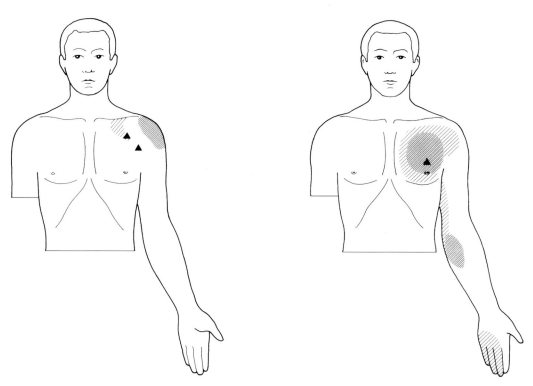

Figure 4.2 The pattern of pain referral from a trigger point or points (▲) in the clavicular section of the pectoralis major muscle.

Figure 4.3 The pattern of pain referral from a trigger point or points (▲) in the sternal section of the pectoralis major muscle.

Palpable bands

A palpable taut band in a muscle has a string-like feel and is frequently detected in the muscles of patients with MPS. There has been much controversy concerning the nature of these bands and their mode of development, particularly as they are not found in all cases. When one is present, however, it is always possible to find a trigger point somewhere along its length. In addition, a transient contraction of muscle fibres (twitch response) can sometimes be produced by sharply plucking, like a violin string, a palpable band in superficial muscle.

Fibrositic nodules

The mode of development of fibrositic nodules is equally enigmatic and it is particularly difficult to explain why they are found mainly in the lumbar region and less commonly, around the neck and shoulders. Awad (1990) has made a careful study of them using both light and electron microscopy. He has shown that they contain large amounts of extracellular, water-retaining, amorphous, mucopolysaccharide material. He is of the opinion that this material, increases the acidity of muscle fibres by impairing their oxygen flow. This activates muscle nociceptors, converting them into pain-producing trigger points.

Associated physical signs

A muscle containing active trigger points becomes shorter and weaker. Any attempt to extend it results in pain before full extension is achieved.

Trigger point activity may also be associated with certain sympathetically mediated changes such as goose flesh, localized sweating and, most troublesome of all, intense coldness of the distal part of a limb. It should also be noted that reflex sympathetic dystrophy and the myofascial pain syndrome may develop concomitantly (Baldry 1994).

Potential, active and latent myofascial trigger points

No discussion concerning the diagnosis of MPS would be complete without drawing attention to the differences between potential, active and latent myofascial trigger points.

Potential myofascial trigger points

A potential myofascial trigger point is estimated by Travell & Simons (1983) to be no more than a few millimetres in diameter. It consists of a number of different types of nerve ending, including nociceptors that are liable to undergo pain-producing activation and sensitization should the muscle in which the myofascial trigger point is located happen to be subjected to trauma. On firm palpation a potential myofascial trigger point in a superficially placed muscle is found to be slightly tender. This distinguishes it from either an active or a latent myofascial trigger point, both of which are so exquisitely tender that the application of firm pressure to them produces an involuntary flexion withdrawal.

Active myofascial trigger points

An active myofascial trigger point is one whose nociceptors have undergone sufficient trauma-induced activation and sensitization to cause pain to be referred to a site some distance from it (the zone of pain referral). Active myofascial trigger points are of three types—primary, secondary and satellite.

Primary active myofascial trigger points are in the muscle or group of muscles that were initially subjected to trauma. In some cases of MPS only these myofascial trigger points are activated. In others, activity develops in secondary myofascial trigger points situated in either synergists or antagonists of the primarily affected muscles, or both. Activity in myofascial trigger points situated in synergistic muscles develops as a secondary event, when these become overloaded as a result of compensating for the weakened primarily affected ones. Activation in the antagonists develops when these muscles become strained from counter-acting the tension and shortening of muscles that are primarily affected.

In addition, myofascial trigger points in muscles within the zones of pain referral of primary and secondary myofascial trigger points are also liable to undergo activation because of pain-induced muscle spasm. When this happens they are known as satellite myofascial trigger points; these in turn cause pain to be referred to still more distant sites, so that over the course of time the pain in MPS may spread to affect an ever-increasingly large area. It is, for example, not uncommon for pain from a primary myo-fascial trigger point in a muscle in the lower part of the posterior chest wall to be referred to the buttock (Fig. 4.4), for satellite myofascial trigger points situated in the gluteal muscles then to become activated, with consequent referral of pain down the back of the leg (Fig. 4.5A,B); and for this in turn to bring about activation of satellite myofascial trigger points in the calf muscles.

For the successful treatment of MPS it is essential that all the primary, secondary and satellite myofascial trigger points present in any individual patient are systematically searched for and then deactivated in an equally sys-tematic manner.

Latent myofascial trigger points

Latent myofascial trigger points are those trigger points whose nociceptors have undergone a limited amount of trauma-induced activation and sensitization, but not enough to cause pain to develop. As the nociceptor sensitization of a latent myofascial trigger point is sufficient to cause it to be as exquisitely tender on firm pal-pation as an active, pain-producing myofascial trigger point, latent myofascial trigger points are liable to be found on routine examination of muscles in symptomless people. Sola & Kuitert (1955), in a survey of 200 fit young people serving in the American Air Force (100 males, age range 17–27; and 100 females, age range 18–35) found that 54 of the females and 45 of the males had myofascial trigger points that, whilst

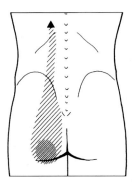

Figure 4.4 The pattern of pain referral from a trigger point (▲) in the longissimus thoracis muscle.

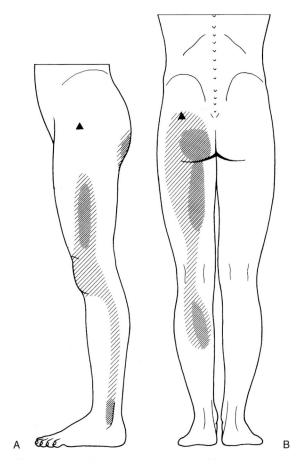

A   B

Figure 4.5 A: The pattern of pain referral from a trigger point (▲) in either the gluteus medius or minimus near to the attachment of these muscles to the greater trochanter. B: The pattern of pain referral from a trigger point (▲) in the posterior part of either the gluteus medius or minimus muscles.

exquisitely tender, were not causing pain and therefore were considered to be in the latent phase. A latent myofascial trigger point is liable to be converted into an active pain-producing one in response to only a relatively small amount of additional trauma.

Finally, it has to be said that histological examination of tissues at potential, active and latent myofascial trigger point sites shows no specific pathological changes. It is partly because of this that myofascial trigger points have not received the attention they so clearly deserve.

DEACTIVATION OF MYOFASCIAL TRIGGER POINTS

As stated earlier, Kellgren (1938) found that he was able to alleviate pain of muscular origin by injecting a local anaesthetic into trigger points. Travell & Simons (1983, 1992) continue to employ this method. Local anaesthetics, however, are occasionally associated with the development of serious adverse reactions, such as syncope, palpitations, cardiac arrest and convulsions (Committee on Safety of Medicine update 1986). It was because of this that Sola and his colleagues (Sola & Kuitert 1955, Sola & Williams 1956) tried normal saline and discovered that they could obtain equally good results. Following on from this Frost, Jessen & Siggaard-Andersen (1980) conducted a double-blind trial in which they compared the pain-relieving effects of injecting trigger points with either mepivacaine or saline. To their surprise, they found that 80% of patients in the saline group but only 52% in the group treated with mepivacaine reported pain relief.

Over the years it has been shown that it is possible to deactivate trigger points by injecting into them one or another of a large number of disparate substances (Lu & Needham 1980). The only reasonable inference to be drawn from this is that the pain relief obtained is not dependent on any specific properties these substances may possess, but rather on the stimulating effect of the needle used for their injection.

Travell & Rinzler (1952) commented on the effectiveness of needling trigger points over 40 years ago, but one of the first physicians to employ dry needling extensively for this purpose was Karel Lewit of Czechoslovakia. Lewit (1979) reported favourably on the use of this technique in a series of 241 patients with musculoskeletal pain. Both he and, since then, Jaeger & Skootsky (1987) have stressed that the effectiveness of the method is dependent not only on inserting the needle deeply into the muscle, but in particular on the precision with which it is inserted into the trigger point itself.

Gunn (1989) also advocates inserting the needle deeply into the muscle. However, such a procedure is liable to give rise to a considerable amount of discomfort for, as he states, 'When the needle enters a muscle band that is in spasm . . . the patient experiences a cramp-like sensation which can be exquisitely painful', and continues, 'The patient's communication of the cramp is the best guide to accurate needling'.

It is certainly essential to locate each trigger point accurately, but there are now grounds for believing that it is not necessary to insert the needle into the trigger point itself and that it is easier, far less pain provoking and just as effective to insert it into the superficial tissues directly overlying the trigger point. My reasons for advocating this method are that some years ago, when attempting to deactivate a trigger point in the scalenus anterior muscle, it seemed prudent to me, in view of the proximity of the apex of the lung, to insert the needle only a short distance under the skin, and found that this was sufficient to relieve the pain referred down the arm from this trigger point. I then tried superficial needling at trigger point sites elsewhere in the body and found this to be equally effective. Not long after this Macdonald et al (1983) confirmed my findings by showing that it is possible to alleviate low back pain by inserting needles to an approximate depth of only 4 mm at trigger point sites.

Bowsher (1987) has now explained why superficial dry needling is all that is required, by pointing out that the Aδ sensory afferents, which are the ones stimulated whenever a needle is inserted into the body, are present mainly but not exclusively in the skin and just beneath it.

Superficial dry needling at trigger point sites

Pain-modulating mechanisms

It is necessary to stress that, when carrying out superficial dry needling (SDN) for the relief of myofascial trigger point pain, each trigger point must be accurately located and then care must be taken to ensure that the needle is inserted into the tissues immediately overlying it. This is in order to make certain that the Aδ nerve fibres stimulated in this manner and the trigger point's C afferent (group IV) fibres project to the same dorsal horn. The needle-induced Aδ afferent activity is then able to block the trigger point's C afferent input to the spinal cord by evoking

activity in enkephalinergic inhibitory interneurons situated on the border of lamina I and II of this dorsal horn by two separate means (Bowsher 1991).

One way in which this occurs is that the Aδ afferent fibres in the outer part of the dorsal horn have branches that project directly to these inhibitory interneurons. The other is that these inhibitory interneurons undergo excitation by the more indirect means of activity developing in the descending inhibitory system. This happens because there is a pathway linking the neo-spinothalamic tract and the upper end of the descending inhibitory system in the periaqueductal grey area of the midbrain, which allows Aδ sensory afferent-generated electrical impulses in this ascending pathway to promote activity in the opioid peptide-mediated serotoninergic fibres situated in the descending dorsolateral funiculus (Fig. 4.6; see also Ch 6).

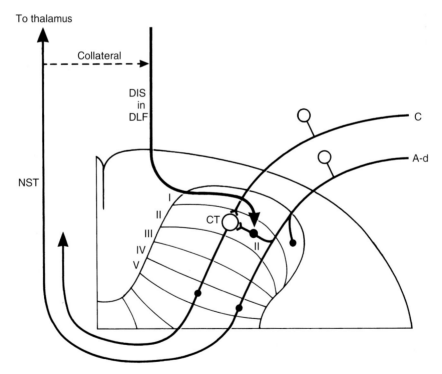

Figure 4.6 Diagram of dorsal horn to show the local intraspinal connection between Aδ nerve fibres and enkephalinergic inhibitory interneuron (II), whose function it is to inhibit activity in C afferent terminal cell (CT). Also, to show the indirect Aδ link with inhibitory interneuron via the collateral connecting the Aδ afferent's ascending pathway—the neospinothalamic tract (NST) with the descending inhibitory system in the dorsolateral funiculus (DIS in DLF).

While this is probably how brief stimulation of Aδ nerve fibres with a dry needle brings about immediate nocigenic pain relief, it does not explain why such relief at times continues to last for weeks, months or even permanently and it is generally recognized that there is still much to be learnt concerning the neural mechanisms responsible for the long-term effects.

SDN technique

It is my current practice when deactivating a myofascial trigger point for the first time, to insert the needle into the tissues overlying the trigger point to a depth of 5–10 mm and to leave it there without any form of manipulation for about 30 seconds. This is because the amount of neural stimulation required is the minimum necessary to abolish the exquisite tenderness at the trigger point site, which before needling had made the patient wince involuntarily (the 'jump sign'). Therefore, on withdrawing the needle, pressure equal to that applied before needling is applied to the trigger point site to see whether abolition has been achieved. One 30-second period of needling is sometimes all that is required, but when it is not the needle is then replaced and left in situ for up to 2–3 minutes. Very occasionally this also proves to be insufficient and the needle is reintroduced and left in place for an even longer period. Also the amount of neural stimulation may have to be increased by means of gently twirling the needle.

The purpose of adopting this step by step approach when determining a patient's individual responsiveness to SDN is because some people are such strong reactors that anything more than a minimal stimulus may cause temporary exacerbation of the pain for 12–24 hours. In cases where there has not been a flare-up of pain following the first treatment, and this should be a majority of cases provided the graduated approach has been followed, the time for which needles are left in situ at subsequent treatment sessions should either be kept the same as on the initial occasion, or increased if the pain relief has not been as good as might have been expected.

FIBROMYALGIA

Fibromyalgia (FM) is a disorder in which generalized musculoskeletal pain develops in association with multiple tender points scattered throughout the body. These tender points, which are mainly in muscles (see Box 4.1), are a mixture of latent and active trigger points. Patients with FM complain of non-restorative sleep, morning stiffness and persistent fatigue. In addition they may have headaches, irritable bowel, irritable bladder, dysmenorrhoea, Raynaud's phenomenon and restless legs (Baldry 1992). For the purpose of standardizing research protocols, the American College of Rheumatology's essential criteria for a diagnosis of FM are widespread pain and 11 or more out of 18 specified tender points (Box 4.1).

It is clinically important to distinguish between MPS and FM as their aetiology, prognosis and management are different. Bear in mind that MPS may mimic FM when two or more regions are affected by it simultaneously. It should also be noted that trauma-induced MPS may be

---

Box 4.1 Diagnostic criteria for Fibromyalgia Syndrome according to the 1990 Multicenter Criteria Committee of the American College of Rheumatology (Wolfe et al 1990)

Widespread pain of at least 3 months duration
Pain in 11 or more of the following 18 tender points when digitally palpated with a pressure of 4 kg.

1. Occiput: at the suboccipital muscle insertions (bilateral)
2. Low cervical: at the anterior aspect of the inter-transverse spaces at C5-C7 (bilateral)
3. Trapezius: at the midpoint of the upper border (bilateral)
4. Supraspinatus: at origins above the scapula spine near the medial border (bilateral)
5. 2nd rib: at the second costo-chondral junctions, just lateral to the junctions on the upper surfaces (bilateral)
6. Lateral epicondyle: 2 cm distal to the epicondyle (bilateral)
7. Gluteal: in upper outer quadrants of buttocks in anterior fold of muscles (bilateral)
8. Greater trochanter: posterior to the trochanteric prominence (bilateral)
9. Knees: at the medial fatpad proximal to the joint line (bilateral)

associated with the subsequent development of FM (Bennett 1986 a,b).

The reason for the activation of C afferent nociceptors at trigger point sites in FM is unknown. It would seem to be due to some as yet unidentified biochemical disorder. There is therefore no specific treatment available and any symptomatic relief of pain obtained by means of stimulation of Aδ nerve fibres is invariably short lived. However, some patients insist that repeated treatment of this type carried out every 3–4 weeks on a long-term basis improves the quality of their lives.

REGIONAL MYOFASCIAL PAIN SYNDROMES

Space permits only a brief discussion of some of these in this chapter. They have, however, been dealt with in greater detail elsewhere (Baldry 1993, Fricton & Awad 1990, Travell & Simons 1983, 1992).

Pain in the head

Persistent headache may occasionally be a manifestation of glaucoma, cranial arteritis or a space-occupying lesion and clearly in every case such disorders have to be excluded. It is far more often, however, due to one of the primary cephalalgias, of which there are four main types—tension headaches, muscle contraction headaches, migraine and migrainous neuralgia (cluster headaches). It is in the treatment of the first three of these that trigger point acupuncture may be of benefit.

Tension headache

This is by far the commonest primary cephalalgia. There is a persistent discomfort, often described as a constricting tight band affecting the whole or any part of the head. In this condition, anxiety causes the muscles of the neck and scalp to be held in a state of persistent tension, and as a result of this trigger points in these muscles become activated.

Muscle contraction headache

In this disorder a persistent pain, localized to one or more parts of the head, develops as a result of trauma-induced activation of trigger points in muscles of the neck. With trigger points in the upper posterior cervical muscles, the pain is often referred along one side of the head (Fig. 4.7). With trigger points in the sterno-cleidomastoid muscle, the pain may be referred to one or more of three sites: behind the ear, over the eye and the top of the head (Fig. 4.8).

Migraine

Migraine is one of the few painful disorders where acupuncture is mainly carried out pro-

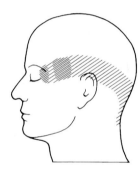

Figure 4.7 A commonly occurring pattern of pain referral from the posterior cervical muscle trigger points.

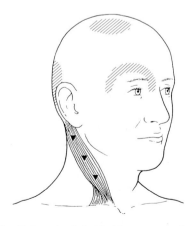

Figure 4.8 Referred pain behind the ear, over the eye and on top of the head: trigger points (▲) in the sternocleidomastoid muscle.

phylactically in between attacks in an attempt to reduce their incidence, rather than at the time of an attack for the purpose of alleviating the pain itself.

The neural mechanisms responsible for the prophylactic effect of acupuncture on migraine are not clearly understood. One seemingly relevant observation is that a large number of patients with migraine have tender points in the muscles of the neck and scalp. Loh et al (1984), in a trial comparing acupuncture with drug therapy for migraine, found tender points in these muscles in no less than 34 out of 41 cases. And furthermore they noted that acupuncture was helpful in preventing migrainous attacks from developing only in those patients in whom these points were present.

From this it might seem that one of the reasons for migraine developing in some patients is a build-up of nociceptor activity at tender points in the neck muscles. In favour of this hypothesis are the clinical observations that overzealous needling of these points is liable to bring on an attack of migraine and conversely that deactivation of these points by the brief insertion of needles into superficial tissues overlying them in between attacks of migraine is often helpful in preventing migraine from developing. However, the situation is far from straightforward, for it is also possible to achieve this prophylactic effect by inserting needles into traditional acupuncture points situated locally in the neck and at distal sites some distance from it. Points commonly used are GB-20 and GB-21 in the neck, Gall Bladder points in the temporal region, LI-4 in the hand and LR-3 in the foot (Dowson, Lewith & Machin 1985, Loh et al 1984). Moreover, Jensen, Melsen & Jensen (1979) have even reported achieving successful prophylaxis by means of stimulating LR-3 in the foot alone!

In view of these diverse, but seemingly comparable, successful prophylactic techniques there is an urgent need for controlled clinical trials to compare their relative efficacy, and in turn to compare their effectiveness with that of a placebo for, as Matthews (1983) has said: 'The placebo effect in migraine is so marked that virtually any

form of treatment administered with sufficient aplomb, as for example, acupuncture, will produce a remission in a high proportion of patients.'

Pain in the neck

Persistent pain in the head, neck and shoulder girdle with or without restricted movements of the neck, and with or without pain down the arm, may occasionally be due to malignant disease infiltrating nerve roots or vertebral bodies; to fractures, infective lesions and rheumatoid arthritis affecting the spine; or to polymyalgia rheumatica. A detailed history together with a neurological examination, and some basic investigations including an erythrocyte sedimentation rate (ESR) and cervical radiographs are therefore essential.

In most cases the ESR is within the normal range and radiographs either show no abnormality or, if the patient is 40 or over, may reveal evidence of the degenerative changes in the discs and facet joints that together comprise the disorder known as cervical spondylosis. The patient is then liable to be told that the pain is due to this disorder giving rise to pressure on a nerve root, and in an attempt to minimize the supposed effect of this is frequently advised to keep the neck as still as possible by wearing a surgical collar. Such an assumption in the majority of cases is, however, unwarranted as the radiographic changes produced by cervical spondylosis are frequently seen in people from middle age onwards irrespective of whether they have a history of neck pain (Friedenberg & Miller 1963, Heller et al 1983, Pallis, Jones & Spillane 1954). A diagnosis of nerve root entrapment brought about by this or any other disorder should therefore be made only in the relatively small number of patients with objective neurological signs and myelographic evidence of it. In the remainder, the radiographically demonstrable degenerative changes are no more than a chance investigatory finding of no clinical significance and the pain is not due to nerve root entrapment, but rather to trauma-induced primary activation of myofascial trigger points.

Acute wry neck

Sudden acute neck pain developing in association with such considerable muscle spasm as to cause the neck to be pulled over to the affected side may occur as a result of a prolapsed disc, but most often it is due to trauma or cold air-induced activation of myofascial trigger points. And when due to the latter the response to acupuncture is often dramatic.

The search for neck and shoulder girdle myofascial trigger points

In order not to overlook trigger points it is essential to palpate in turn the following structures: the ligamentum nuchae and the paravertebral muscles (Fig. 4.9); also the sternocleidomastoid muscle at its upper, middle and lower parts (Fig. 4.8); the scalenus anterior muscle in the front of the neck (Fig. 4.10); the levator scapulae, especially in its mid-part at the angle of the neck and at its insertion into the superior angle of the scapula (Figs 4.11 and 4.12); the trapezius, particularly along its upper free border (Fig. 4.13); the supraspinatus (Fig. 4.1, p 36); the infraspinatus (Fig. 4.14) and the rhomboids (Fig. 4.15).

Pain in and around the shoulder's glenohumeral joint

Pain in this joint may be due to some form of arthritis, of which the rheumatoid form is the commonest. It may alternatively be due to infective arthritis, or, rarely, osteoarthritis. In addition, bony lesions, including metastatic and myelomatous deposits in the upper humerus, scapula, ribs or clavicle, may give rise to pain in the region of the shoulder.

All these therefore have to be excluded but, in over 90% of cases, pain in the shoulder and restriction of the movements of the glenohumeral joint is due to a lesion in the soft tissues (Hazelman 1990).

These soft tissue lesions include rotator cuff tendinitis, bicipital tendinitis, adhesive capsulitis, and the periarticular myofascial trigger point pain syndrome.

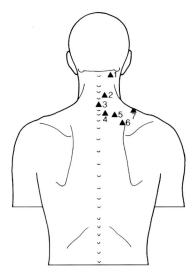

Figure 4.9 To show the positions of some commonly occurring trigger points at the back of the neck and shoulder girdle.
1. Trigger point in a depression between the upper ends of the trapezius and sternocleidomastoid muscles close to the mastoid process and coinciding in position with the traditional Chinese acupuncture point GB-20.
2. Trigger point in a posterior cervical muscle at the level of the 4th cervical vertebra. The particular muscle involved depending on the depth at which the trigger point lies.
3. Trigger point in the ligamentum nuchae.
4. Trigger point in the splenius cervicis muscle at the angle of the neck.
5. and 6. Trigger points in the levator scapulae muscle.
7. Trigger point in the upper free border of the trapezius muscle halfway between the spine and acromion and corresponding in position with the traditional Chinese acupuncture point GB-21.

Rotator cuff tendinitis

The rotator cuff is a composite structure made up of the supraspinatus, infraspinatus and subscapularis tendons. Inflammation may develop in any one of these when the tendon, already weakened by avascular necrotic degenerative changes, is subjected to trauma.

Supraspinatus tendinitis, which is the commonest, causes a persistent aching sensation in the shoulder region at rest. The movements of the joint are full, but pain develops on abduction as the arm passes through the intermediate range of this movement (60–120°), as a result of the inflamed tendon rubbing against the acromion above it. On examination there is

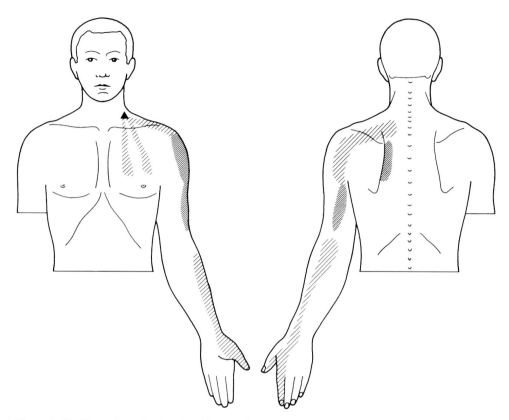

Figure 4.10   The pattern of pain referral from a trigger point or points (▲) in a scalene muscle.

tenderness over the greater tuberosity of the humerus, and abduction of the arm against resistance increases the pain.

Infraspinatus tendinitis and subscapularis tendinitis are distinguished from this by the pain being increased by resisted external or internal rotation respectively.

Rotator cuff tendinitis is traditionally treated by an injection of hydrocortisone (in combination with local anaesthetic) into the point of maximum tenderness. This is symptomatically helpful, but rarely gives long-lasting pain relief and is unlikely to shorten the weeks or months taken for the underlying lesion to undergo spontaneous resolution. As repeated steroid injections are liable to cause tissue damage, there is much to be said for providing short terms of pain relief by periodically needling Aδ nerve fibres at the point of maximum tenderness in the skin and subcutaneous tissues.

Biceps tendinitis

Tendinitis of the long head of biceps, a disorder in which there is inflammation of both the synovial sheath enveloping the tendon and the peri-tendinous connective tissue, is much less common than lesions affecting the rotator cuff. In this disorder, pain in the region of the bicipital groove often extends downwards towards the elbow. On examination, there is tenderness along the length of the bicipital groove and the pain is made worse by restricted elbow flexion. Traditionally treatment again consists of injecting hydrocortisone in combination with local anaesthetic. Injection is along the long axis of the tendon, but care has to be taken not to inject hydrocortisone into the tendon itself as this may cause it to rupture. This procedure may have to be repeated, so dry needling of Aδ nerve fibres at points of maximum tenderness is a suitable alternative.

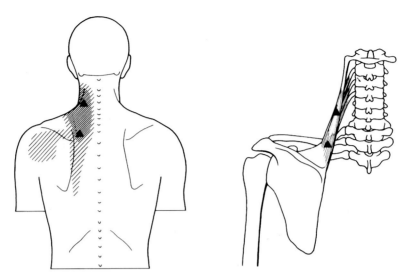

Figure 4.11   The pattern of pain referral to the neck, shoulder and inner border of the scapula from a trigger point or points (▲) in the levator scapulae muscle. Pain in this distribution occurs as a result of activity in either a trigger point at the angle of the neck or one near to the insertion of this muscle into the superior angle of the scapula, or in both.

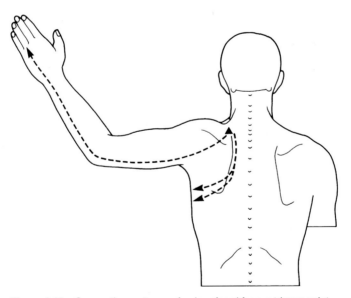

Figure 4.12   Some other patterns of pain referral from a trigger point (▲) in the levator scapulae near to its insertion into the superior angle of the scapula. These include referral down the inner side of the arm to the ring and little fingers. And referral around the chest wall along the course of the 4th and 5th intercostal nerves.

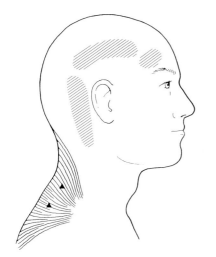

Figure 4.13   Trigger points (▲) in the trapezius muscle.

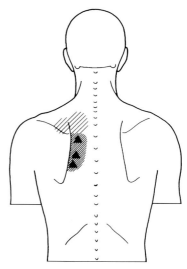

Figure 4.15   The pattern of pain referral from a trigger point or points in the rhomboid muscles.

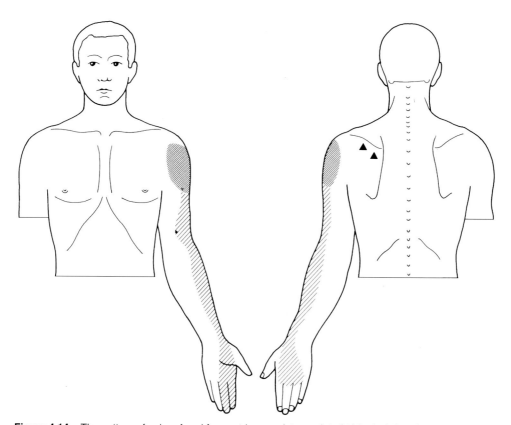

Figure 4.14   The pattern of pain referral from a trigger point or points (▲) in the infraspinatus muscle.

Adhesive capsulitis (frozen shoulder)

Frozen shoulder, a disorder in which there is severe inflammation of the glenohumeral joint capsule, may develop spontaneously or following trauma. There is invariably considerable pain both at night and during the day. In addition, there is marked restriction of *all* movements of the shoulder joint. The natural history of the condition is that the pain remains severe for 3–6 months and then gradually abates, but the restriction of movements persists for 1–2 years. Non-steroidal anti-inflammatory drugs, systemic corticosteroids, local hydrocortisone injections and ultrasound all have their advocates, but there is little to suggest that any of them influence the natural history of the disorder. This has led Bruckner (1982) to suggest that, in the majority of cases, reassuring the patient that it is a self-limiting condition, advising the use of simple 'pendulum' mobilizing exercises and in the early stages of the condition controlling the pain by some simple means is as much as can be hoped for. It is in the alleviation of the pain during this initial phase of the disorder that acupuncture has a place. My approach to this is to palpate systematically all round the periarticular soft tissues in order to locate a number of exquisitely tender points that are invariably found to be present, and then to needle them superficially at each site. This procedure, repeated at regular intervals, usually provides some worthwhile analgesia until such time as the pain spontaneously disappears.

Periarticular myofascial pain syndrome

Trauma to the shoulder is liable to activate trigger points in muscles at or near their insertions into the upper part of the humerus in the region of the glenohumeral joint and also at times in the bellies of these muscles some distance from it.

The muscles liable to be involved in this process include the supraspinatus, infraspinatus, subscapularis, the latissimus dorsi, teres major, the clavicular section of the pectoralis major, the triceps, biceps and deltoid.

Trigger point activity in these muscles causes them to shorten, which, together with pain, causes considerable restriction of some, but not all, of the movements of the joint, as with adhesive capsulitis. Moreover, with the periarticular myofascial pain syndrome, unlike adhesive capsulitis, treatment with trigger point acupuncture eventually results in the movements returning to normal as the pain disappears.

Shoulder pain with full movements of the glenohumeral joint

Pain may develop in the shoulder in the absence of any disorder in or around the joint, and with full normal joint movements, by referral from myofascial trigger points some distance away. The muscles in which trigger point activity may give rise to such pain include the supraspinatus (Fig. 4.1 p 36), infraspinatus (see Fig. 4.14 p 47), subscapularis (Fig. 4.16A,B), latissimus dorsi (Fig. 4.17), teres major (Fig. 4.18A,B), the clavicular section of the pectoralis major (Fig. 4.2 p 36), the triceps (Fig. 4.19), the biceps (Fig. 4.20A,B) and the deltoid (Fig. 4.21A,B). Finally, pain in the shoulder may be referred to that site as a result of cardiac, diaphragmatic or upper abdominal viscus disorders.

Pain around the elbow

Two common painful disorders affecting the elbow region are lateral and medial epicondylitis.

Lateral epicondylitis (tennis elbow)

With this trauma-induced lesion there is inflammation of the common forearm extensor tendon at or near its attachment to the lateral epicondyle, which is thus usually extremely tender. In addition, there are often a number of frequently overlooked, exquisitely tender, trigger points in the vicinity of the elbow, in muscles such as the supinator, brachioradialis, extensor carpi radialis longus, extensor digitorum and the lateral border of the medial head of the triceps. In order to locate these trigger points, palpation should be carried out

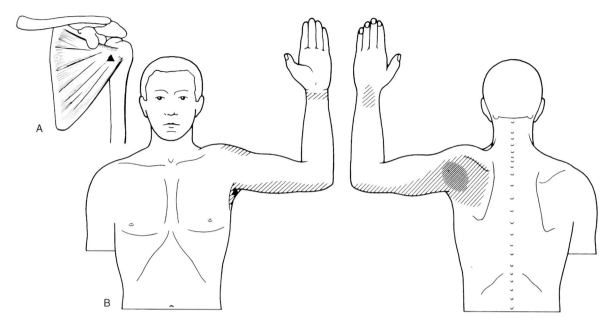

Figure 4.16   A: The subscapularis muscle with a trigger point (▲) near to the insertion of this muscle into the humerus. B: The pattern of pain referral from a trigger point or points (▲) in the axillary part of the subscapularis muscle.

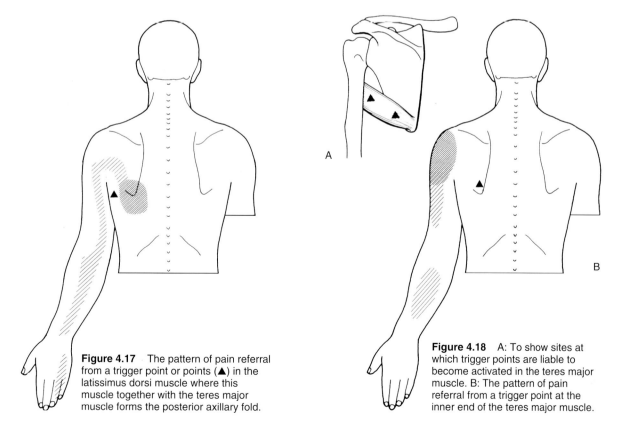

Figure 4.17   The pattern of pain referral from a trigger point or points (▲) in the latissimus dorsi muscle where this muscle together with the teres major muscle forms the posterior axillary fold.

Figure 4.18   A: To show sites at which trigger points are liable to become activated in the teres major muscle. B: The pattern of pain referral from a trigger point at the inner end of the teres major muscle.

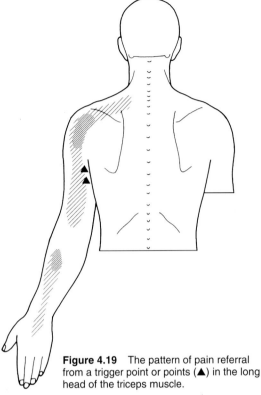

Figure 4.19 The pattern of pain referral from a trigger point or points (▲) in the long head of the triceps muscle.

first with the forearm supinated and then pronated.

Medial epicondylitis (golfer's elbow)

This is a similar type of lesion, except that the inflammation affects the common forearm flexor tendon at or near its attachment to the medial epicondyle. There are also, in addition, activated myofascial trigger points in this locality.

Treatment

The standard treatment for these two conditions is to inject hydrocortisone (with a local anaesthetic) into the point or points of maximum tenderness at or in the vicinity of one or other of these epicondyles. It is sometimes necessary to repeat this two to three times at monthly intervals. Such treatment may not only give rise to considerable pain for 24 hours following it, but

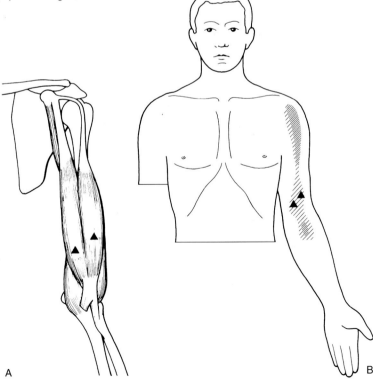

Figure 4.20 A: To show the usual location of trigger points in the lower part of the biceps muscle just above the elbow. B: The pattern of pain referral from trigger points (▲) in the lower part of the biceps muscle.

A

B

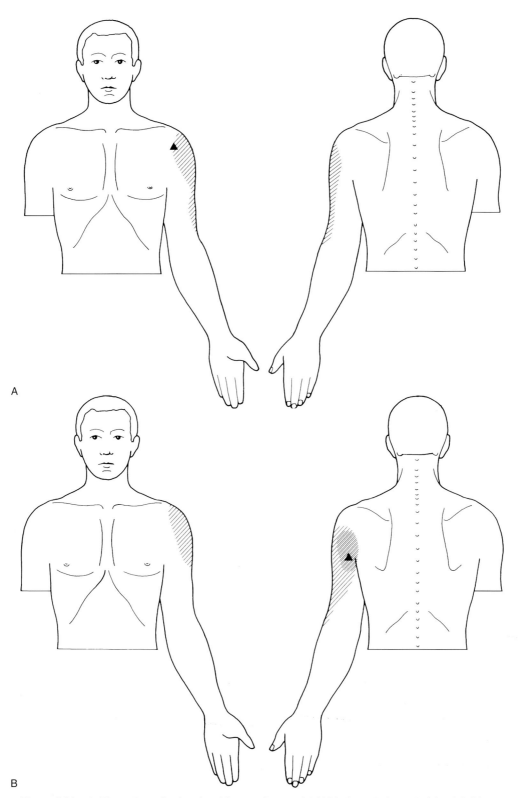

A

B

Figure 4.21   A: The pattern of pain referral from a trigger point (▲) in the anterior part of the deltoid muscle. B: The pattern of pain referral from a trigger point in the posterior part of the deltoid muscle.

may also frequently not give lasting relief. Repeated needling of the tissues overlying a tender epicondyle and nearby myofascial trigger points is at times a very worthwhile alternative. In some cases it proves necessary to employ a combination of acupuncture and hydrocortisone injections.

Low back pain

Chronic non-mechanical low back pain

In cases where persistent low back pain develops insidiously, particularly if the pain bears no relationship to physical activity so that it is as severe whilst resting in bed at night as it is during the day, various investigations including radiography of the spine are mandatory in order to exclude neoplastic, infective, inflammatory and metabolic disorders. However, this non-mechanical type of low back pain is relatively uncommon.

Chronic mechanical low back pain

Far more frequently chronic low back pain is of a mechanical type and is thus aggravated by movement and relieved by rest. All investigations including the ESR are normal, with the exception that radiographs of the spine, particularly from age 40 upwards, may show evidence of lumbar spondylosis—a disorder in which there is first degenerative change in the discs and ultimately degeneration in the facet joints.

It has for all too long been mistakenly assumed that these radiographically demonstrable degenerative changes are the main cause of chronic, mechanical-type, low back pain. The reasons for disputing this are as follows. The pain, unlike the degenerative changes in the spine, does not become progressively more marked with age (Urban & Maroudas 1980). Also, numerous comparative studies have shown that these degenerative changes are as frequently present in those who have never had low back pain as they are in those with it. They have also demonstrated that there is no quantitative relationship between low back pain and

lumbar spondylosis, so that a person with only slight radiographic changes may have severe pain, and conversely a person with advanced degenerative change may give no history of back pain (Fullenlove & Williams 1957, Horal 1969, Hult 1954, Hussar & Guller 1956, La Rocca & McNab 1969, Magora & Schwartz 1976, Splithoff 1952, Torgeson & Dotter 1976).

It is now apparent that, apart from a minority of cases where chronic, mechanical-type, low back pain does develop as a result of degenerative changes in the spine giving rise to nerve root entrapment, this type of pain does not emanate from the spine, but rather from trauma-induced activation and sensitization of nociceptors at trigger point sites in muscles. For this reason a systematic search for myofascial trigger points is essential.

Chronic, *nociceptive*, low back pain developing as a result of the primary activation of myofascial trigger points may respond fairly quickly to acupuncture, but often the latter provides only short-term, symptomatic relief and has to be continued at regular intervals on a long-term basis.

Chronic, mechanical-type pain in the back and down the leg is occasionally *neurogenic*, occurring with spondylolisthesis and when degenerative changes in the spine give rise to central canal or lateral root canal stenosis.

Degenerative spondylolisthesis, a disorder in which there is forward displacement of a vertebra relative to the one below it, affects mainly females and occurs predominately at the L4/5 level. It gives rise to low back pain and pain down the leg in the distribution of a nerve root, with physical examination revealing a motor and sensory deficit. In some cases there is bilateral numbness, tingling and weakness of the legs (Nelson 1987).

Central canal stenosis affects mainly middle-aged males, who usually have a long history of low back pain and a more recent one of vice-like claudication-type pain brought on by exertion, relieved by resting and in particular by bending forwards. The pain, together with numbness, tingling and heaviness, may affect one or both legs. On physical examination there may be a positive straight-leg-raising test and a neurological deficit, but often there is a remarkable paucity of physical signs (Porter 1992).

Lateral root canal stenosis gives rise to low back pain and pain down the leg in the distribution of a nerve root, usually the fifth lumbar or first sacral. The sciatic pain is in the same distribution as with a disc lesion (see below), but, unlike with the latter, it is not relieved by lying down. Physical signs are widely variable. A neurological deficit may or may not be present and, perhaps most surprisingly of all, the straight-leg-raising test is normal (Porter 1992).

In all these disorders secondary activation of myofascial trigger points may take place and a certain amount of symptomatic relief may be obtained as a result of deactivating them with dry needles. However, in addition, specialized investigations such as electromyographic studies and computerized axial tomography (CAT) scanning or magnetic resonance imaging are essential, in order to confirm the diagnosis and to help decide whether or not some form of surgical intervention is required.

Acute mechanical-type low back pain

Acute mechanical-type low back pain is mainly nociceptive. The commonest cause is trauma-induced activation and sensitization of C afferent nociceptors at trigger point sites in muscles. Occasionally it may develop as a result of trauma-induced posterior dislocation of a vertebra impinging on nociceptors on the anterior aspect of the dura mater; or a partially prolapsed intervertebral disc may be either doing the same, or pressing on nociceptors in the dural sleeve, which surrounds nerve roots in their intervertebral foramina (Wyke 1980). The pain produced when nociceptors in the dura mater are stimulated by one or other means is associated with the development of muscle spasm and this in turn gives rise to the secondary activation of myofascial trigger points.

In all cases of acute nocigenic low back pain, dry needle deactivation of myofascial trigger points affords considerable symptomatic relief, no matter whether they had been primarily or secondarily activated.

Acute nociceptive mechanical-type low back and leg pain

The dull, aching, nociceptive-type pain that emanates from myofascial trigger points in the lumbar region may be felt not only in the lower back, but also down the leg, and when this happens there are liable to be satellite trigger points in the zone of pain referral.

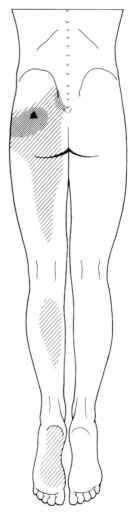

Figure 4.22 The pattern of pain referral from a trigger point in the piriformis muscle.

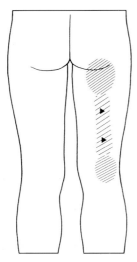

Figure 4.23 Composite pain patterns referred from trigger points (▲) in the right hamstring nucleus.

When trigger point activity develops in muscles such as the glutei (Fig. 4.5A,B p 38), the piriformis (Fig. 4.22) or hamstrings (biceps femoris, semimembranosus and semitendinosus (Fig. 4.23) with consequent production of pain in the buttock and referral down the back of the leg, there is often associated spasm of the muscles in the upper posterior part of the thigh and restriction of straight-leg raising. This often leads to the erroneous assumption that the pain is due to sciatic nerve root entrapment, but it does not have the burning, shooting, electric shock-like characteristics of true sciatica, and also, unlike the latter, there is no neurological deficit.

Acute neurogenic mechanical-type low back and leg pain

In no more than 1% of patients, acute low back pain is neurogenic and shoots down the leg in the distribution of the sciatic nerve as a result of a prolapsed intervertebral disc impinging upon it (Waddell 1987).

In all such cases marked restriction of straight-leg raising develops in association with a neurological deficit. In addition, the pain leads to the development of considerable low back muscle spasm with secondary activation of myo-fascial trigger points. In most cases the pain subsides spontaneously with bed rest and a certain amount of symptomatic relief may be obtained by means of dry needle deactivation of the trigger points. However, when after a few weeks the sciatic pain is as bad as ever or is getting worse, surgical decompression of the nerve root should be carried out, after confirming by magnetic resonance imaging (MRI) scan the level at which this is occurring. There should never be undue delay in performing surgery, as irreversible neural damage and consequent intractable pain may develop whenever a nerve root is chronically compressed (Wynn Parry 1989)—a disorder now known as chronic intrinsic radiculopathy (La Rocca 1992).

Laminectomy carried out at a propitious time in carefully selected cases relieves the sciatic pain in approximately 75% of cases (Nelson 1976), but it fails to relieve the associated back pain in up to 45% of them (Hanley & Shapiro 1989). Much of this postlaminectomy, persistent, low back pain emanates from myofascial trigger points, so in all such cases these should be looked for and deactivated.

The search for myofascial trigger points responsible for low back pain

The search for trigger points in patients with low back pain should always be started in the lower dorsal region in order to find any that may be present in the muscles of the posterior chest wall which, as may be seen from Figure 4.4 (p 38), are liable to cause pain to be referred to the buttock.

As elsewhere in the body, it is essential for the search to be carried out in a systematic manner. So, starting at about the level of the ninth dorsal vertebra, palpation should be continued down the length of the spine and down vertical lines parallel to this from the midline to the periphery. Palpation of the muscles should be carried out with the patient lying first on one side and then on the other, with in each case the upper arm extended above the head. In addition, a pillow should be placed under the head and another under the flank.

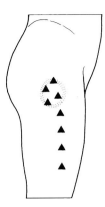

Figure 4.24 Trigger points in and around the greater trochanter and along the tensor fasciae latae.

The search should be continued down the posterior and lateral aspects of the thigh and in particular along the length of the iliotibial tract, as secondarily activated trigger points are frequently found there in patients with low back pain (Fig. 4.24). As low back pain occasionally develops by referral posteriorly from trigger points in either the anterior abdominal wall muscles or muscles in the upper anterior thigh, no examination is complete without also palpating these.

Summary

In summary, it has to be said that in general too much emphasis is placed on disorders of the spine as the cause of mechanical-type, low back pain. The degenerative changes in facet joints and discs, so commonly found radiographically in people from the age of 40 upwards, occur just as commonly and extensively in those without back pain as in those with it. And although of course there is no argument that disorders such as prolapse of a disc, spondylolisthesis, central and lateral canal stenosis are causes of mechanical-type low back pain, they are nevertheless comparatively uncommon.

It needs to be more widely recognized that, in the majority of cases, mechanical low back pain is predominantly muscular in origin and emanates from myofascial trigger points that can be identified only by means of a skilled, systematic, physical examination of the muscles.

It is clearly necessary to carry out a radiographic examination to exclude non-mechanical disorders of the spine, plus a CAT scan and/or MRI in cases where the history and/or physical signs suggest the possibility that the pain may be neurogenic. Regrettably, however, expensive procedures such as these are now increasingly being carried out in the routine investigation of such musculoskeletal pain disorders as chronic low back pain, without a far simpler physical examination of the muscles first being carried out to ascertain whether or not the pain is emanating from myofascial trigger points.

Pain from trigger points in muscles of the chest wall

Pain may develop as a result of trauma-induced activation of trigger points in any of the chest wall muscles. Lack of space, however, limits discussion to pain referral from trigger points in the pectoralis major muscle.

The pectoralis major has clavicular, sternal and costoabdominal sections, which converge laterally to form the anterior axillary fold, before being inserted into the humerus. Trigger points in the clavicular section cause pain to be referred to the shoulder, as do trigger points in the muscle near its insertion into the humerus (Fig. 4.2 p 36).

Trigger points in the costoabdominal section may lead to the development of pain and tenderness in the breast (Fig. 4.25). In women this pain and tenderness is often attributed to mastitis.

Trauma-induced activation of trigger points in the sternal section, gives rise to widespread anterior chest wall pain and pain down the inner side of the arm (Fig. 4.3 p 36), so that on the left side the pattern of pain referral is similar to that of coronary heart disease. And, to add to the confusion, pain in this distribution resulting from coronary heart disease may activate trigger points in the pectoralis major as a secondary event. It is essential, therefore, to search for trigger points in all cases of pain in the praecordial region and inner side of the left arm, and when present to decide whether they have undergone primary or

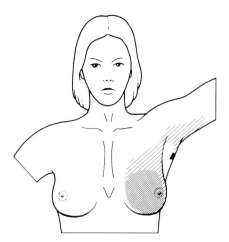

Figure 4.25 The pattern of pain referral from a trigger point or points (▲) in the lateral free margin of the pectoralis major muscle.

secondary activation. This can be done only by careful history taking and in some cases by carrying out a full range of cardiological investigations.

Pain from trigger points in the anterior abdominal wall muscles

Abdominal pain is not, as most doctors believe, invariably visceral in origin. It commonly develops as a result of trauma-induced activation of trigger points in the abdominal wall. Sites where this may occur include the rectus abdominis, the external oblique, and surgical incision scars in the skin (Baldry 1989).

The trauma to muscle may be due to domestic, occupational or sporting activities, but may also be inflicted during the course of surgical operations, principally as a result of the maladroit use of muscle retractors.

Trigger points may become activated in the bellies of these muscles although this occurs more frequently at or near to muscle attachment sites such as the lower ribs, inguinal ligament and pubic bone.

When examining a patient with abdominal pain, the abdomen should be palpated first with the abdominal muscles totally relaxed and then in a state of contraction. The reason for this is

that tenderness produced by palpation of a diseased viscus is reduced when the muscles overlying it are held rigid and, conversely, trigger point tenderness is increased.

Pelvic pain

Much seemingly inexplicable pelvic pain comes from trauma-induced activation of trigger points in one or more of the many muscles present in the pelvic floor.

In addition, a not uncommon and widely overlooked cause of vaginal pain in women and testicular pain in men, together with pain down the inner side of the leg in both sexes, is activation of trigger points in the adductor longus muscle near its attachment to the pubic bone.

In women this may occur as a result of the legs being excessively abducted during the course of gynaecological operations. In both sexes it is also liable to develop as a result of the muscle becoming sprained during sporting activity.

Pain in the leg and foot

Pain in the lower leg and foot may develop as a result of trauma-induced activation of trigger

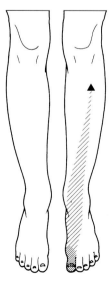

Figure 4.26 The pattern of pain referral from a trigger point (▲) in the tibialis anterior muscle.

points in various muscles including the tibialis anterior (Fig. 4.26), the peronei (Fig. 4.27), the gastrocnemius (Fig. 4.28) and the soleus (Fig. 4.29). It should be noted that with the last two muscles the pain is felt in both the back of the leg and the sole of the foot. Sometimes, however, the pattern of pain referral is predominantly to the sole of the foot. It therefore follows that pain affecting the plantar surface of the foot need not necessarily be arising from a disorder

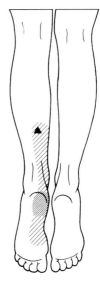

Figure 4.29   The pattern of pain referral from a trigger point (▲) in the soleus muscle.

of the foot itself, and it is thus essential to exclude the presence of trigger point activity in the calf muscles in such cases.

Plantar fasciitis

Pain in the sole of the foot may be due to plantar fasciitis. If so, on examination there is marked local tenderness on the medioanterior aspect of the calcaneum to which the plantar fascia is attached. It is sometimes, but not always, associated with the development of a calcaneal spur. An injection of hydrocortisone (with a local anaesthetic) into the point of maximum tenderness is often helpful but may need to be repeated on several occasions. In such cases a useful alternative is to needle Aδ nerve fibres in the superficial tissues over the tender point.

Achilles tendinitis

Trauma-induced inflammation of the Achilles tendon with pain around the heel is common. Examination reveals local tenderness along the length of the tendon with slight swelling. When the pain is sudden in onset and intense, an injection of hydrocortisone (with local anaesthetic) into a tender area is standard practice.

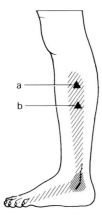

Figure 4.27   The pattern of pain referral from a trigger point (▲) in (a) the peroneus longus muscle (b) the peroneus brevis muscle.

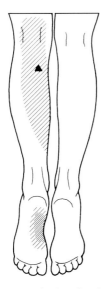

Figure 4.28   The pattern of pain referral from a trigger point (▲) in the gastrocnemius muscle.

There is always, however, the risk that should the steroid injection enter the tendon itself it may cause a rupture. When this happens the patient feels a sudden, severe pain behind the heel and it is essential to repair the tendon as quickly as possible.

Achilles tendinitis may also at times be insidious in its development, with low-grade but persistent pain. In such cases, repeated dry needle stimulation of Aδ nerve fibres at points of maximum tenderness in the superficial tissues along both sides of the tendon is often all that is required to abolish the pain.

OSTEOARTHRITIC PAIN

Alleviation of osteoarthritic pain arising from the metacarpophalangeal joint of the thumb, the finger joints and the ankle joint may be obtained by systematically palpating the soft tissues around these joints and needling at points of maximum tenderness.

Pain from osteoarthritis of the knee is also usually much relieved by acupuncture. Points of maximum tenderness are present in the peri-articular tissues. Most commonly they are found on the medial aspect of the knee, particularly over the upper aspect of the tibia at what is somewhat fancifully known as the 'pes anserinus' or 'goose's foot', a site where the lower part of the medial collateral ligament and, superficial to this, the tendons of the sartorius, gracilis and semitendinosus muscles attach to the tibia.

Tender points may also be found in the fat pads on either side of the quadriceps tendon, in the vastus medialis joint above the knee, and in the popliteal fossa, particularly on its medial border. Tender points may, in addition, be found on the lateral aspect of the knee, but this is less common.

In osteoarthritis of the hip, tender points are often to be found in the tissues around the greater trochanter, in the adductor longus and in the iliopsoas muscle near its insertion into the lesser trochanter. With relatively early osteoarthritis, needling at these points is often helpful. At a later stage of the disease it is far less rewarding.

Pain around the hip region, however, does not necessarily come from the hip joint itself, but from trigger points in the surrounding muscles. Deactivation of these with the dry needle technique then usually affords considerable relief.

CONCLUSIONS

MPS is a very common disorder and one that is liable to affect any region of the body. It is, however, all too often misdiagnosed and, because of this, inappropriately treated as a result of a widespread failure to appreciate the importance of carrying out a systematic search for myofascial trigger points in all cases where there is persistent pain but no obvious pathology to account for it.

The deactivation of a myofascial trigger point may be achieved by a number of different methods. These include injecting into the myofascial trigger point one of a number of disparate substances or inserting a dry needle into it (deep dry needling). Alternatively, the effect may be achieved by stimulating with a dry needle the Aδ nerve fibres situated in the tissues immediately overlying the myofascial trigger point (superficial dry needling). Because the latter is effective and simpler, safer and less pain-provoking than the first two, its use is recommended.

REFERENCES

Awad E A 1990 Histopathological changes in fibrositis. In: Fricton J R, Awad E A (eds) Advances in pain research and therapy, Vol 17. Raven Press, New York, pp 249–258

Baldry P E 1989 Acupuncture in the alleviation of abdominal pain. Acupuncture in Medicine 6(1):2–7

Baldry P E 1992 Fibromyalgia. A review of current knowledge. Acupuncture in Medicine 10(1):13–17

Baldry P E 1993 Acupuncture, trigger points and musculoskeletal pain, 2nd edn. Churchill Livingstone, New York

Baldry P E 1994 Concomitant sympathetically mediated pain and myofascial trigger point pain. Acupuncture in

Medicine 12(1):29–33

Bennett R M 1986a Current issues concerning management of the fibrositis/fibromyalgia syndrome. Americal Journal of Medicine 81 (suppl 3A):15–18

Bennett R M 1986b Fibrositis: evolution of an enigma. Journal of Rheumatology 13(4):676–678

Bennett R M 1987 Fibromyalgia. Journal of the American Medical Association. 257(20):2802–2803

Bowsher D 1987 Mechanisms of pain in man. ICI Pharmaceuticals

Bowsher D 1990 Physiology and pathophysiology of pain. Acupuncture in Medicine 7:17–20

Bowsher D 1991 The physiology of stimulation-produced analgesia. Acupuncture in Medicine 9(2):58–62

Bruckner F E 1982 Frozen shoulder (adhesive capsulitis). Journal of the Royal Society of Medicine 75:688–689

Committee on Safety of Medicine (CSM) Update 1986 Anaesthetists and the reporting of adverse drug reactions. British Medical Journal 292:949

Dowson D I, Lewith G T, Machin D 1985 The effects of acupuncture versus placebo in the treatment of headache. Pain 21:35–42

Fischer A 1988 Documentation of myofascial trigger points. Archives of Physical Medicine and Rehabilitation 69:286–291

Fricton J R, Awad E A 1990 Myofascial pain and fibromyalgia. Advances in Pain Research and Therapy, vol 17. Raven Press, New York

Friedenberg Z B, Miller W T 1963 Degenerative disc disease of the cervical spine. A comparative study of asymptomatic and symptomatic patients. Journal of Bone and Joint Surgery 45A:1171–1178

Frost F A, Jessen B, Siggaard-Andersen J 1980 A controlled double-blind comparison of mepivacaine injections versus saline injections for myofascial pain. Lancet 1:499–501

Fullenlove T M, Williams A J 1957 Comparative roentgen findings in symptomatic and asymptomatic backs. Journal of American Medical Association 168:572–574

Gunn C C 1989 Treating myofascial pain. University of Washington, Seattle

Hanley E N Jr, Shapiro D E 1989 The development of low-back pain after excision of a lumbar disc. Journal of Bone and Joint Surgery 71A:719–721

Hazelman B 1990 Musculoskeletal and connective tissue disease. In: Souhami R L, Moxham J (eds) Textbook of medicine. Churchill Livingstone, New York, p 1031

Heller C A, Stanley P, Lewis-Jones B, Heller R F 1983 Value of X-ray examinations of the cervical spine. British Medical Journal 287:1276–1278

Horal J 1969 The clinical appearance of low-back pain disorders in the city of Gothenberg, Sweden. Acta Orthopaedica Scandinavica suppl 118:8–73

Hult L 1954 Cervical dorsal and lumbar spinal syndromes. A field investigation of non-selected material of 1200 workers in different occupations with special reference to disc degeneration and so-called muscular rheumatism. Acta Orthopaedica Scandinavica suppl 17:1–102

Hussar A E, Guller E J 1956 Correlation of pain and the roentgenographic findings of spondylosis of the cervical and lumbar spine. American Journal of Medical Science 232:518–527

Jaeger B, Skootsky S A 1987 Double-blind, controlled study of different myofascial trigger point injection techniques. Pain suppl 4S292

Jensen L B, Melsen B, Jensen S B 1979 Effect of acupuncture on headache measured by reduction in number of attacks and use of drugs. Scandinavian Journal of Dental Research 87:373–380

Kellgren J H 1938 Observations on referred pain arising from muscle. Clinical Science 3:175–190

Kraft G H, Johnson E W, La Ban M M 1968 The fibrositis syndrome. Archives of Physical Medicine and Rehabilitation 49:155–162

La Rocca H 1992 The failed back. In: Jayson M I V (ed) The lumbar spine and back pain, 4th edn. Churchill Livingstone, New York, pp 435–437

La Rocca H, Macnab I 1969 Value of pre-employment radiographic assessments of the lumbar spine. Canadian Medical Association Journal 101:383–388

Lewit K 1979 The needle effect in the relief of myofascial pain. Pain 6:83–90

Loh L, Nathan P W, Schott G D, Siekha K J 1984 Acupuncture versus medical treatment for migraine and muscle tension headaches. Journal of Neurology, Neurosurgery and Psychiatry 47:333–337

Lu G D, Needham J 1980 Celestial lancets. Cambridge University Press Cambridge

Macdonald A J R, Macrae K D, Master B R, Rubin A P 1983 Superficial acupuncture in the relief of chronic low-back pain. Annals of the Royal College of Surgeons of England 65:44–46

Magora A, Schwartz A 1976 Relation between the low-back pain syndrome and X-ray findings. 1. Degenerative osteoarthritis. Scandinavian Journal of Rehabilitation Medicine 8:115–175

Matthews W B 1983 Headache. In: Weatherall D A, Ledingham J G G, Warrell D A (eds) Oxford textbook of medicine. Oxford University Press, Oxford, pp 145–149

Nelson M A 1976 Surgery of the spine. In: Jayson M V (ed) The lumbar spine and back pain, 2nd edn. Pitman, London, p 476

Nelson M A 1987 Indications for spinal surgery in low-back pain. In: Jayson M I V (ed) The lumbar spine and back pain, 3rd edn. Churchill Livingstone, New York, pp 321–352

Pallis C, Jones A M, Spillane J D 1954 Cervical spondylosis. Incidence and implications. Brain 77:274–289

Porter R W 1992 Spinal stenosis of the central and root canal. In: Jayson M I V (ed) The lumbar spine and back pain, 4th edn. Churchill Livingstone, New York, pp 313–332

Raja S, Meyer J N, Meyer R A 1988 Peripheral mechanisms of somatic pain. Anesthesiology 68:571–590

Rang H P, Bevan S, Dray A 1991 Chemical activation of nociceptive peripheral neurones. British Medical Bulletin 47(3):534–548

Sola A E, Kuitert J H 1955 Myofascial trigger point pain in the neck and shoulder girdle. North West Medicine 54:980–984

Sola A E, Williams R L 1956 Myofascial pain syndromes. Neurology 6:91–95

Splithoff C A 1952 Lumbosacral junction. Roentgenographic comparison of patients with and without backaches. Journal of the American Medical Association 152:1610–1613

Torgeson W R, Dotter E E 1976 Comparative roentgenographic study of the asymptomatic and symptomatic lumbar spine. Journal of Bone and Joint Surgery 58A:850–853

Travell J, Rinzler S H 1952 The myofascial genesis of pain. Postgraduate Medicine II:425–434

Travell J G, Simons D G 1983 Myofascial pain and dysfunction. The trigger point manual, vol 1. Williams & Wilkins, Baltimore

Travell J G, Simons D G 1992 Myofascial pain and dysfunction. The trigger point manual, vol 2. Williams & Wilkins, Baltimore

Urban T, Maroudas A 1980 In: Graham R (ed) Clinics in Rheumatic Diseases vol 6, no 1. Saunders, Philadelphia, p 51

Waddell G 1987 A new clinical model for the treatment of low-back pain. Spine 12(7):632–644

Wolfe F, Smythe H A, Yunus M B et al 1990 The American College of Rheumatology. Criteria for the classification of fibromyalgia: report of the multicenter criteria committee. Arthritis and Rheumatism 33:160–172

Woolf C J 1991 Generation of acute pain: central mechanisms. British Medical Bulletin 47(3):523–533

Wyke B 1980 The neurology of low-back pain. In: Jayson M I V (ed) The lumbar spine and back pain, 2nd edn. Pitman, London, p 307

Wynn Parry C B 1989 The failed back. In: Wall P D, Melzack R (eds) Textbook of pain, 2nd edn. Churchill Livingstone, New York, pp 341–353

5

A new system of acupuncture

Felix Mann

I studied acupuncture in 1958 with several well-known teachers, primarily with Professor Johannes Bischko. At that time the writings and translations of Soulié de Morant were the main fount of wisdom in the West, though the translations of Chamfrault and Ung Kan Sam, Hübotter and a few others were very helpful. Most other books, as far as I was aware, were permutations with reinterpretations and additions of the works of the few well-known authors. Therefore, when I wished to expand and deepen my knowledge, I was compelled to learn to read Chinese, so as to have access to the original and also to modern Chinese texts.

Whatever the opposite of a natural linguist is—I am it. It will therefore be clear that I invested a great deal of time and enormous effort in traditional Chinese acupuncture. Picture then my dismay when it gradually became clear to me from clinical experience that the ancient Chinese system got results, but not for the reasons or in the way postulated by the tradition. It worked rather like the pre-Copernican flat Earth world view, which was sufficient for building houses, roads and even great cathedrals, but not for accurate navigation, the exploration of space or many concepts of modern physics. Even the later, simplified European version, practised by several thousand Western doctors, which added a veneer of scientific medicine to the ancient tradition, fell into the same trap.

What follows in this chapter is primarily the result of my own, very simple observations, a method of investigation I had learnt during my time as assistant to Dr Jean Schoch of Strasbourg. It depends on:

1. listening carefully and unhurriedly to the patient
2. not imposing the concepts of Traditional Chinese Medicine nor of Western medicine on what the patient says, which is not easy
3. thinking about what I heard and collating it with many years' experience.

This is the way the early scientists, such as Charles Darwin, made their discoveries: by careful observation, with only a minimum of laboratory investigation, and by having the courage to think the doctrinally unthinkable.

CORE CONCEPTS

Acupuncture points do not exist

This is apparent from casual observation:

1. Initially, when I studied acupuncture, I occasionally observed doctors who had learnt acupuncture at different schools in various countries. Sometimes the positions they used for specific acupuncture points varied by 1, 2 or even 3 cm, yet their results seemed more or less equally good.

2. A GP colleague used the well-known point Stomach-36 (ST-36), on the tibialis anterior, frequently, for it was one of his favourite points. One day he suddenly realized that, all these years, he had been needling Gall Bladder 34 (GB-34), at the neck of the fibula. From then onwards, of course, he used the correct position of ST-36, which is some 5 centimetres distant. The doctor found, to his surprise, that the effects, clinically, of needling ST-36 and GB-34 were the same, even though they are on different meridians. This was an ideal experiment, difficult to reproduce in acupuncture, for the doctor in both instances thought he was giving the correct treatment.

3. The State Administration of Traditional Chinese Medicine (1990) has standardized the position of acupuncture points, based largely on a variety of historical documents, in which the position of the same points often differ from one another by a centimetre. If there were a clinical difference between stimulating one position of a point with another position, presumably it would be stated (as in orthodox medicine with different drugs), but as it is not, I take it there is no difference.

4. One of my favourite, non-existent, acupuncture points is Liver 3 (LR-3). However, I use a position proximal to that commonly used, (i.e. where the penetrating part of the dorsalis pedis artery dives down between the two heads of the first dorsal interosseous muscle). This position is more frequently tender than the traditional position, which is why I prefer it.

Instead of using the above position, I have frequently tried the following: (a) the end of the big toe; (b) the dorsal surface of the medial cuneiform; (c) the varicose ulcer area, which covers almost the entire length of the medial surface of the tibia (posterior half) and the soft tissue 1 to 3 cm posterior to the medial border of the tibia— a large area.

I find that, on most occasions, there is little to choose between a traditional position of LR-3, the end of the big toe and the dorsal surface of the medial cuneiform. Usually a tender area within the varicose ulcer area (which varies in position) has the same effect, but not always.

I have investigated, in a similar way to LR-3, other acupuncture points in the back, abdomen, thorax, arm, neck and head, with similar results— results which I routinely demonstrate at my acupuncture courses.

5. There exists a system of Korean hand acupuncture in which there are about 150 separate acupuncture points on each middle finger. The late Yoshio Manaka once wrote to me wondering if there was any skin left which was not an acupuncture point!!

Neither these considerations, nor my other ideas not mentioned here, suggest that the use of classical, modern or microsystem acupuncture points does not alleviate or cure disease, for I know that it does. They merely suggest that acupuncture points in the normally accepted physical sense do not exist.

Meridians do not exist

The meridians are invisible structures like the meridians of geography. At one time, various investigators thought they could measure a reduced electrical skin resistance or impedance along the course of the meridians. I investigated this in my practice with three commercially available sets of apparatus. Later, a sophisticated apparatus was made at the Department of Electronics of St Bartholomew's Hospital. With none of these were we able to record meridians, or, for that matter, acupuncture points.

Some doctors think they can demonstrate the existence of meridians by needling, say, the region of the sacroiliac joint, which is on the Bladder meridian. This, if done appropriately, in a patient with sciatica, may produce radiation down the back of the thigh and calf, which are both traversed by the Bladder meridian. Hence these doctors say the radiation follows the course of the Bladder meridian, showing that meridians exist. In reality, the radiation (if one observes carefully) does not follow the course of the Bladder meridian for it does not follow the major zigzag at the back of the knee nor the minor zigzag in the calf. There is also a tendency for the radiation to go in the direction of the pain in the leg, which may not coincide with the position of the Bladder meridian. The Bladder meridian, in the lower part of its course, goes along the lateral border of the foot to end on the little toe, whereas the radiation from the region of the sacroiliac joint goes to any part of the foot.

I have frequently tried needling other parts of the body in an attempt to produce radiation, which I can do more frequently with periosteal acupuncture. Only rarely do the courses of the radiation and of a meridian coincide over more than a modest proportion of their paths.

Strong Reactors and Normal Reactors

The first discovery I made in acupuncture concerning a subject on which the traditional literature did not shed much or any light was that some patients, largely irrespective of their disease, respond to acupuncture like magic, whilst others respond in comparison in a slow and dreary way. (I am not referring to those in whom acupuncture has no effect.) I call these patients 'Strong Reactors' and 'Normal Reactors':

Strong Reactors

Strong Reactors respond amazingly quickly to acupuncture—they may notice a response within a few seconds of treatment. This response may be a feeling of relaxation, sleepiness, euphoria, crying, laughter, increased awareness of sound and colour and, above all, just feeling 'good'.

The response happens with relatively gentle needling, often one thin needle inserted for 1 second to a depth of 1 mm being sufficient. These same patients require fewer treatments than the average patient. The percentage of patients who are cured or helped by acupuncture is greater among Strong Reactors. The degree of improvement in the patient is also higher. They may require smaller than average doses of drugs.

The most difficult diseases may respond to treatment in a Strong Reactor, but not in a Normal Reactor. This should affect the selection of appropriate patients for treatment, for usually it is useless to treat a difficult disease in a Normal Reactor.

The most responsive of all the Strong Reactors I call Hyper-Strong Reactors. Acupuncture analgesia (often misnamed anaesthesia), in so far as it works at all, is usually confined to these Hyper-Strong Reactors.

Normal Reactors

Normal Reactors are the reverse of everything described above. A smaller percentage of patients is cured. They require a larger number of treatments. Needling should sometimes be somewhat more aggressive (i.e. more needles, thicker needles, manipulation of needles). They do not notice an immediate response and radiation occurs less frequently. They require normal doses of drugs and have fewer adverse reactions to these drugs.

There is no laboratory or physical test, as far as I know, that differentiates a Strong Reactor from a Normal Reactor. Identification is based on a purely clinical appraisal of the patient.

It is important to distinguish a Strong Reactor from a Normal Reactor, for, if a Normal Reactor is treated too gently, his symptoms will not be alleviated. In reverse, a Strong Reactor treated too strongly may likewise not get better, or may have a 'reaction', which is a temporary worsening of symptoms or a temporary feeling of general malaise. The 'reaction' is the acupuncture equivalent of the effect of an excessive dosage of a drug, though in the case of acupuncture it is always temporary.

I think by far the commonest cause of failure in acupuncture is the failure to distinguish the Strong Reactor from the Normal Reactor. Anyone can look up in an acupuncture 'cook book' where to place the needle, but how strongly or gently to needle the patient is an art rather than a science or statistic. I have included a whole chapter on the phenomenon in my most recent book, (Mann 1992) but it can only really be learnt by watching an experienced practitioner in action.

NEEDLE TECHNIQUES
Microacupuncture

In most respects this is a gentle form of treatment.

A fine needle, 0.2 mm in diameter, is used. It should have a finely tapered point and be polished so that it is as atraumatic as possible. A length of 15 mm is convenient. Disposable needles are best, particularly as, with my technique, many patients require only one needle.

As a rule the needle is inserted to a depth of 2 or 3 mm, though occasionally deeper. The needle can also be inserted intracutaneously only, for 1 or 2 mm, in which case it should be inserted nearly horizontal to the skin. Normally the needle is inserted at right angles to the skin. The needle is left in place for 1 to 5 seconds and then immediately withdrawn: it is not manipulated.

With this gentle technique the patient rarely has radiation. However, all the other effects of acupuncture, such as relaxation, euphoria, etc., occur in the normal way.

I usually make one, two or sometimes a few more insertions, not the dozen insertions frequently seen in traditional acupuncture. Formerly I thought that such a gentle needle technique was suitable only for Strong Reactors. I have since found, to my initial surprise, that perhaps 50% of patients respond well to this gentle technique.

Periosteal acupuncture

This potentially (but not necessarily) more powerful technique is appropriate for Normal Reactors and even sometimes for Strong Reactors with certain diseases, particularly for the local treatment of musculoskeletal disease.

A needle which is finely pointed and polished, and of appropriate length, is used. A diameter of 0.25 mm is normally enough, though it may be 0.3 mm if a deep insertion is required.

The needle is inserted slowly and gently through the skin, fatty layer and muscle until it reaches the periosteum. I have now found that, normally, only one single gentle tap of the periosteum is sufficient. Nowadays I rarely use multiple periosteal pecking.

One can study the effect of periosteal needling best in those sensitive patients who notice an acupuncture effect within a second of needling. Usually this type of patient is a Hyper-Strong Reactor and hence requires only micro-acupuncture. However, when periosteal treatment is appropriate, the needle is inserted very slowly through the skin and deeper tissues. Then, just as the needle gently touches the periosteum, the doctor suddenly feels 'something happening' and, at the same time or a few seconds later, the patient feels the usual acupuncture response.

As in microacupuncture, one or very few needle insertions are all that is required.

Single-needle technique

When I first practised acupuncture, I naturally adopted the technique commonly used in China and Europe. This involved using, say, 10 needles which were inserted subcutaneously or intramuscularly, perhaps twisted to and fro or otherwise manipulated, and left in place for, say, 10 minutes.

I have gradually evolved a single-needle technique whereby many patients have only a single needle insertion, though some need two, three or, rarely, even more. The single-needle technique applies equally to microacupuncture, periosteal acupuncture or, for that matter, to intramuscular acupuncture. In all instances the needle, as described before, is left in place for only 1 to 5 seconds.

I have met some doctors who have a single-needle technique in which they manipulate the needle for, say, 30 seconds, but I have not heard previously of such a gentle technique as that described in this section. I have found that with my single-needle gentle technique my results are better than those I achieved formerly.

AREAS OF STIMULATION

The degree of specificity required in acupuncture varies considerably: sometimes it is necessary to needle an area as small as a pea whilst, rarely, it may be sufficient to needle literally anywhere in the body (or at least in the appropriate limb), though usually it is between these two extremes. Hence, I normally do not use the word 'acupuncture point', but rather 'acupuncture area'.

I regard the non-existent acupuncture points much as we all regard McBurney's point in appendicitis, which may vary in position by, say, 15 cm and in size from that of a pea to that of a dinner plate. For instance, the pain and tenderness one has in cervical disease may stretch from the lambdoid suture to the tip of the shoulder (say 30 cm) and possibly even further or elsewhere. If a patient has pathological changes at, say, C5, the pain or tenderness in this 30 cm area is not always at the same place; it may just as easily be in the upper, middle or lower part of the area, varying from patient to patient.

In traditional acupuncture there is a 'point' called Bladder 57 (BL-57) (see Fig. 5.1). If the average patient is examined, whether or not he has a disease, not only is BL-57 tender but also an area some 15 cm long and 3 cm wide, which I have called the gastrocnemius tendon

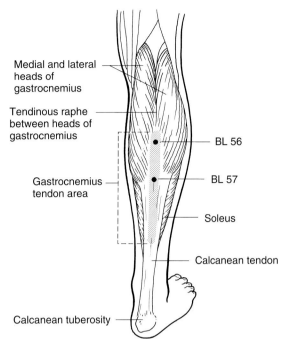

Medial and lateral heads of gastrocnemius

Tendinous raphe between heads of gastrocnemius

BL 56

BL 57

Gastrocnemius tendon area

Soleus

Calcanean tendon

Calcanean tuberosity

Figure 5.1 Gastrocnemius tender area. (From Mann F 1992, with permission, Butterworth Heinemann)

area (see Fig. 5.1). Sometimes the gastrocnemius tendon area can include the whole area covered by the gastrocnemius, the soleus and the tendocalcaneous. On rare occasions the whole leg is affected.

The 'areas' mentioned above, whether they be small or large, may contain one or several smaller areas which are even more tender on palpation. Even these smaller areas have no particular or necessary connection with putative acupuncture points.

Acupuncture may be effective if one needles an acupuncture point, my type of acupuncture area, or for that matter literally anywhere in the same region of the body. As a rule, but by no means always, tender areas like the ones mentioned above are the most effective. Considerable clinical experience is required to make the most effective choice.

RADIATION NOT MERIDIANS

If one needles the region of the head of the radius, the patient may experience radiation. This radiation is more likely to occur if the periosteum is needled (to be done only if it would not constitute an excessively strong treatment for the patient, with possible adverse effects).

The radiation may follow a narrow path, like the putative 'meridians'. It may also encompass the whole limb, or anything in between these two extremes. The sensation of radiation is hard to define; only very rarely is it pain.

As the head of the radius is in the region of the Lung meridian, a traditionalist would expect the radiation to follow the course of this meridian from the shoulder to the thumb along the anterolateral surface of the arm—which it certainly does in a number of patients. In other patients the radiation may go along the medial side of the arm to the little finger. It may also go up the arm, in any position, or over the lateral side of the neck to any part of the face and head on the same side. It may also go anywhere in the thorax.

The radiation which a patient experiences is an indication of which diseased regions may be treated. In the above example, needling the head of the radius, anteriorly, may treat any disease amenable to acupuncture in the arm, thorax, neck or head—though it is far from necessarily the best treatment. If, to take another example, the cervical articular pillar area on the lateral side of the neck is needled, one may have radiation to various regions of the body, including the anterior chest wall and hence, under appropriate circumstances, it may be used to treat mild chest pains—but not serious disease.

SUMMARY

It is apparent, I hope, that in acupuncture there are many roads to Rome. Over the years, I have tried a plethora of methods, some exhaustively, until I evolved the various ideas and methods described in this chapter. For me this system works best and is intellectually more satisfying than the more traditionally orientated approach. I believe it may also prove to be a pointer toward the future evolution of acupuncture knowledge and hope that it may stimulate discussion and the development of further new ideas.

REFERENCES

Mann F 1992 Reinventing acupuncture. Butterworth-Heinemann, Oxford (In German published by A. M. I.-Verlag, Giessen. In Italian published by Editore Marrapese, Rome)

State Administration of Traditional Chinese Medicine 1990. State standard of the People's Republic of China. Foreign Languages Press, Beijing

Theory and basic science

SECTION CONTENTS

6

Mechanisms of acupuncture

David Bowsher

Acupuncture has been used for more than two thousand years in China and Japan; the earliest literary reference is in The Yellow Emperor's book of internal medicine, dating from the second or third century BC. Acupuncture reached Japan in the sixth century of the Christian era, and was introduced into Europe by ten Rhijne (1683), who had learnt about it in Japan. As a therapy, it spread very slowly in Europe. The first European and American publications on acupuncture treatment appeared in the early nineteenth century (Bache 1826, Berlioz 1816, Churchill 1821, Cloquet 1826). Although acupuncture was used to a considerable extent in conventional medical practice in Europe throughout the nineteenth century, attracting such mainstream giants as Osler, its use gradually died out.

While some pioneers such as Felix Mann in the UK and a number of practitioners in France were using acupuncture extensively from the middle of the present century, it was really only in the 1970s that acupuncture captured the public interest and came to be widely practised. Films of acupuncture anaesthesia for operative surgery coming out of China following President Nixon's visit in 1972 fired the public imagination. Acupuncture received full scholarly treatment in the West in the magisterial treatise of Lu & Needham (1980).

In addition to classical acupuncture, a number of variations exist. Notable among these are Ryodoraku (Hyodo 1990, Nakatani & Yamashita 1977, Yoshio 1969) and auricular acupuncture, introduced in France by Nogier (1972). Auricular acupuncture has been further studied by Johnson et al (1991).

Eventually, acupuncture in Western medicine came to be mainly used for pain relief (Mann et al 1973), and much later for the treatment of postoperative nausea and vomiting (Dundee et al 1986). The present chapter will be concerned entirely with an attempt to explain acupuncture in relation to pain relief.

The fact that not all subjects respond to acupuncture appears to present great difficulties to some medical scientists. Acupuncturists divide the population into responders and non-responders. Many animals may also be classed as non-responders, for instance, some rats show no prolongation of the tail-flick response latency following acupuncture (Takeshige et al, 1980a).

As will be more fully discussed below, acupuncture analgesia in people and animals is reversed or abolished by naloxone under most conditions, showing that its mechanism is opioidergic. In human subjects in whom pain was relieved by acupuncture, an increase in cerebrospinal fluid (CSF) β-endorphin level was noted (Clement-Jones et al 1980). Although CSF met-enkephalin levels did not appear to be changed in this study, it has recently been observed in the rat (Bing et al 1991) that met-enkephalin-like material is in fact released in the substance of the spinal cord itself by acupuncture-like stimulation. Recently, Takeshige et al (1990) have shown that non-responsive animals (as measured by non-prolongation of tail-flick latency) can be rendered responsive by treatment with D-phenylalanine, which inhibits the enzyme that degrades met-enkephalin. Attribution of response failure in rats to differences in enzyme mechanisms is reminiscent of the observation that humans who fail to respond to morphine for the relief of nociceptive pain appear to have differences in the enzymatic mechanisms for its glucuronidation (Bowsher 1993).

ACUPUNCTURE POINTS AND MERIDIANS

Experiments showing that, when a nerve is blocked by local anaesthesia, acupuncture is ineffective in the territory supplied by that nerve prove that the acupuncture effect is conducted along nerves (Chiang et al 1973). From the standpoint of modern neurophysiology, this is perhaps the most important and fundamental piece of information on acupuncture.

Acupuncture points

Acupuncture is said to be effective only at certain points on the body surface, known as acupuncture points. In fact, comparison with an anatomical atlas (e.g. Williams et al 1989) shows that many of these points correspond with the points at which small nerve bundles penetrate the fascia; Chan (1984) cites two Chinese studies showing that 309 acupuncture points are situated on or very close to nerves, while 286 are on or very close to major blood vessels, which are of course surrounded by small nerve bundles (nervi vasorum).

That sympathetic nerves may also be involved was first demonstrated by Goulden (1921), who showed that acupuncture points along the sciatic nerve and its branches have a lower impedance than does the surrounding skin. Yoshio (1969) has shown that Ryodoraku points have similar properties. Many acupuncture points are of course deep within the skin. Melzack, Stillwell & Fox (1977) have shown that many of them correlate closely with Travell's 'trigger points' (Travell & Simons 1983), while Liu, Varela & Oswald (1977) have demonstrated that other points correspond to the motor points of muscles, where the nerves enter or leave them. The Hoku point (LI-4), of course, has long been known to correspond to the superficial branch of the radial nerve in the anatomical 'snuff-box'; but the foregoing demonstrates that all acupuncture points examined correspond to small nerve bundles, either cutaneous (purely sensory, or sensory plus sympathetic), vascular (mixed sympathetic and sensory), or muscular (mixed sensory and motor).

While segmental acupuncture is undoubtedly the most effective form for pain relief, acupuncture at distant points has been found empirically also to be effective. In order to demonstrate this, ancient practitioners drew up illustrations in which 'points' were joined by lines that in Western practice are called 'meridians'; the intention was to show that stimulation at a particular point may have an effect elsewhere on the meridian, or in a viscus after which the meridian was named.

This raises two distinct issues:

1. Are the 'points' fixed entities?
2. How are 'meridians' to be interpreted in terms of modern anatomical and physiological knowledge?

If in fact the points are small nerve bundles, then of course their precise position will vary from individual to individual in accordance with normal biological variation.

Most practitioners of acupuncture find that effective points, when needled, give rise to a subjective feeling of warmth in the patient and are often revealed to the therapist as a red flare in the skin. This of course is the axon reflex, brought about by stimulation of C and A delta (Aδ) fibres. Its absence merely indicates that the needle has not hit nerve fibres, and therefore has not been inserted into an effective 'point'.

While a needle may mechanically stimulate nerve fibres of many types, it is most important to establish which peripheral nerve fibre type is responsible for the acupuncture effect. It was suggested some time ago (Bowsher 1976) that Aδ fibres were involved, because the adequate stimulus is needleprick, while the response frequency is 2–3 Hz; these are both properties of Aδ primary afferents. This theoretical hypothesis has been confirmed practically in two different ways. First, it has been demonstrated beyond doubt, by microneurographic stimulation in conscious human volunteers, that stimulation of Aδ fibres gives rise to a pricking sensation, like that of being stimulated with a needle. Secondly, Wang et al (1985) showed that Aδ fibres from muscle conveyed various sensations which Chiang et al (1973) had shown were essential for the acupuncture effect.

An interesting corollary arises in a disease state: Levine, Gormley & Fields (1976) found that acupuncture was ineffective when applied to areas of skin affected by postherpetic neuralgia (PHN). In 1990, Nurmikko & Bowsher showed that, in areas of skin affected by PHN, pinprick sensation is usually absent.

Thus it may be regarded as established beyond reasonable doubt that Aδ sensory units *must* be stimulated in order to produce the acupuncture effect. It should, however be mentioned that, in a number of recent papers, Kawakita and his colleagues (e.g. Kawakita 1991) have suggested that C polymodal nociceptors should also be considered as a physiological substrate of the acupuncture effect. While it cannot be excluded that stimulation of such sensory units may contribute in some measure to the acupuncture effect, both the parameters of stimulation and the perceived sensation following needle stimulation appear to us to militate strongly against the possibility that C polymodal nociceptors are the sole, or even the principal, substrate. Indeed, earlier work on suppression of the jaw-opening reflex in rats by both electroacupuncture and selective Aδ stimulation (Kawakita & Funakoshi 1982) strongly support the notion that Aδ fibres are principally concerned in the acupuncture effect. It may also be added that, unlike the situation with respect to Aδ fibres (see below), there are no known central connections of C fibres that could explain inhibition of (other) C fibre input. Table 6.1 correlates the different sensory fibre types with their physiological functions and with their role in acupuncture analgesia and the TCM phenomenon 'De Qi'. Note that, whilst superficial acupuncture involves Aδ nerve fibres, deep (muscle) acupuncture also stimulates Aδ fibres. The 'soreness' component of acupuncture is the result of stimulating C fibres.

Meridians

The second issue—that of the 'correct' acupuncture points and their relation to meridians—is more complex. Some effect may be produced at any point where a nerve bundle containing Aδ fibres is stimulated, owing to central effects from descending inhibitory controls (DNIC) (Bing, Villanueva & Le Bars 1991). However, powerful

Table 6.1 Neurophysiology of needling (after Thompson 1994)

Sensory Fibre ABC type	Sensory Fibre I–IV type	Diameter μm	Velocity m/s (mph)	Function	Role in analgesia*	Role in De Qi[†]
Aα	1a	15–20	70–120 (155–270)	Annulo-spiral muscle spindles [length]		
	1b			Golgi tendon organ [load]		
Aβ	II	5–12	30–70 (70–155)	Touch		
Aγ	II	3–6	15–30 (35–70)	Flower spray muscle spindles [length]	+	Numbness
Aδ	III	2–5	12–30 (25–70)	Pinprick sensation (= first or fast pain), cold, pressure	+	Aching, distension, heaviness
C	IV	0.4–1.2	0.5–2 (1–4.5)	Aching pain (= second or slow pain), itch, heat		Soreness

References: Guyton 1991, Ganong 1993. * Bowsher 1988, Pomeranz & Paley 1979, Toda & Ichioka 1978, [†] Wang et al 1985, Thompson 1994.

effects are produced only following stimulation at particular non-segmental points on a meridian. As pertinently suggested by Baldry (1993), it is likely that, at least in part, we are dealing with the as yet ill-understood mechanisms of referred effects, as studied by such workers as Kellgren and Lewis before World War II (see Baldry 1993 for details). While such explanations appear to depend entirely on interactions within the somatic nervous system, attention should also be given to pathways travelling in the autonomic nervous system and interactions between the autonomic and somatic nervous systems. There is a considerable body of evidence implicating the sympathetic nervous system in acupuncture effects: the first report (Matsumoto & Hayes 1973) demonstrated a fall in blood pressure and intestinal vasodilation following electroacupuncture in rabbits. More recently, transient skin vasoconstriction followed by a longer-lasting warming effect has been demonstrated in normal human volunteers following both manual and electrical acupuncture stimulation (Ernst & Lee 1985), again revealing autonomic effects elicited by acupuncture. In fact, as early as 1977, Nakatani & Yamashita had drawn attention to the fact that Ryodoraku acupuncture points are in areas of skin containing sweat glands, and modern Ryodoraku theory attributes the heterosegmental effects of acupuncture to interactions between sympathetic and somatic nervous systems. Ogata et al (1993) have demonstrated that sweat production in humans is reduced by acupuncture. Interestingly, it is frequently observed that patients sweat profusely during treatment with acupuncture.

It has recently been suggested (Iguchi & Sawai 1993, Yamada, Hoshino & Watari 1993) that at least some meridians may correspond to lymphatic channels. Like blood vessels, lymphatics are accompanied by fine nerve fibres, as evidenced, for example, by the pain felt following untreated hand infection that travels up the arm to the axillary lymph glands.

SPINAL SEGMENTAL MECHANISMS

Acupuncture analgesia is blocked or reversed by naloxone (Cheng & Pomeranz 1980, Mayer, Price & Rafii 1977, Sjölund & Eriksson 1979). Melzack, Stillwell & Fox (1977) have identified many of Travell's trigger points with acupuncture points. It is therefore of great interest that pain relief by trigger point injection with bupivicaine is also reversed by naloxone (Fine, Milano & Hare 1988). Han, Ding & Fan (1986) have also shown that intracerebroventricular or intrathecal injection of cholecystokinin octapeptide (CCK-8), which is an endogenous opioid antagonist, antagonizes analgesia produced both by morphine and by electroacupuncture in the rat. All these lines of evidence clearly point to an opioidergic mechanism of action for acupuncture. Table 6.2 summarizes

Table 6.2 Neuropharmacology: the role of some neurotransmitters in acupuncture analgesia (after Han 1984)

Substance	Brain (PAG)	Spinal cord
Monoamines		
5-hydroxytryptamine (5-HT)	+	+
noradrenaline (NAD)	–	+
Peptides		
met-enkephalin	+	+
dynorphin A & B	0	+
β-endorphin	+	0
substance P (SP)	+	–
cholecystokinin octapeptide (CCK-8)	–	–
Amino-acids		
γ-amino butyric acid (GABA)	–	0

Key: + potentiation, – antagonism, 0 no effect, PAG periaqueductal grey.

the role of some neurotransmitters in acupuncture analgesia and compares the action of each on the brain and spinal cord.

It therefore behoves us to examine the intraspinal connections of Aδ primary afferent terminals (Fig. 6.1). Kumazawa & Perl (1978) showed that Aδ primary afferents in the primate end principally in the most superficial zone (lamina I) and neck (lamina V) of the dorsal horn of the spinal grey matter. In the region of the large superficial cord cells, there are other very small cells, called 'stalked cells' demonstrated in the cat by Bennett et al (1982) and in humans by Abdel-Maguid & Bowsher (1984); these suppress activity in the subjacent cells of the substantia gelatinosa (SG), on which the small unmyelinated 'pain fibres' end (Sugiura,

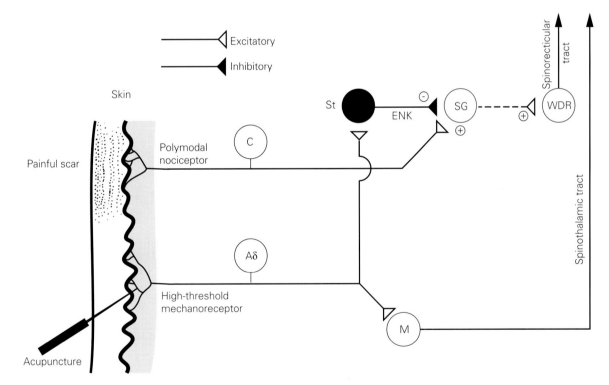

Figure 6.1 Mechanism of segmental acupuncture. The C primary afferent polymodal nociceptor projects to substantia gelatinosa (SG) cells in the superficial dorsal horn; these generate further impulses that pass to, or perhaps disinhibit, wide dynamic range (WDR) (or convergent) cells whose axons pass up to the brain in the spinoreticular tract where they are eventually interpreted as painful.
The Aδ primary afferent pinprick receptors project both to marginal cells (M), which project up to the brain in the spinothalamic tract carrying information about pinprick that will become conscious, and to enkephalinergic stalked cells (St), which can release enkephalins (ENK) that inhibit SG cells, thus preventing information generated by noxious stimulation being transmitted further. (After Thompson & Filshie 1993, derived from Bowsher 1992.)

Table 6.3 Effect of stimulation frequency (from Thompson 1994)

Frequency	Low (2–5 Hz)	High (20–200 Hz)
Technique	Manual or electrical	Electrical: electroacupuncture
Type	High intensity/low frequency	Low intensity/high frequency
Predominant pharmacology	met-enkephalin β-endorphin	Dynorphins 5-HT + NAD
Naloxone	Blocks effect	Unaffected

Lee & Perl 1986). It has been shown that stalked cells do not react to frequencies of stimulation above about 3 Hz (Bowsher et al 1968, Harper & Lawson 1985), which is the optimal frequency at which acupuncture analgesia stimulation is performed. The stalked cells inhibit SG cells by releasing on to them the inhibitory opioid transmitter enkephalin (Ruda, Coffield & Dubner 1984). Stalked cells also receive a direct input from Aδ pinprick fibres (Gobel et al 1980). It has recently been directly demonstrated (Bing et al 1991) that acupuncture-like stimulation in the rat induces release of enkephalin-like material in the spinal cord. Very recently, Sjölund and his colleagues (personal communication) and Hashimoto & Aikawa (1993) have shown that manual acupuncture in the rat induces inhibition in the wide dynamic range (WDR) cells, which project up to the brain, conveying impulses that will be consciously interpreted as painful. WDR cells are influenced by SG cells (Fig. 6.1), thus completing the circuit. Table 6.3 illustrates the effect of stimulation frequency on the predominant pharmacological response of the primary afferent input (Aβ and Aδ nerve fibres).

Thus, the intraspinal terminals of primary afferent Aδ (pinprick) fibres branch to supply the large Waldeyer cells in the marginal layer (lamina I) and the enkephalinergic stalked cells at the border between laminae I and II (SG) of the dorsal horn. Since Aδ primary afferent fibres stimulate the stalked cells, and these in turn enkephalinergically inhibit the SG cells, we have an adequate explanation of the mechanism for segmental acupuncture interrupting the pain pathway from C fibres to the WDR cells.

HETEROSEGMENTAL ACUPUNCTURE

There is no doubt that, in clinical practice, acupuncture at certain points can relieve pain in distant regions supplied by nerves from totally different segments. It is therefore necessary to consider the physiological mechanisms that may underlie these phenomena. To do this, two distinct, but sometimes anatomically intermingled, ascending pathways must be examined, as well as the descending pathways that may inhibit the upward transmission of impulses generated by noxious stimulation.

In the spinal cord WDR, or convergent, cells (Giesler et al 1976, Willis & Coggeshall 1978) respond to most stimuli in a graded manner; noxious stimulation in the periphery causes them to fire at highest frequency. All types of peripheral afferent can therefore excite WDR cells, after relaying through variable numbers of interneurons in the dorsal horn of the spinal grey matter; WDR cells do not receive monosynaptic connections from primary afferents. Some WDR cells are to be found in lamina V, in the neck of the spinal dorsal horn, but most of them are to be found in the deeper layers (laminae VII and VIII) of the intermediate spinal grey matter. These cells send their axons to the opposite side of the spinal cord, where they ascend in the anterolateral funiculus as the spinothalamic and spinoreticular tracts (Kuru 1949, Bowsher 1957). Essentially, the spinoreticular pathway carries information generated by the stimulation of nociceptors to the reticular formation, the intralaminar thalamus and the hypothalamus (Fig. 6.2) (Burstein, Cliffer & Giesler 1987); the spinothalamic tract, on the other hand, carries information generated by thermal and pinprick receptors to the ventroposterior thalamus (Willis & Coggeshall 1978, Willis 1985). Many of the cells projecting into the spinothalamic tract lie in the marginal zone (lamina I), and are activated by Aδ pinprick receptors. It is thus of great interest that the heterosegmental acupuncture effect in the rabbit is abolished by section of the anterolateral funiculus, but not by destruction of other long ascending spinal cord pathways (Chen et al, 1975). We must therefore enquire what collateral connections of the spinothalamic pathway may be responsible for the activation, directly or indirectly, of descending inhibitory pathways. In addition, physiological research (Takeshige 1992, Tsai, Chen & Lin 1993) has shown that two transmitter systems—serotonergic and noradrenergic—are involved (Figs 6.2, 6.3), and Tsai, Chen & Lin (1993) have recently shown that central adrenergic, as well as serotonergic, neurons are excited by acupuncture stimulation.

We shall therefore consider heterosegmental acupuncture effects under these two physio-pharmacological headings and finally mention a third system that may contribute to the acupuncture effect.

The serotonergic system

It has been known for some time that spino-thalamic collaterals reach the midbrain peri-aqueductal grey matter (PAG) in the primate (Mantyh 1982a), and Zhang et al (1990) have recently shown that these axons originate from cells in lamina I.

It was in 1964 that Tsou & Jang demonstrated that the PAG is the most effective spot in the whole nervous system for the abolition of pain by microinjection of morphine. As the PAG was known *not* to send messages upwards to the cerebral cortex so that these messages did not become conscious, this amazing finding was conveniently overlooked by most researchers. However, in 1968 Reynolds showed that painless surgery could be carried out in the rat during electrical stimulation of PAG, and this led to intensive research on possible mechanisms.

Investigations by Mayer & Liebeskind (1974) showed that a descending inhibitory pathway passing down from the caudoventral part of the PAG to the spinal cord was responsible for the inhibition of neurons with ascending axons that carry messages generated by painful stimuli in the periphery (Fig. 6.2). There is evidence that there is a somatotopic organization within this part of the PAG (Soper & Melzack 1982); this might explain why heterosegmental acupuncture effects cannot be obtained from *any* acupuncture point, but only from particular points that are not necessarily within the dermatome in which it is desired to obtain pain relief.

The pathway descending from the PAG, whose transmitter substance is probably neurotensin (Beitz 1982), relays in the nucleus raphe magnus (NRM) of the medulla oblongata. From the NRM, fibres whose transmitter substance is mainly serotonin (5-hydroxytryptamine, 5-HT) descend in the dorsolateral funiculus (DLF) of the spinal cord to terminate directly on the stalked enkephalin-containing interneurons in the spinal dorsal horn (Glazer & Basbaum 1984), which were discussed above. There are also serotonin-containing nerve terminals ending freely in the superficial part of the spinal cord grey matter (Hammond, Tyle & Yaksh 1985, Leranth, Maxwell & Verhofstad 1984, Maxwell, Leranth & Verhofstad 1983). This could explain the 'hormonal' or generalized type of acupuncture effect, as opposed to the point-to-point or neural type. Increased serotonin levels in mast cells and platelets have been reported following acupuncture (Souvannakitti et al 1993, Wu & Deng 1993). Both these latter phenomena might (but very cautiously) be considered an explanation of those acupuncture effects that outlast direct synaptic inhibition.

Finally, as mentioned earlier, the PAG receives fibres containing the naturally occurring morphine-like substance β-endorphin (Bloom et al 1978); these fibres descend from the arcuate region of the hypothalamus (Mantyh 1982b), a primitive but essential part of the forebrain concerned not only with regulation of bodily functions but also with emotion. In humans, the

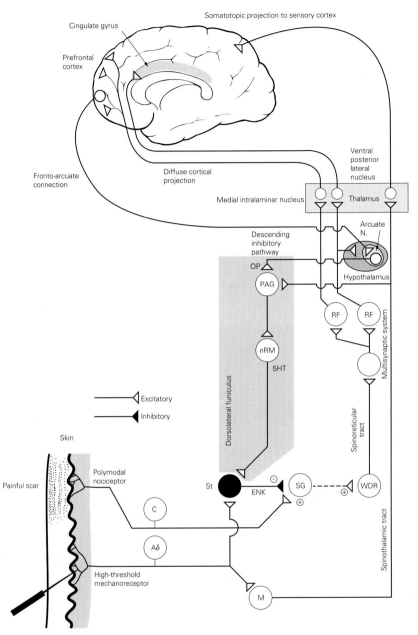

Figure 6.2 Serotonergic mechanism of acupuncture. Pinprick information is carried up from marginal cells (M) (see also Fig. 6.1) to the ventroposterior lateral thalamic nucleus, whence it is projected to the cortex and becomes conscious; but in the midbrain these axons give off a collateral branch to the periaqueductal grey matter (PAG). The PAG projects down to the nucleus raphe magnus (NRM) in the midline of the medulla oblongata, and this in turn sends serotonergic (5-HT) fibres to the stalked cells (St). The latter inhibit substantia gelatinosa cells (SG) by an enkephalinergic mechanism (ENK), and so prevent noxious information arriving in C primary afferent nociceptors from being transmitted to wide dynamic range (WDR) cells deep in the spinal grey matter, which send their axons up to the brain (reticular formation, RF). OP = opioid peptides.

The PAG is also influenced by opioid endorphinergic fibres descending from the arcuate nucleus in the hypothalamus, and the hypothalamus in turn receives projections from the prefrontal cortex. (After Thompson & Filshie 1993; derived from Bowsher 1992 see Fig. 11.3 p 188.)

hypothalamus is under the control of the prefrontal cortex, a region whose blood flow is increased by painful stimuli (Lassen, Ingvar & Skinhöj 1978, Tsubokawa et al 1981). It is because the pathway from hypothalamus to PAG is endorphin-containing that pain relief in humans can be obtained by stimulating electrodes implanted in the PAG or in the periventricular region anterior to it (Richardson 1982) in which the hypothalamo-PAG fibres run. This morphine-like pain relief is reversed by naloxone (Hosobuchi, Adams & Linchitz 1977, Richardson & Akil 1977).

Within the PAG itself, there are inhibitory interneurons that are themselves inhibited by the long-descending β-endorphin-containing hypothalamo-PAG fibres, which accounts for the release of activity in the PAG–NRM pathway and thus inhibition in the spinal cord via the inhibitory NRM–spinal pathway.

Modulation of pain perception through the emotional or psychic state of the individual may depend on the projection from the prefrontal cortex through the hypothalamus to the PAG.

Because the type of acupuncture effect descending through PAG is eventually serotonergic, it is antagonized by methysergide (Takeshige, Sato & Komugi 1980).

The noradrenergic system

In the cat and monkey, lamina I of the spinal grey matter, in addition to projecting to PAG, also sends collaterals to the locus coeruleus in the pons (Craig 1992), which is the principal brainstem source of noradrenergic axons. Unlike the serotonergic axons descending from the NRM, noradrenergic fibres do not operate through enkephalinergic interneurons (stalked cells) in the spinal cord, but bring about direct inhibition on the many types of spinal cell with which they make synaptic contact (Fig. 6.3).

A massive spinal projection, ascending in the anterolateral funiculus, to the gigantocellular reticular region has long been known in humans (Bowsher 1957). Takeshige and his colleagues (1992) have also implicated the paragigantocellular reticular nucleus in the descending adrenergic system whose activity is elicited by acupuncture

stimulation, because the inhibitory effects of direct stimulation of this structure are antagonized by phentolamine. However, they point out that the paragigantocellular reticular nucleus does not itself contain any noradrenergic cells; nor does it project directly to the spinal cord. It must therefore relay to a noradrenergic structure before directly influencing spinal activity. This may be the locus coeruleus, or some other noradrenergic lower brainstem cell group whose axons project into the spinal cord. For example, in the primate, Carlton et al (1991) have identified noradrenergic cells in the C1 area of the medulla and pontomedullary junction whose axons descend on the edge of the lateral white funiculus of the spinal cord to the superficial dorsal horn, the intermediate and the circumcanalicular grey matter. Takeshige (1992) believes that the descending noradrenergic system, like that descending from PAG, is ultimately controlled from the prefrontal cortex and the arcuate nucleus of the hypothalamus.

Diffuse noxious inhibitory controls

Diffuse noxious inhibitory controls (DNIC) (Fig. 6.3) is the name given to a powerful pain-suppressing system described by Le Bars (Le Bars, Dickenson & Besson 1979) and his collaborators. Much research by this group has shown that DNIC is an opioidergic mechanism acting on spinal cord WDR neurons (see above), which transmit pain-generated information toward the brain. Direct input of Aδ-generated information elicited by acupuncture to the subnucleus reticularis dorsalis in the caudal medulla has been demonstrated in the rat and monkey (Villanueva et al 1988, 1990); this is probably the same region as was shown to receive convergent nociceptive information in the cat by Bowsher (1970). The subnucleus reticularis dorsalis projects downward through the dorsolateral funiculus to the dorsal horn of the spinal cord at all levels (Bernard et al 1990). Bing, Villanueva & Le Bars (1991) have shown that this mechanism is brought into play by needle stimulation at both acupoints and non-acupoints on the body surface. The fact that stimulation at non-acupoints elicits

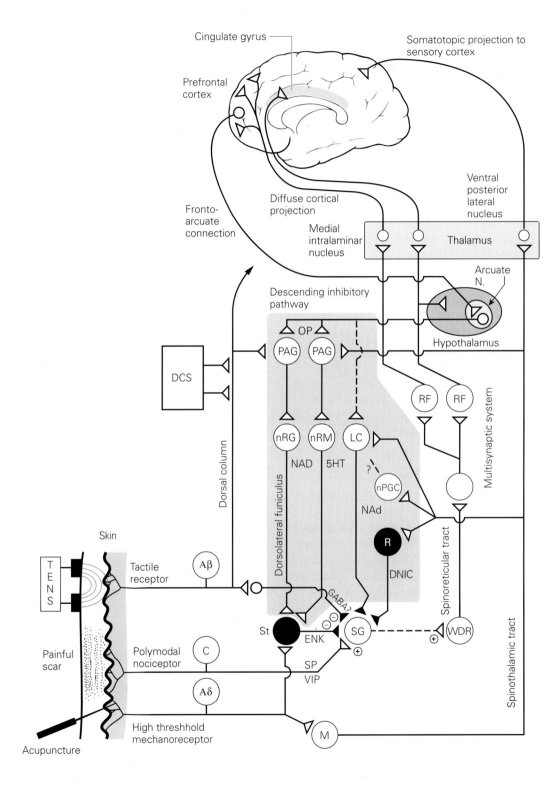

Figure 6.3 (*facing*) Adrenergic mechanism of acupuncture. Marginal cells (M), activated by Aδ pinprick receptors, in addition to their projections to the ventral posterior lateral nucleus and the PAG, also send axon branches to the following: (a) Subnucleus reticularis dorsalis (R) in the caudal medulla oblongata. Descending projections from this structure bring about inhibition of noxiously generated information arriving at the spinal cord (SG) in C nociceptors. This is the DNIC mechanism (see text). (b) Nucleus paragigantocellularis lateralis (PGC), which indirectly (? via the locus coeruleus LC, see (c) below) brings about noradrenergically mediated inhibition at spinal cord level. (c) The locus coeruleus at the junction of medulla oblongata and pons. Its noradrenergic axons (NAD) are directly inhibitory to those spinal neurons with which they enter into synaptic contact. OP = opioid peptides, DCS = dorsal column stimulation.

Note: The figure also includes the Aβ primary afferent tactile receptor, which projects to the dorsal column and in addition, via an interneuron to the SG cells. Thus activation of the tactile receptor sends impulses to the dorsal column and also, via the interneurone, leads to an inhibition of the SG cells, probably through the release of γ-aminobutyric acid (GABA). The latter action will prevent information generated by noxious stimulation being transmitted further; this is believed to be the principal mechanism of transcutaneous electrical nerve stimulation (TENS) (see Ch. 11). (After Thompson & Filshie 1993, derived from Bowsher 1992)

DNIC does not mean that when stimulation is performed at acupoints DNIC does not contribute to the acupuncture effect, particularly the short-term effect, as has recently been emphasized by Hashimoto & Aikawa (1993). The involvement of DNIC in the human acupuncture effect receives support from the recent research of Marchand & Li (1993), who reported pain reduction in *all* skin locations by electroacupuncture.

CONCLUSION

1. Acupuncture stimulates Aδ or Group III small myelinated primary afferents in skin and muscle.

2. Segmental acupuncture operates through a circuit involving inhibitory enkephalinergic stalked cells in the outer part of lamina II (SG) of the spinal grey matter, which are directly contacted by Aδ/Group III primary afferents.

3. Heterosegmental acupuncture is brought about by both a generalized neurohormonal mechanism, involving the release of free β-endorphin and apparently also of met-enkephalin, and by two descending neuronal mechanisms, the first of which is serotonergic and the second adrenergic. A third descending system (DNIC)

may also contribute in a minor way to the acupuncture effect:

(a) The system is influenced by the prefrontal cortex and descending through the hypothalamus (arcuate nucleus) and the PAG to the NRM of the medulla oblongata and thence to the spinal cord, where enkephalinergic stalked cells are activated. This system has discrete but ill-understood somatotopy, which may depend on classical referral of stimuli, on viscero-somatic interactions, and/or on a somatotopic organization existing within the PAG.

(b) Noradrenergic cells in the lower brainstem are excited both by influences ascending directly from the spinal cord, and also relaying through the nucleus paragigantocellularis, and by influences descending from the prefrontal cortex through the hypothalamic arcuate nucleus.

(c) Cells of the subnucleus reticularis dorsalis are influenced by high-intensity inputs from both acupuncture and non-acupuncture points; axons descending from the subnucleus reticularis dorsalis bring about widespread inhibition (DNIC effect).

REFERENCES

Abdel-Maguid T E, Bowsher D 1984 Interneurons and proprioneurons in the adult human spinal grey matter and general somatic afferent cranial nerve nuclei. Journal of Anatomy 139:9–20

Bache F 1826 Cases illustrative of the remedial effects of acupuncturation. North American Medical and Surgical

Journal 1:311–321

Baldry P E 1993 Acupuncture, trigger points and musculoskeletal pain, 2nd edn. Churchill Livingstone, Edinburgh

Beitz A J 1982 The sites of origin of brainstem neurotensin and serotonin projections to the rodent nucleus raphe magnus. Journal of Neuroscience 2:829–834

Bennett G J, Ruda M A, Gobel S, Dubner R 1982 Enkephalin-immunoreactive stalked cells and lamina IIb islet cells in cat substantia gelatinosa. Brain Research 240:162–166

Berlioz L V J 1816 Mémoires sur les maladies chroniques, les évacuations sanguines et l'acupuncture. Croullebos, Paris

Bernard J F, Villanueva L, Carroue J, Le Bars D 1990 Efferent projections from the subnucleus reticularis dorsalis (SRD): A *Phaseolus vulgaris* leucoagglutinin study in the rat. Neuroscience Letters 116:257–262

Bing Z, Cesselin F, Bourgoin S, Clot A M, Hamon M, Le Bars D 1991 Acupuncture-like stimulation induces a heterosegmental release of Met-enkephalin-like material in the rat spinal cord. Pain 47:71–77

Bing Z, Villanueva L, Le Bars D 1991 Acupuncture-evoked responses of subnucleus reticularis dorsalis neurons in the rat medulla. Neuroscience 44:693–703

Bloom F E, Battenberg E, Rossier J, Ling N, Guillemin R 1978 Neurons containing β-endorphin in rat brain exist separately from those containing enkephalin: Immunocytochemical studies. Proceedings of the National Academy of Sciences USA 75:1591–1595

Bowsher D 1957 Termination of the central pain pathway in man: The conscious appreciation of pain. Pain 80:606–622

Bowsher D 1970 Place and modality analysis in caudal reticular formation. Journal of Physiology 209:473–486

Bowsher D 1976 Role of the reticular formation in response to noxious stimulation. Pain 2:361–378

Bowsher D 1988 Introduction to the anatomy and physiology of the nervous system, 5th edn. Blackwell, Oxford

Bowsher D 1992 The physiology of stimulation-produced analgesia. Pain Clinic (Tokyo) 12:485–492

Bowsher D 1993 Paradoxical pain. British Medical Journal 306:473–474

Bowsher D, Mallart A, Petit D, Albe-Fessard D 1968 A bulbar relay to centre médian. Journal of Neurophysiology 31:288–300

Burstein R, Cliffer K D, Giesler G J 1987 Direct somatosensory projection from the spinal cord to the hypothalamus and telencephalon. Journal of Neuroscience 7:4159–4164

Carlton S M, Honda C N, Willcockson W S, Lacrampe M, Zhang D, Denoroy L, Chung J M, Willis W D 1991 Descending adrenergic input to the primate spinal cord and its possible role in modulation of spinothalamic cells. Brain Research 543:77–90

Chan S H H 1984 What is being stimulated in acupuncture: evaluation of the existence of a specific substrate. Neuroscience and Biobehavioral Reviews 8:25–33

Chen Y C, Jen Y L, Teh H C, Yao H P, Shu C C 1975 Studies on spinal ascending pathway for effect of acupuncture analgesia in rabbits. Scientia Sinica 18:651–658

Cheng R S S, Pomeranz B H 1980 Electroacupuncture analgesia is mediated by stereospecific opiate receptors and is reversed by antagonists of Type I receptors. Life Sciences 26:631–638

Chiang C Y, Chang C T, Chu H L, Yang L F 1973 Peripheral afferent pathway for acupuncture analgesia. Scientia Sinica 16:210–217

Churchill J M 1821 A treatise on acupuncturation, being a description of a surgical operation originally peculiar to the Japanese and Chinese, and by them denominated zin-king, now introduced into European practice, with directions for its performance, and cases illustrating its success. Simpkins and Marshall, London

Clement-Jones V, McLoughlin L, Tomlin S, Besser G M, Rees L H, Wen H 1980 Increased beta-endorphin but not metenkephalin levels in human cerebrospinal fluid after acupuncture for recurrent pain. Lancet 2:946–949

Cloquet J G 1826 Traité de l'acupuncture. Becket-Jeune, Paris

Craig A D 1992 Spinal and trigeminal lamina I input to the locus coeruleus anterogradely labeled with Phaseolus vulgaris leucoagglutinin (PHA-L) in the cat and the monkey. Brain Research 584:325–328

Dundee J W, Chestnutt W N, Ghaly R G, Lynas A G A 1986 Traditional Chinese acupuncture: a potentially useful anti-emetic? British Medical Journal 293:583–584

Ernst M, Lee M H M 1985 Sympathetic vasomotor changes induced by manual and electrical acupuncture of the Hoku point visualized by thermography. Pain 21:25–33

Fine P G, Milano R, Hare B D 1988 The effects of trigger point injections are naloxone reversible. Pain 32:15–20

Ganong W F 1993 Review of medical physiology, 16th edn. Appleton & Lange, Connecticut, p 53

Giesler G, Ménétrey D, Guilbaud G, Besson J-M 1976 Lumbar cord neurons at the origin of the spinothalamic tract in the rat. Brain Research 18:320–324

Glazer E J, Basbaum A I 1984 Axons which take up [^{3}H] serotonin are presynaptic to enkephalin immunoreactive neurons in cat dorsal horn. Brain Research 289:389–391

Gobel S, Falls W M, Bennett G J, Abdelmoumène M, Hayashi H, Humphrey E 1980 An E. M. analysis of the synaptic connections of horseradish peroxidase filled stalked cells and islet cells in the substantia gelatinosa of the adult cat spinal cord. Journal of Comparative Neurology 194:781–807

Goulden E A 1921 The treatment of sciatica by galvanic acupuncture. British Medical Journal 1:523–524

Guyton A C 1991 Textbook of medical physiology, 8th edn. WB Saunders, Philadelphia, pp 499–500

Hammond D L, Tyle G M, Yaksh T L 1985 Effects of 5-hydroxytryptamine and noradrenaline into spinal cord superfusates during stimulation of the rat medulla. Journal of Physiology (London) 359:151–162

Han J S 1984 Progress in the pharmacological studies of acupuncture analgesia. In: Paton S W, Mitchell J, Turner P (eds) Proceedings IUPHAR Ninth International Congress of Pharmacology, vol 1. Macmillan, London, pp 387–394

Han J S, Ding X Z, Fan S G 1986 Cholecystokinin octapeptide (CCK-8): Antagonism to electroacupuncture analgesia and a possible role in electroacupuncture tolerance. Pain 27:101–115

Harper A A, Lawson S N 1985 Electrical properties of rat dorsal root ganglion neurones with different peripheral nerve conduction velocities. Journal of Physiology (London) 359:47–63

Hashimoto T, Aikawa S 1993 Needling effects on nociceptive neurons in rat spinal cord. Proceedings of the 7th World Congress on Pain IASP, Seattle, p 428

Hosobuchi Y, Adams J E, Linchitz R 1977 Pain relief by electrical stimulation of central gray matter in humans and its reversal by naloxone. Science 197:183–186

Hyodo M 1990 Ryodoraku treatment. Japanese Society of Ryodoraku Medicine, Osaka

Iguchi K, Sawai Y 1993 Correlationship between the meridians and acute lymphangitis. Proceedings of the 3rd world conference on acupuncture, Kyoto, p 270

Johnson M I, Hajela V K, Ashton C H, Thompson J W 1991. The effects of auricular transcutaneous electrical nerve stimulation (TENS) on experimental pain threshold and autonomic function in healthy subjects. Pain 46:337–342

Kawakita K 1991 Role of polymodal receptors in the peripheral mechanisms of acupuncture and moxibustion stimulation. In: Manchanda S K, Selvamurthy W, Mohan Kumar V (eds) Advances in physiological sciences. New Delhi, pp 731–739

Kawakita K, Funakoshi M 1982 Suppression of the jaw-opening reflex by conditioning A-delta fiber stimulation and electroacupuncture in the rat. Experimental Neurology 78:461–465

Kumazawa T, Perl E R 1978 Excitation of marginal and substantia gelatinosa neurons in the primate spinal cord: indications of their place in dorsal horn functional organization. Journal of Comparative Neurology 177:417–434

Kuru M 1949 Sensory paths in the spinal cord and brain stem of man. Sogensaya, Tokyo

Lassen N A, Ingvar D H, Skinhöj E 1978 Brain function and blood flow. Scientific American 239:50–59

Le Bars D, Dickenson A H, Besson J-M 1979 Diffuse noxious inhibitory controls (DNIC). I—Effects on dorsal horn convergent neurones in the rat; II—Lack of effect on non-convergent neurones, supraspinal involvement and theoretical implications. Pain 6:283–327

Leranth C S, Maxwell D J, Verhofstad A A J 1984 Ultrastructure of serotonin-immunoreactive boutons in the substantia gelatinosa of the rat's spinal cord. Journal of Physiology (London), 355, 20P

Levine J D, Gormley J, Fields H L 1976 Observations on the analgesic effects of needle puncture (acupuncture). Pain 2:149–159

Liu Y K, Varela M, Oswald R 1977 The correspondence between some motor points and acupuncture loci. American Journal of Chinese Medicine 3:347–358

Lu G D, Needham J 1980 Celestial lancets: a history and rationale of acupuncture and moxa. Cambridge University Press, Cambridge

Mann F, Bowsher D, Mumford J, Lipton S, Miles J 1973 Treatment of intractable pain by acupuncture. Lancet 2:57–60

Mantyh P W 1982a The ascending input to the midbrain periaqueductal gray of the primate. Journal of Comparative Neurology 211:50–64

Mantyh P W 1982b Forebrain projections to the periaqueductal gray in the monkey, with observations in the cat and rat. Journal of Comparative Neurology 206:146–158

Marchand S, Li J 1993 The effect of electro-acupuncture on perceived heat pain at different body locations. Proceedings of the 7th World Congress on Pain, p 427

Matsumoto T, Hayes M F 1973 Acupuncture, electric phenomenon of the skin, and post-vagotomy gastrointestinal atony. American Journal of Surgery 125:176–180

Maxwell D J, Leranth C S, Verhofstad A A J 1983 Fine structure of serotonin-containing axons in the marginal zone of the rat spinal cord. Brain Research 266:233–260

Mayer D J, Liebeskind J C 1974 Pain reduction by focal electrical stimulation of the brain: An anatomical and behavioral analysis. Brain Research 68:73–93

Mayer D J, Price D D, Rafii A 1977 Antagonism of acupuncture analgesia in man by the narcotic antagonist naloxone. Brain Research 121:368–372

Melzack R, Stillwell D M, Fox E J 1977 Trigger points and acupuncture points for pain: correlations and implications. Pain 3:3–23

Nakatani Y, Yamashita K 1977 Ryodoraku acupuncture. Ryodoraku Research Institute, Osaka

Nogier P F M 1972 Traité d'Auriculothérapie. Maisonneuve, Moulins-les-Metz

Nurmikko T, Bowsher D 1990 Somatosensory findings in postherpetic neuralgia. Journal of Neurology, Neurosurgery and Psychiatry 53:135–141

Ogata A, Umeyama T, Ogawa T, Kobayashi S, Sugenoya J, Kugimiya T, Hanaoka K 1993 Effects of low-frequency electro-acupuncture on psychological sweating. Proceedings of the 3rd World Conference on Acupuncture, Kyoto, p 157

Pomeranz B, Paley D 1979 Electroacupuncture hypalgesia is mediated by afferent nerve impulses: an electrophysiological study in mice. Experimental Neurology 66:398–402

Reynolds D V 1968 Surgery in the rat during electrical analgesia induced by focal brain stimulation. Science 164:444–445

Rhijne W ten 1683 Dissertatio—de Acupunctura. Leers, Den Haag

Richardson D E 1982 Analgesia produced by stimulation of various sites in the human β-endorphin system. Applied Neurophysiology 45:116–122

Richardson D E, Akil H 1977 Pain reduction by electrical brain stimulation in man. Journal of Neurosurgery 47:178–194

Ruda M A, Coffield J, Dubner R 1984 Demonstration of postsynaptic opioid modulation of thalamic projection neurons by the combined techniques of retrograde horseradish peroxidase and enkephalin immunocytochemistry. Journal of Neuroscience 4:2117–2132

Sjölund B H, Eriksson M B E 1979 The influence of naloxone on analgesia produced by peripheral conditioning stimulation. Brain Research 173:295–302

Soper W Y, Melzack R 1982 Stimulation-produced analgesia: evidence for somatotopic organization in the midbrain. Brain Research 251:301–312

Souvannakitti L, Akasereenont P, Ketsa-ard K, Chotewuttakorn S, Thaworn A 1993 Platelet serotonin in headache patients treated by new trend acupuncture. Proceedings of the 7th World Congress on Pain, p 429

Sugiura Y, Lee C L, Perl E R 1986 Central projection of identified, unmyelinated (C) afferent fibers innervating mammalian skin. Science 234:358–361

Takeshige C 1992 Synaptic transmission in acupuncture analgesia. Showa University, Japan

Takeshige C, Murai M, Hachisu M 1980a Parallel individual variation in effectiveness of electro-acupuncture, morphine analgesia and dorsal PAG-SPA and its abolishment by d-phenylalanine. Acupuncture and Electro-Therapeutics Research 5:251–268

Takeshige C, Sato T, Komugi H 1980b Role of periaqueductal central gray in acupuncture anaesthesia. Acupuncture and Electro-Therapeutics Research 5:323–337

Takeshige C, Sato T, Mera T, Hisamitsu T, Fang J 1992 Descending pain inhibitory system involved in acupuncture analgesia. Brain Research Bulletin 29:617–634

Takeshige C, Tanaka M, Sato T, Hishida F 1990 Mechanism of individual variation in effectiveness of acupuncture analgesia based on animal experiment. European Journal of Pain 11:109–113

Thompson J W 1994 Acupuncture: current ideas on mechanisms of action. Summary from lecture to meeting of Pain Society. April 14th–16th, UMIST, Manchester

Thompson J W, Filshie J 1993 Tens and acupuncture. In: Doyle D, Hanks G, MacDonald N (eds) Oxford textbook of palliative medicine. Oxford University Press, Oxford, ch. 4.2.8

Toda K, Ichioka M 1978 Electroacupuncture: relations between forelimb afferent impulses and suppression of jaw opening reflex in the rat. Experimental Neurology 61:465–470

Travell J G, Simons D G 1983 Myofascial pain and dysfunction. The trigger point manual. Williams and Wilkins, Baltimore

Tsai H-Y, Chen Y-F, Lin J-G 1993 Studies of mechanism of electroacupuncture analgesia in the central monoaminergic neurons. Proceedings of the 3rd World Conference on Acupuncture, Kyoto, p 194

Tsou K, Jang C S 1964 Studies on the site of analgesic action of morphine by intracerebral microinjection. Scientia Sinica 13:1099–1109

Tsubokawa T, Katayama Y, Ueno Y, Moriyasu N 1981 Evidence for involvement of the frontal cortex in pain-related cerebral events in cats: increase in local cerebral blood flow by noxious stimuli. Brain Research 217:179–185

Villanueva L, Bouhassira D, Bing Z, Le Bars D 1988 Convergence of heterotopic nociceptive information onto subnucleus reticularis dorsalis neurons in the rat medulla. Journal of Neurophysiology 60:980–1009

Villanueva L, Cliffer K D, Sorkin L S, Le Bars D, Willis W D 1990 Convergence of heterotopic nociceptive information onto neurons of caudal medullary reticular formation in monkey (Macaca *fascicularis*). Journal of Neurophysiology 63:1118–1127

Wang K M, Yao S M, Xian Y L, Hou Z 1985 A study on the receptive field of acupoints and the relationship between characteristics of needle sensation and groups of afferent fibres. Scientia Sinica 28:963–971

Williams P L, Warwick R, Dyson M, Bannister L H (eds) 1989 Gray's anatomy, 37th edn. Churchill Livingstone, Edinburgh

Willis W D 1985 The pain system. Karger, New York

Willis W D, Coggeshall R E 1978 Sensory mechanisms of the spinal cord. Plenum Press, New York

Wu J, Deng X 1993 The mast cell biologically-active substances and electroacupuncture analgesic effect. Proceedings of the 7th World Congress on Pain, p 429

Yamada K, Hoshino T, Watari N. 1993 Histological study of acupoint. Proceedings of the 3rd World Conference on Acupuncture, Kyoto, p 274

Yoshio N 1969 Introduction to Ryodoraku. Acupuncture Digest 3:70–78

Zhang D X, Carlton S M, Sorkin L S, Willis W D 1990 Collaterals of primate spinothalamic tract neurons to the periaqueductal gray. Journal of Comparative Neurology 296:277–290

7

Acupuncture's non-segmental and segmental analgesic effects: the point of meridians

Alexander J. R. Macdonald

Two puzzling features of acupuncture's practice are examined in this chapter. There is a well-documented paradox that acupuncture performed in a noxious manner tends to produce analgesia in regions of the body far distant from the site of the needle. This is acupuncture's non-segmental analgesic effect. On the other hand, a comparatively unexpected and unexplored phenomenon occurs when a needle is inserted into a tender region. Such an action tends to initiate a lasting reduction in tenderness in the immediate vicinity of the needle; this may be said to be acupuncture's segmental effect.

ACUPUNCTURE'S NON-SEGMENTAL EFFECTS

The idea that an acupuncture stimulus may be applied to one region of the body to relieve pain in another is very old. Yang Jizhou wrote in AD 1601:

Behold now the way of the golden needle! A method so nimble and rare . . . First distinguish the context of the trouble, Next decide on the quality of the points. If the head is troubled, select those on the feet, If the left is troubled, then select the right . . .
(Transl Bertschinger 1991)

It also seems not a little paradoxical that to elicit non-segmental analgesic effects the practitioner must be prepared to use the needle as an instrument designed to produce noxious stimulation in its own right. Indeed over the two millennia that acupuncture has been practised in

China, a variety of vigorous needling methods have been codified in descriptive traditional terms such as 'mountain-burning fire', 'penetrating heaven coolness', 'dragon and tiger joined in battle' and 'green dragon wags its tail' (Shanghai College of Traditional Medicine 1981). Practitioners learn how to manipulate the needles by certain twisting, pushing and pulling movements, yet most claim not to inflict unnecessary pain on their patients.

The author's method is to insert a sterile 30 gauge acupuncture needle vertically to a depth of a centimetre or so into the subcutaneous tissues of any convenient muscular region—for example, the forearm extensors. The needle is rotated approximately 360° around its long axis; this action tends to cause the tissues to grip the needle. While maintaining this angle of rotation, the needle is then pulled partially out of the body; the deep tissues are still gripping the rotated needle, so this action causes them to be forcibly stretched. While maintaining the angle of rotation, the upward pull on the needle is then released for a moment, and then reapplied. This manoeuvre is repeated once or twice a second.

Although manipulation of the needle in this manner tends to produce a good deal of pain in normal subjects, patients who are already suffering pain in some distant region of the body (e.g. retention of urine) hardly notice it. In other words the more pain a patient suffers elsewhere, the less he is aware of the effects of such vigorous needling. Furthermore, needling of this kind when applied for a few minutes tends to produce considerable relief of nociceptive pain arising in other parts of the body, be they visceral or musculoskeletal tissues. Such relief may persist for several hours.

Bing et al (1991) have described a mechanism for the above phenomenon; they found that an increased release of opioids or met-enkephalin-like material occurred in rat CSF in the cervical region, when either a 'true' acupuncture point (Zuzanli, ST-36) or an adjacent 'non-acupuncture point' was stimulated by manual twisting of an acupuncture needle. Identical effects occurred whether a true or false point was

stimulated in this manner. Both of these points lie in the hindlimb, yet three times as much opioid release occurs in the CSF in the cervical area of the spinal cord as in the lumbar region, where the primary afferent fibres of the hindlimb project.

Thus it appears that stimulating one region of the body by manual acupuncture tends to increase opioid release in the CSF from segments of the spinal cord placed far away. This produces widespread, extrasegmental, non-selective analgesia. Indeed the distance between those segments of the cord that innervate the regions where the acupuncture is applied and those where the outflow of opioids is increased precludes the involvement of segmental effects in this phenomenon.

Why a needle?

Noxious mechanical stimulation has similar heterosegmental effects to manual acupuncture (Le Bars et al 1987). However, in contrast both noxious thermal (Cesselin et al 1989) and chemical stimulation (Bourgoin et al 1990) produce a segmental increase in opioids. Furthermore Sjölund, Terenius & Eriksson 1977 demonstrated a segmental increase in CSF opioids when they employed a form of electrical stimulation via surface electrodes called 'acupuncture like'—where bursts of 100 Hz pulses are repeated at a rate of 0.5–3 Hz to mimic the firing rates of α motor neurones.

Why different forms of noxious stimulation should stimulate opioid production in different parts of the spinal cord is not known. Perhaps the difficulties encountered during our evolution, when we were naked or at best poorly protected by clothing, made us develop strong reactions to the presence of anything that threatened the tissues. A very common event that must have occurred on a day to day basis was puncture by thorns. In other words it is more likely than not that the insertion of an acupuncture needle, which is effectively a sterile thorn, would elicit profound reactions in the CNS, especially if such a needle continued to be stimulated in a noxious manner.

Bing, Villanueva & Le Bars (1990) demonstrated that manual acupuncture applied via a single needle to a point (either a 'real' or false acupuncture point) in the hindlimb is as effective as noxious heat applied to the entire limb, both producing inhibitory effects on convergent neurons lying within the spinal tract of V that are stimulated by C fibre firing in the trigeminal nerve. This idea that manual twisting of an acupuncture needle is interpreted by the CNS as a noxious stimulus has been explored in the rat by Bing, Villanueva & Le Bars (1991). These authors paid particular attention to the function of neurons lying in the reticular formation in the medulla oblongata. The properties of the reticular formation as far as noxious stimuli are concerned had already been investigated for many years (Bowsher 1976, Bowsher et al 1968). Bing, Villanueva & Le Bars (1991) demonstrated that manipulation of an acupuncture needle in many parts of the body, particularly the contralateral side, increased the firing rates of neurons lying in a bulbar structure called the subnucleus reticularis dorsalis. These neurons play an important role as a relay in pain pathways. Their activity is depressed by systemic morphine in a dose-related, naloxone-reversible manner (Bing, Villanueva & Le Bars 1989). They are driven by neural traffic caused by noxious stimulation (such as acupuncture) ascending the anterolateral tracts from any segment of the cord (Bing, Villanueva & Le Bars 1991). They project rostrally to many supraspinal structures (see below). They also project caudally in the descending pain-inhibiting dorsolateral tracts to terminate in the dorsal horns at all levels of the spinal cord.

Han et al (1979) showed these descending pain-inhibiting pathways to be mediated by 5-HT. Shen, Ts'ai & Lan (1975) had already demonstrated that non-segmental effects of acupuncture are mediated via these pathways. Han et al (1979) found that the turnover rate of 5-HT in the CNS is greatly increased by acupuncture; furthermore, acupuncture's analgesic effects are reduced when 5-HT is depleted (Chiang et al 1979). From a practical point of view, when a patient is depressed, acupuncture works less well; by the same token, acupuncture itself may be used to treat depression (Han 1986a).

The discovery of neurons in the medulla that are driven by signals (reaching them from the ascending anterolateral tracts) arising as a result of noxious stimulation, which are at the same time capable of initiating pain-inhibiting processes that descend the spinal cord in the dorsolateral tracts, may be the explanation we require to begin our understanding of the phenomenon that the noxious stimulus of an acupuncture needle tends to inhibit pain arising elsewhere.

Electroacupuncture

Manual stimulation of needles has been replaced in many centres by electroacupuncture. Peter Nathan (personal discussion) pointed out that electroacupuncture provides one of the few examples of Europeans practising an important development in the field of acupuncture before the Chinese.

In 1774, Jesuit missionaries introduced acupuncture into France. Here the method has not only survived to this day to be practised by over a thousand physicians, but it is still being actively investigated. Salandière, who had been introduced to acupuncture in 1812 by the physician son of the composer Berlioz, was the first to practise electroacupuncture. He attached his needles to a source of direct or galvanic current in order to treat gout and arthritis (Light 1967). Salandière (1825) claimed his method: '. . . Introduces shock into the very place I wish'.

Magendie, an even bolder physician, plunged needles into muscles and nerves; he even inserted them through the eyeball into the optic nerve and then connected them to an electric battery. He mentions remarkable cures, but never his failures or accidents.

Duchenne (1849) found that he could admit more current in a comfortable manner into the body via moistened surface electrodes. Furthermore, only 18 years after Faraday had discovered how to induce alternating currents, Duchenne announced that the medical use of induced (or faradic) current was safer than that of direct or galvanic current, which he proscribed as a result of the dangers of electrolytic effects.

In order to investigate the electrolytic effects caused by direct current in the immediate vicinity of acupuncture needles, Omura (1975) suspended two needles in molar saline containing pH indicator, and passed a direct current from a 3 V battery. Within half a minute, bubbles appeared around both needles: oxygen formed near the anode, while bubbles given off at the cathode contained hydrogen. The saline in the vicinity of the anode is acid (HCl). The region of the cathode becomes alkaline (NaOH). These reactions to direct current cause necrosis in the tissues. Furthermore, the metal forming the anode ionizes and migrates to the cathode, causing the needle to break, and the portion that still receives current to disappear. Despite these dangers, the direct current method is still used in Japan in a form of acupuncture called Ryodoraku.

In electroacupuncture stimulators available in China and the West today, the current is usually interrupted in the form of square-wave mono-phasic pulses that are brief enough to avoid the dangers of electrolytic effects, yet are sufficiently broad in duration to excite not only Aβ, but also Aδ and C afferent fibres as the amplitude is increased. The electrical parameters of these electroacupuncture stimulators are as follows: a pulse width in the region of 700 μs is employed at a low frequency of 2–20 Hz at an amplitude sufficiently high to produce pain close to the patient's tolerance. The duration of treatment need be maintained only for sufficient time to produce an analgesic effect (from 2–40 minutes).

Fortunately for the patient, Le Bars et al (1991) describe the importance of stimulating the Aδ fibres when employing electroacupuncture, rather than increasing the amplitude to the point where C fibres are excited. Although both Aδ and C fibre stimulation tend to reduce the activity in convergent neurons lying in the dorsal horn elsewhere in the spinal cord, Aδ fibres are able to produce a more synchronized input to the spinal cord than are the slower C fibres.

While studying the inhibitory effects on spinothalamic tract cell responses to maximal stimulation of a primate sural nerve, Chung et al (1984) gradually increased the amplitude of the ipsilateral tibial nerve stimulation while maintaining the frequency at 2 Hz. While it is true that when they increased the amplitudes sufficiently to recruit C fibres total inhibition was produced, the most dramatic increase in inhibition of spinothalamic tract cells occurred as soon as the tibial nerve-conditioning stimulus amplitude was increased sufficiently to recruit Aδ fibres.

C fibres can initially follow a stimulus train of high frequencies such as 100 Hz for a very short period of time. However, after displaying an initial burst of relatively high-frequency activity to suprathreshold stimulation, C fibres quickly adapt to a low-level firing rate (White & Levine 1991); in this adapted state, they cannot produce impulse trains that exceed a frequency of approximately 2 Hz. Furthermore, Bowsher (1975) notes that a striking property of reticular formation neurons is their inability to respond to peripheral stimulation above 3 Hz. On this basis, if we intend to perform electroacupuncture it would seem sensible that, whatever the amplitude, the frequency should remain at 2 Hz.

However, Chung et al (1984) maintained the pulse amplitude at a level sufficiently high to recruit Aδ fibres without exciting C fibres in the ipsilateral tibial nerve, and explored the effects of altering frequency. At this amplitude, they found that a frequency of 20 Hz produced a total inhibition of the effects of maximal sural nerve stimulation on the spinothalamic tract cells. So, provided the amplitude is at a level lying between pain threshold and tolerance, this evidence suggests the most effective electroacupuncture frequency for producing non-segmental analgesia to be at least as high as 20 Hz. Indeed when a commercial transcutaneous electrical nerve stimulation (TENS) unit was applied in this model by Lee, Chung & Willis (1985), inhibition of C fibre-evoked potentials occurred only when the intensity of TENS stimulation was increased sufficiently to recruit Aδ fibres.

Frequency responses

There is still a good deal of controversy and many questions to answer in the search for the most effective frequency of electroacupuncture stimulation. Chung et al (1984) stated:

With current knowledge, it is difficult to define acupuncture and TNS based on either their characteristics or mechanisms ... Undoubtedly, peripheral nerve stimulation produced analgesia through multiple mechanisms. One set of stimulating parameters may merely favor one mechanism, whereas other sets may elicit other mechanisms.

Cheng & Pomeranz (1979) were the first to report that analgesia was produced when needles were inserted into mice both when low-frequency (4 Hz) and when high-frequency (200 Hz) electroacupuncture was employed, but the administration of naloxone (2 mg/kg) blocked only the analgesic effects of low-frequency electroacupuncture. They proposed that low-frequency electroacupuncture was mediated by an opioid system, whereas that of high frequency was not.

Cheng (1989) suggested that signals arising from high-frequency electroacupuncture take a comparatively direct path to the midbrain to stimulate the descending serotonin- and catecholamine-mediated pain-inhibiting dorso-lateral tract, and that this is the route of the non-opioid pathway. It is interesting to note that Xie, Tang & Han (1981) have shown that the presence of both 5-HT and catecholamines in the spinal cord facilitates the effects of acupuncture. But in the brain, on the other hand, the two sub-stances oppose each other: here 5-HT facilitates acupuncture, while catecholamines suppress its effects.

Cheng (1989) believes that low-frequency stimulation has a more circuitous route and produces an effect on many higher centres, including, in the midbrain, the raphe nucleus and various reticular nuclei, and that they in turn stimulate the pain-inhibiting descending dorsolateral tracts that modify or 'gate' the incoming nociceptor signals.

Han (1986b, 1989) has reviewed the evidence that a number of higher centres work together as an integrated system, and that furthermore their ablation or stimulation affects acupuncture. They include centres in the lower brainstem that

stimulate the descending dorsolateral tracts. These are the nuclei raphe dorsalis and magnus, and the locus coeruleus; the latter initiates the release of catecholamines, while the effects of the former are mediated by 5-HT. The peri-aqueductal grey matter also lies in the brain-stem. Its activities are affected by the nucleus habenula and nucleus arcuatus hypothalami lying in the diencephalon. These nuclei, together with those lying in the brainstem, are affected by the following nuclei in the limbic system: the caudate, the amygdala, the septum and accumbens. Hypothalamic nuclei, such as the centrolateral and centromedian, also have an effect on the lower brainstem nuclei. The cerebral cortex projects to the caudate nucleus in the limbic system.

Han et al (1984a) confirmed the work of Cheng & Pomeranz (1979) that the analgesic effects of high-frequency (100 Hz) electro-acupuncture in the rat are not reversed by low doses of naloxone. But Han et al (1984a) found that high doses of naloxone (10–20 mg/kg) did reverse these effects. Furthermore their work suggests that the reason why the analgesia of low-frequency electroacupuncture is readily reversed by naloxone is that it is mediated by μ-receptors, which are particularly susceptible to naloxone blockade.

In order to explore this phenomenon further, Fei, Xie & Han (1987) subjected rats to spinal perfusion. Met-enkephalin was released during low-frequency electroacupuncture, but dynorphin A was found during high-frequency stimulation: its analgesic effects (which are six to 10 times more potent than those of morphine when administered intrathecally to the rat) are mediated via k-receptors that are less responsive to naloxone than μ-receptors (Han & Xie 1984b,c). Furthermore the analgesic effect of high-frequency electroacupuncture is easily reversed by k-receptor antagonists (Han, Ding & Fan 1986).

Han et al (1991) have repeated this work in humans. In order to compare the effects of low (2 Hz) and high frequencies (100 Hz) in a more consistent manner, surface electrodes rather than needles were employed, so in a sense we are looking at high-amplitude TENS rather than electroacupuncture.

Patients under investigation for neurological disorders in two Beijing hospitals volunteered to have two lumbar punctures, one before and the other after stimulation. In order to avoid placebo effects, the stimulation was described as being diagnostic rather than therapeutic.

At a pulse width of 300 μs, stimulation of each kind (2 Hz or 100 Hz) was applied for 30 minutes via surface electrodes attached to the hand and lower leg. The amplitude of each type of stimulation was maintained at a level of 26–30 mA, sufficient to produce visible contractions of the underlying muscles.

Two classes of peptides were measured by radioimmunoassay before and after each type of stimulation: met-enkephalin derived from preproenkephalin on the one hand, and dynorphin A derived from preprodynorphin on the other. Those patients who received low-frequency stimulation produced a significant 367% rise in met-enkephalin with only a modest 29% rise in dynorphin A. In contrast, those patients who received high-frequency stimulation sustained a moderate but significant rise of 49% in release of dynorphin A, whereas their met-enkephalin fell, though not significantly.

In studies of specific antibodies to various endogenous opioids, Han and colleagues (Han 1984, Han et al 1984b) have shown that the presence of [Met^5]enkephalin and dynorphins A and B are necessary for acupuncture's effects in the spinal cord, whereas [Leu^5]enkephalin, and β-endorphin are not necessary. However, reversal of the effects of β-endorphin at supraspinal levels in the periaqueductal grey by a specific antiserum does reduce the effect of acupuncture (Xie, Zhou & Han 1981).

This blurring of the distinctions between electroacupuncture and TENS has led to the development of a new type of stimulator that combines the properties of low- and high-frequency stimulation. Its purpose is to stimulate the release of both met-enkephalin and dynorphin simultaneously. Han (1989) has designed a device (AcuTENS) that delivers 300 μs pulses at 2 Hz and then 100 Hz alternately for 5 second periods. This may be delivered to the patient via either needles or surface electrodes.

Counterirritation

An important concept in the management of patients by acupuncture is the idea that this method is an ancient but refined form of counterirritation. If a patient presents with a bothersome headache, then if you insert a needle into his foot he will soon forget whatever is happening in his head. Conversely, a classical prescription for haemorrhoid pain is the insertion of acupuncture needles in the scalp at the vertex.

Counterirritation regimens were reviewed by Le Bars et al (1989). For instance, binding a tight noose or twitch around a horse's protruberant upper lip produces analgesia during castration or docking of the tail. Le Bars et al (1984) reviewed the medical use of cupping, scarification of the skin, cautery, blistering, and the use of rubefacients such as mustard and oil of turpentine—perhaps all of these are but Western forms of acupuncture-type counterirritation.

Willer (1977) recorded responses in the biceps femoris muscle to sural nerve stimulation in humans. In this study, the amplitude of stimulation was increased gradually; when the pain threshold was reached an additional, somewhat delayed, response developed in the biceps femoris. The magnitude of this nociceptive reflex response correlated with the subject's awareness of pain. This apparently objective method of measuring changes in spinal processing of an experimentally induced noxious electrical stimulus has been employed in a number of studies.

Le Bars, Willer & de Broucker (1992) performed a study in humans, and observed how the moderately noxious thermal stimulus of hot water (at about 46°C) applied to the contralateral hand strongly reduced the nociceptive reflex response elicited by electrical stimulation of the sural nerve. This reduction, however, is itself abolished by low doses of morphine, but is readily regained following the administration of naloxone.

To account for these findings, they have proposed the idea of diffuse noxious inhibitory controls (DNIC) within the CNS. The concept of such controls was earlier described by Le Bars, Dickenson & Besson (1979a,b), and are proposed to function in the following manner. There are interneurons in the dorsal horn called convergent neurons, or wide dynamic range (WDR), multi-receptive or class 2 neurons, since they respond not only to noxious, but also to innocuous inputs arising in skin, deep soft tissues and viscera. There are also spinal interneurons called non-convergent, or nociceptive specific or class 3 neurons, as they respond to noxious stimulation only. When a noxious stimulus is applied to a particular part of the body, these two types of interneurons (lying in the affected segment of the spinal cord) together excite a spino-bulbo-spinal loop. This involves ascending pathways lying in the anterolateral tract that pass upwards to the supraspinal centres, which in turn trigger descending pathways lying within the dorso-lateral tracts of the spinal cord. These descending tracts inhibit the activities of all the convergent interneurons lying in segments of the spinal cord innervated by the unaffected regions of the body.

The effect of this spino-bulbo-spinal loop activity (which Le Bars has called DNIC) produces a contrast between the increased firing rates in the convergent interneurons in the affected segments of the spinal cord compared with the decreased activity everywhere else. As the DNIC increase this contrast, the patient's awareness of pain tends also to be increased. Conversely, anything that decreases DNIC tends to reduce pain.

Bing, Villanueva & Le Bars (1990) have proposed that DNIC is a substrate of acupuncture's non-segmental effects. The essence of the acupuncture approach (Le Bars, Willer & de Broucker 1992) is that the DNIC produced by one source of noxious stimulation may be reduced by applying a second noxious stimulus: the latter is provided by vigorous acupuncture applied to a remote region of the body. They explain this phenomenon by the idea that the second source of pain, provided by the acupunc-

ture, sets up a second set of DNIC that competes with the first.

Low-dose morphine reduces DNIC, as it has an inhibitory effect on cells in the bulbar portion of the loop—the subnucleus reticularis dorsalis (Bing, Villanueva & Le Bars 1991). These cells are responsible for initiating the descending pain-inhibiting effects on the dorsal horns of the remainder of the spinal cord.

Le Bars et al (1984) reviewed the difficulties inherent in studying counterirritation phenomena. One of the difficulties lies in determining an appropriate balance between the two inputs into the central nervous system—on the one hand from the noxious electrical stimulus that elicits the nociceptive reflex, and on the other the conditioning stimulus provided by a means such as manual acupuncture. Both of these inputs are experimentally induced. Imagine how difficult it is to design a meaningful experiment when one of the inputs arises from organic disease. Many find it difficult to imagine that any useful material can be derived from employing experimentally induced pain in a study of the extent of organic pain.

Nevertheless Willer et al (1987) discovered that organic pain has an effect on nociceptive reflexes. They selected patients suffering acute unilateral sciatica associated with disc protrusion; however, these patients were pain free when lying in a resting position. When Lasègue's manoeuvre was performed on the affected side, pain was produced. This had the effect of reducing the response to noxious electrical stimulation of the sural nerve on both sides. When Lasègue's manoeuvre was performed on the unaffected side without causing pain, the nociceptive reflexes were not altered.

In a sense, every time an acupuncturist tries to relieve pain, he is engaging in the difficult study of balancing the effects of organic disease with those provided by the needle (Chang 1978) and tries to provide a sufficient stimulus to have a beneficial effect on the changes that have occurred in the CNS as a result of the patient's condition. Such studies are necessarily incomplete, as many of these changes are as yet unknown.

But there are practical applications of this work in a clinical setting.

An example is the treatment of renal colic. Lee et al (1992) performed a prospective randomized study comparing acupuncture (both manual and 3 Hz electroacupuncture) with a drug regimen: Avafortan (Camilofin and noramidopyrine) an analgesic-containing dipyrone. They found the two were equally effective in relieving the severe, acute pain of renal colic associated with urolithiasis. In the acupuncture group, they inserted needles (both segmentally and non-segmentally) into the back region and the hand. The acupuncture stimulus was sufficient to render 19 of the 22 patients (86.4%) pain free, whereas the analgesic drug relieved pain in 62.5%—a smaller percentage, but not significantly so. However, acupuncture had a significantly more rapid onset of analgesic action (within 1–10 minutes) as compared with 10–30 minutes for Avafortan), and produced none of the side-effects that occurred with the drug (tachycardia, rash or drowsiness).

Some of the underlying neurophysiological mechanisms of this counterirritation phenomenon perhaps explain the adage, 'One must be cruel to be kind'.

ACUPUNCTURE'S SEGMENTAL EFFECTS

Hitherto we have been looking at the results of inserting needles and stimulating them vigorously in regions remote from the origin of the patient's nociceptive pain.

Tender regions

What happens if we insert a needle into the vicinity of the tender region itself? For want of a better term, we may call this 'segmental acupuncture'. However we need to be cautious about the word 'segmental', for, as we shall see, pathological pain of somatic origin is by no means always confined to segmental boundaries.

Dung (1984) believes the Chinese were the first to systematically map the location of frequently occurring tender regions. However, in a particular individual, points indicated in their acupuncture charts may or may not be abnormally tender to palpation. Indeed few tender points are found in a healthy subject when $1–1.5 \, \text{kg/cm}^2$ pressure is exerted. But in patients suffering an illness, tender points are found in number and location according to the nature and severity of the disease. From Dung's observations, the fewer the tender points that can be found in a patient, the more likely it is that the acupuncture will be a success.

This paper was a turning point in acupuncture's long history. We are no longer challenged by the idea that one of the world's oldest forms of medical practice is so mysterious that it is quite beyond our understanding. Rather we are encouraged to start, as the original medical scholars began 2000 years ago, by examining our patients carefully for tender regions. As Wang (1986) stated: 'Through the repeated practice of searching for tender spots, people gradually discovered the reaction-points on the body surface, including the tender points ... .' 'Pain should be cured when the needle reaches the point of pain.' As a well-known physician in the Tang dynasty (AD 618–907) Sun Szu-miao so pithily put it: 'Puncture wherever there is tenderness'. Another saying, 'Where the pain is there is the point', informs us that the tender region was where the noxious stimulus, such as acupuncture, moxibustion or blood letting was performed in ancient times (Wang 1986).

Mann (1977) was the first to connect the practice of acupuncture with studies in the West on the location of trigger points, by Travell, and the maps of tender points noted by Kellgren (1938, 1939a,b) and Sola & Williams (1956). Other Western studies on sources of tender points include Lange (1931). Melzack, Stillwell & Fox (1977) described a 71% correlation between acupuncture points frequently chosen by Chinese practitioners and trigger points described by Western practitioners such as Travell, Simons and Sola in association with particular pain states. Although at that time neither group had any knowledge of the other's work, and differed in their understanding of the mechanisms and methods of practice, there were enough similarities to make one think they were both describing the same phenomenon:

Trigger points are firmly anchored in the anatomy of the neural and muscular systems, while acupuncture points are associated with an ancient conceptual but anatomically non-existent system of meridians ... despite the different origins, however, it is reasonable to assume that acupuncture points for pain relief, like trigger points, are derived from the same kind of empirical observation: that pressure at certain points is associated with particular pain patterns, and brief, intense stimulation of the points by needling sometimes produces prolonged relief of pain. These considerations suggest a hypothesis: that trigger points and acupuncture points for pain, though discovered independently and labelled differently, represent the same phenomenon.

The paper by Melzack, Stillwell & Fox (1977) represents an important stepping-stone for Western-trained practitioners of acupuncture. The idea that trigger or acupuncture points are the same entities is most valuable, particularly when one is trying to search for the most likely position of such a tender region, and one can consult well-illustrated descriptions of trigger points provided by Travell & Simons (1983, 1992) with renewed insight.

Referred pain

The vexed question of referred pain is one of the difficulties that every investigator has to come to terms with in this field of treating somatic pain. Reynolds (1983) described the realization in many authors' minds that pain is referred not only from viscera but also from somatic tissues. Hockaday & Whitty (1967) reviewed the doubts expressed by many that referred pain of somatic origin is always referred segmentally. The difficulties facing the diagnostician trying to discover the source of pain, too dependent on a knowledge of dermatomes, are described by Inman & Saunders (1944):

A problem which often confronts the physician in clinical diagnosis is the meaning of the obscure pain found in association with traumatic or inflammatory lesions involving the bones, ligaments, tendons, fasciae and other mesodermal structures of the body.

On questioning the patient, pain of this nature is often described as of a dull, aching or boring nature which he usually finds difficult to localize with any degree of accuracy. The patient frequently contends that this pain lies deep to the skin and that it frequently radiates proximally or distally to a varying extent. In spite of the fact that the patient often gives a history of deadness or numbness, in the part, nonetheless the physician, on examination of skin sensation, is unable to discern anything of an objective nature except perhaps occasionally a slight hypalgesia. There is no diminution of peripheral sensation and no anesthesia, no hypesthesia, no muscle weakness and no definite reflex changes. A puzzling feature to the physician is the fact that the distribution of the patient's pain is frequently constant in direction and position but yet fails to correspond to the area of supply of any known peripheral nerve or nerve root ...

Torebjörk, Ochoa & Schady (1984) showed that muscle pain need not be referred segmentally. Noxious stimulation of a single afferent fascicle arising from a muscle in the hand, performed via a microelectrode inserted into the median nerve at the elbow, sometimes caused pain to be referred as far afield as the thorax in the regions of serratus anterior and pectoralis major.

Kellgren (1938, 1939a, 1978) described a painful but harmless and repeatable procedure that produces consistent responses in individual subjects: he injected an algesic substance, 6% (hypertonic) saline, into muscles and ligaments of normal subjects, and produced maps of referred pain. However, he noted (Kellgren 1977) how important it is when studying referred pain patterns arising from deep injections of this kind, for the skin and subcutaneous tissues to be infiltrated with local anaesthetic adequately to prevent the onset of local pain arising in the superficial tissues as a result of the hypertonic saline backtracking along the path of the needle. Earlier he had found (Kellgren 1939b) that when he injected muscles with hypertonic saline the pain was frequently referred to joints that are moved by the injected muscles: for example, in the case of tibialis anterior, pain was referred to the ankle, while an injection into the long extensors of the forearm produced pain felt maximally in the region of the wrists and knuckles. When structures in the vicinity of a joint were injected in this way, the localization of pain was more accurate; the region of maximum pain was the joint itself. This localization was most obvious in the case of the foot and hand, but less so in the case of the hip or shoulder.

Many of us were taught that the invariable cause of muscle pain is hypoxia brought about by spasm, maintained by increased 'γ-tone'. On the contrary, Mense & Skeppar (1991) have reported the unexpected finding that artificially induced inflammation in cat muscle produces a marked reduction in γ-motorneuron activity. They suggest that such fusimotor inhibition (accompanied by disfacilitation of α-motor neurons) may offer an explanation for the apparent weakness that is often found in tender muscles. This might also confer the advantage of reducing the tension acting on the damaged tissue. Certainly Macdonald (1980) found that in humans increased pain was produced by any movement or manoeuvre that increased either the length or isometric tension within a tender muscle. In other words, if muscles are tender, when an active or passive movement is painful the antagonist muscles are the likely source, but when a forced resisted manoeuvre is painful it is the agonist.

This knowledge is of practical use in the search for tender muscle regions. Often referred pain is placed some distance away from the tender region, particularly in the case of limb muscles. For example, a patient wakes up complaining of diffuse pain in the hand, particularly when trying to flex the fingers fully. In this instance, examination may reveal only minimal tenderness in the hand, while exquisitely tender regions are found in the long extensors of the forearm (i.e. the antagonists of active flexion). Flexing the fingers causes the tender long forearm extensors to lengthen—and increase the pain. Even though it arises in so proximal a group of muscles, this pain is referred in a deep diffuse fashion to the hand. In this case, employing the ideas of Kellgren (1978), the best analgesic site for the local anaesthetic infiltration would be the forearm extensors not in the fingers where the patient is complaining of pain:

Anaesthetizing the deep tender spot from which the pain is arising produces a dramatic and complete abolition of the symptoms. Anaesthetizing referred tender spots naturally abolishes the tenderness, but has little effect on spontaneous pain, and any limitation of movement . . . remains unchanged.

However, as we will see, the insertion of a needle alone without any accompanying local anaesthetic also relieves pain, particularly when it is inserted into a tender region.

On other occasions the referred pain overlaps the tender region, particularly in the trunk, or when it involves ligaments, especially in the limbs. Thus the diagnostician is often faced with a difficulty in deciding whether a particular region is part of a referred area of pain or the tender region itself. The most practical way of deciding the issue is to employ palpation.

Palpation

According to Travell & Simons (1983) (pp 59–63), palpation is the key to finding the source of tenderness in soft tissues. (As palpation of a tender region may cause an exacerbation of pain for several days, the practitioner must be prepared to treat the region adequately after examination.) For diagnostic purposes, the real object of palpation is to elicit specific responses such as the 'jump sign', described by Kraft, Johnson & La Ban (1968), as follows: 'We palpate the area and watch his reaction, pressure over an involved muscle almost invariably produces a characteristic flinching not seen in other diseases. The patient tends to recoil in a manner out of proportion to the amount of pressure produced by the examining finger.'

In China, regions tender to palpation are often called 'Ah Shi' (oh yes) points, as patients often call out in this polite fashion, as they are so exquisitely tender.

Kellgren (1978) described palpation as a method of distinguishing the source of a pain from its referred region. He concentrated on a particular aspect of the patient's reaction to palpation: when the examining finger is placed with gradually increasing firmness over the source of the pain, the pain engendered is increased out of all proportion to the amount of pressure exerted. Meanwhile the referred area of pain behaves in a different way: the pain elicited by this procedure (although at first is moderately greater than normal) increases only in proportion to the amount of pressure exerted. Thus if a patient complains of pain in the medial aspect of the knee, the practitioner gently increases the pressure of his palpating finger or thumb over this location. If the patient does not show much sign of distress, this region is likely to be part of a referred area. Inserting a needle in this region tends not to relieve the pain, and may actually increase it.

Meanwhile, examination of regions proximal to the knee joint may well uncover exquisitely tender regions: in the case of pain felt deeply in the medial aspect of the knee, the most common tender region is to be found in vastus medialis. Here the tender region is usually a hand's breadth or so proximal to the knee joint. As mechanical pressure exerted by palpation is gradually increased in this region, the patient reacts out of all proportion to the increase in pressure, and often cries out or grimaces. If this is the most tender region, then this is the site for needling.

However, in the case of anterior knee pain, when palpation fails to elicit abnormal tenderness in the leg itself the most tender region may be found as far distant as the quadratus lumborum. So, in the case of anterior knee pain, the examiner should start by examining the upper lumbar region and work his way downwards to the knee itself.

In similar fashion, pains felt in the lower back without radiation to the leg are often associated with tenderness in the quadratus lumborum. In the absence of neurological deficit, pains radiating down the posterior aspect of the leg are often associated with tender gluteal muscles.

Do trigger/acupuncture points exist?

Those who wish to follow progress on naming acupuncture points may find it useful to refer to a new standard nomenclature (World Health Organization 1984). To provide a rapid way of discovering the location of points and a descrip-

tion of many traditional terms mentioned in Chinese articles, an alphabetical dictionary has been compiled by Zhang, Wu & Wang (1985). Baldry (1993) has produced a very extensive and readable review of the literature describing the location of trigger and acupuncture points delineated by practitioners in both Western and Eastern disciplines.

Although one learns a great deal from these small tender spots and their patterns of referred pain, the reader must not be tempted to make too much of either the trigger or acupuncture point concept. For, in practice, patients suffering moderate or severe disability of somatic origin rarely present with just 'points' of tenderness. There may be points of maximal tenderness, but careful palpation reveals large surrounding regions of abnormal tenderness whose surface area often compares in size with that of the referred pain area. The surface area of these regions varies from 16 to 200 cm^2. Thus in these patients the concept of tenderness being represented merely by small points (be they 'acupuncture' or 'trigger') is increasingly difficult to defend. Observations of large tender regions form the modern approach. This concept has been explored by Mann (1992).

Patterns of referred pain or 'algotomes'

Why abnormally tender soft tissue regions, described by Kellgren, Travell and others, should so often be separated anatomically from the referred pain area is a mystery, particularly when the predominant causes of both phenomena are likely to lie in altered central pain processing. In the author's experience, however, each tender somatic tissue region and its referred area of pain tend to be mutually related in commonly occurring fields that often overflow dermatomal boundaries. Why these particular referred pain patterns appear so frequently is a mystery, but, once observed and appreciated, knowledge of the extent and anatomical disposition of these referred pain patterns speeds up the practitioner's quest for the tender regions that require needling.

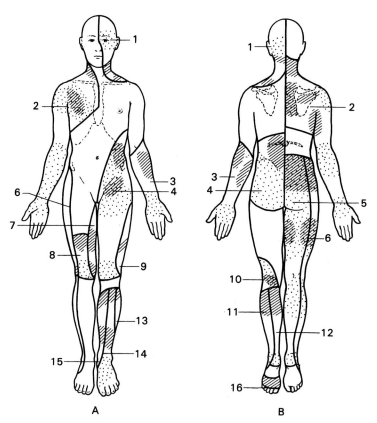

Figure 7.1 A, B   Patterns of referred pain or 'algotomes': although on the whole these are segmentally based, they often overflow segmental boundaries—particularly algotomes 1 and 2. Pain may be referred from anywhere to anywhere within the boundaries (represented by thick black lines) of each numbered algotome. Shading indicates the most common sites for tender regions, which require painless, local needling. The usual referred pain areas are covered in dots. Where tenderness and the feeling of pain coincide, particularly on the trunk, dots and shading are printed together. Where algotomes overlap each other, they are represented on either side of the body.

For convenience we may call these referred pain patterns 'algotomes'; they are illustrated in Figure 7.1. In Figure 7.1, the extent of the surface area of each referred pain pattern or algotome is depicted on the body by means of thick, solid lines. For convenience they have been numbered rostrocaudally from 1 to 16. Regions of shading indicate the commonly occurring locations of abnormally tender regions. Part or the whole of these regions is often found to be abnormally tender to palpation. Pain may be felt or referred from a particular tender region anywhere within the boundaries of its algotome. The most com-

mon areas of referred pain are indicated by a series of dots.

Once a tender region has been found by palpation, this is the most effective region to needle if segmental acupuncture is employed. In the case of the limbs and trunk, the referred areas of pain usually lie distal to the tender regions. In the limbs, pains are most often referred to joints. On the trunk, however, there is a greater likelihood of patients complaining of pain at the site of the tender region.

As we proceed rostrally, pains in the jaw and periorbital regions are often associated with tender regions lying inferiorly in the region of C2–4, or even upper and middle trapezius. Here the most rostral referred pain pattern (algotome 1) has clearly transgressed the segmental concept of referred pain, as it has overflowed from cervical to trigeminal territory. Furthermore, algotome 2 shows that tenderness found in the anterolateral (or subclavian triangle) region of the neck may be linked to referred pain in the posterior thorax in the interscapular (rhomboid) region—thus embracing both lower cervical and midthoracic segments.

In some instances, algotomes overlap each other. To avoid confusion they are drawn separately on each side of the body. So, whichever side the pain actually presents in a patient, it is necessary to look at both sides of the body in Figure 7.1. For example, a patient may present with posterior knee pain. In this condition, the tender region may commonly be found locally in popliteus muscle (algotome 10); or tenderness may be elicited in the more proximal gluteal or upper hamstring regions (algotome 5). Pains in the heel, on the other hand, may arise either in gastrocnemius (algotome 12), or in the gluteal region (algotome 5).

Is muscle fascia one of the most tender layers?

Capsular and ligamentous structures are often tender. But, in many conditions, tender areas are to be found in muscle regions. In such regions, however, it is not known which tissues are the most likely source of tenderness. In severe conditions, it is likely that mechanical pain thresholds are reduced in all the tissue layers in a given region.

Kawakita, Miura & Iwase (1991) explored this question in healthy volunteers who happened to have a few muscular regions that were abnormally tender to palpation. However, mechanical pressure algometry failed to show significant differences in the mechanical thresholds in tender compared with non-tender regions. They then explored the effects of electrical stimulation—incorporating trains of 500 Hz pulses lasting 1 ms, repeated at a frequency of 2 Hz, whose amplitude was increased at a constant rate until

the pain threshold was reached. The anode was connected to a large surface electrode (in order to reduce sensation), while the cathode comprised a 180 μm diameter acupuncture needle, completely insulated except for at the tip. This needle was inserted slowly through the skin and subcutaneous tissues into muscular regions. The depth of the bare needle tip and the nature of the tissues it encountered were determined by ultrasonic tomography. As they explored various depths of insertion into various layers, a significantly low pain threshold (in the tender regions compared with the non-tender) was found in muscle fascia, not in the body of the muscle itself.

The reader may like to perform a similar experiment, and experience the sensation of a needle stimulating muscle fascia. Insert a 30 gauge needle very slowly through the skin overlying the belly of the first dorsal interosseous muscle of the hand. At the level of muscle fascia, at a depth of a few millimetres, small movements of the hand begin to induce equivalent movements in the needle. As the needle tip penetrates the muscle fascia layer, unusual sensations are often experienced. From classical times, according to Lu & Needham (1980), there have been Chinese records of 'needle sensations' arising from deep tissues. The sensations are believed by many to play an important role in therapy. They are called 'De Qi' or Qi (obtaining the Qi (Chi), or energy). The patient feels 'Suan' (an ache that one might experience in muscular fatigue), 'Ma' (numbness), 'Chang' (distension, as if the needled region has become oedematous), 'Chung' (heaviness) or any combination of these. In addition, soreness, tingling and warmth have been described.

Possible mechanisms of segmental acupuncture

Inhibitory or pain-relieving mechanisms may be initiated by either low- or high-threshold afferent activity at both spinal and supraspinal levels. The relationship between these inhibitions and the way in which the tissues are stimulated are very complex (PM Headley, personal communication, 1992). As we know from the TENS literature, Aβ fibre stimulation raises the pain threshold segmentally. And, as discussed earlier, Aδ and C fibre activation may cause non-segmental and segmental pain threshold elevation via ascending and descending loops involving supraspinal structures. What is not so commonly known is that, under certain circumstances, a noxious stimulus produces segmental analgesia.

Lund, Hansen & Kehlet (1990) studied the effect of cutaneous sensitivity and somatosensory evoked potentials to segmental electrical stimulation (of the L1 dermatome) in patients undergoing hysterectomy. In contrast to many animal studies, where a decrease in sensory threshold has been reported after injury, a marked increase was found 48 hours after surgery.

The idea that surgical trauma has an inhibitory or analgesic effect on pain processing has also been explored by Clarke & Matthews (1990); here the segmental surgical effects of preparing a cat for stereotaxic procedures increased the threshold for the jaw opening reflex induced by tooth pulp stimulation. The mechanism of this trauma-induced depression of responses to noxious stimulation is unknown. However, Clarke (1985) showed that this segmental analgesic effect was not affected by ablation of any of the structures mediating DNIC. Furthermore it is not reversed by opioid or 5-HT antagonists.

Clinical experience in humans shows that the insertion of a needle into a region of low mechanical threshold tends to reset the threshold to more normal values, and produces lasting pain relief. This unexpected phenomenon has been investigated in formal studies. Frost, Jessen & Siggaard-Andersen (1980), for example, compared pain relief caused by injection into tender regions in two groups of patients. Group 1 had normal saline injections; group 2 had 0.5% mepivacaine (a local anaesthetic) injection. These injections were administered in double-blind fashion in focal regions of tenderness (myofascial trigger points) on three occasions 2 or 3 days apart and the final assessment was made 1 week after the third injection. The results showed no significant difference between con-siderable or complete relief obtained in the two groups (44% in the saline group; 43% in the mepivacaine group). The authors concluded:

A similar result might perhaps be achieved by merely inserting the needle at the site of pain . . . There is much to suggest that injection therapy of myofascial pain is one form of acupuncture.

In a randomized, double-blind study, Garvey, Marks & Wiesel (1989) found no significant difference between the improvement rate with acupuncture (63%) and the 42% improvement produced by injections of medication (lidocaine or lidocaine-containing steroid) in the management of low back pain.

Macdonald et al (1983) found a significantly superior result of segmental acupuncture versus placebo in a single-blind, randomized study; here the needles were inserted in painless fashion subcutaneously in tender regions found in patients suffering chronic back pain. In the placebo control group, surface electrodes connected to dummy electrical apparatus were attached to the tender regions. (The unsolved difficulties in finding suitable controls for double-blind trials of acupuncture have been reviewed by Macdonald (1989). Pomeranz (1989), Richardson & Vincent (1986) and Vincent & Richardson (1986).)

Little if anything is known about the underlying analgesic mechanisms of acupuncture's local or segmental effects. In this form of acupuncture, many practitioners employ a swift and virtually painless insertion of the needle so significant changes in the release of opioids are not to be expected. Its mechanism is likely to be in a different domain.

Treede at al (1992) have reviewed the factors that cause hyperalgesia. While a good deal is known about both primary and secondary hyperalgesia caused by noxious thermal stimulation (Coderre & Melzack 1991), on the whole less is known about the effects of noxious mechanical stimulation. Yet this is the main clinical feature of so many chronic pathological pains of somatic origin, if mechanical injury is believed to be the cause.

Nevertheless Treede at al (1992), Woolf & King (1990) and Woolf (1991) favour the idea that mechanical hyperalgesia is predominantly central in origin. Following injury, central pain-signalling neurons, usually of the convergent or multireceptive type, become more sensitive to innocuous mechanical pressure. Furthermore, their receptive fields increase (Laird & Cervero 1989). These changes suggest an 'unmasking' (or summation) of convergent afferent inputs that had been relatively ineffective in inducing action potentials in central pain-signalling neurons before injury (Hu et al 1992).

How does a local needle insertion affect tenderness?

As there is still a great deal to be known about the actual mechanisms involved in changing the receptive fields of dorsal horn neurons, one may conjecture that the 'unmasking' that occurs when receptive fields of convergent neurons have increased as a result of sensitization is in effect a removal of a pre-existing inhibition. Furthermore, one may postulate that what has been removed is a part of the afferent or surround inhibition, which in the normal state tends to reduce receptive fields. In the normal state, such inhibitory mechanisms are required to locate the source of external stimuli. In that sense, when afferent inhibition has been reduced in the face of pain, a form of disinhibition presents.

Also we know that in pathological pain the sensitivities of various groups of receptors can become dissociated. Raja, Campbell & Meyer (1984) found that a noxious heat stimulus decreases heat thresholds in the injured region only, while it reduces mechanical thresholds both locally and in surrounding areas. Thus, in the regions surrounding the burn, there is a dissociation between heat thresholds, which are still normal, and the mechanical thresholds, which have become reduced.

It is difficult to imagine a more highly localized stimulus than that caused by needle insertion. Is it possible that such a localized stimulus calls into play afferent inhibitory mechanisms that tend to limit convergence? If so, such action would reduce mechanical disinhibition in a

beneficial manner. Another feature is that the very nature of the stimulus caused by a needle insertion is likely to activate a different group of mechanoreceptors from those whose abnormally low thresholds are associated with tenderness.

The dissociated sensitivity of mechanoreceptors of various kinds in the tender region may be an important factor in this story; for example, it is paradoxical that a patient with an abnormally tender somatic region has a low mechanical threshold, yet in the same region displays an increased threshold to cutaneous thermal and needleprick stimulation. (Sensitivity to needleprick may be conveniently measured with weighted needles, as described by Chan et al (1992).) These patients hardly feel an acupuncture needle, when it is inserted swiftly into a tender region. In effect, in such a mechanically tender region, patients find it difficult to pay attention to or localize the punctate stimulus of a needle.

It seems also to be a paradox that, as their pain conditions begin to resolve, patients begin to complain of more discomfort when needles are inserted. A possible explanation for this phenomenon of increasing awareness of the insertion of a needle is that, as the painful condition improves, disinhibition has started to be lifted and the normal afferent or surround inhibition has begun to return.

Exploring these observations in a formal manner may be the basis of rewarding clinical studies in the future.

Treatment

The first treatment

Segmental acupuncture should be performed with a gentle technique. Palpation is used to reveal the location and size of tender regions. Here, a needle is inserted into each region swiftly with the minimum twisting in an almost painless manner that can scarcely be felt. (Note that if a large tender area is to be treated then multiple needles may be necessary.) No further stimulation is required, and the needle is removed after a few minutes. This is sufficient to produce a localized vasodilatation (Rayman et al 1986) that lasts for several days.

Often palpation reveals the fact that much of the tenderness has resolved immediately after removal of the needle. However, the patient may not experience pain relief for a few hours; often the onset of relief is delayed by 10–48 hours.

Patients should be warned that if the needling is performed in too vigorous a manner then a dramatic worsening of the pain may occur. This flare-up or increase in pain occurs occasionally during the treatment itself, but is more usually delayed by some 10–48 hours. It may last 1–4 days. However, a flare-up may be relieved within a few minutes by reinserting the needle into the tender region for a second or so. This is altogether a puzzling phenomenon, which might itself eventually provide us with further clues about acupuncture's mechanisms.

A course of treatment

Although the first treatment produces a duration of relief that may last but a few hours, on average the second visit will produce 24 hours' relief, while the third produces 48 hours, etc. A chronic condition usually demands five to seven treatments, given at weekly or 2-weekly intervals, to achieve a sustained result of 60% or more pain relief for 6 months or more (Lu & Needham 1980).

The number of treatments required tends to vary with the duration of the illness: an acute condition may need only one treatment, while a subacute requires two to three, and a chronic condition often requires five to seven or even more treatments. If a patient's condition has not begun to regress in the manner described above by the third treatment, then acupuncture therapy should be abandoned in favour of another approach.

Indications and contraindications

In order to be sure one is obtaining significantly better results than placebo, the above figures should remain the goal of every practitioner. If a

practitioner fails to obtain them in 60% or more of his patients (i.e. a significantly greater proportion than the placebo classically provides), perhaps he should question the selection criteria, or take further instruction!

One may apply this thinking when comparing the results obtained in different categories of painful conditions: very severe pain requiring surgery often does not respond. Some forms of neurogenic pain such as postherpetic neuralgia do not often respond well to acupuncture. Certainly there is no place for acupuncture in psychogenic pain; on the contrary, it is a positive contraindication. Emotional disorders and anxiety about matters that are not related to the illness often mitigate against the effects of acupuncture. These patients often develop bizarre side-effects. Those patients who not only subconsciously find physical pain a welcome distraction from their emotional troubles, but also have defeated many a good practitioner before they see you, may either benefit not at all, or have flare-ups on every occasion. Do not persist with these patients without counselling first.

The Chinese were congratulated by Lu & Needham (1980) as being the first to be aware of referred visceral pain and its production of somatic tenderness: 'There can be no question that traditional Chinese medicine deeply appreciated the complex viscero-cutaneous relationships ... Surely the ancient Chinese discovery of such relationships was as brilliant as anything we owe to Hippocratic medicine or Alexandrian physiology.' Gu (1992) noted that, within 30 minutes, electroacupuncture relieves acute visceral pain in 89% of 245 cases of acute abdomen. His diagnoses included such conditions as dysmenorrhoea, appendicitis, and biliary and renal colic. Those who have not seen acupuncture in action will be sceptical about such a report but, if even a fraction of this claim is true, one should be wary of employing acupuncture in the absence of appropriate investigations designed to exclude acute emergencies that require immediate orthodox surgical or medical intervention. Another visceral effect attributed to this form of stimulation is the fear that acupuncture may induce premature labour, so pregnancy forms another relative contra-indication that has to be carefully considered.

The ideal patient has little evidence of emotional disorder and has tenderness arising in somatic (rather than visceral) tissues that has persisted after injury. Provided that there is no ongoing physiological pain caused by inflammation from active rheumatic disease or mechanical input that requires surgery (as one finds in advanced degenerative mechanical spinal conditions or in osteoarthritis of the weight-bearing joints such as the hip or knee) a good long-term result may be expected following a course of treatment.

If in pain relief clinics, where difficult problems present in both emotional and physical terms, acupuncture provides relief in no more than 40% of patients, it may be asked should one continue with this method? The only way to answer this is to compare the results from acupuncture with those obtained by the other pain-relieving techniques, many of which carry greater risk of sequelae.

Nevertheless in pain relief clinics, these low success rates present us with a challenge to see if we can learn from acupuncture and perhaps devise some other equally safe method that is more successful, or find a way of augmenting or improving acupuncture's success when dealing with very intractable painful conditions.

IS THERE A WAY FORWARD?

We need to reassess this ancient medical method in the light of our hard-won knowledge of today. Yet the way forward in the clinical setting will not be easy.

We have seen how acupuncture has both non-segmental and segmental effects. This phenomenon may explain the difficulties encountered by practitioners trying to investigate the topology of analgesic effects caused by needling a particular site. Until these two effects can be separated one from the other, it is hard to see how best to pursue this particular form of enquiry.

Furthermore, one only has to look at modern charts to realize there is hardly a site on the body that is not an acupuncture point. Figure 7.2 is a sample of the 386 extra points (not lying in

the path of a meridian) added by the Shanghai College of Traditional Medicine (1981) to the 361 'classical points' that are distributed over the course of the meridians. This impasse gives us the freedom to break away from the rigours of attempting to learn the location of every point, and concentrate our minds on seeking the sites of tender regions that are unique to each patient.

Yet, when one looks at the modern drawings of trigger points, almost all of which also appear in ancient Chinese charts, and at the distribution of their referred areas of pain (carefully observed by Travell & Simons 1983, 1992), one can not help noting how many of these referred pain patterns resemble portions of meridians, running in a linear fashion and boldly crossing segmental boundaries. Fig. 7.3A,B gives an example of this.

So the meridian (or channel) concept in acupuncture was a scholarly way of reminding the student of important features of pain and its relief. Meridians were thought to flow in certain directions, as pain is so often referred (albeit in a diffuse and imprecise manner) for varying distances along their paths. Thus learning the route of the meridians had a practical use. By this means the ancients, who had no knowledge of the nervous system, were readily encouraged to look for needle sites that are local to the tender region, even when they are anatomically placed at some distance from the referred area of pain. Meanwhile the idea that the entire length of a meridian connects the upper thorax or head region to the hand or foot may have been intended to be no more than a reminder of the long-range, non-segmental analgesic effects of vigorous needling.

These apparently contradictory, yet intertwined and often ill-understood, strands that form the substrate of acupuncture may explain many of the present, almost insuperable difficulties in obtaining meaningful and verifiable clinical data. Yet this fascinating subject that is so old still finds itself at the sharp end of pain research. Well may the sages say in their paean of praise to the properties of the needle:

Although one and a half inches long it embraces a doctrine of Mystery. Though its shaft be as fine as a single hair it may penetrate the many pathways as one.

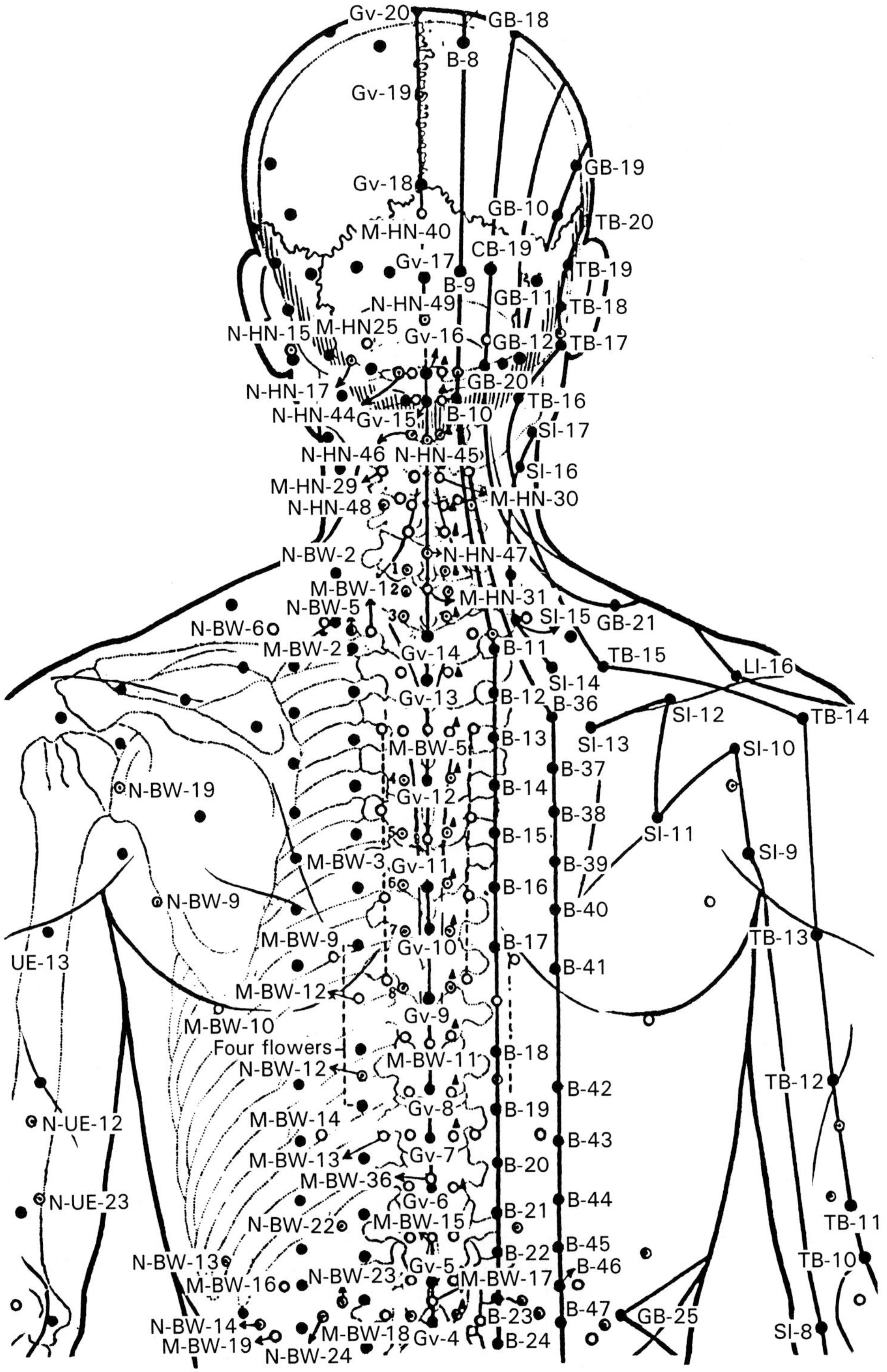

Figure 7.2 Old (●) and new (○ or ◉) acupuncture points in the back and neck region. (From Shanghai College of Traditional Medicine 1981.) Abbreviations for non-meridian points: N, new point; M, miscellaneous point; UE, upper extremity; HN, head and neck; BW, back. See Appendix 3 (p 439) for an explanation of abbreviations for meridian points.

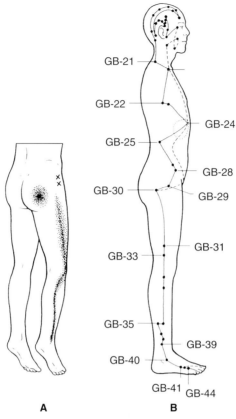

Figure 7.3   The referred areas of pain arising from trigger points (marked by X's) in the gluteus minimus (A) (noted by Travell & Simons 1992) appear to traverse the lower part of the 'gall bladder' meridian (B). (After Zhang et al 1986.)

REFERENCES

Baldry P E 1993 Acupuncture, trigger points and musculoskeletal pain 2nd edn. Churchill Livingstone, Edinburgh

Bertschinger R 1991 The golden needle. Churchill Livingstone, New York

Bing Z, Cesselin F, Bourgoin S, Clot A M, Hamon M, Le Bars D 1991 Acupuncture-like stimulation induces a heterosegmental release of Met-enkephalin-like material in the rat spinal cord. Pain 47:71–77

Bing Z, Villanueva L, Le Bars D 1989 Effects of systemic morphine upon Aδ- and C-fibre evoked activities of subnucleus reticularis dorsalis (SRD) neurones in the rat medulla. European Journal of Pharmacology 164:85–92

Bing Z, Villanueva L, Le Bars D 1990 Acupuncture and diffuse noxious inhibitory controls: naloxone reversible depression of activities of trigeminal convergent neurones. Neuroscience 37:809–818

Bing Z Villanueva L, Le Bars D 1991 Acupuncture-evoked responses of subnucleus reticularis dorsalis neurons in the rat medulla. Neuroscience 44:693–703

Bourgoin S, Le Bars D, Clot A M, Hamon M, Cesselin F 1990 Subcutaneous formalin induces a segmental release of Met-enkephalin-like material from the rat spinal cord. Pain 41:323–329

Bowsher D 1975 Characteristics of central non-specific somatosensory systems. In: Kornhuber A H (ed) Somatosensory systems. Thieme, Stuttgart, pp 68–77

Bowsher D 1976 Role of the reticular formation in responses to noxious stimulation. Pain 2: 361–378

Bowsher D, Mallart A, Petit D, Albe-Fessard D 1968 A bulbar relay to the centre median. Journal of Neurophysiology 31:288–300

Cesselin F, Bourgoin S, Clot A M, Hamon M, Le Bars D 1989 Segmental release of met-enkephalin-like material from the spinal cord of rats, elicited by noxious thermal stimuli. Brain Research 484:71–77

Chan A W, MacFarlane I A, Bowsher D, Campbell J A 1992 Weighted needle pinprick sensory thresholds: a simple test of sensory function in diabetic peripheral neuropathy. Journal of Neurology, Neurosurgery and Psychiatry 55:56–59

Chang H-T 1978 Neurophysiological basis of acupuncture analgesia. Scientia Sinica (Engl transl) 21:829–846

Cheng R S S 1989 Neurophysiology of electroacupuncture analgesia. In: Pomeranz B, Stux G (eds) Scientific bases of acupuncture. Springer-Verlag, Berlin, pp 119–136

Cheng R S S, Pomeranz B 1979 Electroacupuncture analgesia could be mediated by at least two pain-relieving mechanisms: endorphin and non-endorphin systems. Life Sciences 25:1957–1962

Chiang C Y, Tu H X, Chao Y F, Pai Y H, Ku H K, Cheng J K, Shang H Y, Yang F Y 1979 Effect of electrolytic or intracerebral injections of 5,6 dihydroxytryptamine in raphe nuclei on acupuncture analgesia in rats. Chinese Medical Journal 92:129–136

Chung J M, Lee K H, Hori Y, Endo K, Willis W D 1984 Factors influencing peripheral nerve stimulation produced inhibition of primate spinothalamic tract cells. Pain 19:277–293

Clarke R W 1985 The effects of decerebration and destruction of nucleus raphe magnus, periaqueductal grey matter and brainstem lateral reticular formation on the depression due to surgical trauma of the jaw-opening reflex evoked by tooth-pulp stimulation. Brain Research 332:231–236

Clarke R W, Matthews B 1990 The thresholds of the jaw-opening reflex and trigeminal brainstem neurons to tooth-pulp stimulation in acutely and chronically prepared cats. Neuroscience 36:105–114

Coderre T J, Melzack R 1991 Central neural mediators of secondary hyperalgesia following heat injury in rats: neuropeptides and excitatory amino acids. Neuroscience Letters 131:71–74

Duchenne G B A 1849 A critical examination of instruments. Comptes Rendus de l'Académie des Sciences

Dung H C 1984 Characterization of the three functional phases of acupuncture points. Chinese Medical Journal (Engl transl) 97:751–754

Fei H, Xie G X, Han J S 1987 Low and high frequency electroacupuncture stimulation release met 5-enkephalin and dynorphin A and B in rat spinal cord. Chinese Science Bulletin 32:1496–1501

Frost F A, Jessen B, Siggaard-Andersen J 1980 A controlled, double-blind comparison of mepivacaine injection versus saline injection for myofascial pain. Lancet i:499–500

Garvey T A, Marks M R, Wiesel S W 1989 A prospective, randomized, double-blind evaluation of trigger-point injection therapy for low back pain. Spine 14:962–964

Gu Y 1992 Treatment of acute abdomen by electroacupuncture—a report of 245 cases. Journal of Traditional Chinese Medicine 12:110–113

Han C-S, Chou P-H, Lu C-C, Lu L-H, Yang T-H, Jen M-F 1979 The role of central 5-hydroxytryptamine in acupuncture analgesia. Scientia Sinica (Engl transl) 22:91–104

Han J S 1984 Antibody microinjection technique as a tool to clarify the role of opioid peptides in acupuncture analgesia. Pain (suppl 2): 667

Han J S 1986a Electroacupuncture: an alternative to antidepressants for treating affective diseases? International Journal of Neuroscience 29:79–92

Han J S 1986b Physiologic and neurochemical basis of acupuncture analgesia. In: Cheng T O (ed) The

international textbook of cardiology. Pergamon, New York, pp 1124–1132

Han J S 1989 Central neurotransmitters and acupuncture analgesia. In: Pomeranz B, Stux G (eds) Scientific bases of acupuncture. Springer-Verlag, Berlin, pp 7–26

Han J S, Xie G X, Ding Z X, Fan S G 1984a High and low frequency electroacupuncture analgesia are mediated by different peptides. Pain (suppl 2):543

Han J S, Xie C 1984b Dynorphin: potent analgesic effect in spinal cord of the rat. Scientia Sinica (series B, Engl transl) 27:169–177

Han J S, Xie G X, Zhou Z F, Folkesson R, Terenius L 1984c Acupuncture mechanisms in rabbits studied with microinjection of antibodies against β-endorphin, enkephalin and substance P. Neuropharmacology 23:1–5

Han J S, Ding Z X, Fan S G 1986 The frequency as the cardinal determinant for electroacupuncture analgesia to be reversed by opioid antagonists. Acta Physiologica Sinica 38:475–482

Han J S, Chen X H, Sun S L, Xu X J, Yuan Y, Yan S C, Hao J X, Terenius L 1991 Effect of low- and high-frequency TENS on Met-enkephalin-Arg-Phe and dynorphin A immunoreactivity in human lumbar CSF. Pain 47:295–298

Hockaday J M, Whitty C W M 1967 Patterns of referred pain in the normal subject. Brain 90:481–496

Hu J W, Sessle B J, Raboisson P, Dallel R, Woda A 1992 Stimulation of craniofacial muscle afferents induces prolonged facilitatory effects in trigeminal nociceptive brain-stem neurones. Pain 48:53–60

Inman V T, Saunders J B de C 1944 Referred pain from skeletal structures. Journal of Nervous and Mental Disease 99:660–667

Kawakita K, Miura T, Iwase Y 1991 Deep pain measurement at tender points by pulse algometry with insulated needle electrodes. Pain 44:235–239

Kellgren J H 1938 Observations on referred pain arising from muscle. Clinical Science 3:175–190

Kellgren J H 1939a Some painful joint conditions and their relation to osteoarthritis. Clinical Science 4:193–201

Kellgren J H 1939b On distribution of pain arising from deep somatic structures with charts of segmental pain areas. Clinical Science 4:35–46

Kellgren J H 1977 The anatomical source of back pain. Rheumatology and Rehabilitation 16:3–12

Kellgren J H 1978 Pain. In: Scott J T (ed) Copeman's textbook of rheumatic diseases. Churchill Livingstone, New York, pp 62–67

Kraft G H, Johnson E W, La Ban M M 1968 The fibrositis syndrome. Archives of Physical Medicine and Rehabilitation 49:155–162

Laird J M, Cervero F 1989 A comparative study of the changes in receptive-field properties of multireceptive and noireceptive rat dorsal horn neurons following noxious mechanical stimulation. Journal of Neurophysiology 62:854–863

Lange M 1931 Die Muskelharten (Myogelosen). J F Lehmann's Verlag, München

Le Bars D, Dickenson A H, Besson J-M 1979a Diffuse noxious inhibitory controls (DNIC). I. Effects on dorsal horn convergent neurones in the rat. Pain 6:283–304

Le Bars D, Dickenson A H, Besson J-M 1979b Diffuse noxious inhibitory controls (DNIC). II. Lack of effect on non-convergent neurones, supraspinal involvement and theoretical implications. Pain 6:305–327

Le Bars D, Calvino B, Villanueva L, Cadden S 1984 Physiological approaches to counter-irritation phenomena. In: Tricklebank M D, Curzon G (eds) Stress induced analgesia. John Wiley, New York, pp 67–101

Le Bars D, Bourgoin S, Clot A M, Hamon M, Cesselin F 1987 Noxious mechanical stimuli increase the release of Met-enkephalin-like material heterosegmentally in the rat spinal cord. Brain Research 402:188–192

Le Bars D, Willer J C, de Broucker T, Villanueva L 1989 Neurophysiological mechanisms involved in the pain-relieving effects of counterirritation and related techniques including acupuncture. In: Pomeranz B, Stux G (eds) Scientific bases of acupuncture. Springer-Verlag, Berlin, pp 79–112

Le Bars D, Villanueva L, Willer J C, Bouhassira D 1991 Diffuse Noxious Inhibitory Controls (DNIC) in animals and in man. Acupuncture in Medicine 9:47–56

Le Bars D, Willer J-C, de Broucker T 1992 Morphine blocks descending pain inhibitory controls in humans. Pain 48:13–20

Lee K H, Chung J M, Willis W D 1985 Inhibition of primate spinothalamic tract cells by TENS. Journal of Neurosurgery 62:276–287

Lee Y-H, Lee W-C, Chen M-T, Huang J-K, Chung C, Chang L S 1992 Acupuncture in the treatment of renal colic. Journal of Urology 147:16–18

Light S 1967 History of electrotherapy. In: Light S (ed) Therapeutic electricity and ultraviolet radiation. Elizabeth Light, New Haven, pp 1–70

Lu G-D, Needham J 1980 Celestial lancets: a history and rationale of acupuncture and moxa. Cambridge University Press, Cambridge

Lund C, Hansen O B, Kehlet H 1990 Effect of surgery on sensory threshold and somatosensory evoked potentials after skin stimulation. British Journal of Anaesthesia 65:173–176

Macdonald A J R 1980 Abnormally tender muscle regions and associated painful movements. Pain 8:197–205

Macdonald A J R 1989 Acupuncture analgesia and therapy. In: Wall P D, Melzack R (eds) The textbook of pain, 2nd edn. Churchill Livingstone, Edinburgh, pp 906–919

Macdonald A J R, MacRae K D, Master B R, Rubin A P 1983 Superficial acupuncture in the relief of low back pain: a placebo-controlled randomised trial. Annals of the Royal College of Surgeons of England 65:44–46

Mann F 1977 Scientific aspects of acupuncture. William Heinemann, London, pp 63–73

Mann 1992 Reinventing acupuncture. Butterworth Heinemann, Oxford

Melzack R, Stillwell D M, Fox E J 1977 Trigger points and acupuncture points for pain correlations and implications. Pain 3:3–23

Mense S, Skeppar P 1991 Discharge behaviour of feline gamma-motoneurones following induction of an artificial myositis. Pain 46:201–210

Omura Y 1975 Electro-acupuncture: its electrophysiological basis and criteria for effectiveness and safety—Part 1. Acupuncture and Electrotherapeutics Research 1:157–181

Pomeranz B 1989 Acupuncture analgesia for chronic pain: brief survey of clinical trials. In: Pomeranz B, Stux G (eds) Scientific bases of acupuncture. Springer-Verlag, Berlin, pp 197–199

Raja S N, Campbell J N, Meyer R A 1984 Evidence for different mechanisms of primary and secondary hyperalgesia following heat injury to the glabrous skin. Brain 107:1179–1188

Rayman G, Williams S A, Spencer P D, Smaje L H, Wise P H, Tooke J E 1986 Impaired microvascular hyperaemic response to minor skin trauma in type 1 diabetes. British Medical Journal 292:1295–1298

Reynolds M D 1983 The development of the concept of fibrositis. Journal of the History of Medicine and Allied Sciences 38:5–35

Richardson P H, Vincent C A 1986 Acupuncture for the treatment of pain: a review of evaluative research. Pain 24:15–40

Salandière 1825 Mémoires sur l'electropuncture considérée comme moyen nouveau de traiter efficacement la goutte, les rhumatismes et les affections nerveuses. Paris

Shanghai College of Traditional Medicine 1981 Acupuncture a comprehensive text. Eastland, Chicago

Shen E, Ts'ai T, Lan C 1975 Supraspinal participation in the inhibitory effect of acupuncture on viscero-somatic reflex discharges. Chinese Medical Journal (Engl transl) 1:431–440

Sjölund B H, Terenius L, Eriksson M B E 1977 Increased cerebrospinal fluid levels of endorphins after electroacupuncture. Acta Physiologica Scandinavica 100:382–384

Sola A E, Williams R L 1956 Myofascial pain syndromes. Neurology 6:91–95

Torebjörk H E, Ochoa J L, Schady W 1984 Referred pain from intra-neural stimulation of muscle fascicles in the median nerve. Pain 18:145–156

Travell J G, Simons D G 1983 Myofascial pain and dysfunction: the trigger point manual, vol 1. Williams and Wilkins, Baltimore

Travell J G, Simons D G 1992 Myofascial pain and dysfunction: the trigger point manual. Vol 2, the lower extremities. Williams and Wilkins, Baltimore

Treede R-D, Meyer R A, Raja S N, Campbell J N 1992 Peripheral and central mechanisms of cutaneous hyperalgesia. Progress in Neurobiology 38:397–421

Vincent C A, Richardson P H 1986 The evaluation of therapeutic acupuncture: concepts and methods. Pain 24:1–13

Wang X 1986 Research on the origin and development of Chinese acupuncture and moxibustion. In: Zhang X (Chang H-T) (ed) Research on acupuncture, moxibustion and acupuncture anesthesia. Science Press, Beijing, pp 783–799

White D M, Levine J 1991 Different mechanical transduction mechanisms for the immediate and delayed responses of rat C-fiber nociceptors. Journal of Neurophysiology 66:363–368

Willer J-C 1977 Comparative study of perceived pain and nociceptive flexion reflex in man. Pain 3:69–80

Willer J-C, Barranquero A, Kahn M-F, Sallière D 1987 Pain in sciatica depresses lower limb nociceptive reflexes to sural nerve stimulation. Journal of Neurology Neurosurgery, and Psychiatry 50:1–5

Woolf C J 1991 Generation of acute pain: central mechanisms. British Medical Bulletin 47:523–533

Woolf C J, King A E 1990 Dynamic alterations in the cutaneous mechanoreceptor fields of dorsal horn neurons in the rat spinal cord. Journal of Neuroscience 10:2717–2726

World Health Organization 1984 Standard acupuncture nomenclature (ed Wang D). World Health Organization Regional Office for the Western Pacific, Manila

Xie C W, Tang J, Han J S 1981 Central norepinephrine in acupuncture analgesia. Differential effects in brain and spinal cord. In: Takagi H, Simon E J (eds) Advances in Endogenous and Exogenous Opioids. Kodansha, Tokyo, pp 288–290.

Xie G X, Zhou Z F, Han J S 1981 Electroacupuncture analgesia in the rabbit was partially blocked by anti-β-endorphin antiserum injected into periaqueductal gray, but not its intrathecal injection. Acupuncture Research (Engl abstr) 6:278–280

Zhang R-F, Wu X-F, Wang N S 1985 Illustrated dictionary of Chinese acupuncture. Sheep's publications. Hong Kong, and People's Medical Publishing House, China

8

Segmental acupuncture

Rob Bekkering
Robert van Bussel

INTRODUCTION

As many symptoms and acupuncture effects can often be explained in a neurophysiological way on the basis of segmental innervation, this chapter will deal with the neuroanatomy and the neurophysiology of the segments, with segmental relations, symptoms and diagnosis focused around segmental acupuncture therapy.

Formerly obscure relations between symptoms, which are usually overlooked, can often be explained via segmental interactions. Furthermore, a segmental diagnosis can be a great help in finding perpetuating factors, which can maintain existing pathology, and without a correct understanding of segmental interactions it is difficult to understand why a disease will persist after 'correct' treatment.

MacKenzie, in 1917, described three sorts of symptoms:

- **structural symptoms**: changes that are visible and/or palpable, e.g. scar tissue, fractures or stomach ulcers
- **functional symptoms**: symptoms that are alterations in functions, e.g. hypertonic muscles, active trigger points, palpitations, dyspnoea and irritable bowel
- **segmental symptoms**: symptoms that are the result of pathology in one of the parts of a segment (dermatome, myotome, sclerotome or viscerotome), affecting the other parts of the segment, e.g. referred pain, hyperalgesia, trigger points, hypertonic muscles and vasomotor changes

Segmental therapies should, in our opinion, be used mainly in treating functional and segmental symptoms, and in the modulation of pain and the symptomatic treatment of structural symptoms. This chapter clarifies how to build up a correct segmental diagnosis, and how to decide which one of the segmental therapies will offer the best therapeutic option for a particular disease or patient.

SEGMENTAL NEUROANATOMY AND NEUROPHYSIOLOGY

The segments

A segment consists of a dermatome, a myotome, a sclerotome and a viscerotome. All these parts are inter-connected via the same shared innervation, and via this innervation every part of a segment is able to influence any other part of the same segment.

In this way, for instance, visceral pathology (viscerotome) can manifest itself in the skin (dermatome) (Figs 8.1, 8.2), in the muscles (myotome) and in the joints (sclerotome) (Figs 8.3, 8.4) via viscerocutaneous and visceromotor reflexes. Conversely, stimulation of the skin or muscle can influence internal organs with the same segmental innervation via cutaneovisceral and musculovisceral reflexes, which is the basic principle of segmental therapies like acupuncture.

Because of their migration during embryonic development, different parts of the same seg-

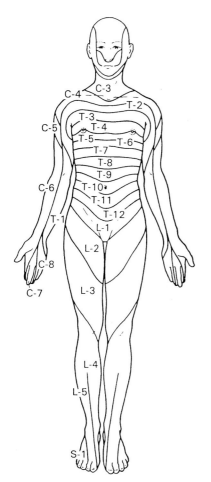

Figure 8.1   Dermatomes (anterior view). (After Hansen & Schliack 1962.)

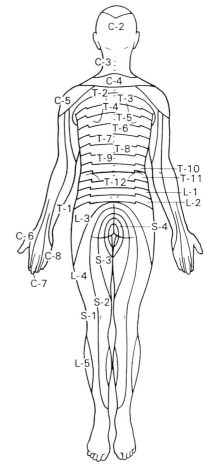

Figure 8.2   Dermatomes (posterior view). (After Hansen & Schliack 1962.)

ment do not always overlap one another neatly. Although they are neuroanatomically connected, they can be situated anatomically far away from each other. Usually a dermatome is situated lower (more caudally) than the corresponding sclerotome, and usually the corresponding viscerotome is situated even lower (Fig. 8.5).

At present there is more or less common agreement on the outlines of the dermatomes, myotomes, sclerotomes and viscerotomes; however, depending on the method of examination, there will always be some variation. Different authors therefore draw different maps of the dermatomes: for example, Head studied referred hyperalgesia, and found dermatomes with a minimal overlap, while Sherrington and Foerster studied discriminative touch, and found zones with much less distinct borders, overlapping each other halfway (Hansen & Schliack 1962; (Figs 8.1 and 8.2).

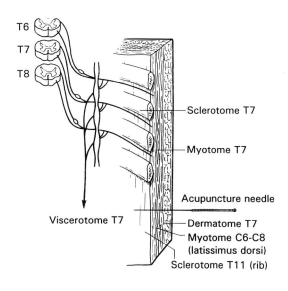

Figure 8.5 Topographical relations between the different parts of the segment T7. Depending on the depth, a stimulus will influence different segments.

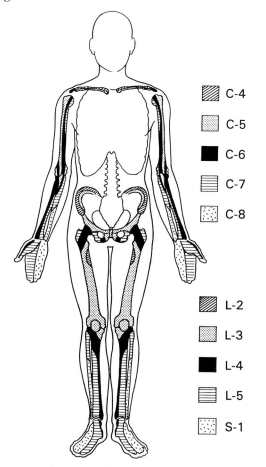

Figure 8.3 Sclerotomes (anterior view). (After Chusid 1982.)

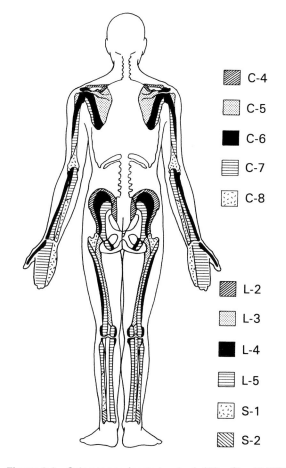

Figure 8.4 Sclerotomes (posterior view). (After Chusid 1982.)

Because the dermatome, myotome and sclerotome of a segment usually do not overlap each other, a stimulus given into a certain part of the body will frequently influence different segments, depending on the depth of the stimulus (see Fig. 8.5). Obviously this is of the utmost importance for the segmental therapies.

Anatomy and physiology of the segments

The sensory posterior horn is the first processing centre for afferent sensory information. From here the sensory information is conveyed in three main directions: via ascending fibres to the central nervous system and via intrasegmental fibres to the anterior and lateral horns of the spinal cord. Processing of afferent information in the posterior horn is constantly being modulated by intersegmental reflexes and by descending stimuli from the higher relay centres.

The anterior motor horn is responsible for the motor innervation of the striatal muscles. The autonomic lateral horn (intermediolateral nucleus) deserves special attention, because it plays an extremely important, but as yet poorly recognized, role in many segmental reactions.

The autonomic lateral horn forms the origin of the sympathetic innervation. From only a limited part of the spinal segments (C8–L2), the whole body is innervated by the sympathetic nervous system. Functionally we can divide the lateral horn into 3 columns (Table 8.1):

- the **medial column** consists of the cell bodies of preganglionic fibres to the internal organs
- the **middle column** consists of the cell bodies of preganglionic fibres to the trunk
- the **lateral column** consists of the cell bodies of preganglionic fibres to the head and extremities.

As we see, there is one column for the internal organs, one for the trunk and another separate column for the head and extremities. This last column needs some further explanation. The autonomic innervation of the head is derived from C8–T4, the upper extremities from T5–T9, and the lower extremities from T10–L2 (Bennet

Table 8.1 Schematic representation of the neuroanatomical relations between the various parts of a segment

Posterior horn	Anterior horn	Lateral horn Medial	Middle	Lateral
—	C1	—	—	–
C2–C7	C2–C7	—	—	–
C8–T2	C8–T2	C8–T2	C8–T2	C1–C2
T2–T4	T2–T4	T2–T4	T2–T4	C3–C4
T5–T6	T5–T6	T5–T6	T5–T6	C5–C6
T7–T9	T7–T9	T7–T9	T7–T9	C7–C8
T10–T11	T10–T11	T10–T11	T10–T11	L3–L4
T12–L2	T12–L2	T12–L2	T12–L2	L5–S2
L2–L5	L2–L5	—	—	–
S1–S5	S1–S5	—	—	–

et al 1986, Carpenter 1985, Dicke & Schliack 1982, Janig 1990, Kunert 1963, Monnier 1968, Oldfield and McLachlan 1980, Oostendorp 1988, Robertson 1987, Rohen 1985). The efferent fibres from this lateral column ascend or descend inside the sympathetic chain to the segments of their destination.

Secondary segmental relations

The vast amount of empirical evidence and the large number of interneurons clearly indicate a mutual influential effect between these three columns of the autonomic lateral horn. Many authors mention these 'secondary relations', and it can clarify matters to put these columns and the secondary relations next to each other as in Table 8.1. (The right-hand columns of the table show the origin of the secondary relations.)

For a correct segmental diagnosis and therapy, one should understand both the possible segmental and the secondary relations and interactions. In acupuncture 'distant points' on the distal parts of the extremities are often used to influence problems of the trunk or viscera. The close relationship between the three lateral horn columns in Table 8.1 is helpful in trying to explain their effectiveness.

Large and small afferent nervous fibres

In order to explain segmental symptoms and predict the effect of the various segmental

Table 8.2 Classification of nerve fibres

Classification	Function
The large nerve fibres:	
Aα (Ia)	Position proprioception
Aα (Ib)	Position proprioception
Aβ (II)	Fine, discriminative touch
Aδ (IIIa) (low threshold)	Touch and pressure
The small nerve fibres:	
Aδ (IIIb) (high threshold)	Acute, sharp, well localizable, primary pain
C (IV)	Chronic, dull, secondary pain and temperature perception

therapies, one also has to understand the physiology of nerve fibres. Because there are two classifications in use for the different fibres (Table 8.2), we shall detail both to prevent confusion.

In the various segmental therapies (like acupuncture, physiotherapy, transcutaneous electrical nerve stimulation (TENS) and manual therapy) the characteristic differences in function between large and small fibres can be utilized. For each one of the segmental therapies it can be determined whether one needs to stimulate the large or the small fibres in order to obtain a particular segmental effect. In general, the aim is to try to stimulate the large fibres selectively, because this inhibits the effects of the small fibres, and therefore, as we shall see, suppresses segmental effects like pain, hypertonic muscles and autonomic disturbances. The large fibres are more sensitive to pressure, while the small fibres are more sensitive to local anaesthesia and temperature.

STIMULATION OF NERVE FIBRES

With these basic neurophysiological facts in mind, it is possible to work out how to stimulate selectively a specific group of nerve fibres (Howson 1978, Li & Bak 1976, Lullies & Trincker 1973, Sato & Schmidt 1973). There are a number of ways of doing this, including pressure, muscle stretching, dry and wet needling, and electrical stimulation.

Pressure

On applying mild pressure, at first only the large Aβ (II) and Aδ (IIIa) fibres are stimulated (paraesthesia). However, with greater pressure applied for a longer time, these large fibres become blocked (giving a numb feeling) and the small Aδ (IIIb) fibres are stimulated (felt as acute, sharp pain). Still later, most of these small fibres cease to respond, and only the small C (IV) fibres will be stimulated (felt as secondary dull pain).

Muscle stretching

This technique is one of the main pillars in the treatment of myofascial trigger points. The stretching of a muscle will mainly stimulate muscle spindles, Golgi tendon organs and the large fibres.

Manual acupuncture ('dry needling')

Mild acupuncture needling will stimulate only the large fibres and will result in a needling sensation (De Qi, see Ch 3) while more painful needling will predominantly stimulate the small fibres. Gentle twisting of the needle will 'wrap' the muscle fibres round the needle, stretching them and thus also stimulating large nerve fibres.

In accordance with the reports of Stux & Pomeranz (1986) and many others, the 'numb' aspect of the needling sensation can be generated by stimulating the large afferent fibres from group Aβ (II) and the heavy feeling can be provoked by stimulating large afferent, low threshold fibres from group Aδ (IIIa), (see also Ch 6).

Injections ('wet needling')

Local anaesthetics at a low concentration (e.g. lignocaine 0.25%) will selectively block small fibres, while higher concentrations will also block the larger Aδ (IIIb and IIIa) fibres. Injections with normal saline (or any other liquid) in a myofascial trigger point will stretch the individual muscle fibres, stimulating the muscle spindles and thus the large nerve fibres.

Electrical stimulation

Electrical stimulation via an acupuncture needle at low intensity (itching sensation) and high frequency (50–100 Hz) will mainly stimulate the large fibres, while high intensity (painful sensation) and low frequency (1–4 Hz) will mainly stimulate the small fibres (Howson 1978, Li & Bak 1976, Lullies & Trincker 1973, Sato & Schmidt 1973) (see Ch 10).

The frequencies used in TENS treatment (Ch 11) have a similar pattern of nerve fibre stimulation to those used in electrical stimulation via acupuncture needles.

THE DIAGNOSTIC AND THERAPEUTIC CONSEQUENCES OF INTERACTIONS BETWEEN THE SOMATIC AND SYMPATHETIC NERVOUS SYSTEMS

In some circumstances the somatoafferent fibres and the sympathetic (efferent) fibres can influence each other.

An increased and prolonged activation of small fibres from group C (IV) is one of the causes of increased sympathetic activity affecting especially vasoconstrictor nerve fibres. This growing sympathetic activity in its turn will sensitize the small afferent fibres in the same segment(s), causing them to react abnormally to mechanical, thermal and chemical stimuli (hyperalgesia and hyperaesthesia) (Janig 1990, Brooks 1983, Oostendorp 1988). This can be the onset of a vicious circle, and in time these longer-lasting abnormal reflexes can get 'fixed' in the spinal cord and brainstem (van Cranenburgh 1989a).

In a meticulous study, Sato & Schmidt (1973) showed that stimulation of somatoafferent fibres can clearly influence sympathetic fibres. They confirm the reports from many authors that selective stimulation of the larger somatoafferent fibres, especially Aβ (II) in the skin and Aδ (IIIa) in muscle, can inhibit an existing increased activity of sympathetic fibres in the same segment after a short initial excitation (Koizumi & Brooks 1984, Oostendorp 1988). It is

not surprising therefore that most of the segmental therapies use techniques that stimulate large fibres selectively; as we have seen, this will inhibit the effects of the small fibres, and thereby diminish pain and abnormal autonomic effects.

Central modulation of segmental interactions

Principally there are two major supraspinal relay centres for sensory information, where incoming information is processed and modulated: the reticular formation in the brainstem and the thalamus/hypothalamus (see also Ch 6).

Modulation by the reticular formation

The reticular formation forms a selective filter for information on touch, pain and temperature, as well as for visceral information. It can modulate ascending information, especially from the Aδ (IIIa) and small fibres, and can 'decide' which information to pass on to higher centres. Information on discriminative touch and proprioception bypasses the reticular formation.

Via the ascending reticular activating system (ARAS) the reticular formation determines the 'state of alert' or the 'non-specific arousal' of the nervous system and the given response to stimuli.

When the reticular formation is stimulated by ascending information from the Aδ (IIIa and IIIb) and C (IV) fibres, it can modulate segmental interactions in segments in the vicinity of the original segmental disturbance via the descending reticular activating system (DRAS) and the pain-modulating tracts.

Via the DRAS the reticular formation can activate the spinal cord non-specifically, determining the excitability of skeletal muscles ('predisposition' for hypertonic muscles and trigger points).

Pain-modulating tracts from the nucleus raphe magnus descend to the posterior horn, where they mainly inhibit the transmission of noxious information (Basbaum & Fields 1978, Gray & Dostrovsky 1983, Hu et al 1981). These pain-modulating fibres (which use the neuro-transmitter serotonin 5-HT) are most effectively activated by stimulation of small afferent Aδ (IIIb) fibres (Basbaum & Fields 1978, Bowsher 1983), and this pathway is often used in segmental therapy.

Modulation by the thalamus/ hypothalamus

The thalamus is the subcortical modulation centre for all sensory information to the cortex. *The phylogenetically older, medial parts* of the thalamus, like the nucleus parafascicularis, mainly modulate information from the small fibres (according to many authors these parts have some sort of a gate control mechanism), while *the younger, lateral parts* of the thalamus mainly modulate information from the large fibres. The production of β-endorphin in the hypothalamus, notably in the arcuate nucleus, can explain the effects of general acupuncture analgesia to a large extent, while the production of adrenocorticotrophic hormone (ACTH), which has an anti-inflammatory effect, can partially explain the effectiveness of acupuncture in patients with, for example, asthma or arthritis. As we shall see, we are able to induce these effects electrically by stimulating acupuncture needles at a high intensity and a frequency of 2–4 Hz (Han 1987).

Summary

Depending on the fibres and modulation centres involved, the stimulation of an acupuncture needle can have segmental, more or less segmental, or general effects.

Very generally speaking, one can say that:

1. *mild stimulation* of the large fibres will have mainly segmental effects via segmental interactions; among others via the production of dynorphin and via gate control
2. *moderate stimulation* of the large Aδ (IIIa), small Aδ (IIIb) and C (IV) fibres will give 'more or less segmental' effects via intersegmental interactions, but also via the DRAS and pain-modulating tracts from the reticular formation

3. *strong stimulation* will have more general effects (anti-inflammatory and analgesic) via the production of β-endorphin and enkephalin in the thalamus/hypothalamus (Han 1987, Stux & Pomeranz 1986).

SEGMENTAL SYMPTOMS

An increased, often nociceptive, activity in one part of a segment can affect all the other parts of the same segment, resulting in segmental symptoms like referred pain, hyperalgesia, hypertonic muscles, activated myofascial trigger points and autonomic symptoms such as vasomotor and trophic changes.

Pain in the left arm can sometimes be associated with cardiac pathology, a painful shoulder can be the result of cervical pathology and pain in the shoulders after a diagnostic laparoscopy can be the result of irritation of the diaphragm (referred pain from the phrenic nerve). As we shall see, all these symptoms can be explained by segmental interactions, and they can be of great diagnostic and therapeutic value.

Segmental symptoms can occur in any part of a disturbed segment (dermatome, myotome, sclerotome or viscerotome). The extent to which these segmental symptoms occur is dependent on:

- the duration and severity of the existing pathology
- the amount of central inhibition
- the state of general arousal
- the existence of other pathology in the same segment.

For instance, a long-lasting painful shoulder is more likely to give additional cervical complaints, especially when the person is overanxious for one reason or another. In that case he can have an increased sense of pain, owing to an insufficient central inhibition by his pain-modulating tracts from the nucleus raphe magnus. Because he is in a continual state of alert, his overactive DRAS will raise the excitability of his skeletal muscles, especially the trapezius, one of the stress muscles, which can become hypertonic.

Types of segmental symptoms

The following segmental symptoms can occur (Fig. 8.6):

1. **pain and hyperalgesia** (via the sensory posterior horn and the ascending tracts)
   a local pain
   b referred pain
   c local hyperalgesia
   d referred hyperalgesia
2. **hypertonic muscles** (via the motor anterior horn)
   a hypertonic muscles
   b the activation of trigger points
3. **autonomic symptoms** (via the autonomic lateral horn)
   a vasomotor effects
   b sudomotor effects
   c pilomotor effects
   d visceral effects

e sensitization of the small afferent nerve fibres (referred hyperalgesia).

These segmental symptoms will be discussed separately.

Pain and hyperalgesia

Local pain Pain caused by a nociceptive stimulus in the more superficial layers (skin and superficial muscles) can usually be localized and defined precisely. This pain is seldom referred. Pain in the deeper layers (deeper muscles) is more vague, and is often referred to the more superficial and distal parts of the body. Visceral pain is a diffuse dull and deep pain in the viscera, which is usually also referred to the more superficial parts of the body.

Referred pain This pain is caused by a nociceptive stimulus in a certain part of a segment, but it is projected to other parts of that

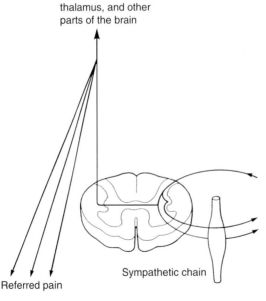

Reticular formation, thalamus, and other parts of the brain

Segmental disturbance
(in: dermatome
      myotome
      sclerotome or
      viscerotome

Segmental symptoms
• *sensory symptoms:*
  local pain
  local hyperalgesia
  referred hyperalgesia
• *motor symptoms:*
  hypertonic muscle
  trigger points
• *autonomic symptoms:*
  homolateral pupil
  dilatation
  vasoconstriction
  pilomotor effects
  sudomotor effects
  visceral effects

Referred pain

Sympathetic chain

Figure 8.6   Segmental symptoms.

same segment (Fig. 8.7). It is the result of the convergence of nociceptive fibres from different parts of a segment (dermatome, myotome, sclerotome or viscerotome) in the same sensory posterior horn.

In general, nociceptive information from a tissue or organ with a relatively low grade of innervation will be projected to those parts of the same segment that are innervated more densely. For this reason, pain usually radiates from the deeper layers to more superficial layers (dermatomes and myotomes) and from proximal to distal, depending on the existing state of alert in the different parts of the segment (locus minoris resistentiae).

Strange patterns of referred pain can result from the convergence of nociceptive information in the reticular formation or in the thalamus. In either case, the brain projects the pain to the most densely innervated parts: the most likely source. So referred pain is truly a misinterpretation of the brain.

Local hyperalgesia Oversensitivity to painful stimuli is caused by the sensitization of the small

afferent nerve fibres, while hyperaesthesia is caused by an increased sensitivity of the large afferent fibres. This sensitization can be the result of either local tissue damage (pain mediators), or segmental hyperactivity of the sympathetic fibres (see below), but also the higher relay centres play an important modulating role (via the ARAS, the DRAS and the pain-modulating tracts).

Referred hyperalgesia Oversensitivity to painful stimuli can also be caused by a disturbance in other parts of the same segment. The most likely explanation is facilitation and summation in the sensory posterior horn, and the sensitizing effect of the sympathetic fibres on the small afferents. Because the small fibres (conveying information on pain and touch), converge to a much larger extent than the large fibres (which convey information on discriminative touch and pressure), referred hyperalgesia is more likely to occur than referred hyperaesthesia. Both symptoms occur predominantly in the more superficial layers (dermatome and myotome) with their higher degree of innervation. In contra-

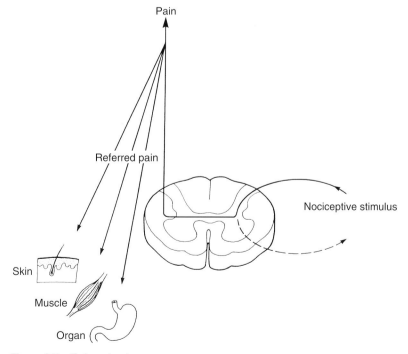

Figure 8.7 Referred pain.

distinction to subjective referred pain, which results from a subjective 'misinterpretation of the brain', referred hyperalgesia and hyper-aesthesia are objective segmental symptoms, resulting from segmental interactions, and more or less bounded by the borders of the segment.

Oversensitivity to pain, touch and pressure is noticed only during examination (showing as tenderness). On examination one can usually find maximum fields (zones of Head) in the skin, while the muscles mainly show maximum points (zones of MacKenzie and trigger points).

Hypertonic muscles and activation of trigger points

Via the motor anterior horn a segmental disturb-ance can result in hypertonic muscles, which, in due time, can turn into irreversible morphological shortening. The muscle zones, with tender hypertonic muscles, described by MacKenzie (1917) are frequent in cases of internal organ pathology (Travell & Simons 1983), for instance the muscle point of McBurney. In these hyper-tonic muscle zones we can often find activated trigger points.

Like every blocked joint, a blocked vertebral joint can be the result of a disturbed segment, and be of great diagnostic value. It is the result of hypertonic small lumbar muscles and trophic changes in the paravertebral structures. As a general rule, in the vertebral column a spinal nerve innervates the muscles and structures of the vertebrae above and below its place of emergence. This means for instance, that a blocked vertebral joint of T5 and T6 can be the result of a disturbed segment T5 (Bogduk & Twomey 1987).

Autonomic symptoms

Via the autonomic lateral horn, a segmental disturbance can produce vasomotor, sudomotor, pilomotor and visceral effects, as well as a sensitization of the small afferent fibres. A longer-lasting vasoconstriction can result in a diminished perfusion of the connective tissue, which will eventually make the connective tissue more rigid, owing to changes in the matrix. In due time these trophic changes can become irreversible.

Sensitization of small afferent fibres (by sympathetic hyperactivity for example) can lead to pain and hyperalgesia (both local and referred), and an increased activity in these small fibres can maintain or intensify a seg-mental disturbance (vicious circles; see p 116).

We shall briefly discuss the most important segmental autonomic symptoms. For more detailed information, we recommend the outline of the autonomic changes in the various tissues, as presented by Oostendorp (1988).

Autonomic symptoms can occur in every part of a segment:

- the **skin** can become pale, cold and clammy, and it can show goose flesh and an increased dermographia
- the **subcutaneous tissue** can show trophic changes (become shiny and oedematous), and its consistency can thicken: the 'subcutaneous connective tissue zones', with their diminished rollability, slidability and pliability (see p 122 and Fig. 8.13)
- the **muscles** can show a diminished stretchability owing to trophic changes, and because trigger points can become activated
- the **joints** can have a painfully restricted range of movement ('blocked joint'), owing to trophic changes of the ligaments and the joint capsule, also to diminished synovia production, resulting in cartilage changes ('sore joints')
- the **organs** can become restricted in their function owing to a diminished circulation, and altered peristalsis can result in spasm.

By noting all the sensory, motor and autonomic symptoms, a segmental diagnosis can be built up with the help of maps of the dermatomes, myotomes, sclerotomes and viscerotomes (see Figs 8.1–8.4 and 8.19–8.24, pp 106–107 and 129–132).

Causes of segmental symptoms

The appearance of segmental symptoms due to visceral pathology, those in the head and neck, and those in the secondary related segments can sometimes be confusing, because the relationship between the cause and the symptoms is more complicated, and because the symptoms can occur in segments that can be at some distance from one another. Nevertheless these groups of symptoms are based on the same segmental principles as mentioned above. We shall now briefly discuss each one of these groups of segmental symptoms.

Visceral pathology

These symptoms are slightly more complicated to understand, because visceral pathology can project to the spinal cord in more than one way. This means that it can be manifest in segments far away from each other. Since visceral afferent information is conveyed by the same routes as is efferent innervation, we can distinguish the following four routes:

- via sympathetic fibres . . . . to the spinal segments C8–L2
- via the phrenic nerve (diaphragm) . .to C3–C5
- via the pelvic nerves . . . . .to S2–S4
- via the vagus nerve . . . . to the brainstem and to C1–C2.

As we can see, some extremity segments are not influenced segmentally by the viscera; these are the 'empty segments' of C5–C8 and L3–S1 (see Fig. 8.24, p 132). This explains why visceral pathology rarely produces referred pain in the extremities.

After we have made a segmental diagnosis, we can use Figure 8.24 on p 132 to make a possible link between these symptoms and the various internal organs. A segmental diagnosis can result in an organ diagnosis, but it can also indicate a possible association between one or more disturbed segments and one or more internal organs. Conversely, in case of clinically clear internal pathology, it is also possible to use the associated segments therapeutically, especially if they show segmental symptoms.

Symptoms in the head and neck

To understand the segmental symptoms and the segmental therapeutic possibilities in the head

and neck, all the possible neurological interactions need to be considered.

The sensory innervation of the head and neck is mainly by the trigeminal and C2–3 spinal nerves. The spinal trigeminal nucleus reaches downwards to the spinal segments C2–4 (Carpenter 1985, Duus 1980, Martinez Martinez 1980, Okamoto et al 1986). There is an extensive interaction between the spinal nerves C1–4, and the trigeminal, phrenic and vagus nerves (Grieve 1988, Oostendorp 1988). Atweh et al (1985) and Oostendorp (1988) describe the possibility of inhibiting nociceptive trigeminal information by stimulating the large fibres of the upper cervical nerves and vice versa.

The sympathetic innervation of the head and neck is derived from the lateral column of the autonomic lateral horns of C8–T4. All autonomic activity (especially visceral) that affects these segments can influence the sympathetic innervation of the head. This can result, for example, in eye, ear, nose and throat (ENT) and other problems due to vasoconstriction or sensitization of the afferent fibres (van Cranenburgh 1989b, Hansen & Schliack 1962).

Segmental symptoms in the head and neck can be truly segmental, because of overactivity in the upper cervical spinal nerves, but they can also be the result of overactivity in the trigeminal, phrenic or vagus nerve. Also, interactions between the three columns of the autonomic lateral horn can explain part of these symptoms (see Table 8.1, p 108). For example: tense suboccipital muscles and trigger points in the trapezius can result in occipital headaches radiating to the forehead, osteopathic mobilization of the cervical vertebrae can sometimes influence eye, ENT and other complaints in the head, and Hansen & Schliack (1962) and others describe distinct zones of referred pain and referred hyperalgesia in the head resulting from visceral pathology.

In everyday practice it is important to remember that head and neck symptoms can be the result of:

- trigeminal pathology
- disturbances in the cervical segments C0–4

- somatic and visceral pathology influencing the segments C8–T4
- visceral pathology irritating the phrenic nerve (C3–5).

Conversely, it is traditionally accepted that acupuncture points in the head and neck can influence pathology elsewhere. The interactions we mentioned in the upper cervical areas, and those between the three columns in the lateral horns of C8–T4, can explain part of these effects.

Symptoms in secondary related segments

We have described above close relationships and interactions between the three columns of the lateral horn, which form the basis of these secondary relations (Table 8.1 p 108). Box 8.1 details relationships that can be found between the dermatomes, myotomes, sclerotomes and viscerotomes in the left column, and those in the right column. A local problem can become segmental, and eventually spread over to the secondary related segments, depending on the severity of the problem and on the same modulating influences as were described for the true segmental symptoms.

To explain these secondary relations, it is necessary to study the relationships and interactions between the segments T5 and C5. A nociceptive irritation, for instance, somewhere in the segment T5 can give segmental symptoms in different parts of this segment, but apart from these symptoms, or instead of them, it is possible to find segmental symptoms in parts of the secondary related segment of C5.

The following segmental interactions can occur:

Box 8.1 Secondary segmental relations
C8/T1/T2 . . . . .C1/C2
T2/T3/T4 . . . . .C3/C4
T5/T6 . . . . .C5/C6
T7/T8/T9 . . . . .C7/C8
T10/T11 . . . . .L3/L4
T12/L1/L2 . . . . .L5/S1/S2

- *via the posterior horn of T5*: pain in parts of T5
- *via the anterior horn of T5*: hypertonic muscles and activated trigger points in parts of T5
- *via the lateral horn of T5*
  a. via the medial column: autonomic symptoms in the viscerotome of T5
  b. via the middle column: autonomic symptoms in the dermatome, myotome and/or sclerotome of T5
  c. via the lateral column: autonomic symptoms in the various parts of C5.

Also, a nociceptive irritation somewhere in the segment C5, will give segmental symptoms in the dermatome, myotome, sclerotome and/or viscerotome of C5, but, because the autonomic segmental interactions of the segment C5 can occur only in the lateral column of the lateral horn of T5, we can also find segmental symptoms in parts of this secondary related segment T5 (Fig. 8.8). If correct manipulative treatment of the vertebral joint C5/C6 does not give a lasting effect, it can therefore be useful to check whether the vertebral joint of T5/T6 is blocked and acting as a perpetuating factor. If segmental acupuncture is only partially successful, it is likewise advisable to look for segmental symptoms in the secondary related segments. If so, treatment of these hitherto unnoticed symptoms can often bring a longer-lasting therapeutic effect.

Vicious circles

Pain, trigger points, joint blockages and other segmental disturbances can become the source of vicious circles that maintain the segmental disturbance, even when the original cause has subsided. Therefore, *a segmental disturbance can maintain itself*. A peptic ulcer, for instance, can give segmental symptoms in the segments of T5–9. Subsequently, hypertonic paraspinal muscles in these segments can give an asymptomatic functional scoliosis (the spine curves around the affected organ), resulting among other effects in a narrowing of the intervertebral foramina and irritation of the spinal nerves. These irritated spinal nerves can have a maintaining effect on the original seg-

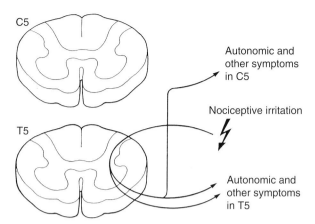

Figure 8.8 Secondary segmental relationships: a nociceptive irritation in the segment of T5 can give segmental symptoms in the segment T5, and secondary segmental symptoms in the segment C5.

mental disturbance, the peptic ulcer (Fig. 8.9) (Gunn 1989).

In addition, *a segmental disturbance can maintain other segmental symptoms*. Attacks of angina pectoris, for instance, can activate trigger points in the pectoralis major muscle. These trigger points can become a new, independent source of segmental disturbance (Fig. 8.10). They can produce symptoms such as shoulder and chest pain, but also somatovisceral (e.g. cardiac) symptoms, even after the original symptoms of angina have subsided (Travell & Simons 1983).

SEGMENTAL DIAGNOSIS

The aim of a segmental diagnosis is to trace the disturbed segment or segments. After classifi-

cation of all the segmental symptoms, we have to translate them into a segmental diagnosis (van Cranenburgh 1987, 1989a,b, Hansen & Schliack 1962). In this way we can often find relationships between apparently independent symptoms. A correct segmental diagnosis enables us to treat the real cause and avoid symptomatic treatment. Segmental symptoms can be found in the dermatome, myotome, sclerotome and viscerotome of a segment (or related segments).

For instance:

- superficial shoulder pain (dermatome) can point to a disturbed C4
- a trigger point in the deltoid muscle (myotome) with referred pain patterns on the upper arm can have a relationship with a segmental disturbance in C5/C6
- an epicondylitis lateralis humeri (sclerotome) can point to a segmental disturbance in C6
- stomach complaints (viscerotome) can be associated with a disturbance in T6.

After making an inventory of the disturbed segment(s) we have to determine which part of the segment (dermatome, myotome, sclerotome or viscerotome) is the most disturbed. This can be important in deciding which segmental therapy will be most appropriate.

Note the difference between a segmental diagnosis and an (internal) organ diagnosis: when we find one or more disturbed segments (*segmental diagnosis*), an organ is not always the cause. If an organ (*organ diagnosis*) is the cause of

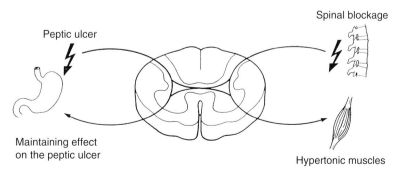

Figure 8.9 Vicious circles: a segmental disturbance can maintain itself.

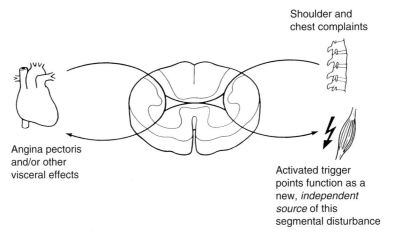

Shoulder and
chest complaints

Angina pectoris
and/or other
visceral effects

Activated trigger
points function as a
new, *independent
source* of this
segmental disturbance

Figure 8.10 Vicious circles: a segmental disturbance can maintain other segmental symptoms, which can become a new independent source of a segmental disturbance.

the segmental disturbance, usually more than one segment will be affected (see Figs 8.17, 8.18 and 8.24, pp 127 and 132).

In drawing up a segmental diagnosis, one has to bear in mind that there are several potential pitfalls:

- Different authors draw different maps of the dermatomes (see p 106).
- The dermatome, myotome, sclerotome and viscerotome of a segment do not necessarily overlap each other anatomically (see p 106); for instance, the dermatome of T7 is situated over the myotomes of C5–8 and T6–8 (the serratus anterior, pectoralis major, latissimus dorsi, intercostal and paraspinal muscles), and over the sclerotomes of T7–11 (7th–11th ribs) (see Fig. 8.5, p 107).
- In the case of visceral pathology, segments are more likely to be disturbed on the homolateral side of the body.
- Segmental symptoms can be due to secondary segmental relations (see p 108 and Fig. 8.8). Consequently, hypertonic muscles, autonomic symptoms and sometimes pain or hyperalgesia can be found in segments other than those expected.

The most important diagnostic procedures for building up a segmental diagnosis will now be reviewed.

Pain and hyperalgesia

Local pain and referred pain are subjective symptoms and can be indicated in the dermatome, myotome, scelerotome or viscerotome, but usually they will be indicated in the more superficial layers (dermatome and myotome), because these layers are more densely innervated (see p 113). First the patient needs to describe very accurately where he feels the pain, and later tenderness to palpation; we can look for locus dolendi in the skin, or trigger points in muscle by palpation.

Local and referred hyperalgesia are more objective symptoms, which are also more often found in the superficial layers. For exact localization of hyperalgesic areas, the patient's cooperation is still needed.

To find hyperalgesic areas in the dermatome, use a blunt needle and test the rollability and pliability of the skin and subcutaneous tissue (for a detailed description of this test see p 122).

In the myotome look for sore muscles, which are usually also hypertonic and which often have trigger points (for detailed description see p 120).

In the sclerotome look for painful joints and painful areas in the ligaments and periosteum (e.g. painful spinous processes).

In translating these symptoms into a segmental diagnosis there are several potentially confusing factors:

- usually painful and hyperalgesic areas will cover more than one segment
- visceral pathology does not give true segmental symptoms like pain and hyperalgesia in the 'empty segments' C6–8 and L3–S1 on the extremities (see Fig. 8.24, p 132), but it can give secondary segmental symptoms (mainly autonomic) in these segments.

For a segmental diagnosis it is important to distinguish whether pain is referred or local. The following methods can be helpful (Macdonald 1983):

- during the palpation of the source of local pain, the pressure of the palpating finger will increase the pain; this does not occur in areas of referred pain
- injection of local anaesthetic in an area of local pain will result in dramatic relief, while an injection in the area of referred pain will result in little pain relief.

After identifying the areas of (referred) pain and hyperalgesia, we can use maps of the dermatomes, myotomes, sclerotomes and viscerotomes (see Figs 8.1–8.4 and 8.17–8.24, pp 106–107 and 127–132) to translate them into a segmental diagnosis.

In everyday practice (referred) pain or hyperalgesia do not always follow the well-known segmental or neuroanatomical patterns. This can be confusing, but when we find other segmental symptoms or, for instance, autonomic symptoms in the secondary related segments, these can help us build up a segmental diagnosis. For instance, when a patient complains of superficial pain in the lower back, there is a diagnostic problem. All the dermatomes between T9 and L2 could be involved. We should examine the myotomes and sclerotomes for other segmental symptoms: if we find a hypertonic quadratus lumborum muscle (T12–L4) and a painful spinous process of T12 (which is situated well above the painful area), this suggests a seg-

mental diagnosis of a disturbed T12 segment (Fig. 8.11).

Hypertonic muscles

Hypertonic muscles will initially correspond accurately with the disturbed segment(s), but in a later phase the muscle hypertonia may become more generalized. Listing the hypertonic muscles, bear in mind that:

- the segmental innervation of the small back muscles (multifidi/bifidi) deserves our special interest because these muscles are easy to localize; consequently the corresponding disturbed segments are easy to find
- hypertonic muscles are not always painful; sometimes they are painful only during palpation
- trigger points in the muscles can be important for a segmental diagnosis
- pathology in the muscles plays an important role in 'vicious circles' (see p 116)

Diagnostic methods to locate hypertonic muscles include the following:

Inspection (Hansen & Schliack 1962)

- **Scoliosis**: hypertonic muscles of the spine can be the cause of a functional scoliosis convex to the healthy side. This effect can be found as a result of internal organ pathology; the spine curves around the affected organ.
- **Asymmetric respiratory movements**: the hypertonic side will show diminished respiratory excursions.
- **Facial asymmetry**: an important sign can be a deeper homolateral nasolabial fold. This is due to increased tone in the homolateral facial muscles. This symptom is present in about 70% of visceral pathology (Hansen & Schliack 1962).

Palpation

Superficial and deep palpation can give information about the skin, subcutaneous tissue and muscles. For a segmental diagnosis based

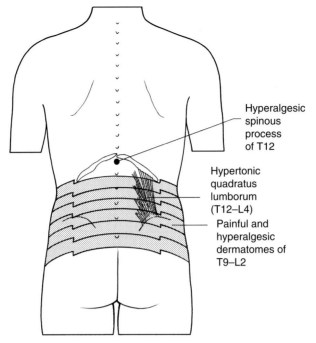

Figure 8.11 Building up a segmental diagnosis: disturbed segment T12.

on the muscles, check muscle tone, trigger points and taut bands. It is important that the patient is comfortable and warm, and the muscles must be relaxed. Palpation can cause (referred) pain.

Travell & Simons (1983) describe several methods to locate trigger points and taut bands in the muscles. To locate taut bands: 'The muscle [has to be] stretched until the fibres of the taut band are under tension and the uninvolved fibres remain slack. The stretch should be on the verge of causing pain, but should evoke only local discomfort and no referred pain'. The taut band feels like, 'A taut cord of tense muscle fibres among the normally slacked fibres'.

The taut bands and the trigger points within them can be located by flat and pincer palpation (Fig. 8.12):

- **flat palpation**: 'refers to a moving finger-tip that employs the mobility of the subcutaneous tissue to slide the patient's skin across the muscle fibres'

- **pincer palpation**: 'is performed by grasping the belly of the muscle between thumb and

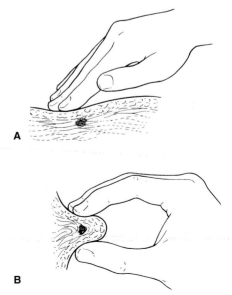

Figure 8.12 A Flat and B pincer palpation. (After Travell & Simons 1983.)

fingers and squeezing the fibres between them with a back and forth rolling motion to locate the taut bands'.

When a trigger point or a taut band is rolled under the fingers, Travell & Simons (1983) describe a 'jump sign' in response to pressure on the trigger point: 'A general pain response of the patient, who winces, may cry out, and may withdraw in response to pressure applied on a trigger point'.

Resistance or pain during movements

Changed resistance during movements; or diminished stretchability due to trophic changes A higher resistance during passive extension of the leg in the hip, for instance, can be due to a hypertonic psoas muscle.

For more information about the diagnosis of trigger points see Baldry (1993) and Travell & Simons (1983, 1992).

Spinal blockage

Hypertonic paraspinal muscles can result in a (secondary) vertebral joint blockage. The diagnostic methods to find a joint blockage will not be discussed here.

A segmental diagnosis based on the hypertonic muscle(s) found during physical examination, can be drawn up with the aid of the myotome tables in Figures 8.19–8.22, pp 129–131.

Autonomic symptoms

Although the body is innervated sympathetically only by the segments C8–L2, these can be the cause of autonomic segmental symptoms in every segment.

For a segmental diagnosis based on autonomic symptoms remember:

- the existence of the secondary segmental relations
- that autonomic symptoms caused by a segmental disturbance can spread over a larger area than somatic effects like pain/hyperalgesia and hypertonic muscles

(van Cranenburgh 1987, 1989a,b, Hansen & Schliack 1962, Oostendorp 1988).

For a list of general autonomic symptoms see p 114. Some autonomic symptoms of special interest are detailed in the following sections (Hansen & Schliack 1962):

Autonomic symptoms of the eyes

In about 90% of visceral pathology, a sympathetic anisocoria can give an indication on which side to expect an affected organ. This homolateral mydriasis is not a structural symptom but a functional one. Consequently it is not continuously present. It can be disturbed by bright light, accommodation and refraction pathology. Note, however, that 8% of healthy persons have an anisocoria. Other autonomic symptoms of the eyes can be: homolateral exophthalmus and a stronger lachrymal secretion.

Autonomic symptoms in the dermatome

- **Sudomotor symptoms**: anisohydrotic areas of the skin can be felt or sometimes seen. These areas may be bilateral, but are usually more distinct on the pathological side.
- **Pilomotor symptoms**: areas of goose flesh can be seen with oblique light. A sudden draught or an application of cold can provoke the onset of goose flesh.
- **Vasomotor symptoms**: zones of vasoconstriction can be noted as changes in colour and temperature of the skin. Some skin symptoms, like dermographia, can be found after provocation. This symptom is more explicit and has a longer onset in the pathological zones. Intracutaneous injections of normal saline are dispersed more quickly in the dermatome of the disturbed segment, possibly because of higher permeability of the capillaries.
- **Changes in the tone or mobility of the skin and subcutaneous tissue**: these can be measured by testing the pliability, slidability and rollability of the skin and subcutaneous connective tissue (Oostendorp 1988) (see below).

Usually we test changes in the skin tone and mobility on the back of the patient, who can either sit in an upright position or lie face down on the examination table.

Rollability This is performed by rolling the skin and subcutaneous tissue between the thumb and index finger in a cranial direction (Fig. 8.13A). This is performed on either side of the midline, comparing the left and right sides. Testing the rollability gives the following information:

- subjective symptoms: this test is normally not painful; hyperalgesic regions can give an indication of which dermatomes are involved
- objective symptoms: regions that feel more 'glued' to the deeper layers can be related to disturbed segments.

Slidability The skin, together with subcutaneous tissue, is pushed towards the head in front of the palpating hand. Regions where the tissue is moved less easily can be detected clearly (Fig. 8.13B).

Pliability The skin and the subcutaneous tissue are picked up between thumb and index finger. Regions where the skin feels more glued to the underlying tissues can indicate a disturbed segment.

In testing rollability, slidability and pliability, always compare left and right, and check for differences in sensation.

These diagnostic tests are relatively easy to do, and can give a lot of information about the dermatome (the skin with subcutaneous tissue). However, there can be some complicating factors:

- in case of hypertonic underlying muscles, the mobility of the subcutaneous tissue can be decreased up to 50%
- in the lumbar region the skin is physiologically more attached to the subcutaneous tissue
- the rollability, slidability and pliability are difficult to classify in quality and quantity, (Oostendorp 1988, Sutter 1983).

Autonomic symptoms in the myotome and sclerotome

Symptoms in the muscles can be caused by disturbances in the somatic nervous system as

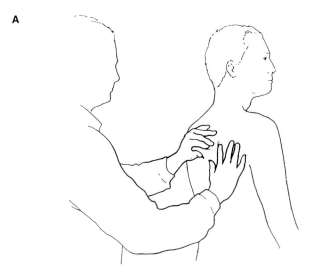

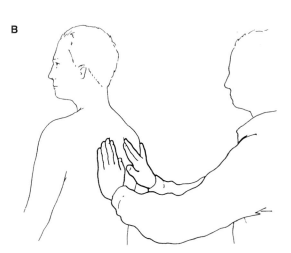

Figure 8.13 A Rollability and B slidability of the subcutaneous tissue.

well as in the autonomic nervous system. The same remarks apply as for the myotome.

Synthesis of the segmental diagnosis

After listing all the symptoms in the dermatomes, myotomes and sclerotomes, we have to determine which segments, and which parts of the segments, are disturbed most. For a correct segmental diagnosis, and consequently for the choice of the best therapy, we have to distinguish whether the symptoms are of a local origin, or whether they are the result or even the cause, of a segmental disturbance, as follows:

- **true segmental symptoms**: these symptoms occur in the segment where the causative disturbance started; sometimes the source of the symptoms may have been unnoticed, or even have vanished (see 'vicious circles' p 116 and Figs 8.9 and 8.10, pp 117 and 118)
- **visceral segmental symptoms**: see p 118.
- **symptoms in the head (and neck)**: see p 115
- **segmental symptoms in the secondary related segments**: the source of the problem can be found in the secondary related segments.

SEGMENTAL ACUPUNCTURE THERAPY

In segmental acupuncture therapy, one aims to use those acupuncture points that are neuroanatomically related to the disturbed segment(s). In principle, these points are situated in the dermatome, myotome or sclerotome of the disturbed segment. When, for instance, segments T3 and 4 are disturbed, and the dermatome is disturbed most, we can make a selection of points with the help of the dermatome charts (Figs 8.1 and 8.2, p 106, 8.14). For example, if the dermatome of the right ventral part of T3 and 4 is disturbed, the following points can be used: PC-1, GB-22 and 23, SP-17, 18 and 19, ST-15 and 16, KI-23, 24 and 25, CV-18 and 19.

Segmental acupuncture therapy is one of the segmental therapies like physiotherapy, manual therapy, therapeutic local anaesthesia (TLA) or neural therapy (Dosch 1986), or trigger point acupuncture. Sometimes one of these therapies can be more effective than segmental acupuncture or vice versa, depending on the clinical situation. It is also possible to use combinations, or switch from one to another. The choice of the most effective therapy largely depends on the clinical situation, and on the part of the segment that is disturbed most.

Before explaining the practical methods in segmental acupuncture therapy, we will comment on suitable techniques for the segmental and neuroanatomical approach.

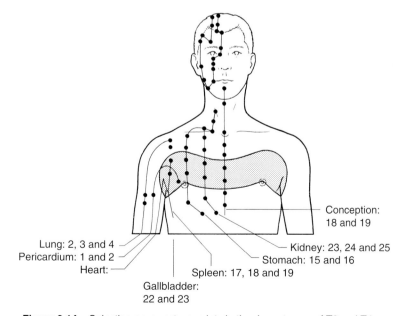

Figure 8.14   Selecting acupuncture points in the dermatomes of T3 and T4.

'Superficial' or 'deep' acupuncture

With the help of the dermatome, myotome and sclerotome maps (e.g. Figs 8.1–8.4, pp 106–107) we can determine which segments will be influenced when a certain acupuncture point is used. By puncturing a point deeply it is possible to influence different segments at the same time, because the myotome and sclerotome situated under the acupuncture point often belong to different segments (see also p 106 and Fig. 8.5, p 107) (van Cranenburgh 1987). Therefore, the depth of the needle determines which segment is stimulated: superficial acupuncture will stimulate only the dermatome, while deep acupuncture will also stimulate the myotome (and the sclerotome) (Fig. 8.15) For example, an acupuncture point like PC-2 is situated in the dermatome T2, while the underlying biceps is part of the myotomes C5 and C6.

'Dry' versus 'wet' acupuncture

Acupuncture is in principle a 'dry' therapy, which means that no pharmacological substances are administered through the needle. The use of segmental acupuncture therapy, however, is strongly related to other segmental therapies. For instance, trigger points can be treated either by 'dry' needling (Baldry 1993) or by the use of local anaesthetic or normal saline (Travell & Simons 1983). For these reasons some details follow about the use of local anaesthetics (which we will call 'wet' acupuncture therapy). Generally speaking, local anaesthetics are mostly injected into locus dolendi and trigger points to treat pain in the musculoskeletal system. However, it is also possible to inject local anaesthetics in painless parts of the body, and still obtain good therapeutic results.

The use of local anaesthetics in segmental therapy

The use of local anaesthetics in the dermatome (locus dolendi) or in the myotome trigger points is only a small part of this therapy. Local an-

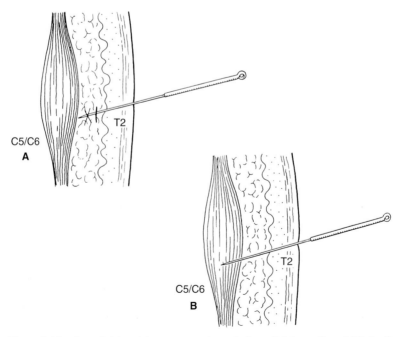

Figure 8.15 Superficial and deep acupuncture. A. Superficial needling of PC-2 will stimulate the segment T2 (dermatome T2). B. Deeper needling of PC-2 will stimulate the segment T2 (dermatome T2), but also the segments C5 and C6 (Biceps: myotomes C5 and C6).

aesthetics can also be injected in the sclerotome (ligaments, joints), in the viscerotome, and especially in the somatic or autonomic nerves and gangliae (Bonica 1984, Dosch 1986). Local anaesthetics can eliminate the (hyper) activity of the nervous system that can develop in any part of the body and can result in a disturbed segment. This will have a more lasting effect than the direct pharmacological action of the local anaesthetic (interruption of vicious circles?).

The therapeutic use of local anaesthetics can be intrasegmental or extrasegmental.

Intrasegmental Injection with local anaesthetic can reduce (hyper)activity in the dermatome, myotome, sclerotome and viscerotome of that same segment. The most generally known use of local anaesthetics is the treatment of locus dolendi and trigger points. This will also influence other parts of the segment, for instance by interrupting vicious circles: sympatholytic effects like vasodilatation, and effects on hypertonic muscles.

Also, non-painful parts of a segment can be treated by using local anaesthetics, as hyperactivity of the nervous system can develop in any structure of the segment, and is not always the result of pain. For instance (painless) scars, or painless hypertonic muscles can be the cause of a continuous segmental hyperactivity. Reducing this hyperactivity with local anaesthetics can have a therapeutic effect. Even the reduction of 'normal' activity (for instance, by using local anaesthetics in painless acupuncture points) in a disturbed segment can be useful.

Take, for example, a patient complaining of neck pain. A segmental diagnosis indicates that the myotome (trapezius) of the segments C2–4 is disturbed most, but treatment of acupuncture points in the trapezius gives no benefit. In the dermatome of C2 we find a scar of a furuncle, and after intra- and subcutaneous infiltration of this scar with a local anaesthetic, acupuncture treatment gives relief.

Extrasegmental Injections with local anaesthetic in the dermatome, myotome, sclerotome or viscerotome of segments other than the disturbed segment can also reduce (hyper)activity of the nervous system in the disturbed segment.

By reducing (hyper)activity in and from other parts of the body, we can also influence the extent of the excitation of the disturbed segment. This may be an explanation of the fact that infiltration of locus dolendi, trigger points, scars or acupuncture points with local anaesthetic in segments anatomically far away from, and not necessarily secondarily related to, the disturbed segment can have a therapeutic effect.

Thus: 'dry' and 'wet' acupuncture work neurophysiologically in quite different ways:

- **'dry' acupuncture** can *increase* segmental inhibition by stimulating the large fibres, and by modulation of central ascending or descending activity
- **'wet' acupuncture** can *decrease* segmental excitation by blocking the small fibres and, depending on the concentration of the local anaesthetic, sometimes also the large fibres.

With acupuncture, different effects occur simultaneously. We can distinguish:

- segmental and general effects
- analgesic effects, autonomic effects and effects on hypertonic muscles.

In segmental acupuncture we usually try to achieve these effects selectively. Thus we have to choose effective points, but also the most effective type of stimulation.

Choice of points

'Local' points

Local points are situated anatomically near the problem. When, for instance, treating a locus dolendi or trigger point, the selection of points often depends on its location, which may be superficial (dermatome) or deep (myotome, sclerotome). In general it is assumed that the rate of success in treating locus dolendi or trigger points depends on the exactness of hitting them (Baldry 1993, Travell & Simons 1983).

Also other, non-painful, problems may benefit from treating points near the complaint.

'Distant' points

Distant points fall into four major groups: in the disturbed segment, in segments related to a pathological organ, in secondary related segments, and other distant points.

'Distant' points in the disturbed segment (segmental diagnosis) Acupuncture points in one part of the segment can influence its other parts. For example, a patient with an epicondylitis lateralis humeri may have a disturbed C6 segment. For treatment one could use the following acupuncture points (shown in Fig. 8.16)

- in the **dermatome** of C6: LU-5–11, LI-1–14 and PC-3–7
- in the **myotome** of C6: all the points that are situated on muscles innervated by C6 (see Figs 8.2, 8.19 and 8.20, pp 106, 129 and 130) but points that are situated on hypertonic muscles are more likely to have a therapeutic effect

- in the **sclerotome** of C6: LU-5–11. PC-2 and 3, HT-3, SI-10 and 11, TE-9, 10, 13 and 14 and LI-1–16 (see Figs 8.22 and 8.23, p 131).

The choice of points in the disturbed segment or its neighbours will depend on the affect desired. To treat pain, acupuncture points in the bordering segments may be used as well as in the affected ones, since nociceptive stimuli also affect the bordering segments. If a sympatheticolytic effect is desired, points in the disturbed segment are most effective, because stimuli via the autonomic nervous system quickly disappear in the bordering segments.

'Distant' points in segment(s) related to a pathological organ (organ diagnosis)
Sometimes, when the affected organ is known, points in the dermatome, myotome or sclerotome of the segment belonging to that organ, like for instance the back (Yu) points (dermatome) on the bladder meridian, can be used.

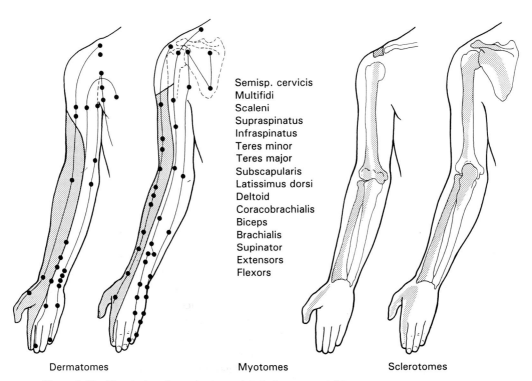

Semisp. cervicis
Multifidi
Scaleni
Supraspinatus
Infraspinatus
Teres minor
Teres major
Subscapularis
Latissimus dorsi
Deltoid
Coracobrachialis
Biceps
Brachialis
Supinator
Extensors
Flexors

Dermatomes   Myotomes   Sclerotomes

Figure 8.16   The choice of acupuncture points in the segment C6.

In traditional Chinese acupuncture the back (Shu) points are used to treat the organs. In segmental acupuncture we use only those back points that correspond with the dermatome of their organs; Bl-14 and 22, Pericardium and Triple Energizer respectively, do not easily fit in the segmental concept (Table 8.3).

The back points BL-15 and 27 are not situated in the segments of their traditionally related organs, although dermatome maps by different authors do vary.

A patient with stomach problems can have segmental disturbances in the segments C3–5 and in T5–9 (Figs 8.17 and 8.18). Any point in the dermatome, myotome or sclerotome of these segments could theoretically be used, so extra diagnostic information is necessary to make the selection.

'Distant' points in segment(s) related to the disturbed segment via secondary segmental rela-

Table 8.3 The correspondence of the back (Yu) points with the dermatome of their organs

Organ	Visveral innervation	Back (Yu) point	Dermatome of (back) Yu point
Lung	T2–T7	BL–13	T3
Heart	T1–T4	BL–15	T5
Liver	T6–T9	BL–18	T7
Gall-bladder	T6–T9	BL–19	T7
Spleen/pancreas	T6–T10	BL–20	T8
Stomach	T5–T9	BL–21	T8
Kidney	T10–L1	BL–23	T10
Large intestine	T9–L2	BL–25	T11
Small intestine	T5–T10	BL–27	L1
Bladder	T12–L2	BL–28	L2

tions For instance, a patient with a disturbed segment C4 can be treated by using points in the dermatome, myotome or sclerotome of T4.

Other distant points Other 'distant' points may be in a segment with a separate problem

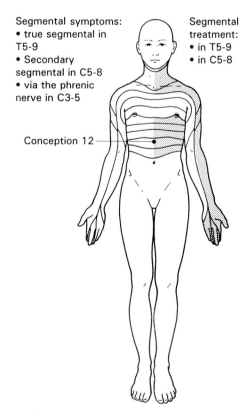

Segmental symptoms:
• true segmental in T5-9
• Secondary segmental in C5-8
• via the phrenic nerve in C3-5

Conception 12

Segmental treatment:
• in T5-9
• in C5-8

Figure 8.17 Segmental diagnosis and treatment of stomach pathology (anterior view).

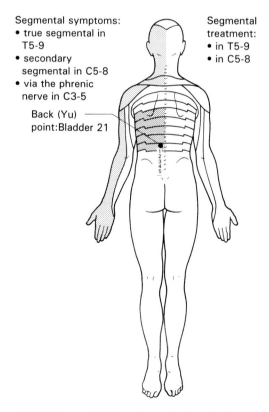

Segmental symptoms:
• true segmental in T5-9
• secondary segmental in C5-8
• via the phrenic nerve in C3-5

Back (Yu) point:Bladder 21

Segmental treatment:
• in T5-9
• in C5-8

Figure 8.18 Segmental diagnosis and treatment of stomach pathology (posterior view).

that is acting as an aggravating factor to the segmental disturbance (see also 'dry' or 'wet' acupuncture). In a patient with a knee complaint (L3) and a 'frozen shoulder' (C4–6) for instance, treatment of the shoulder can improve the knee.

For both 'local' and 'distant' points, bear in mind that points on the homolateral side of the body may be more effective. Differentiation between right and left is not only important for a segmental diagnosis in relation to the organs (Hansen & Schliack 1962), but is also important in therapy.

When it is not suitable to use acupuncture points close to the site of the complaint because it is too painful, or because there is risk of infection (e.g. when treating joints), it is possible to use:

- 'distant' points in the same segment
- 'distant' points in the bordering segments (in case of pain)
- 'distant' points in the secondary related segments
- local anaesthetics.

Choice of stimulation

Depending on the kind of stimulation, we can distinguish:

- a local, a segmental and a general effect
- an effect on the pain, on hypertonic muscles, and on autonomic symptoms.

These effects can not always be separated.
We can also distinguish two kinds of stimulation: manual and electrical.

Manual stimulation

A mild non-painful, stimulation of the acupuncture needle will stimulate large fibres (Aβ and low-threshold Aδ fibres, respectively II and IIIa), resulting in a needling sensation.

- via **segmental interactions (gate control)**: pain, hyperalgesia, hypertonic muscles and autonomic symptoms will be inhibited

- via the **reticular formation**: these segmental symptoms will be inhibited 'more or less segmentally' via both the pain-modulating tracts and the DRAS
- via the **thalamus/hypothalamus**: the production of β-endorphin will result in a general analgesic effect, while the production of ACTH will have an anti-inflammatory action.

In this way it is possible to treat pain, hypertonic muscles and autonomic symptoms (sympatholytic effect) locally and segmentally.

A stronger, more painful stimulation of the acupuncture needle stimulates small fibres (the high-threshold Aδ and the C fibres, respectively IIIb and IV), and has the opposite effect:

- via **segmental interactions (gate control)** we can intensify sensory, motor and autonomic effects; we can also try to inhibit the C (IV) fibres via the stimulation of high-threshold Aδ (IIIb) fibres
- via the **reticular formation** we can 'more or less segmentally' increase the muscle tone (via the DRAS) and sympathetic activity (via the ARAS).

Consequently this form of stimulation can be used to treat hypotonic muscles and autonomic symptoms (sympathomimetic effect).

Electrical stimulation

Electrical stimulation is mostly used for its analgesic effect.

High frequency/low intensity Stimulation at high frequency (50–200 Hz) and low intensity will stimulate the Aβ and the low-threshold Aδ (II and IIIa) fibres, and the effects are comparable with mild manual stimulation. Modulations occur mainly via segmental interactions and in the reticular formation (via the pain-modulating tracts, using serotonin as neurotransmitter). This form of stimulation has a strong segmental analgesic effect; it occurs within a few minutes, and lasts only during the stimulation (Pomeranz in Stux & Pomeranz 1986).

Low frequency/high intensity

Stimulation at low frequency (2–4 Hz) and high intensity (almost painful) will stimulate the high-threshold Aδ (IIIb) fibres. The effects are comparable with painful manual stimulation. This form of stimulation has a more general analgesic effect; it occurs only after 20–30 minutes, but outlasts the time of stimulation.

CONCLUSION

To make a proper segmental diagnosis, we must find the disturbed segments that are related to the complaints/symptoms.

During physical examination this 'checklist' of segmental symptoms can be followed:

● **Pain and hyperalgesia:** Are the pain (medical history) and hyperalgesia (physical examination) located in the dermatome, in the myotome or in the sclerotome? Find the corresponding segments (Figs 8.19–8.24).

Is the pain on one side of the body more distinct? Localize the maximum pain points, and note in which dermatome, myotome or sclerotome they are found.

Differentiate whether the pain is referred or local. Are parts of other segments also painful? (secondary segmental connections).

Look for (local or referred) zones of hyperalgesia in the dermatome, in the myotome or in the sclerotome. Do these zones correspond with the segments already presumed to be disturbed?

● **Hypertonic muscles:** By means of inspection and palpation, find which muscles are hypertonic and/or painful, and the corresponding segments for these muscles (Figs 8.19–8.24). Are there any locus dolendi or trigger points in these muscles?

● **Autonomic symptoms:** Look for autonomic symptoms in the eye. Is there a difference between right and left? (A homolateral mydriasis can give a diagnostic clue.)

Try to provoke and localize autonomic symptoms in the dermatome and in the subcutaneous

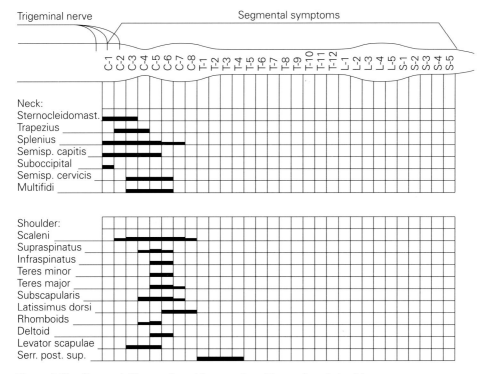

Figure 8.19   Segmental innervation of the muscles of the neck and shoulder.

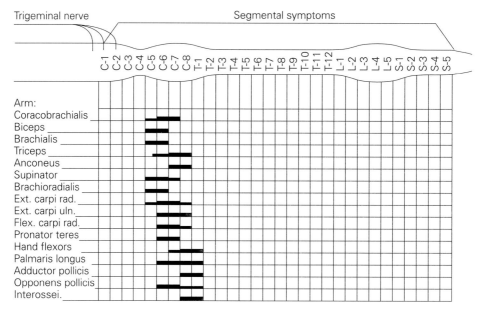

Figure 8.20   Segmental innervation of the muscles of the arm.

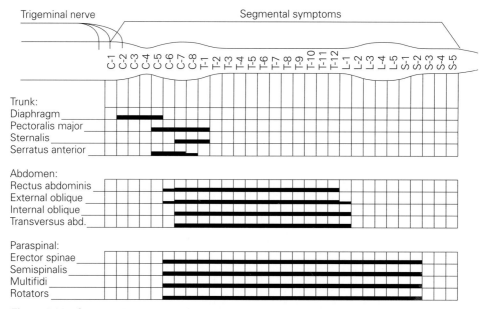

Figure 8.21   Segmental innervation of the muscles of the trunk and abdomen.

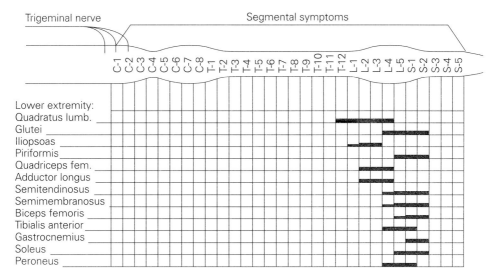

Figure 8.22 Segmental innervation of the muscles of the lower extremity.

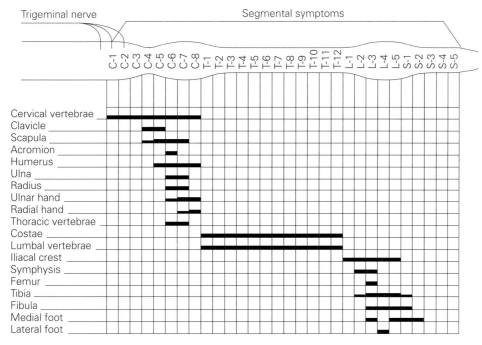

Figure 8.23 Segmental innervation of the skeletal system.

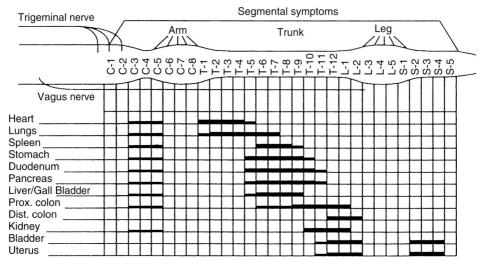

Figure 8.24 Segmental innervation of the internal organs. (Compiled from Brodal 1969, Chandler Elliott 1969, Kunert 1963, Monnier 1968, Rohen 1985).

tissue. With which segments do these symptoms correspond? For the segmental diagnosis, distinguish whether the cause is local or segmental, and which part of the segment is affected most.

- **Symptoms in the head**: Do these symptoms correspond with the presumed segment(s) or organs?

For treatment, first of all distinguish which segmental therapy is the first choice. This will depend on the parts of the segments that are most disturbed (dermatome, myotome, sclerotome or viscerotome). During the first segmental acupuncture treatments, select points in the most disturbed (parts of the) segments. If treatment does not have the expected result, switch to another segmental therapy.

As an example, two case histories are detailed in Boxes 8.2 and 8.3.

Box 8.2   Case study: tension headache and sinus congestion in a 35-year-old woman

A 35-year-old nurse suffered from frequent tension headaches and frequent episodes of sinus congestion. Her doctor prescribed NSAIDs, decongestant nosedrops and other routine medication, every time only with short-term effects. Her friends advised her to look for a less stressful job, while others advised her to try acupuncture treatment. She decided to follow the latter advice first, and made an appointment with a doctor who also practised acupuncture.

When this doctor saw her for the first time, she told him that her problems had started after a whiplash injury some 2 years earlier. The first months were particularly bad, with throbbing headaches, painfully restricted neck movements, vasovagal reactions, etc.; later most of

these complaints subsided, except the headaches and a recurrent sinus congestion.

During physical (segmental) examination, he noticed painful and hyperalgesic areas in the neck and shoulders (C2–4), but also between the scapulae (T2–4). The rollability was especially painful and restricted in these areas. As might be expected, the trapezius muscles were very hypertonic, harbouring active trigger points; the spinous processes of C3, C4 and T3 were painful, and there were some clearly blocked midcervical vertebrae, which could account for the diminished range of cervical movements. His first impression was: disturbed segments of C3 and C4 (dermatomes and myotomes) and possibly also of T3 (dermatome and sclerotome). (cont'd)

Box 8.2 (*Cont'd*)

He decided to use segmental acupuncture, and because Travell & Simons (1983) and also Baldry (1993) clearly indicate that some trigger points in the trapezius muscle (C2–4) can have an influence on sinus congestion, he punctured GB-20, BL-10 and SI-13 (trapezius trigger point), which are all local points in the dermatome and in the myotome of C2–4, and made another appointment for a week later.

At this, she informed him that she had improved a bit, but not much, and that her headaches especially still restricted her work. He punctured the same points, and stretched the trapezius muscle after treatment, he also punctured LR-3 as a distant point with an empirical general relaxing effect and applied an electrical current of high intensity and low frequency to the needle, with the aim of mobilizing central modulation processes like

endorphin production and an increased pain inhibition via the pain-modulating tracts. He also mobilized C3/C4.

The results were much better, but still not good enough. After a successful mobilization of T3/T4 during the fifth consultation, suddenly the complaints responded much better to acupuncture treatment; he then recalled that the autonomic innervation of the head and the neck is derived from C8–T4, and that a disturbed segment of T3 could well have been the maintaining factor of the tension headaches and the sinus congestion. After six treatments the patient was much better, her sinus congestion was gone and, with the help of a physiotherapist who gave her postural exercises, her tension headaches became much less frequent and much less severe.

Box 8.3 Case study: gastric complaint in a 52-year-old man

A 52-year-old maître de cuisine from a well-known restaurant was not exactly a good recommendation to his regular customers, since he was suffering from very bad ˙breath owing to his chronic gastric complaints. He decided that it was about time to visit his GP, who had just completed his course on segmental acupuncture. This doctor first sent him to the nearby hospital for gastroscopic examination, which revealed an old gastric ulcer and gastric irritation. Routine laboratory investigations were all within normal range and standard treatment with antacids and H_2-antagonists showed no lasting effect, so the doctor decided to try out his recently acquired knowledge.

During physical examination he paid close attention to the segments related to the stomach (T5–9) and phrenic innervation (C2–4), and to the secondary related segments of the stomach (C5–T1) (see Figs 8.17 and 8.18). He looked particularly in the dermatomes and myotomes of T5–9 for hyperalgesic areas, hypertonic muscles, trigger points, painful vertebrae and joints that were (painfully) restricted in their function. He then decided to start acupuncture treatment.

The first time he tried appropriate segmental acupuncture points like the back points, ST-19–24, SP-16, BL-16–23 and 45–52, KI-17–21, LR-13, GV-4–9, CV-10–16. He manually stimulated these points in a mild, not painful way, in order to obtain the maximum benefit of the segmental interactions. He also tried PC-6 (as a distant point), which is situated in the secondary related segments, and which is known for its effect on gastric peristalsis.

After two treatments, part of the stomach complaints were relieved, but the overall effect was not really

satisfactory, so he revised his checklist; had he overlooked anything, could he do something about a possible general arousal, had he used the right stimulus for the right acupuncture points, or had he overlooked any perpetuating factors especially in the secondary related segments? Because long-present, visceral disturbances in the same segments, like cholelithiasis, could also be part of one of the vicious circles, he requested an echo of the upper abdomen, 'just to be sure'.

Again he examined his patient. This time, he noticed a slight, but distinct, homolateral pupil dilatation, a deeper homolateral nasolabial fold, and a homolateral area of goose flesh on the back together with a 'spine that curved around the affected organ'. He then looked for hyperalgesic areas, for areas with a diminished rollability, slidability and pliability, for hypertonic muscles with or without myofascial trigger points (all especially on the left side), for joint blockages and for vertebral blockages. He knew that trigger points in the abdominal wall muscles are a known possible maintaining factor in vicious 'myovisceral' circles, so if they were present he should inactivate them.

After a successful midthoracic spinal manipulation of T7/8 (the cook had had slight back problems for so long that he forgot to mention them), and after an injection with lignocaine 0.5% in two myofascial trigger points in the upper third of the rectus abdominis and in the erector spinae muscle (next to the spinous process of T8), the complaints considerably diminished, and the acupuncture points that he had used during the first few sessions became much more effective. Over the next few months, the cook came to his doctor only once in a while, 'more for preventive reasons'.

REFERENCES

Atweh S F, Dajani B D, Saadé N E, Jabbur S J 1985 Supraspinal inhibition of trigeminal input into subnucleus caudalis by dorsal column stimulation. Brain Research 348:401–404

Baldry P 1993 Acupuncture, trigger points and musculoskeletal pain, 2nd edn. Churchill Livingstone, Edinburgh

Basbaum A, Fields H 1978 Endogenous pain control mechanisms: review and hypothesis. Annals of Neurology 4:451–462

Bennett J A, Goodchild C S, Kidd C, McWilliam P N 1986 The location and characteristics of sympathetic preganglionic neurones in the lower thoracic spinal cord of dog and cat. Quarterly Journal of Experimental Physiology 71:79–92

Bogduk N, Twomey L 1987 Clinical anatomy of the lumbar spine. Churchill Livingstone, New York, pp 541–556

Bonica J 1984 Local anaesthesia and regional blocks. In: Wall P, Melzack R (eds) Textbook of pain. Churchill Livingstone, Edinburgh, pp 541–557

Bowsher D 1976 Role of the reticular formation in responses to noxious stimulation. Pain 2:361–378

Brodal A 1969 Neurological anatomy. Oxford University Press, London

Brooks C 1983 Newer concepts of the autonomic systems role derived from reductionist and behavioral studies of various animal species. Journal of the Autonomic Nervous System 7:199–212

Carpenter M B 1985 Core text of neuroanatomy, 3rd edn. Williams & Wilkins, London

Chandler Elliott H 1969 Textbook of neuroanatomy. Blackwell Scientific, Oxford

Chusid J 1982 Correlative neuroanatomy and functional neurology. Lange Medical, California

Dicke E, Schliack H 1982 Bindegewebsmassage. Hippokrates Verlag, Stuttgart

Dosch P 1986 Lehrbuch der Neuraltherapie nach Huneke. Karl Haug Verlag, Heidelberg

Duus P 1980 Neurologisch-topische Diagnostik. Thieme, Stuttgart

Gray B, Dostrovsky J 1983 Descending inhibitory influences from periaqueductal gray, nucleus raphe magnus and adjacent reticular formation. Journal of Neurophysiology 49:932–947

Grieve G 1988 Moderne manuele therapie van de wervelkolom deel 1. De tijdstroom, Lochem

Gunn C C 1989 Treating myofascial pain. University of Washington, Seattle

Han J S 1987 The neurochemical basis of pain relief by acupuncture. Beijing Medical University, Beijing

Hansen K, Schliack H 1962 Segmentale Innervation. Ihre Bedeutung fuer Klinik und Praxis. Georg Thieme Verlag, Stuttgart

Howson D C 1978 Peripheral neural excitability, implications for TENS. Physical Therapy 58:1467–1473

Hu J et al 1981 Functional properties of neurons in cat trigeminal subnucleus caudalis. Journal of Neurophysiology 45:173–192

Janig W 1990 The sympathetic nervous system in pain, physiology and pathophysiology. In: Stanton-Hicks (ed) Pain and the sympathetic nervous system. Kluwer, Boston

Koizumi K, Brooks C 1984 The spinal cord and the autonomic nervous system. In: Davidoff (ed) Handbook of the spinal cord, vols 2 and 3. Marcel Dekker, New York, pp 779–795

Kunert W 1963 Wirbelsaule, Vegetatieves Nervensystem und innere Medizin. Ferdinand Enke Verlag, Stuttgart

Li C L, Bak A 1976 Excitability characteristics of the A and C fibers in a peripheral nerve. Experimental Neurology 50:67–79

Lullies H, Trincker D 1973 Taschenbuch der Physiologie II. G. Fischer Verlag, Stuttgart

Macdonald A J R 1983 Segmental acupuncture therapy. Acupuncture and Electro-Therapeutics Research International 8:267–282

MacKenzie J 1917 Krankheitszeichen und ihre Auslegung. Kabitzsch Verlag, Würzburg

Martinez Martinez P F A 1980 Neuroanatomie. Bunge, Utrecht

Monnier M 1968 Functions of the nervous system, vol 1. Elsevier, Amsterdam

Oldfield B J, McLachlan E M 1980 The segmental origin of preganglionic axons in the upper thoracic rami of the cat. Neuroscience Letters 18:11–17

Oostendorp R 1988 Functionele vertebrobasilaire insufficientie [academic thesis]. Nijmegen

Robertson D R 1987 Sympathetic preganglionic neurons in frog spinal cord. Journal of the Autonomic Nervous System 18:1–11

Rohen J W 1985 Functionelle Anatomie des Nervensystems. Schattauer Verlag, Stuttgart

Sato A, Schmidt R F 1973 Somatosympathetic reflexes: afferent fibers, central pathways, discharge characteristics. Physiological Reviews 53:916–947

Shigenaga Y, Okamoto T, Nishimori T, Suemune S, Nasution I D, Chen I C, Tsuru K, Yoshida A, Tabuchi K, Hosoi M 1986 Oral and facial representation in the trigeminal principal and rostral spinal nuclei of the cat. Journal of Comparative Neurology 244:1–18

Stux G, Pomeranz B 1986 Acupuncture textbook and atlas. Springer Verlag, Berlin

Sutter M 1983 Diagnostische Weichteiltpalpation des Bewegungsapparates. Manuelle Medizin 21:120–122

Travell J G, Simons D G 1983 Myofascial pain and dysfunction. The trigger point manual: the lower extremities, vol 2. Williams & Wilkins, Baltimore

Travell J G, Simons D G 1992 Myofascial pain and dysfunction. The trigger point manual: the lower extremities, vol 2. Williams & Wilkins, Baltimore

van Cranenburgh B 1987 Segmentale verschijnselen. Bohn, Scheltema en Holkema, Utrecht

van Cranenburgh B 1989a Inleiding in detoegepaste neurowetenschappen, deel 1, Neurofilosofie. De Tijdstroom, Lochem

van Cranenburgh B 1989b Inleiding in detoegepaste neurowetenschappen, deel 3, Pijn. De Tijdstroom, Lochem

FURTHER READING

Bonica J 1976 Advances in pain research and therapy, vol I. Raven, New York

Brown A 1982 The dorsal horn of the spinal cord. Quarterly Journal of Experimental Physiology 67:193–212

Cervero F 1982 Noxious intensities of visceral stimulation are required to activate viscerosomatic multireceptive neurons in the thoracic spinal cord of the cat. Brain Research 240:350–352

Cervero F, Iggo A 1980 The substantia gelatinosa of the spinal cord: a critical review. Brain 103:717–772

Elze C 1957 Headsche zonen und dermatomen. Nervenartzt 28:465

Ernst M, Lee M H M 1985 Sympathetic vasomotor changes induced by manual and electrical acupuncture of the hoku point visualized by thermography. Pain 21:25–33

Ernst M, Lee M H M 1986 Sympathetic effects of manual and electrical acupuncture of the tsusanli knee point: comparison with the hoku hand point sympathetic effects. Experimental Neurology 94:1–10

Fields H 1987 Pain. McGraw-Hill, New York

Fitzgerald M, Lynn B 1979 The weak excitation of some cutaneous receptors in cats and rabbits by synthetic substance P. Journal of Physiology 293:66–67

Frost F A, Jessen B, Siggaard-Andersen J 1980 A controlled, double-blind comparison of mepivacaine injections versus saline injection for myofascial pain. Lancet (1):499–501

Kendall F, Kendall E 1983 Muscles, testing and function. Williams & Wilkins, Baltimore

Kerr F W L 1975 Neuroanatomical substrates of nociception in the spinal cord. Pain I:325–356

Macdonald A J R 1980 Abnormally tender muscle regions and associated painful movements. Pain 8:197–205

Melzack R, Stillwell D M, Fox E J 1977 Trigger points and acupuncture points for pain: correlations and implications. Pain 3:3–23

Rexed B 1952 The cytoarchitectonic organization of the spinal cord in the cat. Journal of Comparative Neurology 96:415–496

Schliack H 1963 Die anatomischen Grundlagen einer Segmenttherapie. Therapiewoche 13:1080

Warwick R, Williams P L 1973 Gray's anatomy. Longman, London

Wall P D 1978 The gate-control theory of pain mechanisms: a re-examination and re-statement. Brain 101:1–18

Wall P, Noordenbos W 1977 Sensory functions which remain in man after complete transection of dorsal columns. Brain 100:641–653

9

Acupuncture and the peripheral nervous system

C. Chan Gunn

INTRODUCTION

Western research into acupuncture has focused on the neurochemical basis of acupuncture analgesia and the CNS. In doing so, it has ignored the peripheral nervous system (PNS), and overlooked some important clues to acupuncture's effectiveness.

This paper reviews the relationship of acupuncture to the PNS, and proposes a model based on radiculopathy (which is peripheral neuropathy occurring at the nerve root). This model helps clarify many of the mysteries surrounding acupuncture and how it works in so many different conditions, including chronic pain. The model also shows that many traditional Chinese concepts can be reconciled with today's understanding of physiology.

Before describing the proposed radiculopathy model, the term 'acupuncture' will be examined. 'Acupuncture' is a word of Western origin which was coined in the sixteenth century to describe the Chinese use of a needle to promote healing in certain diseases. The Chinese themselves referred to this technique by many different names (e.g. 'needle effect', 'needle skill', or 'needle therapy') all of which indicate the central role of the needle. 'Acupuncture' can be confusing because it is used in medical literature to refer to a number of related, but not necessarily identical, modalities. The span of acupuncture's effectiveness depends on the modality used, combined with the knowledge and skill of the practitioner.

Varieties of acupuncture

It should be emphasized that classical or traditional acupuncture in China is only part of the whole philosophy of TCM (Sivin 1987). Most Western medical doctors practising acupuncture, or medical acupuncturists, have had training in classical acupuncture, but few practise the ancient principles of TCM, even though they continue to use TCM nomenclature and terminology. Medical acupuncturists, for instance, do not use TCM techniques such as pulse diagnosis for examination. They accept, instead, the neurochemical explanation for acupuncture analgesia; consequently, many of them restrict their practice to pain management. Many medical acupuncturists, in effect, use acupuncture as a form of trigger point therapy (Chapman & Gunn 1990); or as a procedure for electric stimulation (Lee & Liao 1990). Some Western researchers have called electrical stimulation with surface electrodes applied over acupuncture points by the term 'acupuncture', but this is incorrect as acupuncture implies needling. It should be termed instead 'transcutaneous electrical nerve stimulation' (TENS).

Acupuncture becomes perplexing when all versions, despite different methodologies and rationales, are claimed to be effective for a wide range of applications—everything from asthma to allergic rhinitis, from addiction to chronic pain. If these claims are true, how can such a simple procedure have such a prolific range of benefits? By what mechanism is needling effective? Western research, which concentrates on pain, has thrown some light on the neurochemical basis of acupuncture analgesia (Han & Terenius 1982), but has not produced a satisfactory explanation for all of acupuncture's applications.

Intramuscular stimulation

In recent years, more and more medical doctors have replaced TCM concepts to practise a contemporary version that is better attuned to neuroanatomic principles. The Multidisciplinary Pain Center, University of Washington School of Medicine, uses and teaches a system of dry needling that relies entirely on neuroanatomy. Examination, diagnosis and treatment, as well as progress of therapy, are all determined according to physical signs of peripheral neuropathy (Gunn 1989a). The system, referred to as 'intramuscular stimulation' (or IMS) to distinguish it from other forms of needling, is now used at many pain centres throughout the world.

IMS and the proposed model have been developed from the writer's conclusions following clinical observations and research carried out over a period of more than 20 years (first at the Workers' Compensation Board of British Columbia and subsequently at the writer's pain clinic). Some salient conclusions that have led to the radiculopathy model proposed in this paper are:

- acupuncture points are nearly always situated close to known neuroanatomic entities, such as muscle motor points or musculotendinous junctions (Gunn et al 1976)
- points that are found to be effective for treatment belong, more often than not, to the same segmental level(s) as presenting symptoms or the injury (Gunn & Milbrandt 1980)
- these points usually coincide with palpable muscle bands (sometimes called trigger points) that are tender to digital pressure
- tender points are distributed in a segmental or myotomal fashion, in muscles supplied by both anterior and posterior primary rami—indicating radiculopathy (Gunn 1978)
- muscles with tender points are unfailingly shortened from spasm and contracture
- virtually all conditions that respond to needling demonstrate signs of peripheral neuropathy (Gunn 1989b, Gunn & Milbrandt 1978); these signs are not well known, and therefore frequently missed (Gunn & Milbrandt 1978)
- symptoms and signs typically disappear when the tender and tight muscle bands are needled (Gunn & Milbrandt 1980).

IMS practitioners therefore purposely seek out tender and tight muscle bands in affected segments for needling. Following needling, physical signs of peripheral neuropathy such as muscle spasm, vasoconstriction and tenderness often disappear within seconds or minutes, and it is extremely satisfying to see these signs disappear before one's eyes. Other signs, like trophedema, diminish gradually, maybe taking days or even weeks to disappear. Ultimately, however, all signs vanish following successful treatment. IMS practitioners, with extensive training in anatomy and neurophysiology, thus freed from the limited number of empirical points available in classical acupuncture, can be many times more effective than traditional acupuncturists.

Proposed radiculopathy model

This chapter reviews the specific effects of the needle on the PNS, and offers a model in which it is proposed that:

1. the many and various conditions amenable to needle therapy, including chronic pain, are essentially epiphenomena (or signs and symptoms) of abnormal physiology in the PNS that occur with radiculopathy (Gunn 1989b)
2. these various conditions (including any accompanying pain) improve when normal function is restored
3. the needle is a simple, yet unique tool, able to access the PNS to restore normal function.

In other words, although the needle in 'acupuncture' helps *many* conditions, they are but different facets of a *single* underlying condition—that is, radiculopathy. Needle therapy does not treat individual diseases. Rather, it aims to restore homeostasis to the entire patient. It helps many conditions by a single expedient—restoring normal function to the PNS.

SPONDYLOSIS AND RADICULOPATHY

Radiculopathy and denervation supersensitivity

TCM places great emphasis on Qi (Chi), the 'flow of energy' (Sivin 1987). Its physiological

equivalent is probably the flow of nerve impulses in the PNS. When the flow of nerve impulses is blocked, innervated structures are deprived of the trophic factor. This factor (thought to be a combination of axoplasmic flow and electrical input) is normally delivered by the intact nerve. It is needed for the regulation and maintenance of cellular function and integrity. Structures deprived of the trophic factor become highly irritable and develop supersensitivity according to Cannon & Rosenblueth's law of denervation (1949):

When a unit is destroyed in a series of efferent neurons, an increased irritability to chemical agents develops in the isolated structure or structures, the effect being maximal in the part directly denervated.

Not all physicians are familiar with the condition of peripheral neuropathy. It may be defined as a disease that causes disordered function in the peripheral nerve. Although sometimes associated with structural changes, a neuropathic nerve can, deceptively, appear normal. It still conducts nerve impulses, synthesizes and releases transmitted substances, and evokes action potentials and muscle contraction. Muscle cells innervated by the axon, however, become supersensitive and behave as if the muscle had indeed been denervated. They generate spontaneous electrical impulses that can trigger false pain signals or provoke involuntary muscle activity (Culp & Ochoa 1982).

Supersensitivity also affects nerve fibres. These become receptive to chemical transmitters at every point along their length, instead of at their terminals only. Sprouting may occur, and denervated nerves are prone to accept contacts from other types of nerves, including autonomic and sensory nerve fibres. Short circuits are possible between sensory and autonomic (vasomotor) nerves and may contribute to reflex sympathetic dystrophy or causalgic pain.

Cannon & Rosenblueth's original work (1949) was based on total denervation or decentralization for supersensitivity to develop. Accordingly, they named the phenomenon 'denervation supersensitivity'. Today, however, it is known that physical interruption and total denervation are not necessary. Any circumstance that impedes the flow of motor impulses for a period of time can rob the effector organ of its excitatory input, and can cause *disuse* supersensitivity in that organ *and in associated spinal reflexes* (Sharpless 1975).

The importance of disuse supersensitivity cannot be overemphasized. When a nerve malfunctions, the structures it supplies become supersensitive and will behave abnormally. These structures overreact to many forms of input, not only chemical but physical inputs including stretch and pressure. Disuse supersensitivity is basic and universal, yet not at all well known or credited.

Spondylosis and degeneration

It is not unusual for the flow of nerve impulses to be obstructed. Peripheral neuropathy, which is often accompanied by partial denervation, is not exceptional in adults. There are innumerable causes of peripheral nerve damage, such as trauma, inflammation and infection; they may be from metabolic, degenerative, toxic and other conditions. The nerve's response to any agent, however, is always the same: dysfunction of the nerve.

Spondylosis is probably the most common cause of peripheral neuropathy (Gunn 1978). The spinal nerve root, because of its vulnerable position, is notably prone to injury from pressure, stretch, angulation and friction. Because spondylosis follows wear and tear, radiculopathy is typically seen in middle-aged individuals.

Ironically, radiculopathy itself contributes to degenerative conditions (including spondylosis!). Radiculopathy degrades the quality of collagen, causing it to have fewer cross-links: it is therefore more frail than normal collagen (Klein, Dawson & Heiple 1977). The amount of collagen in soft and skeletal tissues is also reduced. Because collagen lends strength to ligament, tendon, cartilage and bone, neuropathy can expedite degeneration in weight-bearing and activity-stressed parts of the body—which include the spine and joints.

EFFECTS OF RADICULOPATHY

This section reviews some of the repercussions of radiculopathy on the PNS. The effects of radiculopathy vary according to the type (sensory, motor, autonomic or mixed) and distribution of nerve fibres involved. All denervated structures can develop supersensitivity (including skeletal muscle, smooth muscle, spinal neurons, sympathetic ganglia, adrenal glands, sweat glands and brain cells).

Contracture and concurrent muscle shortening

Contracture, commonly referred to as 'spasm', is the evoked shortening of a muscle fibre in the absence of action potentials. It cannot be satisfactorily explained without reference to denervation supersensitivity.

Of the structures that develop supersensitivity, the most critical is striated muscle. Neuropathy can cause muscle contracture, with concurrent muscle shortening. These constant companions of musculoskeletal pain can be palpated as ropy bands in muscle (Fig. 9.1). Although shortened muscles are no longer

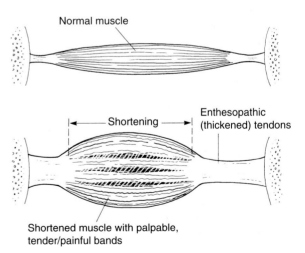

Figure 9.1 Neuropathy can cause muscle contracture, with concurrent muscle-shortening. (From Gunn C C 1996 The Gunn approach to the treatment of chronic pain. Churchill Livingstone, Edinburgh.)

believed to cause pain and tenderness by compressing normal nociceptors (Mense 1993), pain and tenderness may result when nociceptors are supersensitive. Thus, muscle bands, although usually pain free, can become focally tender and painful as trigger points.

When trigger points are numerous and widespread in the body, the condition has been called 'fibrositis', 'fibromyositis', or 'fibromyalgia'. This common condition causes much grief and distress because it is frequently misunderstood and therefore incorrectly treated.

Muscle shortening can cause further pain through mechanical pull. Such syndromes are discussed on pp 143–145.

Contracture is not maintained by volitional contraction, and cannot be ended by voluntary relaxation. When examined in the electromyograph (EMG), it is silent, as in a completely relaxed muscle; there are no motor units. The only findings are miniature endplate potentials (mepps) caused by the release of small packages or quanta of acetylcholine (ACh). This model postulates that these tiny potentials, although incapable of initiating contraction in normal muscle (which is sensitive to ACh only at the endplate region), can indeed initiate contraction in a supersensitive muscle that reacts to ACh along the entire surface of the fibre membrane. ACh slowly depolarizes the muscle membrane, and this induces electromechanical coupling.

Cannon described four types of increased sensitivity:

1. **superduration of response**, where the amplitude of responses is unchanged, but their course is prolonged
2. **hyperexcitability**, where the threshold for the stimulating agent is lower than normal
3. **increased susceptibility**, where lessened stimuli that do not have to exceed a threshold produce responses of normal amplitude and
4. **superreactivity**, where the ability of the tissue to respond is augmented. Contracture may thus represent muscle shortening of superduration, launched by mepps, in a superreactive and hyperexcitable muscle.

Trophedema, or neurogenic oedema, is a frequent companion of underlying muscle contracture. It may result from increased capillary permeability and impaired lymphatic drainage. Trophedema is easily confirmed by the 'peau d'orange' effect, or the matchstick test: trophedema cannot be indented by digital pressure, but when a blunt instrument is used, like the end of a matchstick, the indentation produced is clear cut and persists for many minutes (Gunn & Milbrandt 1978).

Radiculopathy and segmental autonomic reflexes

The actions of the sympathetic and parasympathetic systems are generally mutually antagonistic. The sympathetic system helps maintain a constant internal body environment, or homeostasis. It commands reactions that protect the individual, such as increase of blood sugar levels, temperature regulation, and regulation of vasomotor tone. The parasympathetic system lacks the unitary character of the sympathetic, and its activity increases in periods of rest and tranquillity. The TCM term 'rebalancing the Yin and Yang' (Yin and Yang representing opposing forces) probably parallels restoration of the balance between the two autonomic systems.

Sympathetic fibres in spinal nerves innervate the blood vessels of skin and muscle, pilomotor muscles and sweat glands. In emergency situations, there is a generalized sympathetic discharge and fibres that are normally silent at rest are activated: sweat glands, pilomotor fibres, adrenal medulla and vasodilator fibres to muscles. In radiculopathy, comparable reactions occur in the affected segment, *which indeed behaves as if it were in a state of emergency*. Vasoconstriction gives radiculopathy its cardinal feature—affected parts are discernibly colder, as may be shown by thermography. The pilomotor reflex is alerted, which may be manifested as 'goose bumps' in the involved dermatome; sudomotor activity may be profuse too.

Sympathetic fibres in visceral nerves innervate the intestine, intestinal blood vessels, heart, kidney, spleen and other organs (Fig. 9.2). As

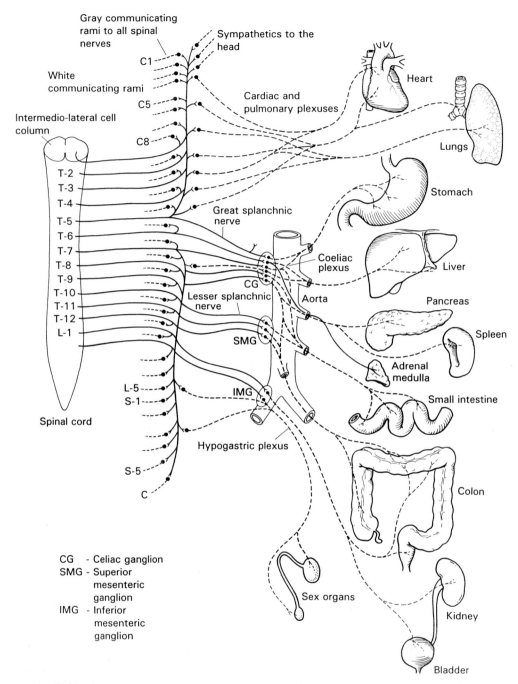

Figure 9.2 Sympathetic division of the autonomic system. (From deGroot J, Chusid G 1991 Correlative neuroanatomy, 21st edn. Appleton & Lange, reproduced with kind permission.)

with the somatic system, afferent impulses from the viscera connect with motor efferent neurons of the autonomic system in the spinal cord and brainstem. Fibres to the different visceral effectors are independent and discrete, and are carried out in reflex fashion. (Early TCM workers undoubtedly noticed the association between the autonomic system and viscera—thus naming meridians after them.)

Although modulation of autonomic reflexes is carried out in the CNS, supersensitive segmental autonomic reflexes can be influenced and restored to normal by releasing muscle contractures in involved segments. For example, epiphenomena (or manifestations) of radiculopathy, such as tension headache, cluster headache, even migraine and allergic rhinitis, improve when supersensitive sympathetic nerve fibres are restored to normal (C1–3, Fig. 9.2).

Upper gastrointestinal complaints are common, but symptoms like heartburn, gastroesophageal reflux, non-ulcer dyspepsia and peptic ulcer disease are often difficult to differentiate from those of the irritable bowel syndrome (abdominal pain, abdominal distention, relief of pain with defaecation, frequent stools with pain onset, loose stools with pain onset, mucus passage and the sensation of incomplete evacuation or tenesmus). The two groups of symptoms may indicate, respectively, dysfunction in the greater and the lesser splanchnic nerves (Fig. 9.2).

Upper gastrointestinal complaints are usually associated with mid-dorsal back pain and signs of spondylotic radiculopathy (such as tenderness and trophedema) in the mid-dorsal back (T2–5). The irritable bowel syndrome is generally associated with the lower dorsal back (T5–L1), but it is not uncommon for a patient to suffer from both groups. Dorsal spondylosis commonly remains silent until symptoms are precipitated by emotional stress or physical strain (lengthy air travel and carrying heavy baggage, for instance).

There is a tendency to overinvestigate these symptoms because they can suggest something benign or something serious. Since these symptoms respond quickly to the release of paraspinal muscle contractures in affected segments, however, it is feasible and probably preferable to try IMS first.

Parasympathetic fibres travelling in the vagus nerve are abundant in the thorax and abdomen; they slow the heart, enhance digestion and produce bronchial constriction. Problems of bronchial constriction and secretion may be relieved with treatment to the cervical and upper dorsal spine.

Radiculopathy and chronic pain

Chronic pain can be the outcome of any (or a combination of) the following: (1) continuous stimulation of Aδ and C fibres from ongoing nociception (such as an unhealed fracture), or from ongoing inflammation (rheumatoid arthritis, for instance); (2) psychogenic factors (which are outside the present discussion), and (3) functional disturbances in the nervous system, when there may be supersensitivity in the pain sensory system, but no actual excitation of nociceptors from extrinsic sources.

Radiculopathic (and neuropathic) pain belongs to category (3); it typically occurs in the absence of ongoing tissue injury, nociception or inflammation. It is secondary to a functional disturbance in the nervous system (radiculopathy), and is always, therefore, accompanied by signs of neuropathy (Thomas 1984), which resolve after successful treatment. When radiculopathic pain involves primarily the musculoskeletal system, it is commonly called myofascial pain.

Radiculopathic pain in this model is deemed to be the *sensory* expression of the mixed manifestations (sensory, motor, autonomic and mixed) that can occur with radiculopathy, and pain is not a feature unless nociceptive fibres are involved. Other features of neuropathic pain (Fields 1987) include: (1) delay in onset after precipitating injury (supersensitivity takes at least 5 days to develop); (2) unpleasant sensations such as dysaesthesiae, or deep, aching pain; (3) pain felt in a region of sensory deficit; and (4) paroxysmal, brief, shooting or stabbing pain. Mild stimuli can be very painful (allodynia). Significantly, additional pain may be produced mechanically by muscle shortening.

The shortened muscle syndrome

Physical force generated by a shortened muscle can give rise to many painful conditions (Gunn 1990), as in the following examples which are *motor* manifestations of neuropathy:

● Shortening gives rise to tension in tendons and their attachments—when protracted, tension can cause such syndromes as epicondylitis, tendinitis, tenosynovitis, or chondromalacia patellae (Box 9.1, and Fig. 9.3). Because these syndromes appear dissimilar and occur at different anatomical sites, they are not currently recognized as having the same aetiology.

● When muscles acting on a joint shorten, they limit the joint's range. An example is acute torticollis, which results from shortening of the splenius capitis and cervicis muscles; an extreme

---

Box 9.1   Common myofascial pain syndromes caused by the shortened muscle syndrome

Muscles shorten on neuropathy and can compress muscle nociceptors to generate primary pain in muscle. Shortened muscles can also cause secondary pain by mechanically overloading tendons and the joints they activate; this increases wear and tear and can eventually lead to degenerative changes in these structures. Musculoskeletal pain syndromes are, therefore, of great diversity. In radiculopathy, muscles of both primary rami are involved, and symptoms can appear in peripheral as well as in paraspinal muscles of the same segment (all of which should always be examined). When paraspinal muscles shorten, they can press upon nerve roots and perpetuate radiculopathic pain. It is also important to note that radiculopathy can involve the autonomic nervous system (see Fig. 9.2). Some common syndromes are:

Syndrome	Shortened muscle
Achilles tendinitis	Gastrocnemii, soleus
Bicipital tendinitis	Biceps brachii
Bursitis, prepatellar	Quadriceps femoris
Capsulitis, frozen	All muscles acting on the frozen shoulder: deltoid, trapezius, levator scapulae, rhomboidei, pectoralis major, supra- and infraspinati, teres major and minor, subscapularis
Carpal tunnel syndrome	The median nerve can be entrapped by the pronator teres, and the tendinous arch connecting the humero-ulnar and radial heads of the flexor digitorum superficialis (the sublimis bridge). Trophedema can compromise the nerve in the forearm and carpal tunnel
Cervical fibrositis	Cervical paraspinal muscles
Chondromalacia patellae	Quadriceps femoris
De Quervain's tenosynovitis	Abductor pollicis longus, extensor pollicis brevis
Facet syndrome	Muscles acting across the facet joint, e.g. rotatores, multifidi, semispinalis
Fibrositis, fibromyalgia, (diffuse myofascial pain syndrome)	Multisegmental radiculopathy
Hallux valgus	Extensor hallucis longus and brevis
Headaches, frontal	Upper trapezius, semispinalis capitis, occipitofrontalis
Headaches, temporal	Temporalis, trapezius
Headaches, vertex	Splenius capitis and cervicis, upper trapezius, semispinalis capitis, occipitofrontalis
Headaches, occipital	Suboccipital muscles
Infrapatellar tendinitis	Quadriceps femoris
Intervertebral disc	Muscles acting across the disc space, e.g. rotatores, multifidi, semispinalis
Juvenile kyphosis and scoliosis	Unbalanced paraspinal scoliosis muscles (e.g. iliocostalis thoracis and lumborum)
'Low back sprain'	Paraspinal muscles: e.g. iliocostalis lumborum and thoracis, multifidi (see also 'Intervertebral disc')
Plantar fasciitis	Flexor digitorum brevis, lumbricals
Piriformis syndrome	Piriformis muscle
Rotator cuff syndrome	Supra- and infraspinati, teres minor, subscapularis
'Shin splints'	Tibialis anterior
Temporomandibular joint (TMJ)	Masseter, temporalis, pterygoids
Tennis elbow	Brachioradialis, extensor carpi ulnaris, extensor carpi radialis brevis and longus, extensor digitorum, anconeus, triceps
Torticollis (acute)	Splenius capitis and cervicis

Reproduced with permission from Gunn C C 1989a

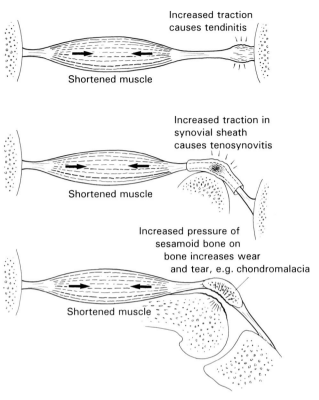

Figure 9.3 Shortening creates tension in tendons and their attachments and can cause such syndromes as epicondylitis, tendinitis, tenosynovitis, or chondromalacia patellae. (From Gunn C C 1996 The Gunn approach to the treatment of chronic pain. Churchill Livingstone, Edinburgh.)

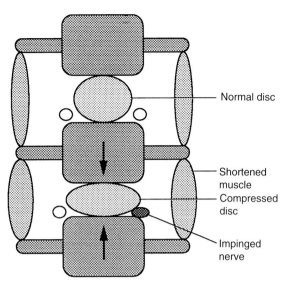

Figure 9.4 Shortened paraspinal muscles across an intervertebral disc space can compress the disc. (From Gunn C C 1996 The Gunn approach to the treatment of chronic pain. Churchill Livingstone, Edinburgh.)

example is the frozen shoulder, in which all muscles acting on the joint have shortened.

• Muscle shortening from contracture can upset joint alignment—hallux vulgus, for example, is due to shortening of the extensor hallucis longus muscle; the bunion is a secondary development.

• Increased pressure on the articular surfaces of a joint can cause arthralgia—as in medial knee joint pain. This pressure can lead also to a torn meniscus.

• Chronic restriction of joint range, misalignment and increased pressure on articular surfaces can eventually lead to degenerative arthritis or osteoarthritis.

• Pressure on a nerve can produce an entrapment syndrome—shortening in the pronator teres or pronator quadratus, for example, can give rise to symptoms of a carpal tunnel syndrome.

• The most critical of all the muscles that can shorten and press on, or pull upon, supersensitive structures to cause pain, are the paraspinal muscles that act across an intervertebral disc space. They draw adjacent vertebrae together, compress the disc, and narrow the intervertebral foraminae. The nerve root can be compressed by a bulging disc; or it can be irritated after it emerges from the intervertebral foramen (Fig. 9.4). A vicious circle can thus arise: pressure on a nerve root causes radiculopathy; radiculopathy leads to shortening in muscles, including paraspinal muscles, and shortening in paraspinal muscles further compresses the nerve root (Gunn 1989a).

The key to treating all radiculopathic conditions is releasing the shortened paraspinal muscles that pull adjacent vertebrae together and cause pressure on the disc and nerve root. *And here is where the acupuncture needle plays its unsurpassed role.*

CENTRAL ROLE OF THE NEEDLE

Acupuncture owes its full capabilities to the needle. The needle is the most effective instrument devised for stimulating the PNS through muscle receptors. (At least 40% of nerve fibres innervating a muscle subserve sensory rather than motor end organs.) A primary object of treatment is to release muscle shortening, and the needle does this more swiftly and precisely than any other physical therapy, including TENS or shallow percutaneous procedures (in which a needle is used to pierce skin to overcome skin resistance).

When the needle is inserted, it is deftly tapped through the skin to avoid alerting $A\delta$ nociceptive fibres located close to the surface. The needle is then eased through subcutaneous tissue and into muscle. The fine, pointed needle (unlike the cutting edge of a hollow needle used for injecting medications) pushes tissues aside and produces minimal tissue injury. Under normal circumstances, when there is no muscle shortening, the patient feels practically no sensation or pain. (C fibres sense pain only when there is cellular damage followed by the release of inflammatory, algogenic substances such as histamine, prostaglandin or bradykinin.)

Acupuncture and the current of injury

When the needle pierces muscle, it disrupts the cell membrane of individual muscle fibres, mechanically discharging a brief outburst of injury potentials referred to as 'insertional activity'. Less insertional activity occurs where muscle tissue has been replaced by fibrosis or necrosis, or where there is trophedema. Insertional activity is greater where muscle cell membrane has become hyperirritable.

Needle injury also generates long-lasting currents that are involved in repair and regeneration. The current of injury, first described by Galvani in 1797, has been shown (using a vibrating probe that can measure steady extracellular currents as small as $0.1\ \mu A/cm^2$) to generate up to $500\ \mu A/cm^2$ in a freshly amputated fingertip (Jaffe 1985). Unlike externally applied, short-lived forms of stimulation like massage or heat, the current of injury can provide stimulation for several days until the miniature wounds heal.

Stimulation by using the body's response to injury is an important resource, as desensitization of supersensitivity can take many days (Lomo 1976, Thesleff & Sellin 1980).

The needle's role in healing

Needle therapy has another unique advantage that other physical modalities do not: it causes local bleeding. Bleeding promotes healing by delivering numerous growth factors, including platelet-derived growth factor (PDGF) (Ross & Vogel 1978). PDGF attracts cells, induces DNA synthesis and stimulates collagen and protein formation; it is, in fact, the principle mitogen responsible for cell proliferation. Body cells are normally exposed only to a filtrate of plasma (interstitial fluid); they do not normally come directly in contact with the platelet factor, except in the presence of injury, haemorrhage and blood coagulation.

Needle-grasp, De Qi and muscle proprioceptors

When the needle penetrates a shortened muscle, it can provoke the muscle to fasciculate and release quickly—in seconds or minutes. A shortened muscle that is not quickly released, however, will invariably grasp the needle. This needle-grasp can be perceived by the physician when an attempt is made to withdraw the needle. Leaving the grasped needle in situ for a further period (typically 10 to 30 minutes) generally leads to objective release of a persistent contracture. Failure of a correctly placed needle to induce needle-grasp signifies that spasm is not present and therefore not the cause of pain—in which case, the condition will not respond to this type of treatment.

When there are several muscles, each with many muscle bands or fasciculi requiring treatment, it may be necessary to hasten contracture release by augmenting the intensity of stimulation. The traditional method is to twirl the grasped needle—a motion that specifically stimulates proprioceptors. All forms of stimuli have their specific receptors: massage excites tactile and pressure receptors; heat and cold activate thermal receptors; traction, exercise or manipulation stimulate muscle proprioceptors, and so on. As an alternative to twirling the needle, heat (moxibustion) or electrical stimulation is sometimes used.

How does twirling the needle work? When a muscle is in spasm, muscle fibres cling to the needle, and twisting causes these fibres to wind around its shaft. This coiling of muscle fibres shortens their length, converting the twisting force into a linear force. Unlike traction or manipulation, this stimulation is very precise and intense because the needle is precisely placed in a taut muscle band.

The needle-twirling manoeuvre vigorously stimulates muscle proprioceptors and gives rise to a peculiar, subjective sensation known in TCM as 'De Qi' (formerly written as Teh Chi) phenomenon. This distinctive sensation is an extreme version of the muscle ache felt in myofascial pain. Patients have variously described the sensation as 'cramping', or 'grabbing', or a 'dull, heavy ache'. De Qi is outside any normal experience of pain, and must be experienced in person in order to fully comprehend the unmistakable quality of myofascial pain. The muscle's grasp on the needle and the sensation the patient feels are both intensified as the needle is twirled to increase stimulation—until some moments later the shortened muscle is released with coincident disappearance of pain.

Twirling the grasped needle elicits the stretch or myotatic reflex (seen clinically in the knee-jerk). The reflex is activated by the muscle stretch and causes a contraction in that same muscle. Twirling the grasped needle is like stretching the muscle: it stretches muscle spindles, causing group-Ia fibres from the annulospiral endings to monosynaptically excite skeletomotor neurons that supply homonymous and synergist muscles. The same afferent volley disynaptically inhibits skeletomotor neurons that supply antagonist muscles.

Group-Ia and group-Ib fibres work together in close association; whereas the muscle spindle signals the velocity of muscle stretch and muscle length, the Golgi tendon organ (GTO) signals the velocity of muscle tension development as well as steady tension. Group-Ib fibres from the GTO make disynaptic inhibitory connections with both homonymous and synergist skeletomotor neurons.

By stipulating the needle-grasp and the De Qi phenomenon as requirements for diagnosis and treatment, TCM has perceptively recognized the central role of muscle proprioceptors in chronic neuropathic pain. Inserting a needle into normal muscle does not produce needle grasp or De Qi. $A\delta$ and C fibres, carriers of injury signals, are not primarily involved in chronic neuropathic pain; their incitement produces nociception, which elicits a different reflex—the flexion or withdrawal reflex.

The important observation is this: when a shortened muscle is released, all associated epiphenomena of peripheral neuropathy (including pain, tenderness and vasoconstriction) vanish from the treated area, and sometimes from the entire segment. Simultaneous resolution of the different epiphenomena by reflex stimulation may be explained by the overlap of neuronal circuits in the periphery (where two reflexes may share the same afferent receptor population), and in the spinal cord (where the same interneuronal circuit and/or motor neuron may serve more than one reflex; Fig. 9.5).

It is important to note too that the end product of any single spinal reflex, such as a muscle contraction, will itself initiate other reflexes.

CHALLENGES OF DIAGNOSIS AND TREATMENT
Clinical diagnosis

Diagnosing pain and dysfunction caused by radiculopathy can be difficult. A history gives little assistance. Pain often arises spontaneously, with no history of trauma; or else the degree of reported pain far exceeds that consistent with the injury. Laboratory and radiologic findings are generally not helpful either. Thermography can reveal decreased skin temperature in affected dermatomes but does not itself indicate pain or identify individual painful muscles.

Stimulus

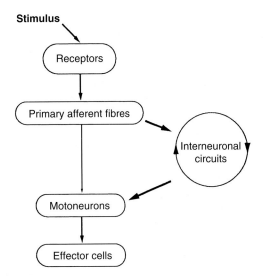

Figure 9.5   Information flow in the nervous system. Receptors transmit information to the CNS via primary afferent fibres, which synapse on to either motoneurons or interneurons. The latter may activate other interneurons, either in the cord or in the brain. Following complex patterns of interactions among these cells, information is fed to motoneurons and effector cells.

Signs of neuropathy are subtle, and differ from those of outright denervation (such as loss of sensation and reflexes). Radiculopathies are difficult to document with routine nerve conduction studies, which measure only the few fastest-conducting and largest fibres and take no account of the majority of smaller fibres. In focal neuropathy, nerve conduction velocities remain within the wide range of normal values, but F wave latency can be prolonged. Electromyography is not specific either.

In view of these considerations, diagnosis depends almost entirely on the examiner's clinical experience and acumen. A careful inspection for signs of motor, sensory, trophic, or autonomic dysfunction in the skin and affected muscles is necessary. Because changes in these conditions are primarily in muscle, even when symptoms appear to be in joints or tendons, signs in the muscles are the most consistent and relevant: increased muscle tone; tenderness over motor points; taut and tender, palpable contracture bands; and associated restricted joint range.

It is important to remember that, in radiculopathy, signs are generally present in the territories of both the posterior primary division and the anterior primary division of the affected nerve root or the formed nerve. Consequently, the symptoms are projected on to the dermatomal, myotomal and sclerotomal target structures supplied by the affected neural structure. Knowledge of the segmental nerve supply to muscles and bones is essential for diagnostic treatment. Each constituent muscle must be palpated and its condition noted. The most effective sites of dry needling are at muscle motor points and musculotendinous junctions. The procedure requires detailed knowledge of anatomy, and clinical skill comes only with practice. Moreover, because many paraspinal muscles are compound (e.g. the longissimus) and extend throughout most of the length of the vertebral column, the entire spine must be examined even when symptoms are localized to one region.

The needle as a powerful diagnostic tool

The needle is more than a therapeutic tool: it is a powerful diagnostic tool as well. Indeed, deep contracture can *only* be discovered by probing with a needle. Contracture is invisible to X-rays, CAT scans, or MRI, and contracture in deep muscles is beyond the finger's reach. The fine, flexible needle transmits feedback on the nature and consistency of the tissues it is penetrating. When it penetrates normal muscle the needle meets with little hindrance, when it penetrates a contracture there is firm resistance and the needle is grasped, and when it enters fibrotic tissue, there is a grating sensation (like cutting through a pear). Sometimes the resistance of a fibrotic muscle is so intense (the hardness can be mistaken for bone) that extreme pressure may be required to force the needle in.

Guided by the needle-grasp and the De Qi, an examiner is able to identify the distressed segment quickly, and with greater accuracy than with X-rays, scans or MRIs. Indeed, radiological findings may mislead by showing older, non-active lesions.

Treatment considerations

When irritation to a nerve is minor, neuropathy can be a transient condition, and releasing shortened muscles may be all that is necessary to restore function while the nerve heals. When shortened muscles are released, pain and joint range improve. Treating the several most painful shortened bands in the muscle is usually followed by relaxation of the entire muscle.

In recurrent or chronic pain, fibrosis generally becomes a feature of the contractures, and response to treatment is then much less dramatic and less effective. The extent of fibrosis is not necessarily correlated with chronological age; scarring occurs after injury or surgery, and many older individuals have less wear and tear than younger ones who have subjected their musculature to repeated physical stress. Treatment of extensive fibrotic contractures necessitates more frequent and extensive needling, and release of the contracture is often limited to the individual muscle band treated. To relieve pain in such a muscle, therefore, *all* tender bands require treatment. In chronic myofascial conditions, the needle can be used to disperse fibrotic tissue entrapping a nerve.

For long-lasting pain relief and restoration of function, it is essential to release shortened paraspinal muscles that are compressing a disc and irritating the nerve root. Surgical intervention is rarely necessary, as the needle can reach almost all shortened muscles.

The efficacy of IMS therapy for chronic low back pain was demonstrated by a randomized clinical trial involving a large group of patients in the British Columbia Workers Compensation Board (Gunn & Milbrandt 1980). At their 7-month follow-up, the treated group was clearly and significantly better than the control group. It is worth noting, however, as examination skill improves, that any physical change in the patient condition becomes self-evident and unmistakable.

DISCUSSION

Many Western researchers are unaware of neuropathic pain. They generally assume chronic pain to be ongoing signals of tissue damage (nociception or inflammation) conveyed to the CNS via a healthy nervous system. As a consequence, they are preoccupied with analgesia and the suppression of nociception. When endogenous opioids were discovered, these researchers assumed that acupuncture worked as a neuromodulating technique, activating multiple analgesia systems in the spinal cord and brain, and stimulating the endogenous pain suppression system to release neurotransmitters and endogenous opioids. However, neurochemicals are most likely to be released under stressful conditions (including drug and smoking withdrawal), which do not even necessarily produce pain. Their role may be to modulate the various homeostatic mechanisms and act as an endocrine–endorphin stress system that complements the neuronal regulatory system.

In fact, acupuncture's suppression of nociception is limited; acupuncture cannot be relied on to block the perception of a noxious input, and even in China it is not a popular choice for surgery.

CONCLUSION

Classical acupuncture is a clever TCM technique, and it is amazing that early workers, centuries ago, appeared to have comprehended so many fundamental principles of health and disease—principles that are often overlooked in today's technological age. These workers, with extraordinary insight, seemed to understand the nature of the trophic factor, the crucial flow of nerve impulses in the nervous system (Qi or Chi), and the need for balance in the parasympathetic and sympathetic autonomic systems (Yin and Yang). They described the critical role of proprioceptors (De Qi), and identified strategic loci (acupuncture points) where these could be accessed.

While many of its ancient philosophic concepts can be reconciled with modern physiology, classical acupuncture does have its limitations. With today's advanced scientific knowledge, however, we can build upon that classical knowledge. In intramuscular stimulation, diagnosis and treatment are correlated with physical signs of peripheral neuropathy, and the medical practitioner, thanks to extensive training in anatomy and neurophysiology, is able to treat any accessible part of the body without constraint by the limited number of traditional points prescribed in classical acupuncture.

The needle is effective in treating many diseases that are resistant to Western methods of treatment by accessing the PNS and reversing peripheral nerve dysfunction. The puzzle of how acupuncture works in so many different conditions is understood when these conditions are seen as being related to radiculopathy.

Because intramuscular stimulation is so effective, it should be taught in all medical schools. Knowledge of IMS can provide an excellent bridge between Eastern and Western medicine. Indeed, not only does IMS bridge the gap between them, it transcends the limitations of both.

REFERENCES

Cannon W B, Rosenblueth A 1949 The supersensitivity of denervated structures, a law of denervation. MacMillan, New York

Chapman C R, Gunn C C 1990 Acupuncture. In: Bonica J J (ed) The management of pain, vol. 2. Lea & Febiger, Philadelphia

Culp W J, Ochoa J 1982 Abnormal nerves and muscles as impulse generators. Oxford University Press, New York

Fields H L 1987 Pain. McGraw-Hill, New York

Gunn C C 1980 'Prespondylosis' and some pain syndromes following denervation supersensitivity. Spine 5(2): 185–192

Gunn C C 1989a Treating myofascial pain—intramuscular stimulation (IMS) for myofascial syndromes of neuropathic origin. HSCER, University of Washington, Seattle

Gunn C C 1989b Neuropathic pain: a new theory for chronic pain of intrinsic origin. Annals of the Royal College of Physicians and Surgeons of Canada 22(5):327–330

Gunn C C 1990 The mechanical manifestation of neuropathic pain. Annals of Sports Medicine 5(3):138–141

Gunn C C 1996 The Gunn approach to the treatment of chronic pain. Churchill Livingstone, Edinburgh.

Gunn C C, Milbrandt W E 1978 Early and subtle signs in low back sprain. Spine 3(3):267–281

Gunn C C, Milbrandt W E 1980 Dry needling of muscle motor points for chronic low back pain. A randomized clinical trial with long-term follow-up. Spine 5:3 279–291

Gunn C C, Ditchburn F G, King M H, Renwick G J 1976 Acupuncture loci: a proposal for their classification according to their relationship to known neural structures. American Journal of Chinese Medicine 4(2):183–195

Han J S, Terenius L 1982 Neurochemical basis of acupuncture analgesia. Annual Review of Pharmacology and Toxicology 22:193–220

Jaffe L F 1985 Extracellular current measurements with a vibrating probe. TINS December:517–521

Klein L, Dawson M H, Heiple K G 1977 Turnover of collagen in the adult rat after denervation. Journal of Bone and Joint Surgery 59A:1065–1067

Lee M H M, Liao S J 1990 Acupuncture in physiatry. In: Kottke F J, Lehmann F (eds) Krusen's handbook of physical medicine and rehabilitation, 4th edn. W B Saunders, Philadelphia

Lomo T 1976 The role of activity in the control of membrane and contractile properties of skeletal muscle. In: Thesleff S (ed) Motor innervation of muscle. Academic Press, New York, pp 289–316

Mense S 1993 Nociception from skeletal muscle in relation to clinical muscle pain. Pain 54:241–289

Ross R, Vogel A 1978 The platelet-derived growth factor. Cell 14:203–210

Sharpless S K 1975 Supersensitivity-like phenomena in the central nervous system. Federation Proceedings 34(10):1990–1997

Sivin N 1987 Traditional medicine in contemporary China. Science, Medicine, and Technology in East Asia Center for Chinese Studies, University of Michigan

Thesleff S, Sellin L C 1980 Denervation supersensitivity. Trends in Neurosciences 3(5):122–126

Thomas P K 1984 Symptomatology and differential diagnosis of peripheral neuropathy: clinical and differential diagnosis. In: Dyck P J, Thomas P K, Lambert E H, Bunge R (eds) Peripheral neuropathy. W B Saunders, Philadelphia, pp 1169–1190

Specialized forms of stimulation

SECTION CONTENTS

10

Electroacupuncture and acupuncture analgesia

Adrian White

INTRODUCTION

'Electroacupuncture' (EA) involves passing a pulsed current through the body tissues via acupuncture needles, for either therapy or analgesia. It came to the attention of the West when American doctors visited China in the early 1970s (Dimond 1971) and were amazed to discover acupuncture apparently being used as the sole analgesic for major operations. The technique had been introduced in 1958, when Chairman Mao had made a pronouncement that 'Chinese medicine and pharmacology are a great treasure-house; effort should be made to explore them and raise them to a higher level' (quoted in Peking Acupuncture Anaesthesia Co-ordinating Group 1973). At first, the anaesthetists had manipulated the needles throughout the procedure, but this was tedious and impeded the surgeon. Electrical pulse generators were therefore developed as a substitute for manual stimulation (Fig. 10.1).

Acupuncture analgesia (AA) was soon used throughout China: there had been 4900 operations under AA in Beijing alone by the time Dimond visited in 1971, and over half a million at the Beijing Children's Hospital by 1975. The technique was being used regularly for craniotomy, ENT surgery, dental extraction, thoracotomy, Caesarean section and limb surgery. Dimond (1971) gives one particularly graphic account in which a thoracic surgeon was himself undergoing a lobectomy under AA. He constantly quizzed the surgeon on his progress, and asked for a short

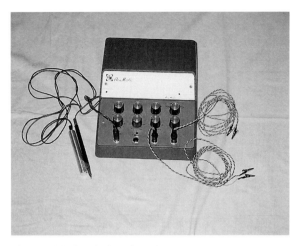

Figure 10.1 A typical modern electroacupuncture apparatus (Acupunctoscope B).

pause so that he could eat some fruit. The moment the lobe had been resected, he started discussing its pathological appearance with the surgeon. He was receiving AA to a single needle in the left arm, and appeared to have been given only 10 mg morphine preoperatively.

Other visitors witnessed similar events; for example, Spoerel (1975) observed AA in different centres and was impressed by the results in 87 operations. He reported that the technique varied considerably among different hospitals, particularly in the frequency of electrical stimulation used. Dramatic documentary films were shown on Western television in the 1970s of wide-awake patients undergoing major surgery under AA, talking to the surgeon and even eating and drinking. These images were a powerful stimulus to the increasing interest in acupuncture in the West.

Andersson (1973) demonstrated the time-course of analgesia from EA in experiments on dental students (Fig. 10.2). However, many Western scientists were resistant to the concept of acupuncture, which initially appeared to be based more on oriental philosophy than on proven anatomy or physiology. A leading article in the Lancet journal (1973) discussed acupuncture analgesia in positive terms, quoting Chinese research that indicated that large-fibre stimulation and an intact nervous system appeared to be

necessary for successful acupuncture analgesia. The proposal of the gate control theory of pain (Melzack & Wall 1965), the discovery of the opioid peptides (Hughes et al 1975) and the evidence for endogenous opioids release by acupuncture (Sjölund, Terenius & Eriksson 1977) provided a possible mechanism for AA and it suddenly appeared more credible to Western researchers.

There remained considerable doubt about the clinical value of AA, however. Modell et al (1976) thought that the selection and preparation of patients were crucial for success. He considered that Chinese anaesthetists were putting their enthusiasm for the technique before concern for their patients, and were asking them to tolerate much higher levels of pain than would be acceptable in the West. Some commentators thought that any genuine effect could be explained by hypnotic suggestion, distraction and political indoctrination. Others reasoned that the Chinese race must have a higher pain tolerance; for example, Johnson (1983) quoted reports from Western missionaries to China in the nineteenth century, who had been astonished at the stoical attitudes of the Chinese and their tolerance of the pain of surgery. On the other hand Knox, Shum & McLaughlin (1977) found no evidence of greater tolerance to pain in Eastern compared with Western individuals.

It is now generally accepted that the original Chinese claims of an 80% success rate were overinflated. Murphy & Bonica (1977) estimated that AA was used in only 10% of operations in China and that, by Western standards, the response was satisfactory in only 30% of these cases. Mann (1974) reported that analgesia was satisfactory in only 10% of subjects. Thus acupuncture is clearly not reliable enough on its own to be a substitute for established anaesthetic techniques in the West. Nevertheless, when combined with general anaesthesia it may have more to offer; this technique evolved in China for children (Peking Children's Hospital 1975), and in Austria and Germany (Hollinger et al 1979) and will be discussed below.

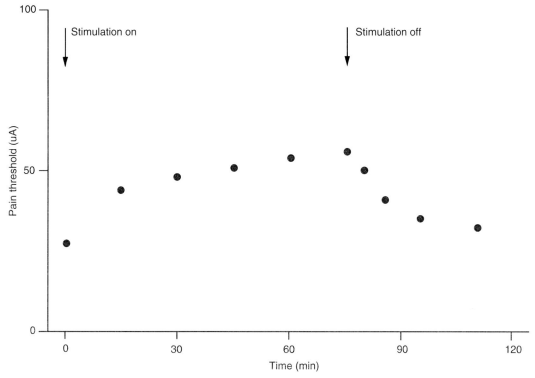

Figure 10.2 Changes in dental pain threshold to painful electrical stimulus induced by electroacupuncture stimulation of LI-4 via needles. (After Andersson et al 1973 with permission of Elsevier Science.)

After reports of the use of EA in surgery appeared, it was soon applied to the treatment of chronic pain. The history of electrotherapy has been well documented by Macdonald (1993). Electrostimulation techniques that do not penetrate the skin with needles, e.g. Ryodoraku (see Ch 3), Voll, VEGA, will not be discussed in detail in this chapter.

MECHANISMS

This brief summary of acupuncture mechanisms is intended only as a background for the following discussion of electroacupuncture analgesia. It is limited to, first, an outline of the direct and indirect effects at the spinal segment, and, secondly, the effects on higher centres. Brief mention will be made of neurotransmitters, and some comparisons will be made with other forms of stimulation-produced analgesia. (See Ch 6 for further details on mechanisms.)

Direct effects on the segment

Acupuncture needles stimulate Aδ nerve fibres in muscle. More precisely, they stimulate the muscle mechanoreceptors, and are probably most effective when they are manipulated to produce needling sensation (De Qi), or electrically stimulated to produce muscle contractions. The Aδ fibres synapse in the dorsal horns of their own and adjacent segments, and proceed to the brain. In the dorsal horn, they release opioid peptides (probably mainly met-enkephalin), which 'close the gate' to pain—that is, they inhibit the transmission of the nociceptive impulses in C fibres. Additionally, the Aδ fibres may influence the autonomic activity of that segment.

Indirect effects on the segment

The Aδ fibres pass on to the cortex where acupuncture stimuli reach the level of awareness. As the fibres travel through the brainstem, they send off collaterals to the medulla, releasing β-endorphin. This in turn sets off a downward influence on all levels of the spinal cord, called 'descending inhibitory control', a process that involves serotonin as a transmitter. The inhibitory effect operates by releasing opioid peptides at the dorsal horn, and so reinforces the local segmental effects of acupuncture, producing widespread analgesia throughout the body.

The full details are still not known, and there is little doubt that other transmitters and other descending inhibitory systems will prove to be relevant to acupuncture analgesia.

Effects on higher centres

Hypothalamus

Aδ fibres send collaterals not only to the brainstem as above, but also to the hypothalamus. Thus acupuncture may produce autonomic effects that strengthen the body's homeostatic responses.

Pituitary

Acupuncture may influence the pituitary via the hypothalamus, and can bring about the release of β-endorphin into the circulation. This does not seem to be an integral part of the mechanism of analgesia, and its clinical importance is still uncertain. Beta endorphin is produced by the breakdown of pro-opiocortin and is therefore accompanied by the release of ACTH. Stress also releases β-endorphin and ACTH, but independently of EA (Willer et al 1981).

Neurotransmitters

Four neurotransmitters have so far been discovered to have a role in acupuncture analgesia: serotonin and the three opioid peptides β-endorphin, met-enkephalin and the dynorphins. Serotonin is involved in descending inhibitory control; β-endorphin and met-enkephalin also inhibit pain, whereas the effect of the dynorphins may be inhibitory or facilitatory depending on the background activity of the CNS. This is a highly complex balance of many factors, and it can be modulated on a short-term basis, or altered more permanently (neuroplasticity), for example in chronic pain, as a result of persistent C fibre stimulation.

The release of different transmitters depends to an extent on the frequency of stimulation. Low-frequency EA releases β-endorphin in the brainstem and hypothalamus, and met-enkephalin and dynorphins in the spinal cord; high-frequency EA releases dynorphins and serotonin. Prolonged electrical stimulation also releases endogenous antagonists to these opioid peptides, such as cholecystokinin (CCK-8).

Other stimuli

Standard (high-frequency) TENS has similar segmental effects to acupuncture, but acts by stimulating the vibration-sensitive Aβ nerve fibres and thus releasing γ-aminobutyric acid (GABA) in the dorsal horn. This analgesic effect of TENS at the dorsal horn is also reinforced by descending inhibitory control in the same way as described above.

Low-frequency TENS has some obvious similarities to EA, and is sometimes called acupuncture-like TENS, although it has been shown to produce different clinical responses. For example Thomas et al (1995) found that the pain of dysmenorrhoea could be prevented by premenstrual treatment with high-frequency acupuncture but not high-frequency TENS. Both modalities were effective at low frequency.

Noxious stimuli can cause profound analgesia over wide regions of the body through a mechanism known as diffuse noxious inhibitory control (DNIC). Terror can produce a similar effect, at least in animals.

The understanding of the enormously complex mechanisms of pain and analgesia has advanced considerably over the last 20 years. Research is complicated by interspecies differences, by genetic variation between individuals, by changes in responses over time and by differential responses to antagonists such as naloxone. Areas of current interest that hold promise are changes in the response of convergent neurons, balance between agonists and antagonists within the neuronal networks, and that between peripheral and central mechanisms of pain and its modification.

STIMULUS PARAMETERS

A number of parameters need consideration in EA. They are summarized in Table 10.1, and individual parameters are discussed below.

Voltage

The voltage must be sufficient to overcome the resistance of the tissues, and deliver a current that will depolarize the nerve endings; this current is typically in the region of 20 mA but depends on the diameter of the nerve (see next section). Ohm's law states that:

$$\text{current (A)} = \frac{\text{voltage (V)}}{\text{resistance } (\Omega)}$$

The skin has a high resistance, so it requires a voltage of 40 V to deliver a current of 20 mA transcutaneously by TENS:

$$20 \text{ mA} = \frac{40 \text{ V}}{2000 \, \Omega}$$

When the skin resistance is by-passed by a needle, a lower voltage is required, so typical figures for EA might be:

$$20 \text{ mA} = \frac{12 \text{ V}}{600 \, \Omega}$$

Table 10.1 Parameters of electroacupuncture stimulation

Voltage	Up to 20 V
Current	10–50 mA
Wave-form	Square wave
Pulse width	0.05–0.5 ms
Polarity	Biphasic
Frequency ranges	Low <10 Hz
	medium 10–100 Hz
	high >100 Hz
	(any combination of the above)

Wave-forms differ in their efficiency at depolarizing nerves, so careful attention to the design of the apparatus will permit the use of the smallest currents.

Current

The analgesia produced by electroacupuncture is virtually an all-or-nothing response, i.e. the current must be above a particular threshold (Fig. 10.3). Experimentally, Pomeranz (1989) showed that analgesia develops as soon as the current is sufficiently strong to stimulate the type II and III muscle afferents, equivalent to Aδ fibres. Schimek et al (1982) recorded the EEG responses to experimental pain while gradually increasing the EA current; EEG pain responses disappeared abruptly at a particular current threshold, at the same moment that the patients felt subjective relief of pain. Mao et al (1980) demonstrated clinically in a crossover trial that high-intensity EA was significantly better at relieving chronic pain in patients than was low-intensity EA.

This high level of stimulation is likely to be accompanied by visible contractions since the needle is inserted into skeletal muscle (Stewart, Thomson & Oswald 1977); muscle twitching was observed in the earliest operations in China (e.g. Dimond 1971). Andersson (1993) has pointed out the interesting parallel between EA and forceful

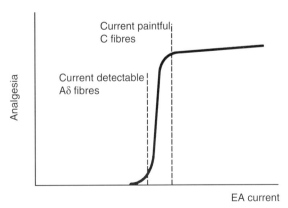

Figure 10.3 Diagrammatic illustration of the relationship between increasing EA current, level of analgesia and strength of sensation as different classes of nerve fibre are recruited.

muscular exercise. Both increase the levels of β-endorphin in the CNS, and both lead to pain relief and improvements in mood. It may be added that both have cumulative effects provided they are repeated frequently enough.

The sensation felt by the patient is strong but not painful. The effective intensity can be identified as just below the pain threshold, and is often associated with a 'pounding' sensation, which seems important for success. Willer et al (1982) and others have emphasized that the analgesic effect was achieved the moment stimulation was increased to a level that would 'induce muscular contractions, as well as cause a painful (but tolerable) sensation described as muscular deep pain mixed with cutaneous prick'. Other descriptions of the sensation are 'good and strong, definite but not painful'.

The different sensations that are felt depend on the tissue being stimulated, as Ishimaru, Kawakita & Sakita (1995) showed in elegant experiments with needles insulated with acrylic resin except at the tip. Needle penetration was monitored by ultrasound, and, interestingly, electrical and manual stimulation at each depth produced similar sensations: in skin, numbness and heat spreading over the surface; in muscle, twitching without any particular sensation, and dull heavy pain, sometimes cramp-like with stronger EA; in fascia, a severe and well-localized uncomfortable sensation; and in periosteum, a heavy unpleasant pain, occasionally sharp.

It should be mentioned here, for the comfort of patients, that Lundeberg et al (1989) showed that analgesia is greatest within the same segment for a given stimulation intensity. It is possible to increase the analgesia further by increasing the intensity above the pain threshold. Chung et al (1984a,b) recorded neuronal activity in the monkey spinal cord and found that increasing the level of stimulation to recruit C fibres does produce some additional analgesia. The mechanisms involved differ from those of EA, and include processes such as DNIC, in which an intensely painful stimulus at any site can induce analgesia (Le Bars, Dickenson & Besson 1979a,b). This observation is the basis of the combined technique (p 166).

Wave-form

The wave-form of the early Chinese stimulators was a spike, but Omura (1987) pointed out that the initial deflection of the pulse should be perpendicular in order to produce the optimal depolarization of nerve fibres. The square wave (Fig. 10.4) is therefore more usual in the West, as it is effective at the lowest possible current.

Pulse width

A pulse width of less than 0.05 ms is insufficient to depolarize nerve endings. Above this threshold level, the greater the pulse width the smaller the current that is required (Woolf 1989). However pulse widths that are greater than 0.5 ms are more likely to stimulate C fibres and cause pain. Most manufacturers therefore fix the pulse width within the range 0.05–0.5 ms. One apparatus, known as HANS, produces a pulse whose width varies from 0.2 ms to 0.6 ms inversely with the frequency (manufacturer's information). Ishiko et al (1978) demonstrated the hyperbolic curve of the strength/duration relationship.

Polarity

A unipolar current (i.e. one whose direction is entirely on one side of neutrality) carries the theoretical risk of causing ionization between the needle and the tissues. This could lead to

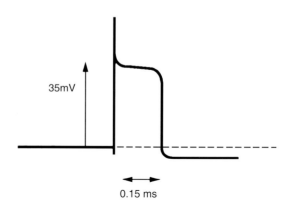

35mV

0.15 ms

Figure 10.4 Typical monophasic square wave (generated by Acupunctoscope system B).

weakening and breakage of the needle and local tissue necrosis from electrolysis, and the formation of hydrochloric acid (Omura 1975). To avoid this, the operator should reverse the direction of current halfway through treatment. More modern apparatus generates a biphasic wave in which there is no significant net flow of electricity. The initial square wave is followed by a negative pulse, commonly produced by the discharge of a capacitance (Fig. 10.5).

Frequency

For descriptive purposes, it is convenient to categorize the frequencies into those below 10 Hz, those above 100 Hz, intermediate and alternating (Fig 10.6). Different transmitters are released preferentially by different frequencies of stimulation, although there is considerable overlap (Chen & Han 1992). An excellent review is provided by Han & Terenius (1982).

It is now generally accepted that low-frequency EA up to about 10 Hz releases β-endorphin in the brain, and met-enkephalin and dynorphins in the spinal cord (e.g. Han & Sun 1990, Pomeranz 1989). Cheng & Pomeranz (1981) showed that

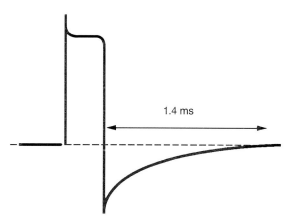

Figure 10.5 Typical biphasic wave-form, showing initial square wave followed by capacitance discharge (generated by KWD-808).

EA at 200 Hz is mediated by serotonin, although Mao et al (1980) detected increased serotonin levels in patients treated with 8–15 Hz.

Low-frequency stimulation of about 3 Hz was originally chosen by the Chinese for surgical analgesia since they were attempting to mimic manual stimulation. This frequency is still commonly used for surgical pain and for experi-

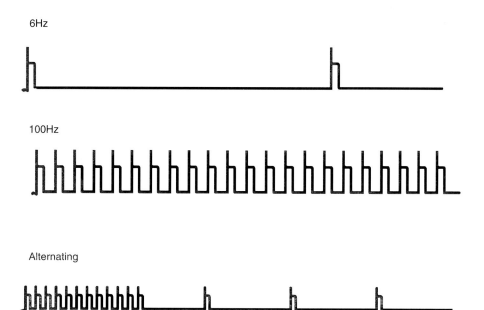

Figure 10.6 Slow, fast and alternating (or dense-dispersed) patterns of stimulation.

mental purposes, although some anaesthetists describe using frequencies up to about 50 Hz (e.g. Christenssen et al 1989, Pauser et al 1976).

When it comes to treatment of chronic pain, Thomas & Lundeberg (1994) have shown that low-frequency stimulation was preferable to both manual acupuncture and high-frequency in producing sustained relief of chronic back pain. However, Lundeberg et al (1989) found 2 Hz and 80 Hz to be equally effective at reducing experimental dental pain, when applied segmentally.

Electroacupuncture has been studied in a variety of other clinical conditions. Dundee et al (1989) explored the effect of 10, 20, 50 and 100 Hz on the reduction of nausea, and found that 10–20 Hz had maximum benefit. Medium frequency has been shown to have a specific effect in reducing experimental itch; Belgrade, Solomon & Lichter (1984) found that 40/80 Hz stimulation of the classical points (LI-10, SP-10, SP-6, unilaterally) significantly reduced the itch intensity produced by a standard injection of histamine. Lundeberg, Bondesson & Thomas (1987) agreed that the maximal effect was with 80 Hz rather than 2 Hz stimulation, but found it to be more effective when given locally rather than heterosegmentally. Itch has some features in common with chronic pain. On the other hand, the improvement in skin-flap survival with EA, as demonstrated by Jansen et al (1989), is the same whether the frequency is 2 Hz or 80 Hz.

Frequencies higher than 100 Hz exceed the refractory rate of muscle fibres, and rates much above 200 Hz exceed that of nerve fibres, although these very high frequencies are not without physiological effect.

Frequencies are often combined in order to release as wide a variety of neurotransmitters as possible, and to reduce the chance of accommodation of nerve endings. For therapeutic EA, for example, low frequency is often interspersed with periods at higher frequencies, alternating in intervals of about 3–6 seconds; the traditional term for this combination was 'dense-dispersed'. Other apparatus offers a sweep of frequencies between 1 and 99 Hz (Deluze et al 1992).

Needle design

Ishimaru et al (1995) explored the possibility of improving analgesia in deep tissues by using insulated needles with bare metal tips. Standard needles were effective at raising pain thresholds in skin and superficial fascia, but only the insulated needles raised pain thresholds in muscle or periosteum. If these findings are confirmed by others they provide an important advance in EA.

PRACTICAL CONSIDERATIONS

Contraindications to EA

Contraindications include:

1. patients who are unwilling to accept the technique
2. those who have a demand pacemaker; Fujiwara et al (1980) clearly showed that EA was capable of inhibiting (but not driving) a demand pacemaker, as shown in Figure 10.7
3. local contraindications.

As examples of the third category, EA should not cross the thorax because of the theoretical danger of interfering with the heart's conducting tissues. However, Hollinger et al (1979) found that maximum strength EA induced an electrical field of only 25–30 mV/cm around the heart, which is estimated to be one-eighth of the level required to cause ventricular fibrillation. (Advice not to connect points across the midline elsewhere in the body are less well founded and may have their origin in traditions of not transferring 'energy' between the two halves of the body.) It is also usually recommended that the region of the carotid body and sinus should be avoided, although Kho et al (1990) reported using LI-18 for thyroidectomy, apparently without complication. The standard restrictions to needling particular sites such as the pregnant uterus, oedematous tissue, etc. also apply.

When setting up EA a careful routine should be developed in order to instil confidence, since patients are often wary of electrical apparatus. The apparatus must be switched off before attaching the leads, with intensity set to zero; the intensity must be increased only slowly because

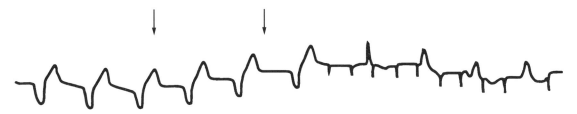

Figure 10.7 Inhibition of cardiac pacemaker by electroacupuncture. EA commenced at the first arrow with gradually increasing intensity. The initial six beats are paced beats, after which only spontaneous beats are seen as EA suppresses the pacemaker. The second arrow indicates elongation of the fifth paced interval, which indicates partial suppression of the pacemaker. (From Fujiwara et al 1980 with permission of *Chest*.)

the thresholds for sensation and pain are close together.

Complications

All the usual complications of acupuncture apply, but there are several that are specific to EA:

1. the result of the muscle contractions: needles may bend or break
2. direct injury from the current: large unipolar currents will increase the risk of electrolysis; local burns have occasionally been reported.

Basic features of EA apparatus

Essential features include:

- robust design, particularly the leads
- electrical reliability, including separation of channels
- clear controls, for easy accurate adjustment
- square impulse, with biphasic wave-form
- frequency range at least 2 to 200 Hz
- facility for automatic alternating or scanning of frequencies (including commonly used combination of 4 and 100 Hz)
- three or four output channels.

Useful options include:

- time-switch
- point-locator (2 mm ball electrode, and sensitivity adjustment)
- digital readout of frequency
- digital readout of current.

EA THERAPY

There are few clinical trials that compare EA and manual acupuncture (MA), and the choice is often a matter of personal preference and experience. Traditionalists dislike EA because it feels unnatural, whereas those with a scientific background may prefer it because it offers greater control and reproducibility, and is backed by neurophysiological research. Patients' opinions are relevant as some refuse any electrical procedure, whereas others find EA very relaxing.

Technique

In point selection, similar needle placements can be used for EA as for MA (e.g. either side of a painful area, within the same or adjacent segments, distally in classical points, or in the auricle). Needle sensation (De Qi, see Ch 3) is usually obtained before starting EA. The apparatus is connected to the needles in pairs, usually in the line of the segment or meridian since nerve fibres are excited at lower currents applied along their length than across their width.

Indications for EA therapy

EA is used most frequently for chronic pain, and clinically it appears to have benefits that outlast the temporary analgesic effect. Price et al (1984) pointed out that good pain relief reduces muscle spasm and permits active movement, improving circulation and encouraging healing. Any patient whose condition has not responded to MA

Table 10.2 Some common indications for electroacupuncture, and references to controlled trials

Category	Condition	Controlled trials
Nociceptive pain	Osteoarthritis and musculoskeletal pain, inc. chronic back pain	Loy (1983), Lehmann et al (1986), Thomas & Lundeberg (1994), Cheng & Pomeranz (1987),
	Gynaecology	Thomas et al (1995)
	Fibromyalgia	Deluze et al (1992)
	Acute renal colic	Lee et al (1992)
	Painful scars	
Neurogenic pain	Trigeminal and other neuralgia	
	Reflex sympathetic dystrophy	
Other	Nausea	Dundee (1989)
	Drug withdrawal	(see Ch 18)
	Stroke	Johansson et al (1993)
	Muscle spasm, e.g. post stroke	
	Depression	Luo, Jia & Zhan (1985)
	Skin disease	

should be considered for a trial of EA. Table 10.2 lists conditions for which EA is commonly used and authors of supporting trials, where these exist.

Results

Chronic painful conditions

Loy (1983) compared EA with physiotherapy in a trial of 60 patients with cervical spondylosis. All of the EA group obtained some relief, and six had complete relief; overall, there was 87% improvement in the EA group, compared with 54% in the physiotherapy group. Lehmann et al (1986) studied 54 patients with chronic back pain who were receiving an inpatient rehabilitation programme which included education and graded exercises. Subjects were randomized into three groups, receiving EA, TENS and dead-battery (placebo) TENS respectively. Pain, disability and range of movement were assessed, and subjects were asked to rate the contribution of each component of the rehabilitation. There was no significant difference between the groups; all participants rated the education as the most important component, which may have overshadowed any benefit of EA or TENS. There were, however, trends to greater improvement in all outcome measures for the EA group compared with TENS or control groups.

Cheng & Pomeranz (1987) randomized 131 patients with chronic pain into a standard EA group and a group who were treated by acupuncture-like TENS. Half of the subjects in both groups gained more than 75% pain relief; after 4 months the proportion had fallen to a fifth. Lee et al (1992) performed a randomized trial of electroacupuncture against a non-opioid/antispasmodic injection for renal colic. The degree of pain relief was similar for both treatments, but acupuncture had a significantly faster onset.

Deluze et al (1992) conducted a randomized single-blind controlled trial of high quality, in 70 patients with fibromyalgia. The active treatment consisted of 4–10 needles stimulated at just below the pain threshold, sufficient to produce visible muscle contractions; the frequency scanned from 1–99 Hz in intermittent pulses. Both patients and assessors were blinded, and tenderness, analgesic intake, pain scores and sleep quality were assessed, as well as global scores (patient and physician). The actively treated group showed significant improvements in seven out of eight parameters, which was significantly better than the control group in five measures. About a quarter of the treated group showed almost complete abatement of symptoms.

In another excellent study, Thomas & Lundeberg (1994) randomized 43 chronic low back pain patients into four groups. Ten subjects remained as waiting list controls, and the remaining 33 were given three initial treatment sessions, one each of manual acupuncture, low-frequency (2 Hz) or high-frequency (80 Hz), starting in random order. After receiving each treatment once, the patients continued with their preferred mode for a total of 10 treatments. Each treatment group showed significant reduction of pain with activity at the end of treatment, but only the 2 Hz group maintained these improvements at the 6-month follow-up. None of the groups showed significant changes in the range of joint movement. This trial introduces a novel attempt at achieving equal placebo effects in all groups, namely maximizing the placebo effects by allowing patients to choose the treatment they preferred. Lundeberg et al (1988) had previously shown the superiority of low-frequency EA in a review of 177 chronic pain patients.

Thomas et al (1995) compared the effect of different modes of acupuncture and TENS in a crossover trial for dysmenorrhoea. Treatment was given 7 and 3 days before menstruation. All modes except high-frequency TENS and sham TENS showed sustained improvement in pain.

Two uncontrolled studies are worth including, as they suggest differential success rates for different kinds of chronic pain, as well as including follow-up studies. Lee et al (1975, 1976) gave four sessions of EA to 533 chronic pain patients with a variety of diagnoses. More than half gained good pain relief (defined as over 75%) at the end of four treatments, although relief was only sustained for 3 months in half of these responders. The results were better for neuralgias (30%) than for osteoarthritis (20%). In a subgroup of 261 patients, there was no difference in outcome whether acupuncture was applied to genuine acupuncture points or to non-acupuncture areas.

In a retrospective report, Waylonis (1976) used a simplified technique with seven standard points and a frequency of 3–10 Hz for the treatment of 179 patients with a variety of painful conditions. Half of his subjects gained at least 50% relief of pain, and this relief persisted for over 3 months in 60% of those who responded to a follow-up questionnaire. The greatest benefits were seen in patients with 'fibrositis' and tension headache.

In summary, EA appears to produce long-term benefit in about 25% of patients with chronic painful conditions, including musculoskeletal pain. The balance of evidence points to low frequency being superior to high frequency. Further trials are needed, of improved design and in particular paying attention to ensuring the adequacy of treatment.

Non-painful conditions

Dundee & McMillan (1991) conducted a small controlled trial of EA treatment of nausea in cancer patients receiving chemotherapy, and a much larger observational cohort study. The active treatment was 5 minutes of EA at 10 Hz to the point PE-6. Ninety-seven percent of patients were either completely relieved of nausea or improved, without any identifiable side-effects.

Johansson et al (1993) used MA and EA in a controlled trial of acupuncture for acute stroke, and found a significant improvement in recovery of health status, together with an increased likelihood of being discharged home within the first year.

Luo, Jia & Zhan (1985) studied 27 patients with endogenous depression, administering EA between GV-20 and Yintang (EX-2) (subcutaneous needles, slanting towards each other) for 1 hour daily. The effect on depression was assessed with the Hamilton Depression Scale, and the results with EA were not significantly different from the comparison group of 20 patients who received standard therapy with amitriptyline. The patients who received EA also recorded a much lower incidence of side-effects.

Other conditions in which successful uncontrolled trials suggest that further study could be worthwhile include nocturnal enuresis (Tuzuner et al 1989), reflex sympathetic dystrophy (Chan & Chow 1981, Hill, Sin & Chandler 1991), neurodermatitis (Liu J 1987), uraemic pruritus (Liu JD 1987), tinnitus (Thomas, Laurell & Lundeberg 1988) and motion sickness (Hu, Stem & Koch 1992). A temporary effect on hypertension was recorded by Williams, Mueller & Cornwall (1991).

ACUPUNCTURE ANALGESIA

The term 'acupuncture analgesia' is used for the control of experimental or surgical pain, and is achieved by EA rather than by MA except for research purposes. The phenomenon was initially called 'acupuncture anaesthesia', but this is not an accurate term because other sensations such as touch and temperature are not reduced. This section is mainly concerned with AA for surgical procedures.

Suitable operations

The literature suggests that AA is currently used in China mostly for head and neck surgery, such as tonsillectomy, thyroidectomy and craniotomy, and for thoracotomy. Windsor (1984) reports that AA is no longer used for cardiac surgery because 'It is easier both for the patient and for the surgeon, particularly in complicated cases, to use general anaesthesia'. AA alone is inadequate for abdominal surgery because the muscles are not relaxed, and traction on the viscera is still painful.

The 'combined' technique has been reported as suitable for an extensive range of surgery: Hollinger et al (1979) presented a large series of open-heart operations in Germany, Kho et al (1991) a series of retroperitoneal lymph node dissection in the Netherlands, and P. Poulain (unpublished work, 1993) described gynaecological surgery in France. As skills improve, confidence grows to tackle other areas, but it is generally agreed that the best results are achieved in operations near the midline and in the upper half of the body, and the least success is with limb surgery. AA is most effective in operations that are completed within 30 minutes, and should not normally be attempted if the operation is likely to last more than 2 hours.

Patient preparation

Suitable patients

Subjects must be psychologically stable and co-operative, and be able to put their confidence in the anaesthetist and surgeon. Higher educational status of the patients improves the effectiveness, and good response to suggestion and distraction are important (Parwatikar et al 1978), but gender is not (Price et al 1984).

Counselling

Patients should be counselled in detail about the proposed procedure. If they are to remain conscious, it is important to prepare them for the strange experience that acupuncture affects only pain, and that touch, pressure, etc. will still be felt normally. Patients managed by the 'combined technique' often report awareness during surgery. They are not usually distressed by this but they should be forewarned (Hollinger et al 1979). In China, only those who are undergoing major surgery receive counselling. Qigong and other specific respiratory exercises (such as breathing with sandbags on the chest for half-an-hour daily!) are taught to patients who are scheduled for thoracotomy.

Assessment

A trial of AA may be conducted before surgery (Wong 1993), by recording the change of skin temperature during EA. A rise of 1°C is associated with an 85% success rate, but if the skin temperature remains constant or falls then the success rate falls to 35%. Skin temperature changes are further discussed by Thomas, Collins & Strauss (1992).

Drug interactions

The possible effects of diet and drugs on neurotransmitter release should be considered. A study by Eriksson, Lundeberg & Lundeberg (1991) showed that diazepam reduced the effect of low-frequency EA on cervical osteoarthritis in humans; and Xu et al (1983) showed that diazepam antagonized AA in rabbits, as did ketamine. The same authors also found that AA was potentiated in rabbits by fentanyl, pethidine, droperidol, perphenazine, metoclopramide, fenfluramine and tetrahydrocannabinol. Xu et al (1983) showed that metoclopramide improved the response to EA in humans undergoing thyroidectomy. In practice, premedication with diazepam and low-dose opioids is satisfactory, and was used successfully by Kho et al (1991).

A diet high in D-phenylalanine or D-leucine enhanced EA in rabbits (Cheng & Pomeranz 1980) but there is no evidence that this is important clinically.

Point selection

A dozen or more points were used in early operations in China, but over time there has been a trend towards fewer needles. A report from Peking Acupuncture Anaesthesia Co-ordinating Group (1973) describes how the number of needles used for pneumonectomy was reduced progressively from over 40 to one. Broedersdorff (1981) also gradually reduced the number of needles to two in each ear, but found this was an irreducible minimum.

Spoerel (1975) described four categories of point that could be used. He suggested that points from at least two categories should be combined, though not all authors agree.

Auricular points

There is wide variation in the auricular points recommended for analgesia, and indeed different systems of nomenclature are incompatible. Three points that are frequently used are the Shenmen, Lung and Sympathetic (Fig. 10.8) innervated by the trigeminal, vagus, and facial nerves re-

spectively. Points named after particular areas of the body are used as well.

Two studies compared the effectiveness of different auricular points. Kitade & Hyodo (1979) tested the level of analgesia to radiant heat at various sites of the body after stimulating various ear points. The results suggested that Lung is the most effective point, followed by Sympathetic, Shenmen and Kidney in that order. Neck point, and needling from Elbow to Arm, produced less analgesia, and a non-acupuncture point produced no analgesia at all. The study was not blinded.

Simmons & Oleson (1993) repeated the above study with blinded subjects and observers. Specific points for dental pain were stimulated by a probe, and a pulp-tester was used to measure analgesia. EA produced an average 18% increase in the pain threshold of the intervention group, which was partially reversed by naloxone. There were no significant changes in the sham group who received stimulation at inappropriate sites.

Broedersdorff (1981) used one needle threaded subcutaneously anterior to the pinna, and another in the helix crus.

Distal points

Several of the classical points are used commonly, particularly those on meridians that pass through the site of the surgery. The following points have been described as having particular attributes, mostly on the basis of clinical observation:

- LI-4 is used for tonsillectomy, dental work, etc.
- LI-4 and PC-6 are combined for thyroidectomy and glaucoma surgery
- ST-36 and SP-6 are used for lower abdominal surgery
- a new point posterior to ST-36 is called 'appendix point' and used for that indication.

In addition, a single needle traversing two points (TE-8 through to PC-4) was used as the sole analgesic for thoracotomy (Spoerel 1975). PC-6 may be added to prevent postoperative nausea and vomiting (Dundee 1989) and TE-9 to produce a vasodilatation in cardiac surgery (Hollinger et al 1979).

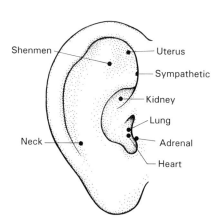

Figure 10.8 Some commonly used points on the auricle, according to a Chinese classification.

Segmental points

Lundeberg et al (1989) found that analgesia occurred at a lower stimulation intensity if the points were chosen from the same segment as the surgical field. Segmental points may be the paravertebral points in the appropriate segments (Inner Bladder line, or Huatuochiachi points), or local points that have the same innervation as the organ (e.g. LI-18 for thyroidectomy) or distal points in the appropriate site in the limbs.

When the patient is to remain supine, flat surface electrodes may be more convenient than needles in the paravertebral region, although needles can be threaded subcutaneously and the handles bent and secured with tape.

Paraincisional points

Analgesia from distal points may not be adequate for the pain of the incision, particularly in the abdomen (Dias & Subramanium 1984); sharp pain is modulated by A fibres, and is less responsive to opioids than is the dull ache of C fibre pain (Rieb & Pomeranz 1992). Long subcutaneous needles on either side of the proposed incision were described by Spoerel (1975), and TENS pads or local anaesthetic infiltration are alternatives.

Point stimulation

Most anaesthetists use a low-frequency current for EA, at the highest intensity that the patient can bear. It is usual to stimulate for about 20 minutes before testing for analgesia. Hyodo & Gega (1977) timed the onset of AA in 30 patients who were in labour: one patient responded within 5 minutes, and 90% within 20 minutes. In the remaining three patients, the onset of analgesia took more than half an hour. Patients often become relaxed when analgesia commences.

Manual acupuncture analgesia

MA releases opioid peptides in different proportions from EA, according to Nappi et al (1982).

It appears that MA may be less effective than EA, although Han, Ding & Fan (1986) suggested that manual stimulation may be preferable for prolonged surgery, since the opioid antagonist CCK-8 can be released by sustained electrical stimulation. Manual AA is still used with success in China; Wong (1993), for example, reported observing MA for pulmonary resection: 11 points were used, and different needles were stimulated according to which tissues the surgeon was working on at the time. However, Ekblom et al (1991) compared MA before or after dental surgery with standard local anaesthesia; the MA patients rated their pain significantly higher and satisfaction lower. Grabow (1994) found that manual stimulation was no more effective overall than placebo, although he stated that 'There is always a fixed proportion of individuals in whom pain can reliably and exclusively be treated by acupuncture as the sole method'.

Standard AA technique

Once the correct positioning of the needle has been confirmed by the sensation of De Qi, low-frequency electrical stimulation is started and increased to the maximum tolerable intensity. The intensity is adjusted as necessary to deal with accommodation, and stimulation is maintained at the same level throughout surgery.

Standard chemical analgesics may be needed in addition, for skin and visceral pain: local anaesthetic may be infiltrated into the skin before the incision, and pain caused by traction on the viscera may need local instillation of procaine. Patients must be observed closely for any indication of pain, and intravenous analgesics given if necessary. In the case of severe distress the anaesthetist should resort immediately to standard general anaesthesia.

Combined technique

The combination of AA and anaesthesia is the method of choice in the West. Good descriptions are given by Grabow & Criveanu (1976), Pauser et al (1976), Hollinger et al (1979) and Kho et al (1991). After premedication with diazepam

10 mg, anaesthesia is induced with thiopentone, and supported by nitrous oxide in oxygen. Muscle relaxants are given if required, then acupuncture needles are inserted and stimulated at a high intensity, to produce strong muscle contractions. The stimulation continues throughout the surgery, and sleep may or may not be maintained depending on the preference of the patient and surgeon. Analgesics are given if indicated.

It is interesting to note that the authors of a review of AA in animals (Janssens, Rogers & Schoen 1988) also reached the conclusion that EA is most useful as an adjunct to standard anaesthesia, and permitted the dose of depressant drugs to be reduced.

Results

Different authors vary in the classification they use for success or failure of the technique. The Chinese use four categories:

1. complete abolition of pain, no supplementary analgesia
2. moderate pain, but tolerated
3. more severe pain requiring additional analgesics
4. failure of the technique, requiring general anaesthetic.

Reports from China often claim that about 80% of cases or more are in categories 1 and 2 (i.e. no further analgesic medication was given) but Murphy & Bonica (1977) recalculated the figures by Western standards and estimated that the correct success rate was about 30%. Table 10.3 gives a summary of published reports of AA, in chronological order, and collates the figures into simple 'success' or 'failure' percentages, as judged solely on whether additional analgesic medication was required, because EA has to prove itself against the highly effective and reliable techniques of general anaesthesia that are available in Western hospitals.

Poulain et al (1993) achieved a notable success with the first double-blind assessment, overcoming the problem of blinding the anaesthetist by using two separate anaesthetic teams. The 'referee'

team inserted needles in auricular points of the treatment group, and covered the area with surgical tape; in the control group, 'dead' leads were fixed to the ear with the tape. Both groups therefore had bandages around the ear, with wires attached to identical-looking stimulators, although the unit used for the placebo group had been inactivated. Baseline interference was created on ECG monitors to disguise the EA impulses. A second anaesthetic team managed the patients during surgery, monitoring vital signs and giving analgesic drugs only if indicated according to a fixed protocol. The referee team then disconnected the patients after surgery, and recovery room staff continued the blinded observations.

Analysis of the results showed a significant and important difference between the groups: every patient in the control group required fentanyl during the operation, compared with only 7% of the EA group. There was no difference in the quality of the anaesthetic, as judged by patients, anaesthetists, or recovery room staff.

Controlled open studies were performed by Kho et al (1991), Li et al (1992), Sun, Li & Si (1992) and Wang, Wang & Chen (1994), all of which showed AA to be as successful as orthodox anaesthesia.

Obstetric analgesia

Martoudis & Christofides (1990) used LI-4 and ear Shenmen for one 20-minute session of EA in labour, and obtained good results in about 50% of patients, but no analgesia at all in 12.5%. Hyodo & Gega (1977) used LI-4, SP-6 and ST-36 with good effect in over 60% of cases; they noted a shortening of the second and third stages of labour. Abouleish & Depp (1975) used 12 points, and had good results in seven patients out of these twelve. A combination of points that is commonly used in China is: Shenmen, Uterus and Endocrine ear points bilaterally, with EA applied to two on each side (Budd, personal communication 1993).

Wallis et al (1974) report the results of acupuncture in labour, given by a Chinese doctor according to traditional diagnosis formulated

Table 10.3 Published reports of acupuncture analgesia

Reference	Operation	n =	Technique	Success %*	Failure %	Main points used[†]
Dimond (1971)	Various	10	Standard	100	0	
Kao et al (1973)	Hernia repair	2	Standard	100	0	GB-27, ST-25, SP-6, GV-2, GV-6, LIV-3
Wallis et al (1974)	Normal labour	12	MA or EA	10	90	
Abouleish & Depp (1975)	Normal labour	12	Standard	75	25	LI-4, ST-25, ST-28, CV-6, CV-4, ST-36, SP-6
Spoerel (1975)	Various	87	Standard	80	20	
Peking Children's Hospital (1975)	Various	412	Standard	35	65	
Peking Children's Hospital (1975)	Various	1062	Combined	31	69	
Shanghai Second Medical College (1975)	Cardiac	107	Standard	92	8	Aur: chest, neck, Lung, Kidney PC-6, LU-7
Grabow & Criveanu (1976)	Various	162	Combined	100	0	
Modell et al (1976)	Plastic surgery	9	Standard	56	44	
Pauser et al (1976)	Tonsillectomy D&C Hernia repair	102	Standard	64	36	LI-4, LI-11 ST-36, SP-6 LR-3, SP-7, local points
Pauser et al (1976)	Various	72	Combined	100	0	
Hyodo & Gega (1977)	Normal labour	32	Standard	47	53	LI-4, ST-36, SP-6
Patel & Nene (1978)	Ectopic pregnancy	1	Standard	100	0	
Hollinger et al (1979)	Cardiac	800	Combined	65	35	Aur: Shenmen, Symp., Heart, trachea, etc. LI-4, TB-9, ST-10, ST-4
Astuti, Vannucci & Caresano (1980)	Gynae.: abdo. surgery e.g. salpingectomy	14	Standard	50	50	Aur: Shenmen, Sedation, Uterus ST-36, SP-6, SP-9, BL-27, PC-6, LI-4, LR-3, CV-12
Astuti, Vannucci & Caresano (1980)	Gynae.: vaginal surgery, e.g. Bartholin's cyst, D&C	47	Standard	70	30	Aur: Shenmen, Ext genitalia ST-36, SP-6, SP-7, CV-3, CV-4
Beijing Group (1980)	LSCS	1000	Standard	76	24	
Vallette et al (1980)	LSCS	14	Standard	60	40	Aur: Uterus, Shenmen, Symp. LI-4, PC-6, SP-6, ST-40 and s/c
Dias & Subramanium (1984)	Lap sterilization	78	Standard	62	38	ST-26–29 s/c
Wang & Jin (1989)	LSCS	40, 920	Standard	?[‡]		
Kho et al (1990)	Thyroidectomy	20	Standard	25	75	Aur: Shenmen, Symp., Neck, Adrenal
Kho et al (1991)	Retroperitoneal lymph node dissection	13	Combined	92	8	Aur: Heart, Shenmen, Symp. paravertebral surface electrodes
Poulain (unpublished work, 1992)	Gynae., abdo. or pelvic	120	Combined	95	5	Aur: Shenmen, SP-6
Wang, Chang & Liu (1992)	Colonoscopy controls	100 ?	Manual Nil	31 13	69 87	Aur: Shenmen, ST-36, ST-37

*Success % indicates the percentage of patients who did not require additional chemical analgesia during the procedure.
[†] Points listed were generally used bilaterally.
[‡] Full breakdown of results not published.
Abbreviations: Aur = auricular points; D & C = dilatation and curettage; LSCS = lower segment caesarean section; s/c = long subcutaneous paraincisional needles; Symp. = Sympathetic.

during periodic consultations through the pregnancy. Treatment was by either manual or electrical acupuncture (0.25–0.75 Hz). Only two of the 21 patients judged their analgesia to be sufficient, and the observers did not consider it sufficient in a single case.

EA is not ideal in labour because of the need to be attached to wires and the unpredictable results. TENS apparatus specially designed for the labour ward is now widely available, and has been found to be more convenient.

Other applications of AA

EA has been used successfully for gastroscopy (Cahn et al 1978), colonoscopy (Wang, Chang & Liu 1992) and extracorporeal shock-wave therapy (Chung et al 1988).

Advantages of AA

The technique is popular with some patients, and one of the major benefits is the reduction in need for opioid drugs. Patients are more likely to be awake when they arrive in the recovery room, they are extubated earlier and suffer less postoperative nausea and vomiting (Dundee et al 1989, Ho et al 1989, Kho et al 1991).

Reduction in postoperative pain

The level of postoperative pain relief after EA is variable. Hollinger et al (1979) and Sun, Li & Si (1992) both found a significant reduction in the need for postoperative analgesics after cardiac surgery, and Vallette et al (1980) found that analgesia sometimes lasted 2 days after Caesarian section. However, Kho et al (1991) found no difference in postoperative analgesic requirement.

EA has also been used immediately after the operation: Christenssen et al (1989) randomized patients to receive either EA or no additional treatment immediately after hysterectomy, while still asleep, in a double-blind controlled study. Postoperative pain was assessed objectively by the dose of pethidine required via patient-controlled analgesia. The active EA group required 40% less pethidine than the placebo group in the first 2 hours after surgery. There was no difference during the following 2 hours. Martelete & Fiori (1985) compared EA with TENS and with pethidine in patients who had undergone abdominal, rectal or lumbar surgery, and found EA to be slightly superior to the two other analgesics, in both effect and duration. However, Christenssen et al (1993) were unable to confirm

their earlier results in a further study, in which EA stimulation was given continuously from 20 minutes before surgery. One possible explanation is that the prolonged EA released opioid antagonists and negated the analgesia.

Wall (1988) and Bush (1993) discuss the importance of pre-emptive analgesia in reducing the incidence of postoperative pain generally, and pathologically prolonged pain in particular. Volleys of noxious impulses arriving at the spinal cord during surgery can cause prolonged hyperexcitability of the local neurons. AA can be established well before surgery, and research into its effects on this problem may be fruitful.

Cardiovascular stability

Hollinger et al (1979) and Kho et al (1991) provide evidence that the pulse and blood pressure remain stable under AA, even during traction on the peritoneum and mobilization of abdominal organs. However, Kho noted that AA did not prevent the pressor response to intubation, and in operations that he observed in China with standard technique (Kho et al 1990) the blood pressure rose during AA, especially in patients who were already hypertensive.

Tayama et al (1984) measured the effects of EA on the cardiovascular system of 25 healthy subjects with impedance cardiography. Stimulating PC-4–6 produced no change in heart rate or blood pressure, but increased the stroke volume and cardiac output, with a significant fall in peripheral resistance compared with placebo. The effect was equivalent to a plasma expander infusion at the rate of 2 ml/kg for 10 minutes. Stimulating LI-4–10 induced a significant increase in radial artery blood flow and vessel diameter, 'Equivalent to the effect of a stellate ganglion block' (Tayama et al 1984). There were no changes in the blood levels of adrenaline or noradrenaline. The effects started about 10 minutes after starting stimulation, and lasted about 30 minutes.

Li (1985) found in animal experiments that EA at PC-6 or ST-36 reduced artificially induced extrasystoles and restored the blood pressure to normal values when it was experimentally raised or lowered. Lee et al (1981) showed that EA reverses the cardiovascular-depressant effect of morphine or halothane in animals. Thus AA may theoretically be useful in cases of shock. Patel & Nene (1978) describe a patient with circulatory collapse from an ectopic pregnancy who was found to have lost 9 pints of blood intra-abdominally. Within 5 minutes of starting auricular and nasal EA, her vital signs improved and peripheral pulses became palpable.

There are anecdotal reports of a reduction in blood loss under AA, though no objective evidence. Klide (1992) commented that veterinary surgeons frequently describe less bleeding with EA than with standard anaesthesia.

Lack of respiratory depression

Kho et al (1991) studied arterial blood gases in spontaneous respiration under AA, compared with fentanyl anaesthesia. They found that there was no difference in the oxygen saturation, but the carbon dioxide saturation remained normal under AA, whereas it was invariably raised after giving fentanyl, a known respiratory depressant.

Facco et al (1981) showed that the vital capacity of patients who were given EA postoperatively remained normal, whereas the capacity of the control group given pentazocine was reduced.

Several authors have suggested anecdotally that the reduced dose of opioids under EA leads to a fall in postoperative chest infections. The Shanghai Second Medical College group (1975) reported only one chest infection in their series of 107 open-heart cases.

Increased rates of healing

There is in-vitro evidence that EA influences the rate of healing. Jansen et al (1989) raised skin flaps and then resutured them, giving different modes of acupuncture through two needles at the base of the flap. The flaps survived significantly better after EA (90%) than after MA or in control animals (50%). The effects were strongest with daily treatment, and higher intensity was more important than whether the frequency was 2 Hz or 80 Hz. Lundeberg et al (1988) applied TENS at 80 Hz to the base of the flap in women who had undergone breast reconstructive surgery for mammary carcinoma. Blood flow in the flaps was significantly increased, as was their survival rate. However, Ekblom et al (1991) found a significantly higher incidence of 'dry socket' (a complication of wound healing) in patients undergoing dental extractions with manual AA compared with standard anaesthetic.

There is no evidence whether EA given at sites distant to the surgery affects tissue healing.

Other reported benefits

Claims have been made that patients recover more quickly after EA than after standard general anaesthesia (e.g. Sun, Li & Si 1992). However, careful measurements by Kho et al (1991) failed to show any significant improvement in time to removal of bladder catheter, resumption of peristalsis, fatigue scores, or length of stay in hospital, compared with moderate-dose fentanyl anaesthesia.

Dias & Subramanium (1984) commented that the technique is cheap, and therefore particularly useful in developing countries; Wei (1977) described its use by barefoot doctors in China.

Disadvantages of AA

The relative disadvantages of the technique are its unreliability, the increased cost in personnel time, and the inconvenience of the attached wires. In addition, staff and patients have doubts about a novel technique, and artefacts are likely to appear on monitors. All these problems can be considered minor, however, and Kho et al (1991) concluded 'The method has no clinically relevant disadvantages'.

There is no doubt that EA does make particular demands on the staff, for example the longer induction period, and the possibility of failure of the technique. Staff need to appreciate that there may be major benefits for the patient in return for some small inconvenience to themselves. The success of the original Chinese method does depend also on excellent surgical technique, and the Shanghai Second Medical

College report (1975) calls for surgeons who are 'steady, definite, light and quick'.

EXPERIMENTAL EVIDENCE FOR ACUPUNCTURE ANALGESIA

Animal research

Analgesia produced by EA has been studied in different species. Han & Terenius (1982) developed the model of the rat's response to radiant heat applied to the nose (head-jerk response) or to the tail (tail-flick latency), and obtained reliable AA in four out of five animals. However, Bossut

and collegues (Bossut & Mayer 1991a,b, Bossut et al 1991) have published evidence that analgesia can be produced reliably only in animals that are used repeatedly for the same experiments; results in acupuncture-naive rats are less consistent. Pomeranz (1989) obtained intracellular recordings from cells in the cat spinal cord to show that EA suppressed the responses to painful stimuli by inhibiting the transmission cell in the dorsal horn. Vierck et al (1974) demonstrated that experimental pain thresholds in monkeys were significantly increased by EA, an effect which persisted for several days. Tseng et al (1981) found a small but significant reduction in

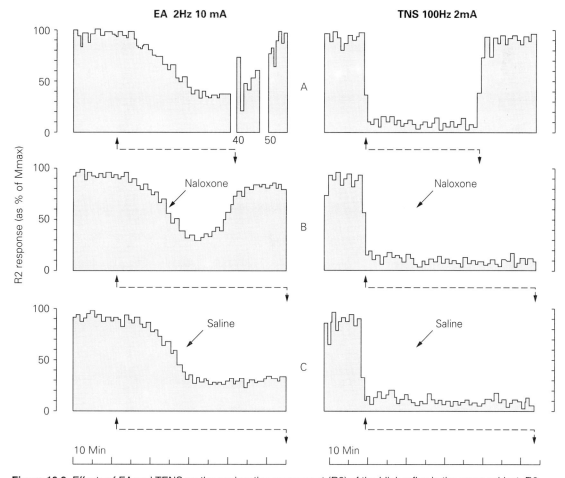

Figure 10.9 Effects of EA and TENS on the nociceptive component (R2) of the blink reflex in the same subject. R2 responses are expressed as percentages of the maximal direct motor response from the orbicularis oculi muscle, elicited by stimulation of the ipsilateral facial nerve. Note left: the progressive and moderate naloxone sensitive depression in the R2 response obtained with EA, and right: the rapid and major depression in the R2 response which is not modified by naloxone. (Reproduced from Willer et al (1982) with permission)

the halothane requirement of anaesthetized dogs when they were also given EA.

Human experiments

A thorough analysis of various analgesic agents was conducted by Parwatikar et al (1978). Twenty volunteers were given EA, wrong-site EA, hypnosis, morphine, aspirin, diazepam or oral placebo. The results showed that hypnosis in good subjects was the most effective agent; morphine and EA at the correct sites had similar effects, although EA produced a significantly greater reduction in the pain of cold water immersion. The pattern of analgesia for EA was thus different from that of hypnosis, and further evidence that they are distinct entities was given by the different EEG recordings, with hypnosis increasing alpha waves whereas EA increased beta waves. The study also showed that EA applied to non-acupuncture points had no significant effect on the EEG.

The assessment of pain is subjective and therefore subject to inaccuracies. Willer et al (1982) devised on objective measurement, namely the blink reflex, which is a brainstem reflex to pain. The blink reflex may be stimulated through the supraorbital nerve, and the threshold is a test of analgesia that is distinct from the subject's awareness. Low-frequency EA gradually suppressed the blink reflex in 12 out of 16 subjects, and could be reversed by naloxone (Fig. 10.9).

Price et al (1984) recruited chronic low back pain patients and assessed the effect of EA both on their chronic pain in the same segment and on artificially induced pain in remote segments. The results demonstrated differences between individuals and over time, which is consistent with theories that two (at least) separate mechanisms are involved. Seven of the 12 subjects reported reduction of pain threshold throughout the body (i.e. reduced back pain and reduced threshold to experimental pain in distant segments); four showed only local relief of their back pain, with no response in distant segments. In some patients the maximum effects were delayed up to 24 hours. When the patients were retested over the following days, only the local segmental effect persisted.

CONCLUSION

Electroacupuncture appears to have a moderate but definite analgesic effect, the strength of which varies from individual to individual. World-wide, innumerable patients can attest to the success of acupuncture analgesia in surgery, particularly in combination with light general anaesthesia. EA has undoubtedly helped a considerable number of patients with chronic pain or other conditions, and further carefully controlled studies are required to define the optimum indications for the technique as an accepted part of orthodox medicine. EA has also proved to be a useful tool for the study of pain pathways and mechanisms.

REFERENCES

Abouleish E, Depp R 1975 Acupuncture in obstetrics: anesthesia and analgesia. Current Researches 54(1):83–88
Andersson S A, Ericson T, Holmgren E, Lindqvist G 1973 Electro-acupuncture. Effect on pain threshold measured with electrical stimulation of teeth. Brain Research 63:393–396
Andersson S 1993 The functional background in acupuncture effects. Scandinavian Journal of Rehabilitation Medicine, Suppl 29:31–60
Astuti R, Vannucci M, Caresano G 1980 L'analgesia mediante agopuntura nella chirurgia ginecologica. Nostre esperienze. Minerva Medica 71:923–925
Beijing Group 1980 Clinical analysis of Caesarian section acupuncture. Chinese Medical Journal 93(4):231–238
Belgrade M J, Solomon L M, Lichter E A 1984 Effect of acupuncture on experimentally induced itch. Acta Dermatologica et Venereologica (Stockholm) 64:129–133
Bossut D F, Mayer D J 1991a Electroacupuncture analgesia in rats: naltrexone antagonism is dependent on previous exposure. Brain Research 549:47–51
Bossut D F, Mayer D J 1991b Electroacupuncture analgesia in rats: effects on brainstem and spinal cord lesions, and role of pituitary-adrenal axis. Brain Research 549:52–58
Bossut D F, Huang Z S, Sun S L, Mayer D J 1991 Electroacupuncture in rats: evidence for naloxone and naltrexone potentiation of analgesia. Brain Research 549:36–46
Broedersdorff C D 1981 Aurikulo-Elektro-Stimulations-Anaesthesie, AESA. Der Akupunkturarzt/ Aurikulotherapeut 5:145–159

Bush D J 1993 Pre-emptive analgesia. British Medical Journal 306:285–286

Cahn A M, Carayon P, Hill C, Flamant R 1978 Acupuncture in gastroscopy. Lancet January 28:182–183

Chan C S, Chow S P 1981 Electroacupuncture in the treatment of post-traumatic sympathetic dystrophy (Sudeck's Atrophy). British Journal of Anaesthesia 53:899–902

Chen X-H, Han J-S 1992 All three types of opioid receptors in the spinal cord are important for 2/15 Hz electroacupuncture analgesia. European Journal of Pharmacology 211:203–210

Cheng R S S, Pomeranz B 1980 Combined treatment with D-amino acids and electroacupuncture produces a greater analgesia than either treatment alone; naloxone reverses these effects. Pain 8:231–236

Cheng R S S, Pomeranz B 1981 Monoaminergic mechanism of electroacupuncture analgesia. Brain Research 215:77–92

Cheng R S S, Pomeranz B 1987 Electrotherapy of chronic musculoskeletal pain: comparison of electroacupuncture and acupuncture-like transcutaneous electrical nerve stimulation. Clinical Journal of Pain 2:143–149

Christenssen P A, Noreng M, Anderssen P E, Nielsen J W 1989 Electroacupuncture and postoperative pain. British Journal of Anaesthesia 62:258–262

Christenssen P A, Rotne M, Vedelsdal R et al 1993 Electroacupuncture in anaesthesia for hysterectomy. British Journal of Anaesthesia 71:835–838

Chung C, Lee W C, Lee T Y, Liang H K 1988 Acupuncture anesthesia for extracorporeal shock wave lithotripsy. American Journal of Acupuncture 16(1):11–18

Chung J M, Lee K H, Hori Y, Endo K, Willis W D 1984a Factors influencing peripheral nerve stimulation produced inhibition of primate spinothalamic tract cells. Pain 19:277–293

Chung J M, Fang Z R, Hori Y, Lee K H, Willis W D 1984b Prolonged inhibition of primate spinothalamic tract cells by peripheral nerve stimulation. Pain 19:259–275

Deluze C, Bosia L, Zirbs A, Chantraine A, Vischer T L 1992 Electroacupuncture in fibromyalgia: results of a controlled trial. British Medical Journal 305:1249–1252

Dias PLR, Subramanium S 1984 Minilaparotomy under acupuncture analgesia. Journal of the Royal Society of Medicine 77:295–298

Dimond E G 1971 Acupuncture anesthesia. Western medicine and Chinese traditional medicine. Journal of the American Medical Association 218(10):1558–1563

Dundee J W 1989 Electro-acupuncture and postoperative emesis [letter]. Anaesthesia 45:789–790

Dundee J W, McMillan C 1991 Positive evidence for P6 acupuncture antiemesis. Postgraduate Medical Journal 67:417–422

Dundee J W, Ghaly R G, Bill K M, Chestnutt W N, Fitzpatrick K T J, Lynas A G A 1989 Effect of stimulation of the P6 antiemetic point on postoperative nausea and vomiting. British Journal of Anaesthesia 63:612–618

Ekblom A, Hansson P, Thomsson M, Thomas M 1991 Increased postoperative pain and consumption of analgesics following acupuncture. Pain 44:241–247

Eriksson S V, Lundeberg T, Lundeberg S 1991 Interaction of diazepam and naloxone on acupuncture induced pain relief. American Journal of Chinese Medicine 19(1):1–7

Facco E, Manani G, Angel A et al 1981 Comparison study between acupuncture and pentazocine analgesic and respiratory post-operative effects. American Journal of Chinese Medicine 9(3):225–235

Fujiwara H, Taniguchi K, Takeuchi J, Ikezono E 1980 The influence of low frequency acupuncture on a demand pacemaker. Chest 78:96–97

Grabow L 1994 Controlled study of the analgetic effectivity of acupuncture. Arzneimittelforschung/Drug Res 44(1) no 4:554–558

Grabow L, Criveanu T 1976 Die kombinierte Akupunktur-Analgesie als Verfahren der allgemeinen Anaesthesie. Anaesthesist 25:231–234

Han J S, Sun S L 1990 Differential release of enkephalin and dynorphin by low and high frequency electroacupuncture in the central nervous system. Science International Journal (NY) 1:19–23

Han J S, Terenius L 1982 Neurochemical basis of acupuncture analgesia. Annual Review of Pharmacology and Toxicology 22:193–220

Han J S, Ding X Z, Fan S G 1986 Cholecystokinin octapeptide (CCK-8): antagonism to electroacupuncture analgesia and a possible role in electroacupuncture tolerance. Pain 27:101–115

Hill S D, Sin M-S, Chandler P J 1991 Reflex sympathetic dystrophy and electroacupuncture. Texas Medicine 87(7):76–81

Ho R T, Jawan B, Fung S T, Cheung H K, Lee J H 1989 Electroacupuncture and postoperative emesis. Anaesthesia 45:327–329

Hollinger I, Richter J A, Pongratz W, Baum M 1979 Acupuncture anesthesia for open heart surgery: a report of 800 cases. American Journal of Chinese Medicine 7(1):77–90

Hu S, Stern R M, Koch K L 1992 Electrical acustimulation relieves vection-induced motion sickness. Gastroenterology 102(6):1854–1858

Hughes J, Smith T W, Kosterlitz H W, Fothergill L A, Morgan B A, Morris H R 1975 Identification of two related pentapeptides from the brain with potent opiate agonist activity. Nature 258:577–579

Hyodo M, Gega O 1977 Use of acupuncture anesthesia for normal delivery. American Journal of Chinese Medicine 5(1):63–69

Ishiko N, Yamamoto T, Murayama N, Hanamori T 1978 Electroacupuncture: current strength–duration relationship for initiation of hypesthesia in man. Neuroscience Letters 8:273–276

Ishimaru K, Kawakita K, Sakita M 1995 Analgesic effects induced by TENS and electroacupuncture with different types of stimulating electrodes on deep tissues in human subjects. Pain 63:181–187

Jansen G, Lundeberg T, Samuelson U E, Thomas M 1989 Increased survival of ischaemic musculocutaneous flaps in rats after acupuncture. Acta Physiologica Scandinavica 135:555–558

Janssens L A A, Rogers P A M, Schoen A M 1988 Acupuncture analgesia: a review. The Veterinary Record 9 April:355–358

Johansson K, Lindgren I, Widner H, Wiklund I, Johansson B B 1993 Can sensory stimulation improve the functional outcome in stroke patients? Neurology 43:2189–2192

Johnson D A 1983 History and the understanding of acupuncture anaesthesia. Southern Medical Journal 76(4):497–498

Kao F F, Sechzer P H, Estrin J, Nghi N V, Darras J-C,

Fang C F, Leung S J 1973 Acupuncture anesthesia in herniorrhaphy. American Journal of Chinese Medicine 1(2):327–328

Kho H G, van Egmond J, Zhuang C F, Lin G F, Zhang G L 1990 Acupuncture anaesthesia. Observations on its use for removal of thyroid adenomata and influence on recovery and morbidity in a Chinese hospital. Anaesthesia 45:480–485

Kho H G, Eijk R J R, Kapteijns W M M J, van Egmond J 1991 Forum. Acupuncture and transcutaneous stimulation analgesia in comparison with moderate-dose fentanyl anaesthesia in major surgery. Clinical efficacy and influence on recovery and morbidity. Anaesthesia 46:129–135

Kitade T, Hyodo M 1979 The effects of stimulation of ear acupuncture points on the body's pain threshold. American Journal of Chinese Medicine 7(3):241–252

Klide A M 1992 Acupuncture-produced surgical analgesia, physiology, indications, techniques, and limitations. Problems in Veterinary Medicine 4(1):200–206

Knox V J, Shum K, McLaughlin D M 1977 Response to cold pressor pain and to acupuncture analgesia in Oriental and Occidental subjects. Pain 4(1):49–57

Lancet 1973 Acupuncture analgesia [leading article]. June 16:1372

Le Bars D, Dickenson A H, Besson J-M 1979a Diffuse Noxious Inhibitory Controls (DNIC). I. Effects on dorsal horn convergent neurones in the rat. Pain 6:283–304

Le Bars D, Dickenson A H, Besson J-M 1979b Diffuse Noxious Inhibitory Controls (DNIC). II. Lack of effect on non-convergent neurones, supraspinal involvement and theoretical implications. Pain 6:305–327

Lee D C, Clifford D H, Lee M O, Nelson L 1981 Reversal by acupuncture of cardiovascular depression induced with morphine during halothane anaesthesia in dogs. Canadian Anaesthetic Society Journal 28(2):129–133

Lee P K, Andersen T W, Modell J H, Sage S A 1975 Treatment of chronic pain with acupuncture. Journal of the American Medical Association 11:1133–1135

Lee P K Y, Modell J H, Andersen T W, Saga S A 1976 Incidence of prolonged pain relief following acupuncture. Anaesthesia and Analgesia: Current Researches 55(2):229–231

Lee Y-H, Lee W-C, Chen M-T, Huang J-I K, Chung C, Chang L S 1992 Acupuncture in the treatment of renal colic. Journal of Urology 147:16–18

Lehmann T R, Russell D W, Spratt K F, Colby H, Liu Y K, Fairchild M L, Christensen S 1986 Efficacy of electroacupuncture and TENS in the rehabilitation of chronic low back pain patients. Pain 26:277–290

Li L, Jian L, Chen Y, Chen X, Chen P 1992 Influence of different types of syndrome on the rising of excellent response rate in hernia repair with acupuncture anaesthesia. Chen Tzu Yen Chiu Acupuncture Research 17(3):147–150 [Engl abstr]

Li P 1985 Modulatory effect of electroacupuncture on cardiovascular functions. Journal of Traditional Chinese Medicine 5(3):211–214

Liu J 1987 Treatment of 86 cases of local neurodermatitis by electro-acupuncture (with needles inserted around diseased areas). Journal of Traditional Chinese Medicine 7(1):67

Liu J D 1987 Electrical needle therapy of uremic pruritus. Nephron 47:179–183

Loy T T 1983 Treatment of cervical spondylosis: electroacupuncture versus physiotherapy. Medical Journal of Australia 2:32–34

Lundeberg T, Bondesson L, Thomas M 1987 Effect of acupuncture on experimentally induced itch. British Journal of Dermatology 117:771–777

Lundeberg T, Hurtig T, Lundeberg S, Thomas M 1988 Long-term results of acupuncture in chronic head and neck pain. The Pain Clinic 2(1):15–31

Lundeberg T, Kjartansson J, Samuelsson U 1988 Effect of electrical nerve stimulation on healing of ischaemic skin flaps. Lancet September 24:712–714

Lundeberg T, Eriksson S, Lundeberg S, Thomas M 1989 Acupuncture and sensory thresholds. American Journal of Chinese Medicine 17(3–4):99–110

Luo H, Jia Y, Zhan L 1985 Electro-acupuncture vs amitriptyline in the treatment of depressive states. Journal of Traditional Chinese Medicine 5(1):3–8

Macdonald A J R 1993 A brief review of the history of electrotherapy and its union with acupuncture. Acupuncture in Medicine 11(2):66–75

Mann F 1974 Acupuncture Analgesia. Report of 100 experiments. British Journal of Anaesthesia 46:361–364

Mao W, Ghia J N, Scott D S, Duncan G H, Gregg J M 1980 High versus low intensity acupuncture analgesia for treatment of chronic pain: effects on platelet serotonin. Pain 8:331–342

Martelete M, Fiori A M C 1985 Comparative study of the analgesic effect of Transcutaneous Nerve Stimulation (TNS), electroacupuncture (EA) and meperidine in the treatment of postoperative pain. Acupuncture and Electro-therapeutics Research 10:183–193

Martoudis S G, Christofides K 1990 Electroacupuncture for pain relief in labour. Acupuncture in Medicine 8(2):51–53

Melzack R, Wall P D 1965 Pain mechanisms: a new theory. Science 150:971–979

Melzack R, Wall P D 1984 Acupuncture and transcutaneous electrical nerve stimulation. Postgraduate Medical Journal 60:893–896

Modell J H, Lee P K Y, Bingham H G, Greer D M, Habal M B 1976 'Acupuncture anesthesia'—a clinical study. Anesthesia and Analgesia: Current Researches 55(4):508–512

Murphy T M, Bonica J J 1977 Acupuncture analgesia and anesthesia. Archives of Surgery 112:896–902

Nappi G, Facchinetti F, Legnante G et al 1982 Different releasing effects of traditional manual acupuncture and electroacupuncture on proopiocortin-related peptides. Acupuncture and Electro-therapeutics Research 7:93–103

Omura Y 1975 Electro-acupuncture: Its electrophysiological basis and criteria for effectiveness and safety—Part I. Acupuncture and Electro-therapeutics Research 1:157–181

Omura Y 1987 Basic Electrical Parameters for safe and effective electro-therapeutics (electro-acupuncture, TES, TENMS (or TEMS), TENS and electro-magnetic field stimulation with or without drug field) for pain, neuromuscular skeletal problems, and circulatory disturbances. Acupuncture and Electro-therapeutics Research 12:201–225

Parwatikar S D, Brown M S, Stern J A, Ulett G A, Suetten I S 1978 Acupuncture, hypnosis and experimental pain—I study with volunteers. Acupuncture and Electro-therapeutics Research 3:161–190

Patel K, Nene M L 1978 An unusual ectopic pregnancy

operated on under acupuncture analgesia. East African Medical Journal 55(2):87–89

Pauser G, Benzer H, Bischko J et al 1976 Klinische und experimentelle Ergebnisse mit der Akupunktur-Analgesie. Anaesthesist 25:215–222

Peking Acupuncture Anaesthesia Co-ordinating Group 1973 Preliminary study on the mechanism of acupuncture anaesthesia. Scientia Sinica 16(3):447–456

Peking Children's Hospital 1975 A clinical analysis of 1474 operations under acupuncture anesthesia among children. Chinese Medical Journal 1(5):369–374

Pomeranz B 1989 Acupuncture research related to pain, drug addiction and nerve regeneration. In: Pomeranz B, Stux G (eds) Scientific basis of acupuncture. Springer-Verlag, Berlin

Price D D, Rafii A, Watkins L R, Buckingham B 1984 A psychophysical analysis of acupuncture analgesia. Pain 19:27–42

Rieb L, Pomeranz B 1992 Alterations in electrical pain thresholds by use of acupuncture-like transcutaneous electrical nerve stimulation in pain-free subjects. Physical Therapy 72(9):658–667

Schimek F, Chapman C R, Gerlach R, Colpitts Y H 1982 Varying electrical acupuncture stimulation intensity: effects on dental pain-evoked potentials. Anesthesia and Analgesia 61(6):499–503

Shanghai Second Medical College, The Third People's Hospital 1975 Intracardiac operations with extracorporeal circulation under acupuncture anaesthesia. Scientia Sinica 18(2):271–280

Simmons M S, Oleson T D 1993 Auricular electrical stimulation and dental pain threshold. Anaesthetic Progress 40:14–19

Sjölund B, Terenius L, Eriksson M 1977 Increased cerebrospinal fluid levels of endorphins after electroacupuncture. Acta Physiologica Scandinavica 100:382–384

Spoerel W E 1975 Acupuncture analgesia in China. American Journal of Chinese Medicine 3(4):359–368

Stewart D, Thomson J, Oswald I 1977 Acupuncture analgesia: an experimental investigation. British Medical Journal January 8:67–70

Sun P, Li L, Si M 1992 Comparison between acupuncture and epidural anesthesia in appendectomy. Chen Tzuy Yen Chiu Acupuncture Research 17(2):87–89 [Engl abstr]

Tayama F, Muteki T, Bekki S et al 1984 Cardiovascular effect of electro-acupuncture. Kurume Medical Journal 31:37–46

Thomas D, Collins S, Strauss S 1992 Somatic sympathetic vasomotor changes documented by medical thermographic imaging during acupuncture analgesia. Clinical Rheumatology 11(1):55–59

Thomas M, Lundeberg T 1994 Importance of modes of acupuncture in the treatment of chronic nociceptive low back pain. Acta Anaesthesia Scandinavica 38:63–69

Thomas M, Laurell G, Lundeberg T 1988 Acupuncture for the alleviation of tinnitus. Laryngoscope 98:664–667

Thomas M, Lundeberg T, Björk G, Lundström-Lindstedt V 1995 Pain and discomfort in primary dysmenorrhoea is reduced by preemptive acupuncture or low frequency TENS. European Journal of Physical Medicine and Rehabilitation 4:71–76

Tseng C-K, Tay A-A L, Pace N, Westenskow D R, Wong K C

1981 Electro-acupuncture modification of halothane anaesthesia in the dog. Canadian Anaesthetic Society Journal 28(2):125–128

Tuzuner F, Kecik Y, Osdemir S, Canakci N 1989 Electroacupuncture in the treatment of enuresis nocturna. Acupuncture and Electro-therapeutics Research 14:211–215

Vallette C, Niboyet J E H, Imbert-Martelet M, Roux J F 1980 Acupuncture analgesia and Cesarean section. Journal of Reproductive Medicine 25(3):108–112

Vierck C J, Lineberry C G, Lee P K, Calderwood H W 1974 Prolonged hypalgesia following 'acupuncture' in monkeys. Life Sciences 15:1277–1289

Wall P D 1988 The prevention of postoperative pain [editorial]. Pain 33:289–290

Wallis L, Shnider S M, Palahniuk R J, Spivey H T 1974 An evaluation of acupuncture analgesia in obstetrics. Anesthesiology 41(6):596–601

Wang B G, Wang E Z, Chen X Z 1994 A study on combined acupuncture and enflurane anesthesia for craniotomy. Chung-Kuo Chung Hsi i Chieh Ho Tsa Chih 14(1):10–13 [Engl abstr]

Wang D W, Jin Y H 1989 Present status of Cesarian section under acupuncture anaesthesia in China. Fukushima Journal of Medical Science 35(2):45–52

Wang H-H, Chang Y-H, Liu D-M 1992 A study in the effectiveness of acupuncture analgesia for colonoscopic examination compared with conventional premedication. American Journal of Acupuncture 20(3):217–221

Waylonis G W 1976 Subcutaneous electrical stimulation (acupuncture) in the clinical practice of physical medicine. Archives of Physical and Medical Rehabilitation 57:161–165

Wei W 1977 Acupuncture anesthesia in China. Comparative Medicine East and West 5(2):185–188

Willer J C, Dehen H, Cambier J 1981 Stress-induced analgesia in humans: endogenous opioids and naloxone-reversible depression of pain reflexes. Science 212(May 8):689–690

Willer J C, Roby A, Boulu P, Boureau F 1982 Comparative effects of electroacupuncture and transcutaneous nerve stimulation on the human blink reflex. Pain 14:267–278

Williams T, Mueller K, Cornwall M W 1991 Effect of acupuncture-point stimulation on diastolic blood pressure in hypertensive subjects: a preliminary study. Physical Therapy 71(7):523–529

Windsor H M 1984 Cardiac surgery in China. Medical Journal of Australia May 12:599–602

Wong C 1993 Acupuncture induced anaesthesia: fiction or fact? Acupuncture in Medicine 11(2):55–60

Woolf C J 1989 Segmental afferent fibre-induced analgesia: transcutaneous electrical nerve stimulation (TENS) and vibration. In: Wall P D, Melzack R (eds) Textbook of pain. Churchill Livingstone, New York, pp 884–896

Xu S, Cao X, Mo W, Xu Z, Pan Y 1989 Effect of combination of drugs with acupuncture on analgesic efficacy. Acupuncture and Electro-therapeutics Research 14:103–113

Xu Z, Pan Y, Xu S, Mo W, Cao X, He L 1983 Synergism between metoclopramide and electroacupuncture analgesia. Acupuncture and Electro-therapeutics Research 8:283–288

11

Transcutaneous electrical nerve stimulation (TENS)

John W. Thompson

HISTORICAL BACKGROUND

Human beings are reactive animals. When confronted with a problem they try to do something about it. Thus, from time immemorial it has been known that when a part of the human body becomes painful it is an intuitive response to stroke, massage or rub the affected part because this tends to relieve the pain. In other words, local stimulation interferes somehow with the perception of pain. When a pain is very severe it may require very intense stimulation, to the extent of producing its own pain, before the original pain is reduced to any useful degree. It is common knowledge that electrical currents can excite the skin and other tissues of the body. The use of electricity for therapeutic purposes (electrotherapy) and especially for the relief of pain (electroanalgesia) also originates in antiquity, as evidenced by stone carvings that date from the Egyptian Fifth Dynasty (circa 2500 BC) and show the use of the electric fish (*Malapterurus electricus*) to treat painful conditions. Over 2000 years later, Hippocrates (400 BC) referred to the use of the electric torpedo fish for the treatment of such conditions as headache and arthritis. Much more recently, different forms of vibration have been used as a means of applying mechanical stimulation to the skin for the relief of various painful conditions. All these foregoing methods are examples of stimulation-induced analgesia, of which electroanalgesia is the most convenient to apply and the easiest to control.

Electroanalgesia

Following this discovery, there has been continuous interest and development in electroanalgesia. Box 11.1 lists some of the milestones over the last four and a half thousand years; as can be seen, up to the twentieth century progress was concerned mainly with identifying those conditions that responded to electroanalgesia and also to developments of the apparatus used to apply electrotherapy. A pivotal point in the history of electrotherapy occurred in 1965 when Melzack & Wall proposed their Gate

Control theory of pain, which, in essence, stated that the input of pain information to the brain is controlled at spinal cord level by a gate mechanism which is itself influenced by the nature and intensity of non-painful information entering the spinal cord. This hypothesis was readily verifiable and was soon put to the test by Wall & Sweet (1967) when they showed that high-frequency (50–100 Hz) *percutaneous* electrical nerve stimulation relieved chronic neurogenic pain. This exciting result received further corroboration when, in the same year, Shealy and his colleagues (Shealy, Mortimer & Reswick 1967) performed the first dorsal column implantation and were able to show that electrical stimulation of the dorsal column was also effective for the relief of chronic pain. Two years later, Reynolds (1969) made a discovery of fundamental importance (although not recognized so at the time), namely that electrical stimulation of the periaqueductal grey area of the rat brain produced surgical anaesthesia. In the meantime, *transcutaneous* electrical nerve stimulation (TENS) was being utilized to select patients for dorsal column implantation. But it was soon realized by Long and his associates (Long, Campbell & Gurer 1979) that TENS *alone* was often effective in relieving chronic pain and thus largely obviated the need for patients to undergo an operation for dorsal column implantation. It was also fortuitous that at this time the development of solid-state electronics was proceeding apace and this made it possible to manufacture small, battery-operated stimulators for TENS, which quickly developed into a branch of medical electronics.

More recently, TENS has been applied for use in obstetric analgesia (Augustinsson et al 1977) and to promote the healing of chronic ulceration (Kaada 1983). The use of different patterns of electrical stimulation such as pulsed (burst), modulation (ramped), random and complex wave forms have all been developed in order to improve the efficacy of TENS, such as the use of acupuncture-like TENS by Eriksson, Sjölund & Nielzen (1979); different forms of TENS are discussed later in this chapter (see also Table 11.3).

Box 11.1 Some milestones in electroanalgesia. Reproduced with permission from the Royal Society of Medicine Services

2500 BC	Egyptian Fifth Dynasty	Stone carvings show electric fish *Malapterurus electricus* used to treat painful conditions
400 BC	Hippocrates	Used electric fish to treat headache and arthritis
1759	Dr John Wesley	In 'Electricity made plain and useful by a lover of mankind and of common sense', described treatment of sciatica, headache, gout, kidney stone, etc.
1965	R Melzack & P Wall	Proposed the Gate Control theory of pain
1967	P Wall & W Sweet	Reported use of high-frequency (50–100 Hz) percutaneous electrical nerve stimulation for relief of chronic neurogenic (neuropathic) pain
1967	C N Shealy et al.	Reported use of dorsal column stimulation (DCS) of spinal cord
1969	D V Reynolds	Discovered that stimulation of (PAG) in the midbrain produces surgical anaesthesia
1973–4	D M Long, C N Shealy	Reported results of (TENS)
1979	M B E Eriksson, B Sjölund & S Nielzen	Reported increased analgesic efficacy of acupuncture-like TENS compared with continuous TENS

In theory, it is possible to stimulate electrically any part of the nervous system, but in practice it has been found that pain relief occurs only when specific parts are stimulated and this applies in particular to the relief of chronic pain (Table 11.1). As discussed earlier, electrical stimulation of a main sensory nerve or some of its cutaneous branches that innervate a painful part of the body may achieve pain relief in the same way that rubbing a painful part 'rubs it better'. Stimulating certain areas of the brain, especially the thalamus and the periventricular grey matter,

can be used as a last resort to relieve intractable pain that has failed to respond to other methods of pain relief.

PRINCIPLES OF USE

TENS can be used successfully to treat a large number of pain conditions, as shown in Table 11.2. Examples of *acute* pain conditions for which TENS has been used effectively include obstetric pain (Augustinsson et al 1977), postoperative pain (Pike 1978) and acute orofacial

Table 11.1 Sites and methods of electrical stimulation used to relieve pain. Reproduced with permission of the Royal Society of Medicine Services

Division of nervous system	Anatomical area	Method of electrical stimulation
Peripheral nerve	Cutaneous	Transcutaneous TENS, TES Percutaneous Electroacupuncture
	Nerve trunk	Transcutaneous TENS, TES Percutaneous Implanted electrodes
Spinal cord	Dorsal column	Implanted electrodes PISCES (percutaneously introduced electrical stimulation of the spinal cord)
Brain	Thalamus (posterior ventrolateral nucleus) Periventricular grey matter Other sites	Implanted electrodes Implanted electrodes Implanted electrodes

Table 11.2 Examples of acute and chronic pain conditions that have been treated with TENS

Speciality	System	Tissue	Acute	Chronic
Medical	Musculo skeletal	Muscles	Sprained or torn muscles, sports injuries	Myofascial pain, fibromyalgia
		Bones	Fractured rib	Rib with neoplastic deposit, osteoarthritis, rheumatoid arthritis
		Joints	Sprained or torn ligaments, arthritis, sports injuries	Osteoarthritis, rheumatoid arthritis
	Nervous system	Peripheral	Herpes zoster infection, Acute vertebral collapse	Postherpetic neuralgia Spinal nerve compression, causalgia
		Central	Acute stroke	Poststroke pain (thalamic pain), multiple sclerosis
	Cardiovascular	Cardiac muscle	Angina pectoris	Raynaud's disease, venous graft scars
	Visceral	Pancreas	Acute pancreatitis	Chronic pancreatitis
		Liver	Acute hepatitis	Enlarged neoplastic liver
Surgical	Integumental	Skin	Trauma, surgical wound pain	Painful scar
Gynaecological	Reproductive	Uterine muscle	Dysmenorrhoea, Labour pains	Pelvic pain, endometriosis
Dentistry	Dental	Teeth	Pulpal infection	Periodontal disease
		Orofacial	Acute orofacial pain	Temporomandibular joint

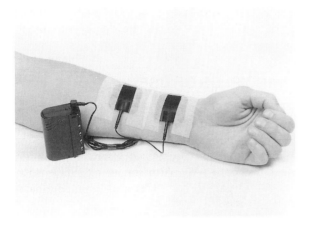

Figure 11.1 TENS unit attached to the forearm.

pain (Hansson & Ekblom 1983). *Chronic* pain conditions for which TENS has been used successfully include peripheral nerve disorders, spinal cord and spinal root disorders, pain associated with neoplastic lesions as well as muscle and joint pain (Woolf 1989). In general, the application of TENS is simple although the positioning of electrodes can be critical (as discussed later). Figure 11.1 shows how TENS can be applied to the forearm for the relief of pain arising in that area.

DIFFERENT TYPES OF TENS

Different types of TENS are now available, of which three are in common use. These are (1) continuous (conventional): high-frequency/low-intensity TENS, (2) pulsed (burst): low-frequency/low-intensity TENS, and (3) acupuncture-like (acu-TENS): low-frequency/high-intensity TENS. The main features of these three types have been summarized in Table 11.3. The application of these different types of TENS is described on p 184.

PRACTICAL USE OF EQUIPMENT

TENS equipment consists essentially of three components:

1. the stimulator
2. the connecting leads
3. the electrodes.

During the past 15 years there has been a steady increase in the number of stimulators world-wide that are designed specifically for TENS therapy. The manufacture of TENS equipment is a profitable exercise, as a consequence of which new models are launched on the market frequently. This situation makes it bewildering

Table 11.3 Types of TENS. Reproduced with permission from Oxford University Press

Form	Pattern of pulses	Pulse frequency	Pulse intensity	Effects
1. *Continuous* high frequency/ low intensity	Continuous	High 40–150 Hz	Low 10–30 mA	Non-painful paraesthesia directed into area supplied by stimulated nerve(s)
2. *Pulsed (Burst)* low frequency/ low intensity	Bursts	Low Bursts of 100 Hz at 1–2 Hz	Low 10–30 mA	As above, but felt in bursts
3. *Acupuncture-like (Acu-TENS)* high intensity/ low frequency	Bursts	Low Bursts of 100 Hz at 1–2 Hz	High 15–50 mA	As above, but accompanied by non-painful phasic twitching of muscles in those myotomes stimulated

Note: (i) On some stimulators pulsed forms of TENS (2 and 3) are available in *modulated or ramped form* so that the amplitudes of each set of shocks making up the pulses or burst are not equal but form a rising staircase of increasing intensity. This pattern of pulsing produces a stroking sensation which is more comfortable for the patient.
(ii) On some stimulators a *randomized* continuous output is available, the purpose of which is to reduce the development of tolerance to TENS, which may occur more readily with a regular pattern of stimulation owing to habituation of the nervous system.
(iii) Stimulators are now available that produce *complex waveforms* designed to operate with a single pair of electrodes (LIKON) or multiple electrodes activated randomly (CODETRON), and it is to be hoped that their role in TENS therapy will soon become clear.

for the would-be purchaser who is unfamiliar with TENS equipment. Before purchasing a particular instrument, the potential buyer should check that it incorporates the following features as a minimum (Thompson & Filshie 1993):

1. The stimulator should be compact, lightweight, conveniently shaped, comfortable to wear and to handle, sturdily built, and easily attachable to belt or pocket.
2. On–off/amplitude (strength) and frequency controls should be of convenient size and shape, easily adjustable yet adequately protected from accidental knocking or disturbance.
3. Availability of pulse patterns: continuous (conventional) and pulsed (burst) patterns are mandatory. A modulation (ramped) pattern is highly desirable, and random pattern is an added advantage.
4. The connecting lead(s) should be lightweight and flexible, comfortable to wear next to the skin, and should connect to all standard types of electrodes.
5. Low battery drain: where necessary (i.e. for intensive use) it should be possible to use the stimulator with rechargeable batteries for which a compatible, compact mains-operated battery charger can be obtained.
6. A simple, lucid and well-illustrated instruction manual is essential.
7. The stimulator should have a minimum 2-year guarantee.
8. The equipment should be reliable, and a helpline and maintenance service should be provided, the latter preferably as a rapid replacement service operated postally or by courier service.

For those who plan to purchase a bank of stimulators (e.g. for use in a pain clinic) it is best to proceed as follows. First, survey the field of those stimulators readily available and select two or three stimulators that possess the essential features listed above. Secondly, request each of the relevant manufacturers to loan one or more instruments of each type under consideration. Thirdly, run a pilot trial of the stimulators on loan in order to determine how effective, reliable and economical each stimulator is likely to be from the point of view both of the patients and of the staff who will be using the equipment. Such an exercise is well worth the time spent on it and is more likely to lead to the purchase of equipment that is appropriate to the clinic for which it is to be used. This is much more satisfactory than the undesirable alternative of haphazard purchasing of several stimulators of different design and manufacture, each of which will be found to possess its own idiosyncracies and electrical incompatibilities with respect to the others.

TREATMENT PLAN (Thompson 1986, Thompson & Filshie 1993)

It is important to work to a treatment plan as follows.

Diagnosis before treatment

As with all other forms of therapy, it is essential to diagnose the cause of the pain before attempting to treat it. However, when dealing with pain it is not always possible to make a precise diagnosis, particularly in the case of chronic pain. Therefore, what must be done, especially when contemplating the use of TENS to control pain caused by a neoplasm, is to ensure that the condition does not require some other form of urgent and/or more radical therapy. It cannot be emphasized too strongly that some pain conditions (including those of neoplastic origin) may demand a considerable amount of time and patience on the part of both patient and therapist to establish the most effective electrode positions. During this investigational phase it is also important to establish that TENS does not aggravate the pain condition; occasionally this occurs and when it does so it usually indicates that this form of treatment is unsuitable for that patient.

Extended trial period

Experience has shown that the best way to find out whether or not TENS will produce effective pain relief is to loan the patient a stimulator for a trial period of, say 1 month, so that it can be given an exhaustive test under normal everyday conditions of the patient's life. The following are typical instructions that should be given to the patient:

1. 'Use all day initially or for a minimum of 1 hour's treatment three times a day.'
2. 'Adjust according to need.'
3. 'Use as much as you like.'
4. 'Try comparing the pain-relieving effect of continuous and burst TENS, and then use which is best for you, including both forms if necessary.'
5. 'You may get a bonus of pain relief after the stimulator has been switched off (post-TENS analgesia), but don't be disappointed if relief is limited to the time that the TENS unit is actually in use.'
6. 'If you have any problems with the treatment, for example with the stimulator or the electrodes, contact the clinic immediately for advice.'

Review

During the month's trial period, the patient is encouraged to contact the clinic in order to report progress. Initially, each patient on TENS therapy should be reviewed at monthly intervals and thereafter according to need.

Choosing the form of TENS

Experience coupled with the results of a recent survey (Johnson, Ashton & Thompson 1991) have made it abundantly clear that the only method by which to discover the optimum form of TENS for each patient is by trial and error. Having said this, continuous (conventional) TENS may be found better for those pains that are predominantly nociceptive, namely skeletal, paravertebral and joint pains and also visceral referred pain. By contrast, pulsed and acupuncture-like TENS may be found to be better for neuropathic (neurogenic) pain, especially where hyperaesthesia and/or dysaesthesia are prominent features (Sjölund, Eriksson & Loeser 1990).

Indications for TENS therapy

Essentially, TENS can be used to treat any localized pain of somatic or neurogenic origin, provided paraesthesia can be generated in the region of the pain or within the same or a closely related dermatome (Woolf & Thompson 1994). TENS can also be used effectively in the treatment of pain of visceral origin such as angina pectoris (Mannheimer et al 1986). TENS is usually least effective for the treatment of pain that is predominantly psychogenic in origin. The practical situation is that not every patient with the same type of pain will respond to TENS. Thus, the response to TENS is a function of the patient rather than the pain. *An important axiom is that no pain should be considered untreatable by TENS until proved otherwise.*

Position of electrodes

Representative electrode positions for TENS are illustrated in Figure 11.2A and B. It is important to appreciate that these are for guidance only and will need to be modified in the light of circumstances and the response of the patient to treatment.

Acute pain

By definition, acute pain is of short duration and therefore self-limiting. Pain that follows minor trauma is usually short lived and, since it often responds to simple analgesics such as aspirin or paracetamol, TENS is not required. On the other hand, in sports clinics it is common practice to use TENS to treat localized pains that are the result of strains or tears of ligaments or muscles. Where multiple traumata are involved, it is not practical to use TENS but instead an appropriate analgesic should be prescribed. Table 11.2 (p 179) gives other examples of acute pain that can be treated effectively by TENS and indicates that these include surgical, gynaecological and dental conditions. Historically, postoperative

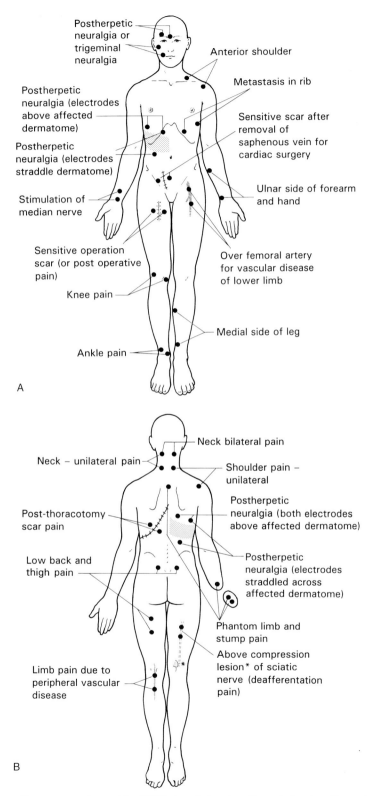

Figure 11.2 Electrode positions commonly used for TENS. A: anterior view. B: posterior view. Reproduced with permission from Oxford University Press.

pain was the first form of acute pain for which TENS was used (Hymes et al 1974) and when used for this purpose constitutes a simple form of what is now known as patient-controlled analgesia (PCA). The use of TENS to control labour pain was first reported by Augustinsson et al (1977), and subsequently by Nesheim (1981), Polden (1984) and Davies (1989), and is now a well-established part of the armamentarium of the community midwife and labour ward.

Chronic pain

TENS has proved to be a useful, effective and non-invasive form of analgesia for the control of many chronic pain conditions, examples of which are shown in Table 11.2 (p 179). As with the use of TENS for acute pain, no pain is untreatable until proved otherwise. Furthermore, neuropathic (neurogenic) pains often respond to TENS whereas they respond little or not at all to primary analgesics, including potent agents such as morphine. The latter observation suggests strongly that neuropathic pains involve non-opioid mechanisms. Widespread chronic pains are perhaps less likely to respond to TENS although these problems can sometimes be overcome by the use of multiple electrodes connected, where necessary, to a multichannel stimulator (see below). It is important to note that certain severe central pain states, for example, brachial plexus avulsion injury (Wynn Parry 1980) and pain that follows injury of the spinal cord (Banerjee 1974, Richardson, Meyer & Cerullo 1980) may respond well to TENS but often much experimentation is required in order to determine the optimum position of the electrodes.

Mode of stimulation

As described earlier (see p 180) present-day TENS equipment makes it possible to vary both the frequency and the pattern of stimulation applied to the body via electrodes. Sjölund & Eriksson (1979) demonstrated that the pharmacological response of the nervous system to TENS is frequency dependent. Thus, low-frequency (1–5 Hz)/high-intensity stimulation

produces analgesia that is blocked by the opioid antagonist naloxone, so demonstrating that this form of stimulation involves opioid mechanisms. By contrast, high-frequency (> 15–150 Hz)/low-intensity stimulation produces analgesia that is unaffected by naloxone, demonstrating that it does not involve opioid mechanisms. The results of experimental work (Duggan & Foong 1985) suggest that high-frequency/low-intensity stimulation may involve the release of GABA an inhibitory neurotransmitter. Thus, there is clear evidence for the existence of at least two types of pain-relieving systems that can be activated by TENS. One might conjecture that there would be a correlation between these two systems and the types of pain relieved by activating them. However, in practice no such correlation has been found and the optimum mode of stimulation to relieve a particular pain in a particular patient must always be found by trial and error, utilizing both modes of stimulation (Johnson, Ashton & Thompson 1991). An important corollary of the foregoing observation is that both modes of stimulation should be tried for every new pain and that, to enable this to be achieved, only stimulators with this dual facility should be purchased. Experience with TENS, coupled with the results of special studies, have made it clear that there is no correlation between the frequency and/or pattern of stimulation that relieves particular pains (Johnson, Ashton & Thompson 1991).

In the past, continuous high-intensity/low-frequency stimulation was employed but was found to cause unpleasant and frequently painful muscle contractions (Andersson, Hahsson & Holmgren 1976, Melzack, 1975.) This problem was overcome by Eriksson, Sjölund & Nielzen (1979) who used *trains* of high-frequency stimuli repeated at a low frequency. This mode of stimulation is referred to as 'acupuncture-like TENS' (see p 180). A modification of acupuncture-like TENS is a modulated or ramped form in which each set of shocks form a rising staircase of increasing intensity. This pattern of pulsing produces a stroking sensation that is more comfortable for the patient (see Table 11.3, p 180).

POST-STIMULATION ANALGESIA

When analgesia induced by TENS persists after the stimulator has been switched off, post-stimulation analgesia is said to occur. Only about 50% of patients are fortunate enough to experience this phenomenon. In those in whom it does occur, the duration varies from less than 30 minutes to over 2 hours and obviously confers a number of advantages. First, it is an added convenience to the patient because it reduces the time needed for electrical stimulation and consequently reduces battery consumption. It also enables the patient to plan his or her treatment in advance and so ensure that analgesia will be available at a particular time (e.g. during an important social event). Secondly, it enables the patient to have intervals unencumbered with TENS apparatus, although modern equipment is so compact that this is not usually a problem. When a patient's pain is found to respond to TENS, it is important to discover whether the bonus of post-TENS analgesia occurs, so that full advantage can be taken of this effect.

CHANGES IN RESPONSE OF THE PATIENT TO TENS

When a patient with chronic pain responds favourably to a trial with TENS, it is not possible to know whether this response is likely to be maintained or is likely to wane. When the latter occurs, it may be due to an increase in the level of pain or due to a change in the response of the patient to TENS, and these different responses must now be discussed.

A change in pain level

It must always be remembered that the intensity of a pain for which TENS is being used may increase, or there may be a change in the emotional response of the patient to the pain. Alternatively, an increased level of pain may be the result of a change in the quality of pain; for example, a neuropathic (neurogenic) component may be added to a primarily nociceptive pain. Another possibility is that one or more new pains have become added to the original pain and this underlines the great importance of monitoring regularly each and every pain, particularly in patients who are suffering from pain associated with advanced cancer.

Causes of change in response

Three main causes must be considered. First, the initially favourable response may have been due to a placebo response, the hallmark of which is that it is likely to fade rapidly or even abruptly within about a week of starting treatment, although sometimes persisting longer (Bates & Nathan 1980). Secondly, the waning response may be due to the onset of tolerance to TENS, a term that conceals much ignorance about its mechanism! When tolerance occurs it usually develops more slowly and insidiously than a placebo response and may not take place for many weeks or months after the start of treatment. It appears to be a similar phenomenon to that of drug tolerance, which may develop over the course of weeks (e.g. opioid tolerance) or over the course of months or even years (e.g. insulin tolerance). The mechanism of tolerance to TENS may involve a number of possible mechanisms that could include some or all of the following: waning neurotransmitter release or downregulation of receptors concerned with neurotransmitters involved in the pharmacology of pain (Thompson 1994) including opioid peptides, 5-HT or noradrenaline, or interference caused by the production of increasing amounts of endogenous opioid antagonists, for example CCK-8, the octapeptide form of cholecystokinin (Wang, Wang & Han 1990). The effectiveness of some of these mechanisms may depend upon the establishment of regular patterns of neuronal activity in the nerve pathways involved, so encouraging the well-known phenomenon of habituation, which the normally regular pulse patterns of TENS may help to establish. It is for this reason that some of the more recently developed stimulators have been constructed with the option of a random pulse output, which discourages the establishment of regular patterns of neuronal activity. This approach has been developed to the furthest degree in the Codetron stimulator, which applies randomly distributed pulses to a set of six electrodes (instead of the usual pair) and is claimed, for this reason, to be more effective than ordinary TENS (Pomeranz & Niznick 1987).

COMPLICATIONS

Complications of TENS therapy may be related to (i) the response of the patient or (ii) the performance of the equipment:

1. TENS therapy is rarely associated with serious complications. The majority of problems arise as a result of skin irritation, allergy to the electrode (this includes the associated conducting jelly, tape or gum) or a skin burn. In a survey of nearly 200 patients who used TENS regularly (Johnson, Ashton & Thompson 1991) the only common problem, occurring in a third of the patients, was skin irritation and this was probably due, at least in part, to drying out of the electrode jelly (Mason & Mackay 1976, Yamamoto, Yamamoto & Akiharu 1986). Irritation of the skin can be minimized by ensuring that the area to which the electrodes are to be applied is kept dry and free from grease and cosmetics. By this means the electrical resistance between the electrode and the skin is kept as low as possible and evenly distributed, thus avoiding 'hot spots' due to the presence of islands of low resistance through which electrical current flow is higher. This situation applies both to carbon rubber electrodes, which require electrode jelly, and to those that are self-adhesive. It is important for all users and prescribers of TENS to be aware of this important and preventable problem.

2. Failure of TENS equipment due to faulty leads, stimulator, battery or charger, is also uncommon. Modern, custom-designed and properly constructed equipment used in accordance with the manufacturer's instructions is very reliable. The leads remain the weakest link in the chain, with failure occurring particularly at the end of the leads where these are joined to the electrodes, usually via a pair of plugs, and where fracture of the leads may occur, or where

lack of careful cleaning may lead to a build-up of dried conductive jelly, resulting in poor contact between the plug and the electrode. It also needs to be remembered that both disposable and rechargeable batteries have a finite life and that the latter cannot be recharged indefinitely.

CONTRAINDICATIONS TO TENS THERAPY

These are relatively few and are most conveniently presented in the form of a list.

1. Do not place electrodes on inflamed, infected or otherwise unhealthy skin.
2. Do not stimulate over the anterior part of the neck. This is to avoid the possibility of stimulating the nerves of the carotid sinus or the larynx, which could produce hypotension or laryngeal spasm, respectively.
3. Do not stimulate over a pregnant uterus (except when TENS is being used for obstetric analgesia where the electrodes are applied posteriorly).
4. Do not use the stimulator in the presence of a cardiac pacemaker. This contraindication applies particularly to an on-demand pacemaker. In order to err on the side of safety, the manufacturers of TENS equipment apply this as a general restriction. Nevertheless, it is not uncommon to operate fixed-rate pacemakers in the presence of a TENS machine, *but this should never be done without the permission of the consulting cardiologist responsible for the patient and also, if necessary, the advice of the manufacturers of both the pacemaker and the TENS equipment.*
5. Do not try to force the use of TENS on a patient who is non-compliant or one who has learning difficulties. In addition, there exists a very small core of patients who have a congenital fear of, or rooted objection to, the use of electricity in any form for medical treatment, including TENS.

OTHER TYPES OF TENS

Since the introduction of TENS, sustained efforts

Table 11.4 Developments of transcutaneous electrical stimulation (TENS)

Type	Description	Comments	References
Acupuncture-like TENS	High-intensity/low-frequency TENS	Increases efficacy; some patients who fail to respond to continuous stimulation will respond to this form	Eriksson, Sjölund & Nielzen (1979)
Codetron stimulator	Uses multiple electrodes, which are excited randomly	Claimed to increase efficacy and to reduce onset of tolerance	Pomeranz & Niznick (1987)
Likon stimulator	Shocks delivered on a complex high-frequency carrier wave	Claimed to increase efficacy by achieving deeper penetration of the tissues by electrical stimulation	Packham & Chandler (1992)
H-wave stimulator	Biphasic wave with exponential decay	Claimed to increase efficacy and to be a more comfortable form of electrical stimulation	McDowell et al (1995)
Microcurrent electrical stimulation (MES)	Very low current (μA) delivered at very high frequency	No sensation of stimulation produced. Unknown mechanism of action. Claimed to be more effective than ordinary TENS	Gersh (1989)
Transcutaneous spinal electroanalgesia (TSE)	High-frequency stimulation (600 Hz)* with very short pulses (4 μs) of high voltage (120 V or more)	Stimulation applied via surface electrodes placed over the spinal cord in one of two locations. Little or no sensation of stimulation. Unknown and novel mechanism of action. Cumulative effect with repeated treatment that can produce analgesia lasting many months	Macdonald & Coates (1995)

have been made to improve every aspect of this method of electroanalgesia, especially its efficacy. Table 11.4 lists some of these developments, from which it can be seen that a number of different modifications have been tried. These are (1) the wave form of the pulse: H wave (McDowell et al 1995), (2) the current/frequency relationship: acupuncture-like TENS (Eriksson, Sjölund & Nielzen 1979) and microcurrent electrical stimulation (MES) (Gersh 1989), (3) addition of a high-frequency carrier wave: Likon (Packham & Chandler 1992) and a multichannel random stimulation: Codetron (Pomeranz & Niznick 1989). The most recent and exciting modification is that of transcutaneous spinal electroanalgesia (TSE) in which high-frequency stimulation (600 Hz)* with very short pulses (4 μs) of high voltage (120 V or more) are applied via surface electrodes placed over the spinal cord (Macdonald & Coates 1995).

MECHANISM OF ACTION OF TENS AND COMPARISON WITH ACUPUNCTURE

During the past two and a half decades, great progress has been made with the study of the neuroanatomy and neuropharmacology of nociceptive systems, including studies on the possible mechanisms of action of both TENS and acupuncture. On the basis of a considerable body of evidence now available, it appears that both peripheral and central neuroanatomical and neuropharmacological mechanisms are involved. Figure 11.3 illustrates diagrammatically the neuro-anatomical and neuropharmacological basis of pain and also the way in which this is modified by TENS and acupuncture. This diagram, which is reproduced from Thompson

*The frequency has been increased to 2000 Hz since this chapter was written.

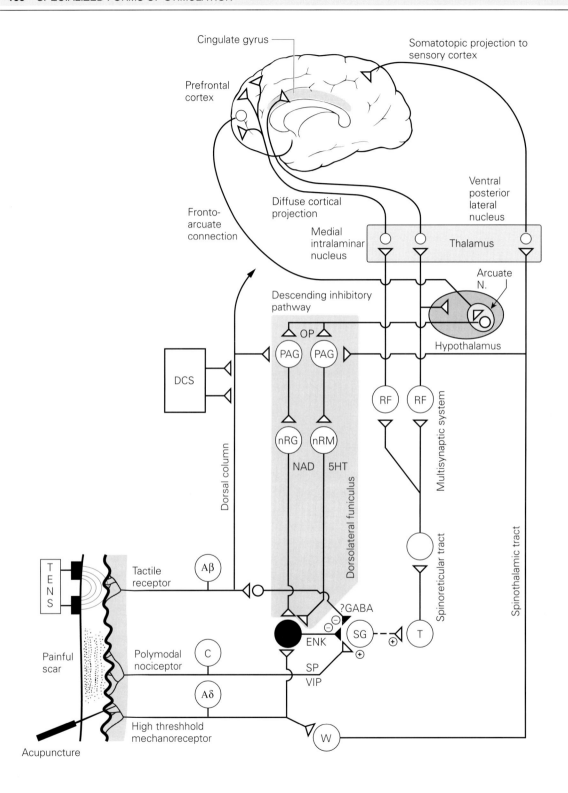

& Filshie (1993), is based on the writings of Bowsher (1985, 1987), Duggan & Foong (1985), Fields & Basbaum (1994), Han & Terenius (1982), Jones et al (1991), Le Bars, Dickenson & Besson (1979) and Pomeranz & Stux (1989).

So-called 'first', 'rapid' or 'aversive' pain is due to the activation of small; myelinated Aδ fibres, whereas 'second', 'slow' or 'tissue-damage' pain is due to the activation of mostly unmyelinated C fibres with the activation of some Aδ fibres (Bowsher 1985). Against this neuroanatomical background there are four conditions that need to be considered:

1. **Pathways for tissue-damage pain**: Peripheral, polymodal, nociceptor afferents are activated as the result of, for example, a painful scar (as shown in Fig. 11.3). The C fibre afferents terminate in the substantia gelatinosa (lamina II) where their axon terminals release substance P or vasoactive intestinal polypeptide (VIP), according to whether they arise from skin or viscera. The substantia gelatinosa cell indirectly excites transmission cells deep in the spinal grey matter whose axons form the spinoreticular tract and which form one component of the crossed anterolateral funiculus which ascends to the brain. The spinoreticular tract sends collaterals to the hypothalamus (triggering autonomic responses to pain) and then synapses in the thalamus. Here it excites other neurons that distribute widely over the cerebral cortex, including the frontal cortex and also the limbic system, giving rise to the conscious sensation and emotional experience of tissue-damage (second) pain.

2. **TENS**: Electrical stimulation excites Aβ afferents connected to tactile receptors. After entering the spinal cord these afferents ultimately ascend in the dorsal columns. At spinal cord level these Aβ afferent fibres give rise to collaterals that synapse with short interneurons that end close to the terminations of the C fibres as the latter synapse with substantia gelatinosa cells. These interneurons probably release γ-amino butyric acid, which causes presynaptic blockade of the C afferents, thereby preventing them from exciting the substantia gelatinosa cells and so blocking the onward transmission of nociceptive information.

3. **Segmental acupuncture**: High-threshold mechanoreceptors connected to small myelinated primary afferents (Aδ) are activated by acupuncture. One central branch of the Aδ afferent excites the inhibitory enkephalinergic interneuron (on the borders of the laminae I and II), releasing enkephalin, which produces postsynaptic block of the substantia gelatinosa cell. This prevents the onward transmission of noxiously generated information. This mechanism would explain the phenomenon of segmental acupuncture.

4. **Extrasegmental acupuncture**: Waldeyer cells in lamina 1 of the spinal grey matter are excited by acupuncture via another central

Figure 11.3 (*Facing page*) Neuronal circuits involved in acupuncture and also in TENS analgesia. The afferent pathways involved in transmitting nociceptive information from a painful scar to the higher centres via the dorsal horn, the ascending tracts and the thalamus are shown. The connections to the descending inhibitory pathways that descend in the dorsolateral funiculus are also shown. The connections to the hypothalamus are indicated. Abbreviations: Aβ, C and Aδ = posterior root ganglion cells of Aβ, C and Aδ fibres; DCS = dorsal column stimulation; ENK = enkephalinergic neuron; GABA = γ-amino-butyric acid; 5-HT = 5-hydroxytryptamine; NRG = cell in the nucleus raphe gigantocellularis; NAD = noradrenaline; NRM = cell in the nucleus raphe magnus; OP = opioid peptides; PAG = periaqueductal grey; RF = reticular formation; SG = cell in the substantia gelatinosa (lamina II); SP = Substance P; T = transmission cell; VIP = vasoactive intestinal polypeptide; W = Waldeyer cell.

Segmental acupuncture pathway: High-threshold mechanoreceptors → Aδ primary afferents → enkephalinergic interneuron (laminae I and II) → postsynaptic block of substantia gelatinosa cell, thus blocking onward transmission of nociceptive information.

Extrasegmental acupuncture pathway: High-threshold mechanoreceptors → Aδ primary afferents→ Waldeyer cells in lamina I → spinothalamic tract (crossed) → periaqueductal grey → [descending] nucleus raphe magnus → dorsolateral funiculus → enkephalinergic interneurons at all levels of spinal cord, so accounting for extrasegmental effects.

TENS pathway (segmental only): Tactile receptors → Aβ primary afferents → GABA-ergic interneuron (+ dorsal columns)→ GABA release → presynaptic inhibition of endings of C primary afferent neuron on substantia gelatinosa cell→ block nociception.

(From Thompson & Filshie 1993, with kind permission of Oxford University Press.)

branch of Aδ primary afferents. The axons of the Waldeyer cells constitute another component (spinothalamic tract) of the crossed anterolateral funiculus and convey pinprick information to consciousness through the ventral postero-lateral nucleus of the thalamus and thence to the somatosensory cortex (where there is soma-totopic representation). Collaterals excite the periaqueductal grey, which in its turn projects to the nucleus raphe magnus situated in the mid-line of the lower brainstem reticular formation. Serotonergic (5-HT) and adrenergic (NAD) axons of nucleus raphe magnus cells descend through the dorsolateral funiculus of the spinal cord to synapse eventually with the cells described above, and so block the onward transmission of noxiously generated information in the same way as does segmental acupuncture. However, *this descending inhibitory pathway gives off these connections at all levels of the spinal cord*, thereby explaining the extrasegmental effect of acupuncture.

Having given the foregoing explanation, it is only fair to point out that the actual mechanism whereby the opioid and serotonergic (5-HT) systems interact to produce their descending inhibitory control is controversial. Indeed, it seems likely that the amount of nociceptive information actually transmitted to the brain depends not simply upon the volume of the nociceptive signal but on the *ratio* of the nociceptive (noxious) signal to the non-nociceptive (non-noxious) signal (i.e. signal to noise ratio). A noxious signal will activate the descending inhibitory system so as to *enhance* the input of the noxious signal at the expense of the non-noxious signals, that is, to *increase* the noxious : non-noxious signal ratio, which will increase the pain perceived (Dickenson 1989). On the other hand, morphine or enkephalin will *reduce* the amount of descending inhibition, which in turn *reduces* the noxious : non-noxious signal

ratio so attenuating the amount of nociceptive information transmitted to the brain, that is, producing analgesia (Willer & Le Bars 1995). It is conceivable that extrasegmental acupuncture and acupuncture-like TENS may produce analgesia by activating the same opioid mechanisms.

A striking and puzzling difference between analgesia produced by TENS and acupuncture is the duration of pain relief. Whereas TENS usually produces analgesia for minutes or hours, acupuncture can, and often does, produce analgesia for days or weeks (certainly after a course of acupuncture). The mechanisms discussed above cannot account for the prolonged analgesia commonly seen after acupuncture, so additional mechanisms (discussed elsewhere in this book) must be involved.

Acknowledgements

The author wishes to thank the coauthor, editors and publishers who have given permission to reproduce material published elsewhere as follows:

Royal Society of Medicine Services Ltd and Dr Derek Doyle, Editor of 1986 International Symposium on Pain Control, to use tables and text from *The role of transcutaneous electrical nerve stimulation (TENS) for the control of pain*; Oxford University Press, the Editors of the *Oxford Textbook of Palliative Medicine* and Dr Jacqueline Filshie, coauthor of our chapter *TENS and Acupuncture*, for permission to use figures, tables and text from this book, Dr Simon Hayhoe, Editor of *Acupuncture in Medicine*, to use Table 4 from *Transcutaneous electrical nerve stimulation for the relief of pain* in *Acupuncture in Medicine: Journal of the British Medical Acupuncture Society* 1995, 13: p 35.

He also wishes to express his grateful thanks to Mrs Margaret Cheek for her excellent secretarial help.

REFERENCES

Andersson S A, Hansson G, Holmgren E, Renberg O 1976 Evaluation of the pain suppressant effect of different frequencies of peripheral electrical stimulation in chronic pain conditions. Acta Orthopaedica Scandinavica 47:149–157

Augustinsson L E, Bohlin P, Bundsen P, Carlsson C A, Forssman C, Sjoberg P, Tyreman N D 1977 Pain relief during delivery by transcutaneous nerve stimulation. Pain 4:59–65

Banerjee T 1974 Transcutaneous nerve stimulation for pain after spinal injury. New England Journal of Medicine 291:796

Bates J W V, Nathan P W 1980 Transcutaneous electrical nerve stimulation for chronic pain. Anaesthesia 35:817–822

Bowsher D 1985 Sensory mechanisms. Clinical Neuropsychology 45:227–244

Bowsher D 1987 The physiology of acupuncture. Journal of the Intractable Pain Society of Great Britain and Ireland 5:15–18

Davies P 1989 An evaluation of transcutaneous nerve stimulation for the relief of pain in labour. Journal of the Association of Chartered Physiotherapists in Obstetrics and Gynaecology 65:2–7

Dickenson A H 1989 Pain transmission and analgesia. In: Webster R A, Jordan C C (eds) Neurotransmitters, drugs and disease . Blackwell Scientific, Oxford, pp 446–464

Duggan A W, Foong F W 1985 Bicuculline and spinal inhibition produced by dorsal column stimulation in the cat. Pain 22:249–259

Eriksson M B E, Sjölund B H, Nielzen S 1979 Long-term results of peripheral conditioning stimulation as an analgesic measure in chronic pain. Pain 6:335–347

Fields H L, Basbaum A I 1994 Central nervous system mechanisms of pain modulation. In: Wall P D, Melzack R (eds) Textbook of pain, 3rd edn. Churchill Livingstone, New York, Ch 12

Gersh M R 1989 Microcurrent electrical stimulation: putting it in perspective. Clinical Management 9:51–54

Han J S, Terenius L 1982 Neurochemical basis of acupuncture analgesia. Annual Review of Pharmacology and Toxicology 22:193–220

Hansson P, Ekblom A 1983 Transcutaneous electrical nerve stimulation (TENS) as compared to placebo-TENS for the relief of acute oro-facial pain. 15:157–165

Hymes A C, Raab D E, Yonchiro E G, Nelson G D, Drintz A 1974 Acute pain control by electrostimulation: a preliminary report. In: Bonica J J (ed) Advances in neurology, vol 4. Raven Press, New York, 761:761–773

Johnson M I, Ashton C H, Thompson J W 1991 An in depth study of long-term users of transcutaneous electrical nerve stimulation (TENS). Implications for clinical use of TENS. Pain 44:221–229

Jones A K P, Brown W D, Friston K J, Qi L Y, Frackowiak R S J 1991 Cortical and subcortical localisation of response to pain in man using positron emission tomography. Proceedings of the Royal Society of London B 244:39–44

Kaada B 1983 Promoted healing of chronic ulceration by transcutaneous nerve stimulation (TNS) and its vasa. Vasa 12(3):262–269

Le Bars D, Dickenson A H, Besson J M 1979 Diffuse noxious inhibitory controls (DNIC). I: Effects on dorsal horn convergent neurones in the rat; II: Lack of effect on non-convergent neurones, supraspinal involvement and theoretical implications. Pain 6:283–304, 305–327

Long D 1973 Electrical stimulation for relief of pain from chronic nerve injury. Journal of Neurosurgery 39:718–722

Long D M, Campbell J N, Gurer G 1979 Transcutaneous electrical stimulation for relief of chronic pain. In: Bonica J J (ed) Advances in pain research therapy, vol 3. Raven Press, New York, pp 593–599

Macdonald A J R, Coates T W 1995 The discovery of transcutaneous spinal electroanalgesia and its relief of chronic pain. Physiotherapy 81:653–661

McDowell B C, Lowe A S, Walsh D M, Baxter G D, Allen J M 1995 The lack of hypoalgesic efficacy of H-wave therapy on experimental ischaemic pain. Pain 61:27–32

Mannheimer C, Carlsson C A, Vedin A, Wilhelmson C 1986 Transcutaneous electrical nerve stimulation (TENS) in angina pectoris. Pain 26:291–300

Mason J L, Mackay N A M 1976 Pain sensations associated with electrocutaneous stimulation. IEEE Transactions on Biomedical Engineering 23:405–409

Melzack R 1975 Prolonged relief of pain by brief transcutaneous somatic stimulation. Pain 1:357–373

Melzack R, Wall P D 1965 Pain mechanisms: a new theory. Science 150:971–979

Nesheim B I 1981 The use of transcutaneous nerve stimulation for pain relief during labour. Acta Obstetrica et Gynaecologica Scandinavica 60:13–16

Packham R J, Chandler C S 1992 A comparison of Likon and transcutaneous electrical nerve stimulation for the relief of pain in patients suffering from ankylosing spondylitis. Clinical Rehabilitation 6 (suppl):36–37

Pike P M 1978 Transcutaneous electrical stimulation: its use in management of postoperative pain. Anaesthesia 33:165–171

Polden M 1984 Transcutaneous nerve stimulation used in labour. Journal of the Association of Chartered Physiotherapists in Obstetrics and Gynaecology 54:13–16

Pomeranz B, Niznick G 1987 Codetron a new electrotherapy device overcomes the habituation problems of conventional TENS devices. American Journal of Electromedicine First quarter:22–26

Pomeranz B, Stux G (eds) 1989 Scientific bases of acupuncture. Springer-Verlag, Berlin

Reynolds D V 1969 Surgery in the rat during electrical analgesia induced by focal brain stimulation. Science 164:444–445

Richardson R R, Meyer P R, Cerullo L J 1980 Neurostimulation in the modulation of intractable paraplegic and traumatic neuroma pains. Pain 8:75–84

Shealy C N 1974 Transcutaneous electrical stimulation for control of pain. Clinical Neurosurgery 21:269–277

Shealy C N, Mortimer J T, Reswick J B 1967 Electrical inhibition of pain by stimulation of the dorsal column: preliminary clinical reports. Anaesthesia and Analgesia 46:489–491

Sjölund B H, Eriksson M B E 1979 The influence of naloxone on analgesia produced by peripheral conditioning stimulation. Brain Reviews 173:295–301

Sjölund B H, Eriksson M B E, Loeser J D 1990
Transcutaneous and implanted electrical stimulation of
peripheral nerves. In: Bonica J J (ed) The management of
pain, vol II, 2nd edn. Lea & Febiger, Philadelphia
1852–1861

Thompson J W 1986 The role of transcutaneous electrical
nerve stimulation (TENS) for the control of pain. In: Doyle
D (ed) International Symposium on Pain Control. Royal
Society of Medicine Services International Congress and
Symposium Series 123. Royal Society of Medicine, London

Thompson J W 1994 Neuropharmacology of the pain
pathway. In: Wells P E, Frampton V, Bowsher D, (eds)
Pain management by physiotherapy, 2nd edn.
Butterworth Heinemann, Oxford

Thompson J W, Filshie J 1993 Transcutaneous electrical nerve
stimulation (TENS) and acupuncture. In: Doyle D, Hanks
G, MacDonald N (eds) Oxford textbook of palliative
medicine. Oxford University Press, Oxford, ch 4.2.8

Wall P D, Sweet W 1967 Temporary abolition of pain in man.
Science 155:108–109

Wang X-J, Wang X-H, Han J 1990 Cholecystokinin
octapeptide antagonises opioid analgesia mediated by
mu- and kappa- but not delta-receptors in the spinal cord

of the rat. Brain Research 523: 5–10

Willer J C, Le Bars D 1995 Electrophysiologic studies of
morphine analgesia in humans. In: Bromm B, Desmedt J E
(eds) Pain and the brain: from nociception to cognition.
Advances in Pain Research and Therapy. Raven Press,
New York, 22:541–557

Woolf C J 1989 Segmental afferent fibre-induced analgesia:
transcutaneous electrical nerve stimulation (TENS) and
vibration. In: Wall P D, Melzack R (eds) Textbook of pain,
2nd edn. Churchill Livingstone, New York, pp 884–896

Woolf C J, Thompson J W 1994 Stimulation induced
analgesia: transcutaneous electrical nerve stimulation
(TENS) and vibration. In: Wall P D, Melzack R (eds)
Textbook of pain, 3rd edn. Churchill Livingstone, New
York, ch 63

Wynn Parry C B 1980 Pain in avulsion lesions of the brachial
plexus. Pain 9:41–53

Yamamoto T, Yamamoto Y, Akiharu Y 1986 Formative
mechanisms of current concentration and breakdown
phenomena dependent on direct current flow through
skin by a dry electrode. IEEE Transactions on Biomedical
Engineering 33:396–404

12

Laser therapy

Peter Baldry

INTRODUCTION

During the 1970s many experienced acupuncturists began to advocate the use of low-power lasers (LPLs) as an alternative for pain relief (Bishko 1980). Lack of certainty, however, as to whether LPLs have any specific influence on the body's pain-modulating mechanisms, and the poor results of those few LPL controlled clinical trials so far conducted, means that much more research remains to be carried out and positive evidence accumulated before their routine employment for this purpose can be confidently recommended (Baldry 1993). In this chapter the various possible mechanisms responsible for LPLs' alleged ability to relieve pain, and the results of controlled clinical trials carried out to show whether or not they have a specific pain-relieving effect, will be reviewed. Before doing this it is necessary to say something about LPLs.

PHYSICAL PROPERTIES OF LPLS

Laser light is an artificially produced electromagnetic radiation; the term LASER is an acronym for 'light amplification by stimulated emission of radiation'. The physical properties of laser light are different from those of natural light and include:

1. **coherence**: i.e. independent atoms emit their radiation concurrently
2. **monochromasy**: i.e. laser light has a single well-defined wavelength, which varies according to the type of laser used

3. **minimal divergence**: i.e. the beam remains focused for a long time
4. **polarizability**: i.e. laser light is readily polarized.

Types of LPL

The most frequently used LPLs for attempting to promote tissue healing and alleviate pain are the visible red light Helium–Neon gas laser with a continuous emission at a wavelength of 633 nm, the infrared gallium–aluminium–arsenide laser and the infrared gallium–arsenide laser. These have pulsed emissions at wavelengths of 830 nm and 904 nm respectively. High-power lasers used surgically have a power density of around 10 W/cm^2; in contrast LPLs have a power density of less than 1 W/cm^2 so that the irradiated tissue is not noticeably heated. For this reason LPL irradiation is referred to as being 'athermic'.

Tissue penetration

First, laser light is no different from natural light with respect to its depth of tissue penetration as neither monochromasy nor coherence enhance penetration.

Secondly, when light, whether it is natural light or artificially produced laser light, penetrates tissues its intensity becomes exponentially reduced. For this reason, just as one refers to the half-life of a drug, so it is helpful to define a 'half-depth' at which 50% of the initial energy is still present. It has been estimated that, for the infrared gallium–arsenide laser with a wavelength of 904 nm and for the visible red light helium–neon laser with a wavelength of 633 nm, the half-depth is less than 1 mm for people with white skin and even less for those with dark skin (Seichert 1991). Thus, even assuming that the half-depth of these LPLs is as much as 1 mm, then at 2 mm (i.e. twice the half-depth) the intensity is reduced to 25% of the original; after 3 mm it is only 12.5% and at a depth of 10 mm (i.e. 10 times the half-depth) no more than 1/1000 of the initial energy is still present. It therefore follows that at a depth of 1 cm or more from the skin surface the intensity is negligible—a state of affairs which clearly has to be taken into account when considering the clinical applications both of natural light and laser light.

REGULATIONS GOVERNING THE USE OF LASER EQUIPMENT

LPLs employed for their possible pain-relieving effect are subject to the same legal restrictions as those governing the use of high-power 'surgical' lasers. The main reason for this is because a LPL beam, when directed at the pupil of the eye from a distance of less than 1 metre, is liable to cause damage to the retina. Space does not permit a detailed discussion of the somewhat complex statutory rules governing the various types of premises in which laser treatment may be carried out and the personnel authorized to use it. Those who wish to know more about the matter should therefore consult White's (1993) comprehensive review of the subject.

THE MODUS OPERANDI OF LPLS
Animal studies

In 1971, Fork reported that it required only an extremely short period of athermic irradiation with an argon laser to bring about a change in the firing pattern of abdominal ganglion cells isolated from *Aplysia californica*—a marine mollusc. Six years later Vizi et al (1977) reported that non-thermal irradiation with a ruby laser enhanced the release of acetylcholine from Auerbach's plexus neurons isolated from guinea pig ileum.

However, despite the fact that these two animal studies seemed to suggest that LPL irradiation may be capable of stimulating activity in neural tissue, another study carried out by Lundeberg, Hode & Zhou (1988) did not agree with this. In that experiment, nociceptive neurons isolated from the medicinal leech (*Hirudo medicinalis*) were irradiated with either a helium–neon laser or a gallium–arsenide laser held 1 cm from the neurons for varying periods of 1, 5 or 10 minutes. A failure to increase neuronal activity by this means led them to conclude that 'The non-existing effect of low-power He–Ne and Ga–As lasers on the nociceptors in the present study indicate that the pain alleviating effects reported in other studies with similar modes of low-power laser cannot be explained by effects on nociceptors'.

In-vivo studies

When light of any type is directed at the skin in in-vivo studies, its intensity quickly falls off as it penetrates the tissues. However, sensory afferent nerve terminals in the skin are only 200–300 μm below the surface (Jarvis, MacIver & Tanelian 1990) and therefore the exponential reduction in the penetrative power of light should not prevent it from stimulating sensory neurons if it should have the intrinsic ability to do so.

The results of a trial carried out by Walker (1983) led her to believe that LPL light applied to the skin overlying a peripheral nerve has, by its action on that nerve, a pain-relieving effect. Her observations also led her to believe that the latter might be brought about as a result of laser irradiation influencing serotonin metabolism, but further work by Hansen & Thorøe (1990) discounted this.

Nevertheless, support for her observation that LPL irradiation of a superficial nerve might have a specific therapeutic effect seemed to be provided by Walker & Akhanjee (1985) reporting that it produces a somatosensory-evoked potential identical in latency to that obtained with electrical stimulation of the same nerve, for, as they stated, this 'indicates that the peripheral nervous system possesses a previously unsuspected degree of photosensitivity and provides the rationale for the therapeutic application of low-power laser'.

However, when Wu et al (1987) conducted similar experiments they were unable to confirm Walker & Akhanjee's findings. Similarly, although Snyder-Mackler, Bork & Fernandez (1985) and Snyder-Mackler & Bork (1988) reported that helium–neon laser irradiation of the skin overlying the radial nerve at a site where it lies superficially in humans produces a notable increase in conduction along the nerve, neither Greathouse, Currier & Gilmore (1985) nor Lundeberg, Haker & Thomas (1987) have been able to confirm this. As Jarvis, MacIver & Tanelian (1990) have commented, 'To date, no two studies have described the same neural effect of He–Ne laser irradiation'. However, this seeming confusion, as Basford (1989) has pointed out, may be due to the techniques employed in these studies being widely different.

As an alternative to directing LPL light at skin overlying a superficial nerve, other clinicians have been directing it at either traditional Chinese acupuncture points or trigger points in the belief that it might have the same effect as needle stimulation at these sites, and some have gone so far as to refer to it as 'laser acupuncture' (Glykofridis & Diamantopoulos 1987).

If LPL light is akin to acupuncture, then its pain-modulating effect should be by the same mechanism the stimulation of Aδ nerve fibres. In order to establish whether this is so, MacIver and Tanelian in Stanford, USA and Jarvis in Adelaide, Australia (Jarvis, MacIver & Tanelian 1990) carried out a large number of sophisticated electrophysiological experiments on the cornea of the rabbit. In these experiments they were unable to determine any activity in the Aδ or C nociceptors as a result of irradiation with a helium–neon (He–Ne) laser over a range of 0–5 mW energy with exposure times of 0–15 minutes. They therefore concluded that any pain relief LPLs may provide is not produced by the same mechanism as that responsible for the development of acupuncture analgesia. On these grounds alone, therefore, besides it being etymologically incorrect, it is wrong to employ the term 'laser acupuncture'.

Athermic irradiation

The question to be addressed next is whether any pain-relieving effect of LPLs is due to an ability to heat the tissues. Devor (1990) has pointed out that a helium–neon laser is no more powerful than the laser pointer used in lecture halls, which 'at close range packs about the same radiation punch as a small flashlight with a piece of red cellophane over the front'. This type of laser is thus certainly not capable of imparting any appreciable heat to irradiated tissues and even the slightly more powerful infrared ones do not raise tissue temperature by more than 0.3–0.62°C (Boussignac, Vielledent & Geschwind 1985). Temperature rises of this order are minimal when compared with rises of 5°C or more with modalities such as hot packs, ultrasound and short-wave diathermy, and for this reason LPLs are said to be athermic. This means that if they have a pain-relieving effect it cannot be due to their ability to deliver heat.

LPLs' tissue-healing effects

The place of LPLs in assisting with the healing of superficial lesions such as leg ulcers, bed sores, burns and irradiation ulcers was first explored by Mester and his co-workers in the early 1970s (Mester, Mester & Mester 1985). Their findings unfortunately were originally published in Hungarian journals and did not come to the attention of those outside that country for some years. More recently, much research on the biological effect of LPLs has been carried out by Dyson & Young (1986) in this country. These workers have confirmed that LPL therapy accelerates tissue healing and that its ability to do so is dependent on the frequency at which light is delivered. The process is enhanced when the LPL irradiation is carried out at a frequency of 700 Hz and inhibited when carried out at a frequency of 1200 Hz (Dyson & Young 1986).

In a review of the subject, Young & Dyson (1993) point out that not only coherent LPL light but also non-coherent natural light is capable of promoting tissue healing (Karu 1988, Young et al 1988) and that natural light and LPL light are particularly effective in doing so when used during the early inflammatory stage of the repair process. This being because of light's stimulating effect on macrophages (Young et al 1988) and mast cells (El Sayed & Dyson 1990).

Various hypotheses have been put forward as to how light of one type or another accelerates the healing of tissues, but the most likely explanation would seem to be the one proposed by Karu (1988). He postulates that the energy provided by light is taken up by cytochromes, which are photoabsorbers present in the mitochondria of all cells, and that the effect of this is to trigger off a series of intracellular events that produce cell membrane permeability changes for a variety of ions, including calcium. In support of this hypothesis is the finding of Young, Dyson & Bolton (1990) that light therapy modifies the calcium intake of macrophages.

Young, Dyson & Bolton (1990) have also shown that these light-induced effects on cells involved in the healing process vary according to the wavelength, energy density and frequency of the light source. Much work therefore has still to be done in order to determine the optimal parameters for the therapeutic use of natural and LPL light.

If it should ultimately be proved that natural light and LPL light afford pain relief then it may well do so, as Hayhoe (1993) has suggested, as a result of its tissue repair-accelerating effect. If this is so then it might be expected that LPL therapy would be more effective than a placebo in alleviating the pain of a predominantly inflammatory soft tissue lesion such as, for example, an enthesopathy. Controlled clinical trials, however, that have been carried out on patients with lateral epicondylitis (referred to in the next section) do not show this to be so. The explanation for this may be that, as stated earlier, light of any type has a negligible intensity in tissues below a depth of 10 mm and that it may thus be realistic to expect its biological effects to be of value only in the treatment of lesions in and just beneath the skin.

CONTROLLED CLINICAL TRIALS

Many of those who have advocated the use of LPLs for pain relief have unfortunately based their claims on anecdotal case histories or the results of uncontrolled trials. As such evidence is liable to be misleading, only controlled clinical trials will be reviewed here.

Neurogenic pain trials

Trigeminal neuralgia

Walker et al (1987a) reported the results of a trial in which LPL therapy and placebo laser therapy were compared in the treatment of trigeminal neuralgia. The treatment group had a statistically greater reduction in pain.

Postherpetic neuralgia

Moore et al (1988), in a double-blind crossover trial comparing laser and placebo therapy in postherpetic neuralgia, found the pain-relieving effect of the LPL to be superior to that of the placebo.

   These two good results with LPLs in the treatment of neurogenic pain are somewhat surprising, particularly as there is not much convincing evidence that acupuncture has any significant effect on pain of this type. It is, of course, possible that the modus operandi of these two types of treatment is different. However, before one can speculate about this there is first an urgent need for further large-scale trials to be carried out to see whether or not these results can be confirmed.

Pain from compression of the median nerve

Ysla & McAuley's (1985) trial in which patients with the disorder were randomly assigned to an infrared laser treatment group, a placebo laser group and a control group showed that the laser had no statistically significant subjective or objective therapeutic effects.

Arthritic joint pain trials

Rheumatoid arthritic pain

The pain of rheumatoid arthritis would seem to be the one exception, in that a number of controlled trials have shown it to be relieved to a greater extent by LPL irradiation than by placebo therapy (Bliddal et al 1987, Colov et al 1987, Goldman 1980, Oyamada & Izu 1985, Walker et al 1987b). Seichert (1991), however, has sounded a warning concerning some of these results, stating that they 'have to be looked upon with some reservation until they are published with a description of the experiments'. Furthermore, Basford (1989) during the course of reviewing the various trials already mentioned, expressed the opinion that, whilst the majority of them seem to confirm that laser irradiation diminishes pain, lessens joint swelling, reduces medication and improves morning stiffness in rheumatoid arthritis, it is not clear that the benefits are large enough to be of clinical significance or the treatment sufficient to replace conventional therapies. He did, however, then go on to say that, in the unlikely event of the USA Food and Drug Administration (FDA) granting its approval for the use of low-energy lasers 'It may well first be as an adjunct to the treatment of rheumatoid arthritis'.

Osteoarthritic pain

In contrast to the seemingly promising results with rheumatoid arthritic pain, controlled trials in patients with osteoarthritic knee pain (Jensen, Harreby & Kjer 1987, McAuley & Ysla 1985) and osteoarthritic thumb pain (Basford et al 1987) showed no subjective or objective differences between the LPL-treated groups and the placebo-treated groups.

Myofascial pain trials

There have been several claims of a 70–80% success rate with LPL treatment for myofascial neck (Kroetlinger 1980) and shoulder pain (Calderhead et al 1982). Such claims have for the most part come from uncontrolled studies: Waylonis et al (1988) state that the presentation of Emmanouilidis & Diamantopoulos to the sixth annual meeting of the American Society for Laser Medicine and Surgery, in which according to Stein (1986) they attributed the rehabilitation of athletes with knee strains, thigh sprains, dislocations and assorted forms of inflammation to the effects of laser therapy, was a good example of the type of anecdotal reporting that has made the scientific evaluation of low-energy lasers' pain-relieving potential so difficult.

Indirect evidence that LPL therapy may have a deactivating and desensitizing effect on myofascial trigger points has come from a study carried out by Pöntinen and his colleagues in Finland (Airaksinen et al 1989). In this trial they divided patients with myofascial trigger points into two groups. Skin overlying the points was irradiated with an infrared laser in one group and with a placebo laser in the other. Immediately following treatment the pressure threshold in the treated group was $0.97 \, \text{kg/cm}^2$ greater than it was in the placebo group and 15 minutes after treatment it was $1.87 \, \text{kg/cm}^2$ greater. However, all they could conclude from this was that the 'results suggest that infrared laser had an effect at the trigger points and that the treatment significantly increased the pressure threshold'. It is much to be regretted that they did not attempt to correlate these pressure threshold measurements with subjective assessments of changes in pain intensity in the two groups. It is similarly regrettable that Snyder-Mackler et al (1986) did not do this in a double-blind study showing that LPL irradiation decreases the electrical resistance of skin overlying myofascial trigger points.

One of the very few controlled trials carried out to assess whether LPL therapy has a successful myofascial pain-relieving effect was most unfortunately not carried out on patients with the myofascial pain syndrome, the pain of which is generally acknowledged to respond well to acupuncture, but on patients with fibromyalgia, the pain of which is known to respond far less well to acupuncture. Furthermore, in this trial carried out by Waylonis et al (1988), the LPL in the treatment group and the non-functioning placebo laser in the control group were not directed at the skin overlying trigger points but at skin overlying 12 arbitrarily selected traditional Chinese acupuncture points in the upper part of the body.

Although Waylonis and his colleagues from a carefully conducted statistical analysis showed no difference with respect to fibromyalgia pain relief in the laser and control groups, their conclusion from this that 'low-power laser therapy is not an effective modality for soft-tissue pain

when applied at conventional acupuncture points' was clearly not justified. It is obviously wrong to draw conclusions about the effectiveness of LPLs in relieving soft tissue pain in general and myofascial trigger point pain in particular from a trial restricted to the treatment of fibromyalgia. Controlled trials to establish whether or not LPL therapy directed either at skin overlying trigger points, or at skin overlying traditional Chinese acupuncture points in patients with the myofascial pain syndrome, have therefore still to be carried out.

Enthesopathy pain trials

These will be considered separately from myofascial pain trials because the pain in an enthesopathy partly develops as a result of an inflammatory process in a tendon at or near to its attachment to bone and partly emanates from trigger points in nearby muscles.

Haker & Lundeberg (1990) and Lundeberg, Haker & Thomas (1987) have conducted controlled trials in patients with lateral epicondylitis. In addition, Siebert et al (1987) have carried out a trial in patients with one or other of a number of different tendinopathies including lateral and medial epicondylitis. In none of these trials was the pain-relieving effect significantly better with laser than it was with placebo treatment. This evidence somewhat contradicts the idea discussed earlier that LPL may relieve pain by an anti-inflammatory action.

Chronic orofacial pain trials

Wilder-Smith (1988), a dental surgeon at the University of Heidelberg Dental School, in a paper entitled 'The soft laser: therapeutic tool or popular placebo?', stated that, although soft laser therapy had been recommended for a variety of different dental conditions, she had found no benefit from augmenting the conventional treatment with LPL irradiation, other than that the use of the latter was associated with a better psychological acceptance of dental procedures. One interesting example of this quoted by her was an experiment involving 20 patients who repeatedly experienced nausea during dental procedures. Each of the 20 patients, before a dental procedure was embarked upon, received soft laser irradiation to skin overlying an acupuncture point on the chin for 3 minutes. Ten of the patients were told this would alleviate the nausea, and in six of them it did. Ten, however, were not told that it might relieve the nausea and in none of them did it do so. From similar observations with the use of a soft laser in a variety of dental disorders, she concluded that this form of therapy is nothing more than a popular placebo.

Hansen & Thorøe (1990), in a trial carried out at the University Hospital and Dental College, Copenhagen, compared the effects of an active infrared laser probe and an inactive placebo probe on a variety of different orofacial pain disorders. Twenty-eight patients had the burning mouth syndrome, five had pain in a single tooth, four had trigeminal neuralgia and three had tension headaches. Treatment effects were evaluated by means of visual analogue scales and global assessments of pain. No statistically significant difference between the analgesic effect of the active and placebo lasers was found. Both forms of treatment gave the traditional placebo response of improvement in 40% of patients.

Meta-analysis

Gam, Thorsen & Lonnberg (1993) carried out a meta-analysis of trials of LPL therapy in patients with musculoskeletal pain of myofascial, arthritic and enthesopathic origin. This included 23 trials culled from the literature, 17 of which were controlled trials. Their conclusion from this was that LPL therapy 'has no effect on pain in musculoskeletal syndromes'.

CONCLUSIONS

The manner in which LPL irradiation might exert a pain-reducing effect remains obscure. LPL irradiation is athermic; it has no influence on serotonin metabolism; above all, it has no stimulating effect on Aδ nerve fibres, and for this reason alone cannot be likened to acupuncture. It is conceded, however, in view of its widely accepted tissue-healing properties, that it could have an effect on pain when the latter develops as a result of soft tissue inflammation.

Pöntinen (1992) has written extensively and enthusiastically about the use of LPL therapy for the alleviation of pain but, as may be seen both from the results of controlled trials reviewed in this chapter and from a recently conducted meta-analysis, there is still considerable doubt as to whether any pain relief obtained with a LPL is greater than that obtained with a placebo. This conclusion is in line with the opinion expressed by Seichert (1991), a physician at the University of Munich who, having herself reviewed the literature, stated 'it seems evident that the clinical use of . . . laser irradiation cannot be recommended either from a scientific or clinical point of view'. This concurs with the opinion expressed by Basford (1986, 1989), a physician at the Mayo Clinic, who, having comprehensively reviewed the literature on two occasions, concluded that controlled studies have shown LPL therapy is of such limited value as to make it unlikely that FDA approval will be granted for its use at any time in the near future.

It is therefore evident that, before LPL therapy can confidently be recommended for use as a pain reliever in everyday clinical practice, more positive evidence is essential. Much work still has to be done to determine the optimum irradiation parameters for the various types of LPL now on the market. Also there is no general agreement as to which pain disorders LPL therapy should be used for.

As light energy is rapidly dissipated as it penetrates the tissues it might be that the most promising use of LPLs, so far as their analgesic effect is concerned, will prove to be for the relief of pain arising in association with disorders that cause structural damage to the outer layers of the body. Certainly there is no evidence to suggest that LPL therapy may be used as an effective alternative to acupuncture for the treatment of myofascial pain syndrome (Ch 4). Before this can be contemplated there is a need for a large-scale trial to be carried out for the purpose of comparing the relative trigger point-deactivating efficacy of these two forms of therapy.

Furthermore, it has to be said that, before doctors and physiotherapists expend large sums of money purchasing highly priced LPLs, they need to be satisfied that such instruments offer significant advantages over equipment supplying cheaper, non-coherent light (Young et al 1988).

Finally, it is salutary to bear in mind the following cogent comments made by Professor Devor (1990), a physician at the University of Jerusalem:

So let's say that the numerous 'open' studies of laser pain therapy amount to a placebo effect. What is wrong with that, as long as it works? Nothing really, but on two conditions. Firstly, the physician must be aware that he is using a placebo. Secondly, there needs to be protection against financial exploitation. If a red flashlight with mystic labels is as effective as a 10 000 dollar laser instrument, who wins when the laser is purchased?

REFERENCES

Airaksinen O, Rantanen P, Pertti K, Pöntinen P 1989 Effects of the infrared laser therapy at treated and non-treated trigger points. Acupuncture and Electro-therapeutics Research 14:9–14

Baldry P E 1993 A review of low-power laser pain-relieving controlled clinical trials. Acupuncture in Medicine. XI(1):2–10

Basford J R 1986 Low-energy laser treatment of pain and wounds: hype, hope or hokum? Mayo Clinic Proceedings 61:671–675

Basford J R 1989 Low-energy laser therapy: controversies and new research findings. Lasers in Surgery and Medicine 9:1–5

Basford J R, Sheffield P T, Mair B A, Illstrup M S 1987 Low-energy helium–neon laser treatment of thumb osteoarthritis. Archives of Physical Medicine and Rehabilitation 68:794–797

Bischko J 1980 Use of the laser beam in acupuncture. Acupuncture and Electro-therapeutics Research. 5:29–40

Bliddal H, Hellesen C, Ditlevsen P, Asselberghs J, Lyager L 1987 Soft-laser therapy of rheumatoid arthritis. Scandinavian Journal of Rheumatology 16:225

Boussignac G, Vielledent C, Geschwind H 1985 Thermal effects of semi-conductor lasers in man (abstr). In: Proceedings of the 6th Congress of the International Society for Laser Surgery and Medicine, p 77

Calderhead G, Oshiro T, Itoh E, Okada T, Kato Y 1982 The Nd YAG and Ga ALAs Lasers: a comparative analysis in pain therapy. Laser Acupuncture 21:1–4

Colov H C, Palmgren N, Jansen G F, Kas K, Windelin M 1987 Convincing clinical improvement of rheumatoid arthritis by soft laser therapy. Lasers in Surgery and Medicine 7:77

Devor M 1990 What's in a laser beam for pain therapy? Pain 43:139

Dyson M, Young S R 1986 Effect of laser therapy on wound contraction and cellularity in mice. Lasers in Medical Science 1:125–130

El Sayed S O, Dyson M 1990 Comparison of the effect of multiwavelength light produced by a cluster of semiconductor diodes and of each individual diode on mast cell number and degranulation in intact and injured skin. Lasers in Surgery and Medicine 10:559–568

Fork R L 1971 Laser stimulation of nerve cells. In: Aplysia Californica. Science, 171:907–908

Gam A N, Thorsen H, Lonnberg F 1993 The effect of low-level laser therapy on musculoskeletal pain: a meta-analysis. Pain 52:63–66

Glykofridis S, Diamantopoulos C 1987 Comparison between laser acupuncture and physiotherapy. Acupuncture in Medicine 4(1):6–9

Goldman J A, Chiapella J, Casey H, Bass N et al 1980 Laser therapy of rheumatoid arthritis. Laser in Surgery and Medicine 1:93–101

Greathouse D G, Currier D P, Gilmore R L 1985 Effects of clinical infrared laser on superficial radial nerve conduction. Physical Therapy 65:1184–1187

Haker E, Lundeberg T 1990 Laser treatment applied to acupuncture points in lateral humeral epicondylagia. A double-blind study. Pain 43:243–247

Hansen H J, Thorøe U 1990 Low-power laser biostimulation of orofacial pain. A double-blind placebo-controlled cross-over study in 40 patients. Pain 43:169–179

Hayhoe S 1993 [Editorial.]Acupuncture in Medicine 11(1):1

Jarvis D, MacIver M B, Tanelian D L 1990 Electrophysiological recording and thermodynamic modeling demonstrate that helium–neon laser irradiation does not affect peripheral A-delta or C-fiber nociceptors. Pain 43:235–242

Jensen H, Harreby M, Kjer J 1987 Is infrared laser effective in painful arthritis of the knee? Ugeskrift Forlaeger 149:3104–3106

Karu T I 1988 Molecular mechanisms of the therapeutic effect of low-intensity laser irradiation. Lasers in Life Sciences 2:53–74

Kroetlinger M 1980 On the use of the laser in acupuncture. Acupuncture and Electro-therapeutics Research 5:297–311

Lundeberg T, Haker E, Thomas M 1987 Effects of laser versus placebo in tennis elbow. Scandinavian Journal of Rehabilitation Medicine 19:135–138

Lundeberg T, Hode L, Zhou J 1988 Effect of low-power laser irradiation on nociceptive cells in *Hirudo medicinalis*. Acupuncture and Electro-therapeutics Research 13:99–104

McAuley R, Ysla R 1985 Soft laser: a treatment for osteoarthritis of the knee? [abstr]. Archives of Physical Medicine and Rehabilitation. 66:577 [NB due to printer's error, title of this paper and one by Ysla & McAuley on trial of laser in Carpal tunnel syndrome have been transposed.]

Mester E, Mester A F, Mester A 1985 The biomedical effects

of laser application. Lasers in Surgery and Medicine 5:31–39

Moore K C, Hira N, Kumar P S et al 1988 A double-blind crossover trial of low-level laser therapy in the treatment of post herpetic neuralgia. Laser Therapy, Pilot issue 1:7–9

Oyamada Y, Izu S 1985 Application of low energy laser in chronic rheumatic arthritis and related rheumatoid diseases (abstr). In: Proceedings of the 6th Congress of the International Society for Laser Surgery and Medicine, p 80

Pöntinen P J 1992 Low level laser therapy as a medical treatment modality. Art urpo, Tampere

Seichert N 1991 Controlled trials of laser treatment. In: Sclapbach P, Gerber N J (eds) Physiotherapy: controlled trials and facts. Rheumatology, vol 14. Karger, Basel, pp 205–217

Siebert W, Seichert N, Siebert B, Wirth C J 1987 What is the efficacy of 'soft' and 'mid' lasers in therapy of tendinopathies? A double-blind study. Archives of Orthopaedic and Traumatic Surgery. 106:358–363

Snyder-Mackler L, Bork C E 1988 Effect of helium–neon laser irradiation on peripheral sensory nerve latency. Physical Therapy 68:223–225

Snyder-Mackler L, Bork C, Fernandez J 1985 The effect of helium–neon laser on latency of sensory nerve (abstr). Physical Therapy 65:737

Snyder-Mackler L, Bork C, Bourbon B, Trumbore D 1986 Effect of helium–neon laser on musculoskeletal trigger points. Physical Therapy 66(7):1087–1090

Stein J (1986)Laser therapy accelerates Rehab lower limb injuries. Orthopedic Product News Sept.:17

Vizi E W, Mester E, Tisza A, Mester A 1977 Acetylcholine releasing effect of laser irradiation on Auberbach's plexus in guinea-pig ileum. Journal of Neural Transmitters 40:305–308

Walker J B 1983 Relief from chronic pain by low-power laser irradiation. Neuroscience Letters 43:339–344

Walker J B, Akhanjee L K 1985 Laser-induced somatosensory evoked potentials: evidence of photosensitivity in peripheral nerves. Brain Research 344:281–285

Walker J B, Akhanjee L K, Cooney M M et al 1987a Laser therapy for pain of trigeminal neuralgia. Clinical Journal of Pain 3(4):183–187

Walker J B, Akhanjee L K, Cooney M M et al 1987b Laser therapy for pain of rheumatoid arthritis. Clinical Journal of Pain 3:54–59

Waylonis G W, Wilke A, O'Toole D, Waylonis D A, Waylonis D B 1988 Chronic myofascial pain: management by low-output helium–neon laser therapy. Archives of Physical Medicine and Rehabilitation 69:1017–1020

Wilder-Smith P 1988 The soft laser: therapeutic tool or popular placebo. Oral Surgery, Oral Medicine, Oral Pathology 66:654–658

White A 1993 Regulations governing the use of laser equipment. Acupuncture in Medicine 11(1):21

Wu W, Ponnudurai R, Katz J et al 1987 Failure to confirm report of light-evoked response of peripheral nerve to low-power helium–neon laser light stimulus. Brain Research 40:407–408

Young S R, Dyson M 1993 The effect of light on tissue repair. Acupuncture in Medicine XI(1):17–19

Young S R, Bolton P A, Dyson M, Harvey W, Diamantopoulos C 1988 Macrophage responsiveness to a light therapy. Lasers in Surgery and Medicine 9:497–505

Young S R, Dyson M, Bolton P A 1990 Effect of light on calcium uptake by macrophages. Laser Therapy 2:53–57

Ysla R, McAuley R 1985 Effects of low-power infrared laser stimulation on carpal tunnel syndrome. A double-blind study (abstr). Archives of Physical Medicine and Rehabilitation 66:553–554 [NB Due to printer's error title of this paper and one by McAuley & Ysla on laser treatment of osteoarthritis of the knee have been transposed.]

Clinical usage and evidence

SECTION CONTENTS

13

The clinical evaluation of acupuncture

George T. Lewith
Charles A. Vincent

INTRODUCTION

Traditional Chinese medicine has developed over a period of at least 3000 years (O'Connor & Bensky 1981), and there is a large and rather daunting literature. The most important early written record is the Yellow Emperor's Classic of Internal Medicine, or Nei Jing (Veith 1972), probably written about 300 BC. The origins of acupuncture, its place in the systems of medicine and philosophy of ancient China, and the application of these traditional ideas to diagnosis and treatment of disease have been discussed in several important books (Kaptchuk 1983, Lu & Needham 1980, O'Connor & Bensky 1981) (Ch 20). Scientific research into acupuncture has a number of different aspects. Experimental studies have sought to demonstrate short-term analgesic effects and examine the biochemical and physiological mechanisms that underlie such effects. (Chung & Dickenson 1980, Price et al 1984). In this chapter, however, we will be primarily concerned with the evaluation of acupuncture as a treatment for chronic pain and other disorders. Even when the scope of the review is narrowed to the clinical evaluation of acupuncture there is still a large literature; certainly many thousands of papers have been published in English. Many of these, however, are primarily descriptive, of poor quality and little value.

The main criticisms revealed against acupuncture are, first, that the theories underlying traditional acupuncture are implausible and irrelevant to modern medicine, and, secondly, that any effects acupuncture has are simply those of an appealing placebo (Vincent & Richardson 1986). We shall only briefly discuss the traditional ideas in any detail; for more information the reader is referred to the books cited above. The approach we shall take is that the traditional ideas need to be understood in outline, but that questions about efficacy can be asked without considering them in detail. The treatment may be effective whether or not the theory is valid.

The most important questions, in our view, are:

1. Does acupuncture have a beneficial effect on any individual disease or disorder?
2. Is this effect primarily, or even partly, due to the action of the needles (and associated treatments), or is it due to psychological processes? To put it another way, is acupuncture just a placebo, or is there some specific treatment effect?

This chapter describes a number of approaches to the evaluation and understanding of the treatment process, pointing out the value of observational studies, single-case designs and controlled trials. There are a large number of descriptive studies of acupuncture (Richardson & Vincent 1986) and some single-case designs (Vincent 1990a). We do not want to dispute the value of such approaches. We will assume, though, that controlled trials are the final arbiter of the efficacy of a therapy (Pocock 1985), and concentrate on their methodology and results.

We begin by sketching the ideas underlying traditional acupuncture, briefly considering their validity and relevance to the evaluation of acupuncture treatment. We then discuss some methodological issues, particularly the definition of an appropriate placebo control for acupuncture. The most urgent task for researchers of acupuncture treatment is to establish an agreed and satisfactory methodology for its evaluation. We will then briefly review controlled trials of acupuncture for chronic pain and a variety of other disorders. A chapter of this length cannot possibly attempt a comprehensive

account and the reader is advised to consult the various review papers that are cited, and from there the individual studies. Finally, we will comment on the small group of studies that do appear to have used a satisfactory placebo control and offer some suggestions for the conduct of future trials.

TRADITIONAL AND NON-TRADITIONAL ACUPUNCTURE

Traditional acupuncture

A thorough understanding of the concepts and theory underlying the practice of traditional acupuncture is not essential to assess individual studies, but certain aspects (such as point location) need to be considered. The reader also needs to appreciate that the diagnosis made by traditional acupuncturists can be quite independent of, and quite foreign to, more orthodox medical approaches.

The core ideas of traditional acupuncture are as follows. Qi, or 'energy' (see also Ch 20) flows within the body along lines known as channels or meridians. There are 14 main channels, most of which are associated with an organ of the body, and a number of subsidiary channels. The state of a person's health is dependent on the balance of energy in the system and the overall level of energy. In the treatment of disease, needles are inserted in the classical acupuncture points located on the channels and are manipulated with the aim of restoring the energy flow to a state of balance, and so restoring the patient to a state of health. Any disease or disorder should be reflected in an imbalance of this system and should, in principle, be amenable to treatment. Traditionally oriented acupuncturists are often prepared to treat a wide range of conditions.

Diagnosis for a traditional acupuncturist will encompass the medical history, the patient's psychological state and the impact of the patient's lifestyle on their complaint. The patient's state of health, and hence the state of the energy system, will also be inferred from subtler signs such as the quality of the pulse, the colour of the tongue, the complexion and the patient's smell. The pulse diagnosis is especially complex as 12 pulses are discerned, each with different qualities, corresponding to the 12 main meridians. The resulting diagnosis is usually couched in terms that are entirely different from orthodox medical diagnosis (Kaptchuk 1983).

A comparison of types of acupuncture

The traditional acupuncturist may treat patients with similar conditions (in orthodox medical terms) in very different ways, according to the (traditional) diagnosis they have made. For instance, 10 different patients with migraine might be treated in 10 different ways. In contrast, many practitioners use orthodox diagnoses and a corresponding prescription or 'formula' of points for each dysfunction or disease. Where this approach is taken, the formula has usually been derived from traditional Chinese ideas, even though the practitioners may no longer subscribe to them. Most clinical trials employ this approach. Only a very few allow the individual approach of traditional acupuncture (Coan et al 1980, Vincent & Richardson 1986).

In some modern forms of acupuncture, classical point locations play no part. The locations can be trigger points, tender areas, points in the same dermatome as the pain, etc. (Melzack 1984), and electrical stimulation is often employed. There are also hybrid techniques such as electro-acupuncture according to Voll (1975) and Ryodoraku therapy (Okazaki 1975), which are derived from traditional acupuncture but have been refined and systematized using electrical methods of diagnosis and treatment. As yet, however, they have not been systematically evaluated. With so many methods available it is obviously crucial that each study specifies its particular methods as closely as possible, as differences in technique may explain apparently discrepant findings.

Practitioners of traditional acupuncture may criticize the formula approach on the grounds that it gives inferior results and is not in keeping with the spirit of traditional acupuncture. The

attention paid to the individual patient during a traditionally based diagnostic session is no doubt valuable, regardless of the validity of the traditional ideas. Whether traditional acupuncture gives superior results or not is an empirical matter, and to our knowledge no study has yet addressed this question.

Validity of traditional ideas

Numerous books have been published about traditional approaches to diagnosis and treatment (Kaptchuk 1983, O'Connor & Bensky 1981), but there have been very few attempts to evaluate these methods of diagnosis. Cole (1975) carried out a series of small studies examining the reliability and validity of the pulse diagnosis. She concluded that the pulse diagnosis 'is not apparently a means of objective analysis, but offers subjective meaning to the practitioner and is a vehicle for a meaningful and helpful interaction with the patient'. Further studies on the process of diagnosis and treatment would be extremely useful. Whether or not the traditional ideas were substantiated, such research would help to rid acupuncture of its reputation for irrationality (Skrabanek 1984).

A considerable amount of work has been carried out, especially in China, on the possible anatomical basis of meridians and points. 'Propagated channel sensation' refers to the sensations experienced by a small proportion of people when acupuncture points are needled; these sensations tend to run along the acupuncture meridians even though patients do not know in advance where the meridian pathways are supposed to be. Changes in skin resistance and temperature have also been suggested as providing evidence for the existence of meridians (Meng, Zhu & Hu 1985). Reviewing this work, Macdonald (1989) acknowledges that sensations may follow meridian lines but suggests that such phenomena can be explained without postulating the existence of a meridian system. Meridians have also been detected by the injection of radiotracers into acupuncture points, but more recent work suggests that the pattern of spread of the radiotracer corresponds to vascular drainage of the tracer (Lazorthes et al 1990). In China, work on research on meridian phenomena continues, but most Western researchers would probably dismiss the idea of a meridian system. At the very least, we must conclude that the existence of meridians remains unproven.

Research on acupuncture points has been more fruitful, and there are definite links between the observations made by acupuncturists and phenomena observed by other clinicians and scientists. As we shall see, a discussion of the existence and location of acupuncture points is crucial for a proper evaluation of the clinical studies. Macdonald (1989) makes a number of comments. First, it is difficult to be precise about the location of acupuncture points. Their position is usually assessed according to the size and shape of the patient, and while there is reasonable agreement about the locations of the fundamental points (Vincent & Richardson 1986), the number of points continues to grow (Macdonald 1989). Secondly, there is evidence that they become tender when a patient is sick, and there is certainly considerable overlap with the independently developed concept of trigger points (Melzack, Stillwell & Fox 1977, Travell & Simons 1983). Thirdly, it is possible that acupuncture locations have some kind of neurophysiological basis, perhaps corresponding to the termination of peripheral nerve endings. For our purposes, it is important to realize that while acupuncture locations may provide useful therapeutic guidelines, it is unlikely they have a precise and constant location. The effect of acupuncture may be stronger at some points than others, but this is unlikely to be an all-or-nothing phenomenon.

METHODOLOGY OF ACUPUNCTURE TRIALS

Many studies of acupuncture treatment are seriously flawed by methodological problems (Vincent & Richardson 1986). Poor design, inadequate measures and statistical analysis, lack of follow-up data and substandard treatment are all too common. The most important problems are the measurement of outcome, design and choice of control group. The main issues addressed here are the question of whether trials of acupuncture should be single blind or double blind, the definition of an appropriate control group, and methods of testing the adequacy of the control. Controlled trials may encompass comparisons of acupuncture with a waiting-list group, an alternative treatment or a placebo. The main methodological problems arise with the placebo control (Vincent 1989a).

Sources of bias in controlled trials

There are various possible sources of bias in all controlled trials (Kramer & Shapiro 1984). Two are particularly important in trials of acupuncture. First, trials of acupuncture have to be single blind. Inevitably, the clinician giving the acupuncture treatment is aware of which is the true treatment and which is the control, and may inadvertently communicate different expectations to the patients in the treatment and control groups. Any advantage shown by a true treatment may then be due to factors other than the specific effect of the needles.

A second difficulty with any control condition, particularly if it is of a different form from the true treatment, is that it may have a different psychological impact. Some trials of acupuncture have used mock TENS, in which electrodes are applied as usual but no current is passed. If mock TENS has a lesser psychological impact than acupuncture, then a significant difference between treatments might simply mean that acupuncture was the more powerful placebo. Whichever control condition is used, the psychological impact of the true treatment and the control needs to be assessed if we are to be confident that the trial is not favouring either the real or control treatment.

Both these problems arise in controlled trials of acupuncture or any other skilled, physical treatment. They do not mean the trials are necessarily flawed or that the methodology is unsatisfactory, but they do suggest that great care must be taken in the choice of placebo control.

Placebo control conditions used in acupuncture trials

A bewildering variety of control procedures have been used in acupuncture trials. In some, all acupuncture procedures are matched with those in the true treatment group except that needles are not inserted; instead they are rubbed against the skin (Borglum-Jensen, Melsen & Borglum-Jensen 1979) or glued to it (Gallachi 1981). These are not really credible, as even patients with no experience of acupuncture treatment are likely to know that needle insertion is involved.

In the most commonly used control treatment, needling is carried out at theoretically irrelevant sites, away from the classical point locations. Depth of insertion and stimulation are the same; only location differs. This procedure, which is termed 'sham' acupuncture, has been used as a placebo in a great many studies (Gaw, Chang & Shaw 1975, Godfrey & Morgan 1978, Henry et al 1985). Sham acupuncture was initially assumed by most investigators to be ineffective, and therefore ideal as a placebo. However, Lewith & Machin (1983) pointed out that sham acupuncture appeared to have an analgesic effect in 40–50% of patients, in comparison with 60% for real acupuncture. Experimental work suggests that stimulation at many different sites, whether or not they be classical point locations, may produce analgesia (Chapman, Wilson & Gehrig 1976, Melzack 1984, Reichmanis & Becker 1977, Stewart, Thompson & Oswald 1977), possibly via diffuse noxious inhibitory control (DNIC) (Le Bars et al 1991). Controlled trials have also shown significant therapeutic benefits from both classical and non-classical locations (Gaw, Chang & Shaw 1975, Melzack 1984, Richardson & Vincent 1986). It is now clear that sham acupuncture cannot be considered a placebo. Real versus sham acupuncture trials for pain therefore provide information only about the role of point location (Lewith & Vincent 1995, Vincent 1993). If precise point location is not important there will be no difference between groups even if the true treatment does have specific effects.

The argument with respect to the treatment of non-painful conditions such as the use of PC-6 to treat nausea is different. Here the clinical trial evidence suggests that point location is important and that acupuncture away from PC-6 has little effect on nausea and is primarily a placebo. Real PC-6 acupuncture or acupressure shows a consistent 60–70% response rate, consistent with it being primarily a real effect of acupuncture versus placebo (Bayreuther, Lewith & Pickering 1994, Dundee & McMillan 1992). It is probable that in non-painful conditions the underlying physiological mechanism is different from that in pain and so sham acupuncture can then act as a valid placebo control treatment (Lewith & Vincent 1995). Nevertheless, in the interests of standardizing the evaluation of acupuncture, one of the options considered below might be preferable as a control condition.

Solutions to the problem of acupuncture control

The basic problem is to find a control condition with small or non-existent specific physiological effects.

Mock TENS

The first plausible solution was the introduction of mock TENS as a control condition in acupuncture trials. In this procedure TENS stimulators are used in the usual way, except that no current actually passes between the electrodes. Patients are sometimes told that they are receiving subliminal pulse therapy and they will therefore not feel the current. This control was developed as a placebo comparison in trials of TENS itself, but first used in 1983 in a trial of acupuncture by Macdonald et al (1983). Mock TENS has also been used in a number of trials of acupuncture including postherpetic neuralgia (Lewith, Field & Machin 1983) and migraine (Dowson, Lewith & Machin 1985).

Minimal acupuncture

In minimal acupuncture (Vincent 1989a,b)

needles are placed away from classical or trigger points, inserted only 1–2 mm and stimulated extremely lightly. This procedure theoretically minimizes the specific effects of the needling while maintaining its psychological impact: it can be almost exactly matched to the real treatment. Minimal acupuncture has been used as a control condition in several studies, though not necessarily described in this way. It is possible that minimal acupuncture might have some therapeutic effect but, even if there is a small effect, the trial is not invalidated; it is just slightly harder to demonstrate a difference between treatment and control.

Either minimal acupuncture or mock TENS may be appropriate as a control, depending on whether it is likely to seem plausible to the patients involved. The choice may depend on the condition being treated, the expectations of the patient and the nature of the real treatment. For instance if very light stimulation is being assessed, minimal acupuncture may be too close to the true treatment and mock TENS should be employed. In other situations it may be preferable to simulate the true treatment very closely and minimal acupuncture may be preferred. The most important matter though, seldom considered in clinical trials, is to find a way of assessing the adequacy of whichever control is chosen. This means ensuring that the psychological impact of the true treatment and the control are equivalent, in essence that they have equivalent placebo power.

The concept of the placebo

Placebo effects are seldom studied in their own right, usually being treated simply as a nuisance variable to be eliminated so that the specific treatment effects can be discerned. This may not matter too much when the placebo has, as in a drug trial, the same form as the true treatment. It is of greater concern with skilled physical treatments on conscious patients where changes to the treatment may be noticed by the patient. In these cases we need to pay a little more attention to the nature of the psychological effects involved.

As Richardson (1989) has pointed out, the placebo is a 'portmanteau' concept, involving the use of a single term to describe a set of quite disparate phenomena. The power of placebo effects is influenced by treatment characteristics (more 'serious' treatments being more powerful) and by therapist characteristics (status, style of treatment administration). A number of different psychological processes may be involved: 'For example many psychological processes influence pain perception. Effective placebo analgesia could conceivably be achieved through the manipulation of any of these processes. One placebo may divert the patient's attention, e.g. mock TENS, while another may reduce anxiety and reassure the patient, e.g. traditional inert tablet or injections' (Richardson 1989). Assessing the power of a placebo, or comparing the placebo effects of two different treatments, or a treatment and a control condition is therefore not a simple matter. A host of non-specific factors may influence response to treatment and it is impossible to assess all potentially relevant factors; there are simply too many variables to take into account. The only solution is to select and assess one of the more important aspects of the placebo response. One of the most valuable approaches has been the assessment of the credibility of a treatment, and hence indirectly the strength of the patient's expectations of improvement. The credibility of a treatment appears to be an important aspect of its power, more credible treatments tending to have greater therapeutic effect (Richardson 1989).

Validating placebo controls in acupuncture studies

The treatment credibility scale was originally conceived and employed by Borkovec & Nau (1972) in a study of the credibility of different forms of psychological treatment; it has since been used in a variety of other psychological treatments as well as in studies of acupuncture (McGlynn & McDonnel 1974, Shapiro 1981, Vincent 1990b). The main questions identified by Borkovec & Nau in their 'Credibility of treatment rating scale' were:

1. How confident do you feel that this treatment can alleviate your complaint?
2. How confident would you be in recommending this treatment to a friend who suffered from similar complaints?
3. How logical does this treatment seem to you?
4. How successful do you think this treatment would be in alleviating other complaints?

The scale is sometimes given a slightly different title such as 'attitudes to acupuncture'. The form of the questions can be slightly amended to take account of the condition being treated and other circumstances of the trial (Borkovec & Nau 1972).

It is usual to ask patients to rate their response to the four questions on a five-point Likert scale ('strongly agree' to 'strongly disagree'). Vincent (1990b) assessed the psychometric properties in a sample of patients receiving acupuncture treatment and found that it had good internal consistency and rest–retest reliability; the questions all relate to the central concept of credibility and patients answer consistently on different occasions.

Petrie & Hazleman (1985) were the first to use the credibility scale in an acupuncture study. They assessed the credibility of acupuncture and mock TENS on their study population before embarking on the clinical trial. Acupuncture and mock TENS were considered to be equally credible treatments for neck pain when demonstrated to patients before treatment began, so justifying the use of mock TENS as a placebo control. The trial demonstrated that acupuncture was significantly more valuable than mock TENS in providing pain relief, but placebo credibility was not reassessed at the end of the study.

Vincent (1990b) used the scale in a controlled trial of the treatment of migraine by acupuncture in which real acupuncture was compared with a minimal acupuncture control. The credibility scale was given to patients at the end of the second and fifth treatments. There were no significant differences between true and sham treatments on any of the credibility measures. The true treatment was seen as slightly more credible (though not significantly so) by the 5th week. In the trial the true acupuncture proved more effective than the control; the difference in credibility late in treatment probably reflects the fact that by then patients receiving the true treatment were deriving greater benefit.

A similar assessment was utilized by Bayreuther, Lewith & Pickering (1994) in a double-blind crossover study of acupressure for the treatment of early morning sickness. Twenty-three patients were given instructions to use a real or sham acupuncture point in a random order. The study showed a significant effect of real over sham treatment (66% of patients versus 33%). The credibility of the real and placebo points was evaluated using two questions from the credibility scale, nos. 1 and 3, at the start of the trial, and a further two at the end of the study, nos. 2 and 4. At the outset, the women were equally confident that acupressure would work at both positions. At the end of the study, they were significantly more confident in the real rather than the sham point. It seemed therefore that the sham point was a credible placebo at the outset. It produced a clinical response compatible with that of a placebo and the opinions of the women changed in response to an effective treatment.

All these studies support the contention that the credibility scale accurately reflects patients' beliefs about the authenticity and efficacy of the acupuncture treatment they received. This in turn suggests that the scale is a useful index of the psychological impact of acupuncture treatment and therefore the credibility of placebo controls within acupuncture studies.

Implications for research: routine assessment of the adequacy of control conditions

There are at least two viable control conditions for acupuncture trials, and the choice of control may vary according to the particular nature of the trial. Whatever the choice of control group it is valuable to check its adequacy. It is not feasible to assess every psychological variable that may be of importance, but it is possible to make some assessment of the adequacy of whichever control procedure one is using. The credibility measure is introduced as a check that the treatment and control are equivalent in their psychological impact. If they prove to be equally credible, this increases our confidence that the control procedure is adequate. If they prove to be different, the difference can be introduced as a variable in the statistical analysis of the results. The fact that minimal acupuncture, acupressure and mock TENS are equally credible to acupuncture or acupressure in one study does not necessarily mean that they will be in all. A different clinician, a different group of patients, and a different setting may all influence the perception of the respective treatments or control procedures. As acupuncture becomes more widely used, patients will be more aware of the sensations of correct treatment and so more liable to detect variations introduced in control procedures. The recommendation must be that credibility, or a similar index of psychological impact, be routinely assessed in trials of acupuncture, in fact in all controlled trials of any physical treatment. Only then can we be sure, in any particular trial, that the treatment and control are adequately matched. Credibility is only one possible parameter of assessment, but it has already been shown to be a simple and useful measure. Routine measures of treatment credibility in trials of acupuncture would mean that arguments about placebo controls in acupuncture trials could in future rely less on speculation and more on evidence.

QUESTIONS ADDRESSED IN CLINICAL ACUPUNCTURE RESEARCH

In the last decade a number of authors have reviewed trials of acupuncture and attempted to establish a coherent and rational methodology for the evaluation of acupuncture (Lewith & Machin 1983, Richardson & Vincent 1986, Vincent & Richardson 1986, Ter Riet, Kleijnen & Knipschild 1990). This chapter re-examines the three areas that have encompassed the major part of clinical trial research within acupuncture:

the use of acupuncture in chronic pain, in addiction (particularly smoking cessation), and in the treatment of nausea and vomiting. We then attempt to integrate neurophysiological work on the mechanisms of acupuncture's action with findings from clinical trial results in order to explain some apparently inconsistent findings and provide a foundation for future research in which clinical and basic research are more closely integrated. Before our hypothesis can be developed it is necessary to clarify the meaning of the results from acupuncture trials. There have been many different questions asked, though generally subsumed under the global term, 'Does acupuncture work for …?' The problems that concern us are particularly associated with placebo-controlled trials.

We are now in a position to disentangle the various questions that have been (knowingly or unknowingly) asked in acupuncture trials. Table 13.1 summarizes the main points. Real versus sham acupuncture trials provide information about the role of point location, and do not indicate whether or not acupuncture is a placebo. Real versus sham trials therefore ask a rather complex second-order question that is concerned with the parameters of the treatment, rather than the primary question of whether there is any (physiological) effect at all. There are a number of different parameters that can be varied: depth of stimulation, rate of stimulation, type of stimulation (manual/electrical), and location (classical/nonclassical, trigger points, motor points) and site of stimulation (same spinal segment versus distant points). The great advantage of beginning to think about the various parameters is that it brings outcome studies closer to mechanism studies; the more we know how effects can be achieved, the more possible it is to home in on the appropriate mechanism.

CLINICAL EVIDENCE
Acupuncture for chronic pain

Several reviews of the use of acupuncture in the treatment of chronic pain have now appeared

Table 13.1   Acupuncture control conditions and their purposes

Control condition	Description	Question addressed	Comments
No treatment	Monitoring of waiting list or no treatment group	Are observed changes simply due to the passage of time?	Possible to show that effects not due simply to passage of time. No information about placebo effects or comparison with other treatments.
Alternative treatment	Usually comparison with standard treatment (e.g. physiotherapy)	Does acupuncture have any advantage/disadvantage over standard treatment in terms of efficacy, adverse effects, cost?	Valuable for assessing direct clinical consequences of different treatment policies
Sham (mock) acupuncture	Like true acupuncture except with altered point location; needles approximately half inch from usual location; depth and stimulation the same	Is point location an important determinant of effect of acupuncture?	Mistakenly used in many trials involving chronic pain as placebo equivalent, with consequent misinterpretation of results. Huge subject numbers needed to detect difference from true acupuncture
Mock TENS	Transcutaneous nerve stimulation with surface electrodes, but no current passing; may be enhanced with additional monitors, etc.	Is acupuncture more effective than placebo?	First attempt to address problems associated with sham acupuncture. Advantage: completely inert, hence excellent placebo. Disadvantage: may be perceived differently from acupuncture by trial subjects
Minimal acupuncture	Acupuncture away from usual locations, very shallow needling, and very slight stimulation	Is acupuncture more effective than placebo? (Strictly speaking more effective than a near-placebo)	Advantage: almost exact semblance of true acupuncture. Disadvantage: may have physiological effect

(Bhatt-Sanders 1985, Lewith & Machin 1983, Patel et al 1989, Richardson & Vincent 1986, Ter Riet, Kleijnen & Knipschild 1990a). All have commented on the poor quality of most of the studies, and all have stated that this severely limits the conclusions that can be drawn from the review. Richardson & Vincent (1986) reviewed all English language controlled trials of acupuncture published before 1986. They concluded that there was good evidence for the short-term effectiveness of acupuncture for low back pain, mixed results for headache, and some encouraging preliminary results for cervical pain and arthritis. The proportion of patients helped varied from study to study but commonly fell in the region 50–80%. Follow-up periods, however, were disappointingly short and evidence for longer-term benefits was weak. They suggested that the response rate and degree of benefit obtained were higher than might be expected from a placebo response, but

cautioned that very few studies used a satisfactory placebo control. The extent to which acupuncture was producing benefit by psychological mechanisms alone such as suggestion, hypnosis and a pure placebo effect had not really been established.

In addition to the basic reviews, two meta-analyses of the literature on chronic pain have been reported. Meta-analysis is a discipline that critically reviews and statistically combines the results of previous research. The purposes of such a procedure include increasing overall statistical power, resolving uncertainty between conflicting reports and improving estimates of the size of the effect being investigated (Sacks et al 1987). However, it should be emphasized that although these techniques have the potential for resolving questions about the efficacy of acupuncture, they cannot compensate for the poor quality of studies they set out to combine. For instance, if the placebo control is unsatisfactory in the original studies, then biased estimates will be produced in the final meta-analysis.

Patel and colleagues (1989) reviewed all randomized controlled trials of acupuncture for chronic pain that measured outcome in terms of the numbers of patients improved. They attempted a statistical pooling of the results and concluded that the results favoured acupuncture, though various methodological problems precluded a definite conclusion. However, combining the results of these studies does not seem very sensible. There are only 14 trials, of very variable standard, they address the treatment of various chronic pain problems, and they

appear to use eight different control groups. It is not clear what any statement about the superiority of acupuncture over a control can mean in these circumstances.

A more comprehensive meta-analysis, and the most recent review available, was produced by Ter Riet, Kleijnen & Knipschild (1990a). They decided not to attempt a statistical pooling of results, arguing that the studies were on the whole too poor and too disparate to allow their results to be combined. Their report is therefore perhaps best considered a critical review. They identified 51 reports of acupuncture for chronic pain involving some kind of control or group for

Table 13.2   Acupuncture for chronic pain: studies with acceptable placebo controls

Authors*	Population	n	Design	Control
Junilla 1982	Musculoskeletal pain	32	Group comparison	Minimal acupuncture
Hansen & Hansen 1983	Facial pain	16	Crossover	Minimal acupuncture
Macdonald et al 1983	Low back pain	17	Group comparison	Mock TENS
Petrie & Langley 1983	Cervical pain	13	Group comparison	Mock TENS
Lewith et al 1983	Post-herpetic neuralgia	62	Group comparison	Mock TENS
Dowson et al 1984	Migraine headache	48	Group comparison	Mock TENS
Petrie & Hazelman 1986	Chronic neck pain	25	Group comparison	Mock TENS
Lehmann et al 1986	Chronic low back	53	Group comparison	Mock TENS
Ballegaard et al 1986	Severe angina	26	Group comparison	Minimal acupuncture
Vincent 1989	Migraine	30	Group comparison	Minimal acupuncture
Dickens & Lewith 1989	Osteoarthritis	13	Group comparison	Mock TENS
Ballegaard et al 1990	Moderate angina	49	Group comparison	Minimal acupuncture

*The original references can be found in Richardson & Vincent (1986).

comparison. Each study was scored on 18 methodological criteria, some weighted more heavily than others, with a maximum possible score of 100. Only 11 studies scored 50 or more points, with the best study obtaining 62% of the maximum score. Positive and negative results were approximately equally divided in the higher-quality studies, whether a cut-off score of 40 or 50 points was taken. Studies were also separated into four categories of pain: headache, musculoskeletal (spine), musculoskeletal (other) and miscellaneous. The pattern of results did not change, however. Results are equivocal for all four groups, though the treatment for musculo-

skeletal problems of the spine (mostly low back pain) show slightly more positive results.

The overall conclusions of all reviewers are similar. Studies are generally methodologically poor. Acupuncture appears to produce some benefits for patients with chronic pain, but it is not clear how long they last or whether they are psychologically mediated. When acupuncture is compared with alternative treatments (such as TENS) the results are equivocal (Richardson & Vincent 1986). When acupuncture is compared with a placebo control the results are also equivocal. However, flaws in the placebo control may bias the results of some of these studies

Table 13.2 (cont'd)

Type of acupuncture	Dependent measures	Follow-up period	Results
Four treatments	Daily pain ratings	4 weeks	22% placebo benefit, 72% acupuncture
Classical 10 daily sessions	Daily pain ratings	4 weeks	66% patient improved, true acupuncture significant > control
Tender areas and trigger points. Some EA. Up to 10 sessions	Various pain VASs, mood, independent clinician's assessment	None	Acupuncture significant > placebo for pain relief, activity, physical signs in pain area
Classical 8 sessions, twice weekly	Self-ratings	None	84% acupuncture group reported good pain relief. Acupuncture significant > placebo
Classical and auricular 6–8 sessions	Daily records sleep, moderation sleep disturbance	2 months	Significant improvement in only 7 patients in each group. No significant difference between groups
Classical 6 sessions	Frequency, duration, intensity, medication	24 weeks	56% acupuncture and 30% placebo showed 33% pain relief; 44% acupuncture and 57% placebo less frequent headaches. No significant difference between groups
8 sessions, twice weekly	Daily diary: pain intensity disability, medication	1 month	45% of acupuncture group and 30% of placebo group show significant response. No significant difference between groups
EA group and TENS group (all groups had additional treatment)	Physician assessment. VRS measures of pain and disability	6 months	EA significant > TENS and mock TENS
Classical 7 sessions over 3 weeks	Exercise tests, pain diaries, medication	3 weeks	Acupuncture significant > control for cardiac work capacity only
Classical 6 weekly sessions	4 × daily ratings of pain and medication	1 year	43% reduction in weekly pain score for acupuncture group, 14% for control. Acupuncture significant > control for pain levels, but not for medication reduction
Classical 6 sessions over 2 weeks	Diaries. VAS pain scores, medication, sleep, grip, tenderness	3 weeks	76% reduction in pain in acupuncture group. 10% in control, but no significant difference between groups
Classical 10 sessions over 3 weeks	Exercise tests, pain diaries, medication, well-being	6 months	Reduction of 50% in attacks and medication. No significant difference between groups

against acupuncture. It appears that the status of acupuncture as a treatment for chronic pain has been assessed exhaustively, although the situation is still very muddled. In order to clarify this confusion, we would now like to consider the studies in two groups: real acupuncture versus placebo and real acupuncture versus sham acupuncture.

Real acupuncture versus placebo

Table 13.2 shows true placebo controlled trials. There are only 12 studies, and they concern the treatment of a variety of disorders. Only five of the studies show a significant advantage of acupuncture over placebo, although several others show a non-significant advantage. The trials are small, however, with four involving less than 20 subjects. It is doubtful whether many of them have sufficient power to conclude that a non-significant result definitely shows acupuncture to be equivalent to placebo. The probability of a type II error—failing to detect an actual difference—is high. A cautious interpretation of these studies is that the results of postherpetic neuralgia and angina suggest that acupuncture is ineffective in these conditions, that it may well be helpful for low back pain, and that its efficacy for migraine remains to be resolved.

Real versus sham acupuncture: the role of point location

The largest and most recent review of acupuncture for chronic pain (Ter Riet, Kleijnen & Knipschild 1990a) did not distinguish the different types of control condition. However, earlier reviews (Lewith & Machin 1983, Richardson & Vincent 1986) suggest that, whereas most studies do not show a significant advantage of real acupuncture over sham (i.e. an effect of point location), there is a tendency for real acupuncture to show superior results. Lewith & Machin (1983) suggested that, in patients suffering with chronic pain, real acupuncture produced a clinical response in approximately 60%, sham acupuncture a response in 40–50%, and placebo acupuncture a response in 30%. Clearer results

seem to have emerged in experimental studies (Reichmanis & Becker 1977). For the purposes of our argument, however, it is only necessary to suggest that point location might be an important variable in the treatment of chronic pain.

Addiction

Ter Riet, Kleijnen & Knipschild (1990b) have suggested that acupuncture provides no benefit in smoking cessation, and their arguments centre around two main factors. The first is that real acupuncture provides no therapeutic advantage over sham acupuncture. Their second argument is that many of the studies are methodologically poor. Overall, approximately 15% of patients have ceased to smoke at the end of 6 months, and this in itself places acupuncture in the realms of a reasonable antismoking treatment. Data from Schwartz (1988) produce a similar picture. In his analysis of eight studies that involved a real versus sham acupuncture model to evaluate acupuncture as an antismoking treatment, the overall cessation rate is 25%. It is very interesting to note that there was absolutely no overall difference between real and sham acupuncture in seven of the eight studies. Therefore, one of Ter Reit's hypotheses—that acupuncture has no effect because real acupuncture provides no therapeutic benefit over sham acupuncture—is confused. It is clear that acupuncture has an effect greater than that expected from doing nothing, but it also is true to say that real acupuncture has the same effect as sham acupuncture—that is, point location is unimportant (Table 13.3).

Nausea

The third group of studies involves the use of PC-6 in the treatment of postoperative nausea, morning sickness and chemotherapy-induced nausea (see also Ch 15). The initial studies were published by Dundee et al (1989) and were largely descriptive and uncontrolled. The studies have been reviewed elsewhere (Turner 1993) and demonstrate that between 60 and 70% of

Table 13.3 Acupuncture in the treatment of smoking cessation: real versus sham

Authors*	Total	Acupuncture technique	Follow-up period	Study model	Cessation rates	
					Real acupuncture (%)	Sham acupuncture (%)
Vandevenne et al 1985	200	Classical body	1 year	Blind randomized controlled trial (RCT)	40	32
MacHovec & Man 1978†	58	Auricular lung point	6 months	Comparative RCT including untreated group	25	0
Gillams & Lewith 1984	87	Auricular lung point	6 months	Comparative RCT including group therapy	18	15
Lamontagne et al 1980	75	Auricular lung point	6 months	Single blind RCT including advice group	8	16
Gilbey & Neumann 1972	93	Auricular lung point	3 months	RCT, single blind	21	15
Parker & Mok 1977	41	Auricular lung point	6 weeks	RCT, single blind	14	15
Lagrue et al 1983	154	Auricular lung point	1 week	RCT, single blind	44	40
Steiner et al 1982	23	Auricular lung point	End of treatment	RCT, single blind	9	8

* These original references can be found in Schwartz (1988) or Ter Riet, Kleijnen & Knipschild (1990a,b).
† If we exclude the MacHovec & Man study, which appears to be the only one showing sham acupuncture has no effect at all, then the average response to real acupuncture is 22.5%, and the average response to sham acupuncture is 20%.

patients benefit from acupuncture in this context. Subsequent, more thorough, investigations have supported Dundee's initial descriptive observations and have also used a real versus sham comparison. The controlled trials have shown that real acupuncture or acupressure provides a 60–70% real treatment benefit, and sham acupuncture and acupressure only a 30% real treatment effect (Table 13.4).

Summary

We therefore have three groups of studies, all providing slightly different answers when a sham versus real trial model is used to evaluate the effects of acupuncture. This implies that point location may be an important determinant of the effect of acupuncture in some conditions but not in others. In chronic pain there may be some difference between sham and real acupuncture. This suggests that some effect may be produced by random needling, but that the effect might be improved by needling at specific locations. In the treatment of addictions, specifically smoking cessation, it appears that there is no difference between real and sham acupuncture. In our present state of knowledge this may mean either that acupuncture is an effective placebo or that its effect relies simply on the general stimulation of a natural opioid-based mechanism. In the treatment of nausea, it appears that there is a significant difference between real and sham stimulation of acupuncture points, and sham stimulation seems to approximate a real placebo effect. The effect appears to rely on stimulation at a particular location, although other locations may also be feasible sites.

Table 13.4 Acupuncture and acupressure at PC-6 in the treatment of nausea: real versus sham

Authors*	n	Condition	Acupuncture technique	Study model	Real acupuncture (%)	Sham acupuncture (%)
Price and Lewith 1991	53	Chemotherapy induced nausea	Acupressure	Randomized single-blind crossover study	54	18
Bayreuther and Lewith 1994	23	Early morning sickness	Acupressure	Randomized double-blind crossover study	69	31
Aloysio and Penachioni 1992	66	Early morning sickness	Acupressure	Randomized controlled study comparing 4 groups of patients	60	30
Dundee et al 1988	120	Early morning sickness	Acupressure	Randomized controlled study with no crossover	58	24
Dundee et al 1991		Postoperative nausea	Acupuncture and acupressure	Comparative randomized study involving comparative groups	Real acupressure 60 Real acupuncture 80	30
Dundee et al 1989	20	Chemotherapy induced nausea	Acupuncture	Comparative groups	Real acupuncture 90 Sham acupressure 10	

*These original references can be found in Turner (1993).

HOW DOES THIS RELATE TO OUR UNDERSTANDING OF NEUROPHYSIOLOGY?

The neurophysiology of acupuncture has been investigated extensively and reviewed in detail elsewhere (Lewith & Kenyon 1984; see also Ch 6); we only discuss those findings that are relevant to our hypothesis. The principal suggestion is that acupuncture operates largely through an endorphin-related mechanism. This argument has been supported almost exclusively by evaluating acupuncture in the context of acute pain within an animal model (Pomeranz 1991). These studies demonstrate conclusively that acupuncture's effects are related to the release of a variety of natural opioids and that this opioid-based effect is naloxone reversible. The very thorough work done by Le Bars and his group in Paris (Le Bars et al 1991) has demonstrated conclusively that any noxious stimulus will result in endorphin release through the neurophysiological mechanism that he describes as DNIC. Therefore, DNIC represents a non-specific physiological mechanism that triggers the

natural opioid system in both humans and experimental animals (Le Bars et al 1991). There are some studies with human subjects that suggest that acupuncture is not always naloxone reversible (Chapman et al 1980), but they do not fit the general weight of evidence available from animal models. Recently, Bowsher (1991) suggested that DNIC plays a relatively minor role in acupuncture analgesia and that other systems, mediated by serotonin and noradrenaline, may be more important (Bowsher 1993). Some types of neurogenic pain, not involving nociceptor stimulation, do not appear to be susceptible to acupuncture treatment and should perhaps be excluded from this analysis (Clement-Jones et al 1980).

It is quite probable that chronic pain has different underlying mechanisms from those involved in acute experimental pain in animals. Those working in pain clinics will be only too aware that empirical manipulation of the autonomic system, such as the use of guanethidine blocks in sympathetic dystrophies, can result in dramatic clinical improvement. In spite of the fact that we do not have a unified theory to explain the mechanism of chronic pain, the empirical evidence available to us would suggest that the autonomic system plays an important, but as yet undefined, role in the complex phenomena involved in intractable pain.

The mechanisms of acupuncture involved in its use as a treatment for addictions almost certainly utilize the endorphin and enkephalin systems. Clement-Jones and colleagues noted this as early as 1980. There are, however, no detailed studies that define the exact mechanisms involved in smoking cessation. It would be reasonable to hypothesize that the withdrawal symptoms experienced in almost any addictive process may be, at least in part, endorphin mediated. The mechanism of acupuncture in internal diseases, such as asthma and irritable bowel, and the treatment of symptoms such as nausea, is as yet unknown. There is no clear coherent hypothesis to suggest how acupuncture may be operating in these conditions. Acupuncturists have hypothesized that the autonomic system plays an important, but as yet ill-defined, part in the underlying mechanisms that are involved in the treatment of such internal problems (Mann 1977), and acupuncture has been shown experimentally to affect blood pressure and heart rate (Bowsher 1993). If we accept that acupuncture might affect the autonomic nervous system in some way, a crucial question now emerges: how is it that needling at some points can affect the autonomic pathways, and needling at others does not, or does so to a much smaller extent?

Trigger points: further light on point location?

While both peptide release and autonomic changes could play a part in explaining acupuncture's action, it is not clear how this work could explain the long-term effects of acupuncture treatment. As Price and colleagues (1984) point out, the release of these peptides into the blood could account for a direct analgesic effect lasting only a few hours. In an ingenious and careful experiment they distinguished two patterns of analgesia after the acupuncture treatment of chronic back pain: a central-inhibitory

pattern affecting the whole body and an origin-specific pattern affecting only the site of stimulation. The central pattern is short acting and, they suggest, probably mediated by a neuro-humoral mechanism. The local analgesia, however, lasted 10–14 days and cumulative effects were observed at 4 months. They argue that the treatment has a direct or indirect effect on the tissues from which the nociceptive stimulus arises and suggest that one possible mechanism might include the reflex relaxation of muscles induced by intense stimulation of trigger points. This hypothesis is consistent with evidence linking acupuncture and trigger point techniques (Lewit 1979, Melzack 1984, Melzack, Stillwell & Fox 1977, Travell & Simons 1983) and suggests another way in which point location might be important.

Hypothesis

It is probable that addictive processes are mediated through the natural opioid systems. Consequently, if we observe clinically that there is no difference between real and sham acupuncture in the treatment of smoking cessation, it is reasonable to suggest that this may be because acupuncture is exclusively endorphin mediated in this clinical context. Non-specific needling may be having as great a clinical effect as specific needling techniques.

In the treatment of nausea, we are probably dealing with a non-endorphin-mediated mechanism. The clinical trial evidence to date suggests that acupuncture has an effect and that point location is important; needling away from PC-6 does not seem to produce as great an effect. It is possible that the theories that underpin TCM relate to an empirical and pragmatic understanding of the autonomic nervous system and its detailed correspondences and effects on the body. If this hypothesis is correct, then we would expect that within the treatment of a purely internal and non-pain-related problem, needling of particular areas, rather than just general stimulation, may be important.

The final group of studies involves chronic pain. Here there is clear evidence that chronic pain is mediated, at least in part, through the natural opioid system, but the empirical evidence suggests that the autonomic system is also important in maintaining a number of chronic pain syndromes. Therefore, clinical trials involving acupuncture as a treatment for chronic pain will provide a mixed picture. Sham acupuncture will have some effect through DNIC and provide a greater effect than that expected from placebo alone. Real acupuncture will utilize the endorphin system as well as a putative autonomic response and local trigger point action to produce additional effects and an increased clinical response when compared to sham acupuncture. A comparison of acupuncture with placebo in a clinical trial will produce the most clear-cut results when attempting to evaluate acupuncture, but point location (real versus sham) may also be important to test the validity of the specific theories concerning point prescription. In essence this hypothesis suggests that the closer one gets to a purely endorphin-mediated effect, the less relevant it is to think in terms of point location and the more misleading a real versus sham acupuncture model is in the context of a clinical trial. Conversely, the more that acupuncture treatment is autonomically mediated, such as in the management of non-painful conditions, the more relevant it may be to use a sham versus real acupuncture model when evaluating its clinical effectiveness.

Implications for research and testing the hypothesis

It is important to clarify the precise question addressed in any trial, as previously different questions have been confounded. There is no one appropriate control; the control condition will vary with the question being asked. Different parameters of treatment may be varied in a trial, perhaps with more than two comparison groups. For instance, the role of both point location and placebo effects could be addressed in a trial of acupuncture for chronic pain comparing: acupuncture at classical sites or trigger points, acupuncture at non-classical sites,

and a placebo (mock TENS) or near-placebo (minimal acupuncture).

Where point location is not thought to be important, such as in studies of smoking, three-arm trials may also be useful but the comparisons will be different. In the treatment of smoking the most important questions are whether acupuncture offers any advantage over conventional treatments and whether it is operating through psychological mechanisms. Three groups could be compared: acupuncture, conventional treatment, perhaps nicotine patches or gum, and a placebo (probably mock ear stimulation). Comparison of acupuncture given at different sites (real versus sham) is unlikely to be illuminating.

Where acupuncture has been found to have a specific physiological effect the parameters of treatment can be investigated. The results of such studies will have clinical implications for optimum effectiveness and may also suggest likely modes of action. For instance, one might compare the 'package' of electroacupuncture given deeply at classical locations with minimal acupuncture; then one could 'unpack' the treatment by comparing electrical stimulation with manual, one set of point locations with another, and so on, though probably in an experimental context looking at short-term effects rather than in a clinical trial. There are a very large number of potential questions once all the parameters are clearly discerned.

Greater attention should be paid to a precise specification of the treatment given. Certainly, to aid replication, the acupuncture points used should be indicated. However, it may also be useful, for both real acupuncture and the control, to specify the site of stimulation in anatomical terms, as this may influence the interpretation of the results. Are most of the points on the limb, back, or lobe of the ear? Are the points generally distant or local to the location of the pain (or other complaint)?

If trigger points are thought to be of interest, concurrent measurement of trigger point sensitivity could be done during treatment trials. Reeves, Jaeger & Graff-Radford (1986) have revived the use of the pressure algometer to record changes in sensitivity at trigger points that produce referred pain. It would seem worthwhile incorporating routine measurements of sensitivity at headache trigger points and points used in acupuncture treatment in subsequent trials. Concurrent measures of trigger point sensitivity might have a role to play both in the understanding of acupuncture's action and the prediction of treatment response.

For conditions in which point location is thought to be important, the validity of traditional Chinese diagnoses could be examined in relation to treatment outcome. The most obvious step would be to take one or two conditions that have shown some preliminary response to acupuncture (such as asthma and irritable bowel syndrome) and compare a point prescription based on a traditional Chinese diagnosis with sham acupuncture. If real acupuncture showed significant benefit, then this treatment could again be unpacked, perhaps by comparing set point prescriptions versus individualized traditional Chinese diagnoses in the treatment of each individual. Again, type and mode of stimulation would be important parameters requiring more detailed analysis. Because of the expense and difficulty of performing large clinical trials, this type of study should probably also be done in an experimental context or in tightly controlled single-case studies.

The hypothesis is necessarily speculative. Physiological understanding of acupuncture is still incomplete, and acupuncture has still not been properly evaluated. Many of the trials are methodologically flawed, and some may consider our fairly critical interpretation of the findings as too generous. In most areas the evidence is at best equivocal. However, the hypothesis does provide a framework that links empirical experience, neurophysiology and the current evidence available from clinical trials. Neurophysiological work should be considered as a background to both the design and interpretation of clinical trials. Clinical trial results should be fed back directly to neurophysiologists, and clinical observations could then be used as a basis for generating further experimental work. Finally, if this theoretical model is proven to be correct, then it provides an excellent vehicle for differentiating between Western acupuncture, which might be purely an endorphin-based treatment, and the more traditional Chinese approaches, which could be more autonomically based.

The suggestions must not be seen as fact, but rather as hypothesis generated by the different clinical responses noted in three areas of clinical trials and correlated with our limited understanding of the underlying neurophysiology in acupuncture and some closely related techniques. Whether or not it proves to be correct, it does, at the present time, provide a coherent theoretical framework that integrates neurophysiology, clinical trial work and some aspects of traditional Chinese medicine.

CONCLUSIONS

Disappointingly little has been achieved by literally hundreds of attempts to evaluate acupuncture. Major methodological flaws are apparent in the vast majority of studies. Some tentative conclusions can be drawn, however. Controlled studies have shown positive findings for low back pain and nausea, and equivocal results for migraine. The results of studies on addiction depend very much on how they are interpreted. Nevertheless, larger-scale studies are warranted for all these disorders, though other types of musculoskeletal pain, tension headache and arthritis are also possible candidates.

Controlled trials of any treatment have become an immensely difficult and technical undertaking. They are expensive, time consuming and ideally require collaboration between practitioners and researchers and consultation with a statistician. It is not really possible for complementary practitioners in private practice to mount such trials, and it is very difficult for a professional association or college. However, it is clear that there is no longer any point in conducting small, preliminary studies of acupuncture treatment. There are dozens of such studies, with some encouraging findings. The only way though that acupuncture can gain full acceptance as a valid form of treatment is through good controlled trials that are large enough to answer the questions they pose.

Recommendations for the conduct of clinical trials are made throughout this chapter, and Ter Riet, Kleijnen & Knipschild's (1990a) list of criteria is a good starting point for anyone designing a trial of acupuncture.

Specific points we would emphasize, after reviewing the existing research on acupuncture, are:

1. Trials should be single blind; it is not feasible to conduct double-blind trials. Some trials are nevertheless incorrectly described as double-blind.

2. A range of outcome measures should be used, preferably with some independent assessment. An adequate follow-up is essential.

3. Considerable care needs to be taken in the choice of control group, especially with placebo controls. For a placebo we suggest either mock TNS or a form of acupuncture treatment that is designed to have minimal effects. It will be the option that is the closest match to the true treatment and avoids the difficulties inherent in randomizing patients to a non-acupuncture treatment.

4. It is very useful to check the adequacy of any control treatment with a measure of credibility, or similar assessment, as the choice of control is frequently a matter for criticism.

5. Trials have generally been too small to permit firm conclusions. Ter Riet, Kleijnen & Knipschild (1990a) imply that 50 patients per group are needed. This may not be necessary. However, preliminary calculations of the necessary size for a reasonable power need to be carried out.

6. The hypothesis we have suggested in relation to different types of controlled trial methodology in different clinical conditions will need to be considered and evaluated.

REFERENCES

Bayreuther J, Lewith G T, Pickering R 1994 Acupressure for early morning sickness: a double blind, randomized controlled crossover study. Complementary Therapies in Medicine 2(2):70–76

Bhatt-Sanders D 1985 Acupuncture for rheumatoid arthritis: an analysis of the literature. Seminars in Arthritis and Rheumatism 14(4):225–231

Borglum-Jensen L, Melsen B, Borglum-Jensen S 1979 Effect of acupuncture on headache measured by reduction in number of attacks and use of drugs. Scandinavian Journal of Dental Research 87:373–380

Borkovec T D, Nau S D 1972 Credibility of analogue therapy rationales. Journal of Behavioral Therapy and Experimental Psychiatry 3:257–260

Bowsher D 1991 Neurogenic pain syndromes and their management. British Medical Bulletin 47:644–666

Bowsher D 1993 Mode of action of acupuncture analgesia. Presented at Third World Congress of Acupuncture and Moxibustion, Kyoto, Japan

Chapman C R, Wilson M E, Gehrig J D 1976 Comparative effects of acupuncture and transcutaneous stimulation on the perception of painful dental stimuli. Pain 2:265–283

Chapman C R, Colpitts Y M, Benedetti C, Kitaeff R, Gehrig J D 1980 Evoked potential assessment of acupuncture analgesia: attempted reversal with naloxone. Pain 9:183–197

Chung S-H, Dickenson A 1980 Pain, enkephalin and acupuncture. Nature 283:243–244

Clement-Jones V, Tomlin S, Rees L H, McLoughlin L, Besser G M, Wen H L 1980 Increased beta-endorphin but not met-enkephalin levels in human cerebrospinal fluid after acupuncture for recurrent pain. Lancet ii:946–949

Coan R M, Wong G, Ku S L, Chan Y C, Ozer F T, Coan P L 1980 The acupuncture treatment of low back pain: a randomized controlled study. American Journal of Chinese Medicine 8:181–189

Cole P 1975 Acupuncture and pulse diagnosis in Great Britain. [Unpublished PhD thesis.] University of Sussex, Brighton

Dowson D, Lewith G T, Machin D 1985 The effects of acupuncture versus placebo in the treatment of headache. Pain 21:35–42

Dundee J W, McMillan C M 1992 P6 acupressure and postoperative vomiting. British Journal of Anaesthesia 68:225–226

Dundee J W, Ghaly R G, Fitzpatrick K T J, Abram W P, Lynch G A 1989 Acupuncture prophylaxis of cancer chemotherapy-induced sickness. Journal of the Royal Society of Medicine 82:268–271

Gallacchi G 1981 Acupuncture for cervical and lumbar syndrome. Schweizerischer Medizinische Wochenschrift 111:1360–1366

Gaw A C, Chang L W, Shaw L C 1975 Efficacy of acupuncture on osteoarthritic pain: a double blind controlled trial. New England Journal of Medicine 293:375–378

Godfrey C M, Morgan P 1978 A controlled trial of the theory of acupuncture in musculoskeletal pain. Journal of Rheumatology 5:121–124

Henry P, Baille H, Dartigues JF, Jogeix M 1985 Headache and acupuncture. In: Pfaffenrath V, Lundberg P O, Sjaastad O (eds) Updating in headache. Springer Verlag, Berlin, pp 29–33

Kaptchuk T 1983 The web that has no weaver: understanding Chinese medicine. Congdon Weed, New York

Kramer M S, Shapiro S H 1984 Scientific challenges in the application of randomized controlled trials. Journal of the American Medical Association 252:2739–2745

Lazorthes Y, Esquerre J-P, Simon J, Guiraud G, Guiraud R 1990 Acupuncture meridians and radiotracers. Pain 40:109–112

Le Bars D, Villanueva L, Willer J C, Bouhassira D 1991 Diffuse noxious inhibitory control (DNIC) in animals and man. Acupuncture in Medicine 9(2):47–57

Lewit K 1979 The needle effect in the relief of myofascial pain. Pain 6:83–90

Lewith G T, Kenyon J N 1984 Physiological and psychological explanations for the mechanism of acupuncture as a treatment for chronic pain. Social Science and Medicine 19:1367–1378

Lewith G T, Machin D 1983 On the evaluation of the clinical effects of acupuncture. Pain 16:111–127

Lewith G T, Vincent C A 1995 On the evaluation of the clinical effects of acupuncture: a problem reassessed and a framework for future research. Pain Forum 4(1):29–39

Lewith G T, Field J, Machin D 1983 Acupuncture compared with placebo in post-herpetic pain. Pain 17:361–368

Lu G-D, Needham J 1980 Celestial lancets: a history and rationale of acupuncture and moxa. Cambridge University Press, Cambridge

Macdonald A J R 1989 Acupuncture analgesia and therapy. In: Wall P D, Melzack R (eds) Textbook of pain, 2nd edn. Churchill Livingstone, New York

Macdonald A J R, Macrae K D, Master B R, Rubin A P 1983 Superficial acupuncture in the relief of chronic low back pain. Annals of the Royal College of Surgeons of England 65:44–46

McGlynn F D, McDonnell R M 1974 Subjective ratings of credibility following brief exposure to desensitization and pseudotherapy. Behaviour Research and Therapy 12:141–146

Mann F 1977 Scientific aspects of acupuncture. Heinemann Medical Books, London

Melzack R 1984 Acupuncture and related forms of folk medicine. In: Melzack R, Wall P D (eds) Textbook of pain. Churchill Livingstone, New York

Melzack R, Stillwell D M, Fox E J 1977 Trigger points and acupuncture points for pain: correlations and implications. Pain 3:3–23

Meng Z W, Zhu Z X, Hu L 1985 Progress in the research of meridian phenomena in China during the last 5 years. Journal of Traditional Chinese Medicine 5(2):145–152

O'Connor J, Bensky D 1981 Acupuncture: a comprehensive text. Shanghai College of Traditional Chinese Medicine, Shanghai. Eastland Press, Chicago

Okazaki K 1975 Ryodoraku for migraine headache. American Journal of Chinese Medicine 3:61–70

Patel M, Gutzwiller F, Paccaud F, Marazzi A 1989 A meta-analysis of acupuncture for chronic pain. International Journal of Epidemiology 18(4):900–906

Petrie J, Hazelman B 1985 Credibility of placebo transcutaneous nerve stimulation and acupuncture. Clinical and Experimental Rheumatology 3:151–153

Pocock S J 1985 Current issues in the design and interpretation of clinical trials. British Medical Journal 290:39–42

Pomeranz B 1991 The scientific basis of acupuncture. In: Stux G, Pomeranz B (eds) The basics of acupuncture. Springer-Verlag, Berlin

Price D D, Rafii A, Watkins L R, Buckingham B 1984 A psychophysical analysis of acupuncture analgesia. Pain 19:27–42

Reeves J L, Jaeger B, Graff-Radford S B 1986 Reliability of the pressure algometer as a measure of myofascial trigger point sensitivity. Pain 24:313–321

Reichmanis M, Becker R O 1977 Relief of experimentally induced pain by stimulation at acupuncture loci: a review. Comparative Medicine East and West 5:281–288

Richardson P 1989 Placebos: their effectiveness and mode of action. In: Broome A K (ed) Health psychology: processes and applications. Chapman & Hall, London

Richardson P H, Vincent C A 1986 Acupuncture for the treatment of pain: a review of evaluative research. Pain 24:15–40

Sacks H S, Berrier J, Reitman D, Ancona-Berk VA, Chalmers TC 1987 Meta-analysis of randomized controlled trials. New England Journal of Medicine 316:450–455

Schwartz J L 1988 Evaluation of acupuncture as a treatment for smoking. American Journal of Acupuncture 16:135–142

Shapiro D A 1981 Comparative credibility of treatment rationales: three tests of expectancy theory. British Journal of Clinical Medicine 20:111–122

Skrabanek P 1984 Acupuncture and the age of unreason. Lancet ii:1169–1171

Stewart D, Thompson J, Oswald I 1977 Acupuncture analgesia: an experimental investigation. British Medical Journal 67–70

Ter Riet G, Kleijnen J, Knipschild P 1990a Acupuncture and chronic pain: a criteria based meta-analysis. Journal of Clinical Epidemiology 11:1191–1199

Ter Riet G, Kleijnen J, Knipschild P 1990b A meta-analysis of studies into the effect of acupuncture on addiction. British Journal of General Practice 40:379–382

Travell J G, Simons D G 1983 Myofascial pain and dysfunction. The trigger point manual. Williams and Wilkins, Baltimore

Turner P 1993 Experimental studies on the anti-emetic effects of acupuncture and its non-invasive alternative techniques. Complementary Therapies in Medicine 1:88–91

Veith I 1972 The Yellow Emperor's classic of internal medicine. University of California Press, Berkeley, CA

Vincent C A 1989a The methodology of controlled trials of acupuncture. Acupuncture in Medicine 6:9–13

Vincent C A 1989b A controlled trial of the treatment of migraine by acupuncture. Clinical Journal of Pain 5:305–312

Vincent C A 1990a The treatment of tension headache by acupuncture: a controlled single case design with time series analysis. Journal of Psychosomatic Research 34(5):553–561

Vincent C A 1990b Credibility assessment in trials of acupuncture. Complementary Medicine Research 4(1):8–11

Vincent C A 1993 Acupuncture as a treatment for chronic pain. In: Lewith G T, Aldridge D A (eds) Clinical research methodology for complementary therapies. Hodder & Stoughton, London, pp 289–308

Vincent C A, Richardson P H 1986 The evaluation of

therapeutic acupuncture: concepts and methods. Pain 24:1–13

Voll R 1975 Twenty years of electroacupuncture therapy using low-frequency current pulses. American Journal of Acupuncture 3:291–314

Zhaowei M, Zongxiang Z, Xianglong H 1985 Progress in the research of meridian phenomena in China during the last five years. Journal of Traditional Chinese Medicine 5(2):145–152

14

The clinical use of, and evidence for, acupuncture in the medical systems

Jacqueline Filshie
Adrian White

INTRODUCTION

This chapter reviews the effects of acupuncture on diseases in the different body systems. The text is based on the existing literature rather than on clinical impressions, but clinical details and suggested point locations have been included whenever they seem to be relevant. Precedence is given to controlled trials, where these exist, and we have included all those we have found, reporting them with as little bias as we are able. However, we do not claim that these reviews are thoroughly 'systematic' in the sense of being totally scientifically rigorous. For example, the selection of studies has had to be restricted somewhat; we therefore attempted to retrieve all the English-language literature listed in the standard databases, but where titles seemed very unpromising they were not retrieved.

The acupuncture literature is dominated by articles from China, which are unanimously positive but regrettably often of poor quality. The faults we found most commonly were:

1. a homogeneous group was not defined by the inclusion and exclusion criteria, so that it was not clear what precise clinical diagnostic group was being treated
2. research was not prospective, and authors did not specify that all consecutive subjects were recruited, leaving the research open to the accusation that there was bias in selecting patients

3. patient bias in favour of acupuncture was not excluded: groups receiving acupuncture were compared with control groups receiving either no treatment or standard medical therapy
4. there was probably bias in assessing the outcome of treatment because the therapist and the observer were often one and the same person
5. the assessments were so ill defined (e.g. 'improved') as to be virtually meaningless
6. the results failed to present the raw data or even means and standard deviations, and there was no mention of the statistical methods used. Thus there is no way of repeating the analysis or otherwise verifying the significance of results.

Readers who are practising acupuncturists may be surprised to find that there is a lack of really rigorous research that supports their own positive clinical experiences. There are several possible reasons for this — apart from our critics' argument that acupuncture doesn't work! In actual practice, acupuncture is often used for subacute conditions rather than chronic diseases, and for those odd symptoms that seem to defy accurate diagnosis. On the other hand, controlled trials have often been performed on a very different group of patients, *viz* chronic cases, which can be clearly defined by strict inclusion and exclusion criteria. Success rates for any therapy in such cases would be expected to be lower. Another reason for lack of success is that the acupuncture may not have been adequate for the condition.

Clearly evidence is crucial and must guide the practice of acupuncture. So far most of our evidence is empirical, and we must strive to produce more watertight studies for every indication.

GASTROINTESTINAL CONDITIONS

Many acupuncturists boast great success in dealing with a plethora of common gastrointestinal disorders. A number of papers have been reviewed here, arranged anatomically from the oesophagus to the rectum and with a short section on the liver, gall bladder and pancreas. The area that has been researched the most is undoubtedly acupuncture treatment for nausea and vomiting, and this has a chapter in its own right in this textbook (Ch 15). This section would be perilously slim if only controlled clinical trials were considered and so it has been expanded to contain selected empirical information.

Cynics may find it paradoxical that the same acupuncture points appear to be recommended for opposite complaints such as constipation and diarrhoea and traditionalists often say that acupuncture is used to bring the body and its functions back into balance. Many of the following 'strong' points: CV-12, ST-25 and 36, LI-14, SP-6, BL-20 and 21, and LR-3 appear as treatment for almost every gastrointestinal complaint. This can also give considerable comfort to novice acupuncturists who want to keep things simple! Present studies on gastrointestinal complaints have been reviewed by Li et al (1992) and Dill (1992) and they support the efficacy of acupuncture in the regulation of gastrointestinal motor activity and secretion through opioid and other neural pathways. However, the reviewers state that, because of the heterogeneity of study design, results are often difficult to compare and sometimes conflict; this conflict may be due to differences in the mode of manual or electrical stimulation employed. Some of their findings are summarized in this section.

OESOPHAGUS

Acupuncture at CV-17, PC-6, ST-36 and extra points including auricular points was reported to have helped seven out of eight patients with dysphagia due to oesophagitis and achalasia (Xia & Huang 1991). One anecdotal paper by Feng (1984) describes the use of acupuncture for patients with carcinomatous obstruction using the principal points BL-17, 21 and 46, and PC-6 or CV-12 and 22, ST-36 and SP-4 plus others. Treatment was on 2 consecutive days with a 3-day gap, repeated for *n* courses of treatment. Acupuncture was given as adjuvant to conventional treatment. In trying to speculate why any relief would occur, the authors suggested that perhaps endogenous ACTH secretion could lead to temporary diminution of oedema around the tumour, which could cause some benefit. Further objective evaluation is recommended.

UPPER GASTROINTESTINAL TRACT

Stomach

Acupuncture has been studied to a varying extent in stomach motility, gastric acid secretion, blood flow and electrical activity.

Motility

A number of physiological studies have shown that acupuncture has an effect on gastro-intestinal motility. Study design can vary widely; much of the animal work has involved implantation of strain gauges and observation for a few hours under anaesthesia. Some conscious animals with chronically implanted strain gauges have also been studied. Li et al (1992) tabulated and summarized much experimental work in both animals and humans. All the studies concluded that acupuncture affected gastric motility, but not necessarily in the same direction! In humans, a promoting effect of electroacupuncture at ST-36 versus a sham point was shown in patients with low initial gastric activity and a suppressing effect was shown in patients with active initial motility during endoscopy (Yuan, Zhu & Zhing 1985). Further studies are desirable and physiological explanations for these findings should be sought.

Iwa & Sakita (1994) studied gastrointestinal motility in mice given acupuncture and moxibustion by measuring carbon transit times. Acupuncture in the abdomen significantly increased intestinal motility compared with acupuncture at points on the back. Moxa on the abdomen significantly reduced gastrointestinal motility compared with moxa on the back. Both acupuncture and moxibustion tended to reverse the increase in motility caused by vasostigmin and the decrease in mobility caused by atropine.

Neither acupuncture nor moxibustion reversed the inhibition of carbon transit times by ephedrine.

One practical application of electroacupuncture in humans may be to reverse the inhibition of intestinal peristalsis induced by epidural or intrathecal opioids. Dai et al (1993) found electroacupuncture to have a peristalsis-sparing action after intrathecal injections of morphine in rabbits. As most opioids inhibit peristalsis to a varying extent, this is an interesting paradox; perhaps endogenous opioids are less active at μ-receptors or act differently in different circumstances. The acupuncture did not reverse or worsen any respiratory depression caused by the opioid. The points chosen were ST-36 and SP-6. This study supports the wider application of acupuncture for reducing postoperative pain and hopefully decreasing the ileus time. A modification of the technique would be required for acute pain management following surgery in patients given epidural local anaesthesia in addition to opioid perioperatively. This is because the local anaesthetic action would be expected to abolish the afferent stimulation at points ST-36 and SP-6 and therefore would most likely negate the benefit. Therefore any acupuncture would need to be given either before an epidural, that is, preoperatively or at different points altogether, proximal to the level of sensory blockade, or else some time postoperatively when the local anaesthetic had worn off over chosen distal acupuncture points.

Gastric acid secretion

Li et al (1992) state that acupuncture can suppress gastric acid output in both animals and humans.

Animals. Dogs with a Heidenhain pouch given acupuncture at GV-20 inhibited both sham-feeding acid output and maximal acid output stimulated by histamine. Acupuncture at ST-36 also significantly suppressed pentagastrin-stimulated maximal acid output. However, conflicting results were described in rats.

Basal acid output was reduced by manual and electroacupuncture at ST-36 in conscious dogs compared with sham electrical stimulation and non-specific acupoints (He, Yie & Gong 1986).

Humans. Six randomized placebo-controlled studies were performed in Hunt's department in Ontario on the effect of electroacupuncture on gastric acid output in healthy volunteers (Tougas et al 1992a).

1. Basal acid output was significantly reduced following electroacupuncture to ST-36 as opposed to identical placebo stimulation on the lateral side of the arm.

2. Electroacupuncture at ST-36 also inhibited sham feeding-stimulated acid output by reducing the volume of gastric secretion. Placebo acupuncture, in contrast, had no effect on secretion volume or gastric acid output.

3. Biphasic electroacupuncture at 8 Hz did not inhibit pentagastrin-stimulated acid output.

4. Local anaesthetic injections of Xylocaine to the acupuncture points prior to stimulation failed to abolish all sensation and, perhaps on account of this, also failed to block the inhibitory effect of electroacupuncture on sham-feeding acid output.

In contrast,

5. Intravenous naloxone completely abolished the inhibitory effect of electroacupuncture on sham-feeding acid output.

6. Neither placebo nor active electro-acupuncture altered plasma gastrin levels, but there was a significant rise in circulating gastrin levels in subjects given naloxone and electro-acupuncture compared with electroacupuncture or placebo acupuncture alone.

The marked effect of electroacupuncture on sham-feeding-stimulated acid output, but not with pentagastin stimulation, was thought to be a vagally mediated effect (Tougas et al 1992b) and further corroborative evidence was provided. They concluded that the antisecretory effects of electroacupuncture do not result from decreased gastrin release or decreased parietal cell sensitivity to gastrin, but are mediated via naloxone-sensitive opioid neural and vagal efferents.

The same authors described a study showing that acid secretion was largely abolished by vagotomy and that additional transection of splanchnic nerves completely prevented the effect of acupuncture. This showed that acupuncture works through a combination of parasympathetic and sympathetic pathways. Autonomic afferents may be stimulated as well as peripheral nerves (Ouyang, Fan & Gong 1987). Why then does the innervation of the placebo point differ from that of ST-36? This needs further elucidation.

The naloxone result is most interesting and is thought to be due to its antagonism of opioid pathways rather than a direct stimulatory effect on acid secretion. These short-term effects of acupuncture suggest a potential therapeutic value for acupuncture in diseases associated with gastric acid secretion (Tougas et al 1992a). Lux et al (1994) studied the effect of classical acupuncture, electroacupuncture, TENS, laser therapy and sham acupuncture on sham-feeding acid secretion. They found that electroacupuncture at 5 Hz at BL-21, ST-36 and CV-12 and TENS at 3 Hz significantly reduced gastric acid secretion in comparison to the other forms of stimulation.

Sodipo & Falaiye (1979), in an uncontrolled study, showed acupuncture to inhibit pentagastrin-stimulated maximal acid output significantly in patients with duodenal ulcer and that acupuncture also statistically significantly decreased basal acid output in patients with duodenal ulcer.

Peptic ulcer. Hsu, Chen & Shen (1987) have shown that 10 days' electroacupuncture at ST-36 prevented stress ulceration in rats. Ouyang, Ding & Fan (1984) in a further study have shown acupuncture to reduce sodium chloride-induced ulcers. A number of uncontrolled studies suggest that acupuncture can heal peptic ulcers. Salvi et al (1983) reported endoscopic healing of duodenal ulcers after a 1–2-month course of traditional acupuncture in four patients who had failed to get relief by conventional medication. In a further study, Zhu, Huang & Zhang (1984) compared the results of endoscopy pre and post traditional acupuncture in 41 patients with peptic ulcer and demonstrated a healing rate of 73%. The most surprising thing of all is the lack of controlled studies for these common conditions.

Gastrointestinal blood flow

In one study, Lee (1974) gave electrostimulation to ST-36 in rats and showed a significant reduction in mesenteric red blood cell velocity in the mesenteric artery, capillary and venule after acupuncture versus sham treatment. This cardiovascular response could not be obtained if the sciatic nerve was cut, therefore afferent stimulation was an integral part of the treatment. This was also accompanied by a reduction in mean carotid blood pressure; the authors suggested that these cardiovascular changes were due to inhibition of sympathetic vasoconstrictor activity. Increased intestinal motility was also observed subjectively during electrostimulation.

Electrical activity

Li et al (1992) summarized experimental data on electromyography and electrogastrogram results, but space does not permit amplification of these details.

Analgesia for endoscopy

A randomized controlled double-blind trial on 90 patients undergoing gastroscopy showed acupuncture to be significantly better as an analgesic than placebo acupuncture treatment (Cahn et al 1978) Electroacupuncture at ST-36 and LI-4 was as successful as diazepam and atropine in a further series (Chu, Zhao & Huang 1987); however, the trial compared an analgesic acupuncture treatment with a sedative.

Epigastric pain and intestinal colic

Visceral pain is often deep, dull and poorly localized and may be referred to deep or superficial structures. Uncontrolled descriptive accounts abound for treatment of epigastric pain of mixed origin using various techniques, for example ST-36 (Zhang 1992), three pairs of paravertebral points from T9 to T12 (Zhao 1991) and a TCM approach (Lu 1990). Even patients with an acute abdomen have been referred from

the emergency room and treated in 245 cases, using a selection of points based on a medical diagnosis and a stimulation time of 20–30 minutes (Gu 1992).

Although risky, conservative treatment has been used successfully with acupuncture for acute volvulus of the stomach by Wan & Yu (1981). Intestinal colic has been helped by ST-36 stimulation (Jiang 1990). In one descriptive, non-randomized series of 70 patients with stomach ache attributed to peptic ulcer, gastritis or gastroenteritis, acupuncture at BL-20 and 21 was significantly more successful at pain reduction than acupuncture at BL-24 and 25 (Yuan et al 1986). The authors also stated that the points BL-20 and 21 correspond to skin and muscle innervation of T9–T12 and are at the approximate level of the sympathetic ganglia that innervate the stomach. When looking for tender points they measured tenderness thresholds with a spring-loaded device before and at a mean of 8.5 days after subtotal gastrectomy in 33 patients around the location of BL-20 and 21 and between these two points. Ninety per cent of points at BL-20 or 21 or between the two were tender with reduced tenderness thresholds prior to surgery, and returned to normal post-operatively. Nodules and cording detected preoperatively also reduced or disappeared post-operatively. Most of this non-rigorous data support the more scientific theories of segmental acupuncture.

LARGE BOWEL

Diarrhoea

Infantile diarrhoea

Infantile diarrhoea is usually a self-limiting condition. It is difficult to identify those who would not get better spontaneously. No randomized controlled trials could be found for this condition. Lin (1987) described 170 infants aged 1 to 29 months, with an average age of 7.8 months, presenting with diarrhoea from four to over 20 times per day for a range of 1–515 days, and given acupuncture daily for 3 days. The points chosen were CV-9 and 6 and ST-25 bilaterally and ST-36 bilaterally. Secondary points sometimes used were SP-3 and 4 plus or minus moxibustion. A 'half puncture' technique was employed with a shallow puncture and fast withdrawal. After 1 course of treatment 86.6% were judged to be cured (i.e. less than two normal motions per day), 7.6% were improved with half the number of motions per day and 3.6% showed no improvement at all. The spontaneous remission rate was not discussed in these cases.

A further series of 1050 cases (Su 1992), in children having more than five to six motions a day using vigorous stimulation at ST-25 and GV-1 at a depth of 0.7 cm, reported 43% success after one treatment, a further 45% success after a second treatment and 7% success after a third treatment. Five per cent failed to respond to three treatments. There would be strong ethical opposition to the use of such vigorous treatment in small children in Western centres.

Two other series of 500 (Zhongxin 1989) and 30 cases (Feng 1989) with similar 'success' have been reported but there was a lack scientific merit; Feng (1989) also recommended dietary modification, which made interpretation of results difficult if not impossible. Infantile toxic intestinal paralysis secondary to infection by various life-threatening organisms was treated using ST-36, PE-6, ST-25, CV-12, ST-44, SP-4, BL-25, GV-20, EX-6 and CV-6 as the main points and was 'cured' in 134 out of 172 cases, 'improved' after one to five treatments in 27 cases and unchanged in six cases, with five deaths also reported in one Chinese series on critically ill children (Li 1987). It is possible that infants who do not get better rapidly are at high risk if acupuncture treatment is continued in the absence of conventional treatment.

Low-level laser therapy was found to give a 65% 'cure' rate and 30.8% 'improved' rate in 415 children with infantile diarrhoea from a variety of causes using ST-36, SP-6, Tian Su and Baheo points (He-Jz 1989).

Escherichia coli-induced diarrhoea

One interesting trial by Hwang & Jenkins (1988) was on 34 preweaning pigs after inoculation with *E. coli* had been used to induce diarrhoea in all animals. They were then allocated to four groups:

1. 11 pigs: electroacupuncture 4 days—100 Hz first treatment and 5 Hz three treatments at GV-1, ST-36 and Baihui (on the pig)
2. 11 pigs: acupuncture to GV-1, ST-36 and BL-20 plus moxibustion at CV-12 and ST-25 and haemoacupuncture at various points
3. 7 pigs: neomycin 2 days
4. 5 pigs: control.

At day 5 postinoculation, 60% of control pigs and more than 80% of pigs in all treated groups recovered from diarrhoea. At day 3 post-inoculation, recovery rates were: group 1: 27%, group 2: 81%, group 3: 71%, and group 4: 20%. The authors concluded that traditional acupuncture, but not electroacupuncture, was effective in controlling the early stages of *E. coli* diarrhoea in pigs.

This paper raises more questions than it answers. First, manual acupuncture was not compared with electroacupuncture at the same points (i.e. the choice of point in this study may have been critical). The mode of electrical stimulation may not have been optimal. Secondly, the contribution of moxibustion and, thirdly, use of points CV-12 and ST-25 could have been critical. Also the haemoacupuncture could be omitted in a future study as it is impossible to assess what, if any, contribution it made to the recovery. In consequence, we consider that the only possible conclusion is that one or more components of the manual/moxa/bleeding sequence was as effective, at these points, as conventional antibiotic therapy. Electro-acupuncture at the other points appeared to be ineffective but has yet to be tested at varying modes of stimulation on the same points. The authors' conclusion that electrical acupuncture may be less effective in modulation of the immune system could be challenged. Electro-acupuncture at a different choice of points and at different modes of stimulation may have had different effects. This should not put off any further serious investigations in this fascinating area. Criticism aside, due credit should go to the authors for attempting to assess these animals objectively for this condition.

Bacillary dysentery

One randomized controlled study on acute amoebic dysentery showed significant benefit following daily acupuncture for 7 days at ST-25 and 37, which cured 94% of 55 patients as opposed to 78% of 50 patients given furazolidone within 14 days (Cheng et al 1979). Success was measured as negative faecal cultures on day 14 and recurrence rates were found to be similar in both groups. A further uncontrolled series of 654 cases given acupuncture as opposed to 281 controls given antibiotics showed superiority of the acupuncture group over the antibiotic group (Qiu, Sheng & Li 1979). A traditional approach to treatment was described by R. Yan (1988); the paper also supported the view that acupuncture may strengthen immune function. A controlled study on rhesus monkeys infected with bacillary dysentery given acupuncture treatments daily at KI-4, 6 and 10, ST-25 and 36 and moxa on KI-8 showed that faecal bacterial cultures cleared, in contrast to the controls, which all remained positive (Zhang, Jin & Li 1979).

No studies have measured antibody formation during acupuncture treatment to support the claims to date.

Constipation

Despite the fact that constipation is a common complaint, there is only one objective study of this problem, in eight patients with colonic marker transit times of over 60 hours, (Klauser et al 1993). Electroacupuncture at 10 Hz was given to LI-4, LR-3, ST-25 and BL-25 on six occasions in a 3-week period. Two patients dropped out and the rest failed to show a significant reduction in colonic transit time following acupuncture. One other paper described habitual constipation due to 'poor bowel habits', with a treatment given to a selection of points based on TCM diagnosis for 'normalization of Qi' (Jiao 1986).

Ulcerative colitis

The treatment of ulcerative colitis is empirical to date and can be performed using two rows of needles, 12 in all, in the lower abdomen and with more severe cases given LR-3, LI-4 and ST-36 or BL-24 to 28. A course of three to six treatments has been said to give the maximum improvement (Campbell 1992). The more traditional approaches reported 65% success in one study (Requena 1981), but the number of cases was sadly omitted. Success was also found in 12 patients who had failed with conventional treatment but given dietary advice and vitamin B12 injections into acupuncture points in addition (Khoe 1975).

Irritable bowel

Although a common and a rather fashionable diagnosis, only one report of acupuncture for this condition has been found to date, with a traditional approach and no patient details (Lewis 1992). This condition is known to give a high placebo response to a variety of pharmacological techniques, which could make study design somewhat difficult.

RECTUM
Prolapse

In a descriptive series, rectal prolapse in children that occurred at least once per day was treated successfully in 94% of 65 children with a peak age of 3 years and average duration of symptoms of 5 months, range 11 days to 5 years (Jin 1987). Moderately vigorous treatment was given to points GV-1, GV-20, BL-35 and 57 and between six and 18 treatments were given in total. The 'cured' patients showed no further recurrence when assessed between 3 months and over 1 year and the best results were obtained in the children with symptoms less than 6 months' duration.

Hirschsprung's disease

A traditional Chinese medical approach to 90 cases of Hirschsprung's disease has been described, including the use of auricular needling, body acupuncture point injection with ginseng solution and adenosine triphosphate and herbs (Wang et al 1987). Unfortunately, this form of combined therapy makes the evaluation of the acupuncture component impossible either to interpret or to recommend.

Anal fissure

In a brief communication describing results from 300 cases with anal fissures treated by points GV-1 and BL-30, encouraging results were found (Yang & Kong 1987). In 82% of patients, pain and bleeding improved after the first treatment and the fissures healed after an average of six daily treatments. Ten per cent improved but were not cured and 87 failed to respond after 18 treatments in total. Twenty-four cases recurred after varying intervals of time between a few weeks and over a year. This promising work deserves further investigation.

Haemorrhoids

The treatment of haemorrhoids by acupuncture remains to be scientifically appraised, and one paper describes TCM principles of point selection but gives no patient details (Su 1987a). Vigorous acupuncture at BL-2, LI-4 and HT-5 or BL-57 and CV-24 were given for postoperative pain relief following haemorrhoidectomy and anal surgery (Xiao, Xie & Dong 1992). Thirty-four per cent of patients had complete pain relief and 53% improved. It is a pity that results of the two groups of acupuncture points were not compared and that points serving the appropriate segments were not used.

LIVER, GALL BLADDER AND PANCREAS
Liver

There are, unfortunately, more references on acupuncture causing hepatitis (see Ch 19) than to its providing relief. As far as treatment is concerned, Schnorrenberger in Germany uses it

but no formal evaluation has so far been performed.

Gall bladder

Auricular acupressure for 365 cases of cholelithiasis using seeds (semen Vaccariae) on the liver, gall bladder and bile duct points, plus or minus others, has been described by Dong et al (1986, 1988). After treatment on alternate days for 1 month, 16 patients (4.4%) expelled all stones according to ultrasound and 56 (15%) had a 50% reduction in stones. The results as presented, however, stated an 81% effective rate as judged by stools containing expelled stones, but less than half of the stones were expelled on ultrasound examination. However, ultrasound examination can miss some stones (possible 9%). The patients were also given advice and told not to overwork and to avoid catching cold. The attempt to compare it with a 'control' group given 'antiphlogistic and cholagogic tablets' (probably herbal treatment) without randomization clearly left the interpretation of the data open to question. Even if the treatment were to be of clinical value, the quality of the analysis is low.

Bilateral extra points from T9–T12 were chosen for a number of patients with cholelithiasis in one anecdotal review by Zhao (1991), and the points GB-25, 26 and 27 were used in another article by Heinzl (1986) who also recommended GB-37, 38 and 40 for biliary colic. The latter reference, by a jovial doctor who carried acupuncture needles everywhere and used them at parties, in the street or even on a plane, warned sensibly that acupuncture could cause a stone to dislodge and cause obstruction in some cases.

Han has shown that acupuncture not only causes an increase in endogenous opioids but also increases endogenous cholecystokinin production (Han, Ding & Fan 1986). Cholecystokinin, an opioid receptor antagonist, is released centrally in the central nervous system. But can its release peripherally, if at all, improve gall bladder function in some way? Cholecystokinin stimulates gall bladder emptying and also decreases gastric contractions but increases intestinal contractions. It also promotes pancreatic se-cretions. Further research is recommended in this area.

Pancreas

Ballegaard et al (1985) performed a randomized crossover trial of active versus sham electro-acupuncture or active versus sham TENS in patients with chronic pancreatitis. Neither electroacupuncture nor TENS brought about the significant pain relief that had been expected from the result of their pilot study. A series of traditional recipe points for acute pancreatitis has been described in a paper by Su (1987b) but gave no patient details and should be treated with due circumspection.

HICCUP

No controlled trials have been described on hiccup to date, but several approaches are out-lined using auriculotherapy and body acupunc-ture; the mechanisms of actions have not been studied. Several uncontrolled reports are described to encourage further work.

Li, Yi & Qi (1990) describe 85 cases of hiccup with 18 postoperative cases, 62 due to cerebro-vascular diseases and five to miscellaneous causes. Auriculotherapy was employed, using a point detector on diaphragm, stomach, spleen and liver points as main points and Shenmen, Sympathetic, Brain and Brainstem points as auxiliary points. Following 10–15 minutes electri-cal stimulation, auriculopressure was maintained by semen Vaccariae on the same acupoint. Fourteen per cent stopped after the first session and 54% after three to five sessions, but the condition may also have been self-limiting.

Li, Wang & Ma (1991) reported a further series of 40 cases treated with manual auriculo-acupuncture using Shenmen, Sympathetic and Erzhong as the main points and Stomach, Liver, Kidney, Duodenum, Lung, Yuanzhong, Thorax and Abdomen as auxiliary points; 83% of cases were 'cured' within three sessions.

Electrostimulation at a neck point close to the phrenic nerve was used, plus CV-22, in another series of 52 patients; this had varying success (Yan 1988). Two cases using PE-6 and ST-36 stimulation stopped immediately after the patients experienced De Qi at ST-36 with manual stimulation (Wong 1983). One paper by Italian researchers included patients with hiccup per-operatively (Bondi & Bettelli 1981). Zhao (1989) described a traditional approach, but no patient details were given.

MECHANISMS

The gut is a sophisticated conveyor belt designed to coordinate onward motility, secretion of diges-tive fluids, absorption of nutrients and fluids and excretion of waste products. Its function is regu-lated by a combination of enteric nerves, afferent and efferent autonomic function and psycho-immunological influences (Gwee & Read 1994).

The subtleties of the interplay between endogenous opioid and CCK secretion, 5-HT and autonomic nerve manipulation by acupunc-ture are only just beginning to be studied. Drug treatment is currently directed at specific targets such as smooth muscle, the enteric nervous system, sensory receptors in the gut, autonomic nerves and the brain. Acupuncture is likely to work at multiple sites simultaneously, utilizing endogenous transmitters at lower and more specific amounts and 'doses' than drug therapy and with fewer side-effects.

CONCLUSION

Li et al (1992), in their review of effectiveness of acupuncture for gastrointestinal function and disorders, stated that no firm conclusions could be drawn because of the lack of properly random-ized controlled trials. One area of potential interest for future studies is the effect of acupuncture on stress. Many gastrointestinal disorders are exacer-bated by stress. In the section of immunological disorders (p 270) it is reported that, if an animal is given a distinctly flavoured drink with an immunosuppressant drug, the same flavoured drink alone at a later stage can suppress the immune reponse (Ader, Cohen & Felten 1995). This Pavlovian response shows that the gastro-intestinal system is eminently responsive to many influences including the higher centres. This strengthens the need for prospective randomized studies. This would reduce the element of treatment bias that may have influenced the previous conclusions drawn from non-randomized studies.

CARDIOVASCULAR CONDITIONS

Research into acupuncture and the cardiovascular system (CVS) has two important applications. First, as a tool for investigating acupuncture mechanisms, the CVS can be monitored accurately and conveniently and may be used to study autonomic effects. Secondly, acupuncture may be useful in the management of diseases of the cardiovascular system itself. We shall consider these two applications separately.

Patients frequently comment that they feel warm after acupuncture. It was observed that patients who responded to EA analgesia tended to show a measurable rise in the skin temperature of the palms, which is consistent with a reduced sympathetic tone (Cao, Xu & Ly 1983). However, some studies failed to show such changes. These inconsistencies may be due to technical difficulties in measuring skin temperature changes reliably. Ernst & Lee (1986) used thermography to overcome these problems in a series of 19 volunteers. They found that EA produced a temporary increase in sympathetic tone locally during stimulation. After the end of stimulation, they recorded a sustained vasodilatation throughout the body, particularly in the hands.

Ballegaard et al (1993) showed that the effect of acupuncture on skin temperature depended on the baseline temperature. In a carefully controlled series of blinded experiments with volunteers, EA was found to reduce skin temperatures that were initially high, raise those that were initially low and have little effect on intermediate values. This is a clear example of acupuncture activating the homeostatic mechanism.

EXPERIMENTAL STUDIES ON THE CARDIOVASCULAR SYSTEM

Li, Sun & Zhang (1983) surgically constructed a permanent carotid artery 'bridge' in dogs in order to monitor the rise in blood pressure (BP) during and after i.v. infusions of adrenaline. EA at ST-36 prevented the adrenaline-induced rise in BP. This effect was inhibited by naloxone, indicating that it involved the opioid peptides.

Yao (1993) compared the effect of EA on two strains of rat with congenital high and low BP respectively. During the period of EA stimulation, the BP initially rose in both groups. Subsequently there was a prolonged fall in BP, which was much more marked in the hypertensive group (Fig. 14.1). This fall was accompanied by a decreased rate of firing in the splanchnic nerve, that is, a reduction in sympathetic tone. Yao (1993) confirmed that this effect was inhibited by naloxone, but also found that it was inhibited by reducing the production of serotonin by pretreatment with parachlorophenylalanine. The mechanism clearly involves both opioid peptides and serotonin.

Acupuncture has the ability to correct abnormally low BP in experimental animals. Sun, Yu & Yao (1983) lowered the BP of rats by withdrawing blood. Simultaneous EA to the sciatic nerve reduced the fall in BP compared with untreated controls. This homeostatic effect of acupuncture has been elegantly demonstrated by Yao (1993) with experiments on the baroreceptor reflex (Fig. 14.2). The curve of the response of mean arterial BP to changes in carotid baroreceptor pressure is shifted downwards when the BP is raised (probably through the release of endorphins and serotonin) and upwards when it is depressed (probably through the release of central acetylcholine and vasopressin).

Ballegaard et al (1993) extended their observations on skin temperature, described above, to include measurements of changes in pulse and BP. The results were similar—that is, acupuncture regulated these values towards normal. This was indicated most clearly by the high correlation between the initial values and changes in the BP–heart-rate product. Results were highly significant ($P < 0.001$) in comparison to placebo.

Tayama et al (1984) used impedance cardiography to measure the effects of EA on the

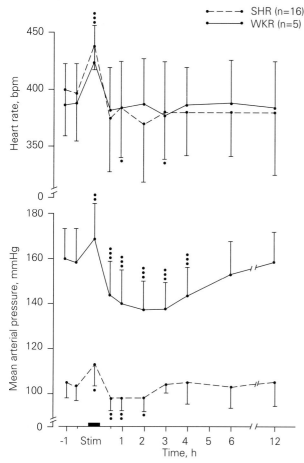

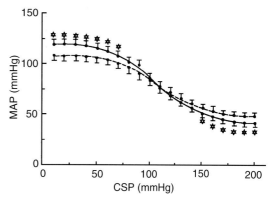

Figure 14.2 Baroreceptor response to acupuncture: effects of prolonged deep peroneal nerve stimulation on the shape and slope of the carotid sinus baroreceptor function curve. Values are the mean arterial pressure (MAP) and carotid sinus pressure (CSP). Dot-and-dash curves are controls before stimulation, solid curves are during stimulation, *$P <$ 0.05. (From Yao 1993, with permission of Scandinavia University Press.)

Figure 14.1 Lower panel: blood pressure is depressed more severely and for longer in hypertensive rats (SHR) than in normotensive rats (WKY) after electroacupuncture stimulation (Stim.). Upper panel shows simultaneous changes in pulse rate. Values are expressed as mean ± SD. Asterisks indicate a significant difference from the control value before stimulation (*$P < 0.05$, **$P < 0.01$, ***$P < 0.001$,) (From Yao 1993, with permission of Scandinavia University Press.)

levels of adrenaline or noradrenaline. The effects started about 10 minutes after starting stimulation, and lasted about 30 minutes.

From the above experimental evidence it appears that EA is capable of producing profound changes in the CVS, acting to regulate it towards normal, probably through the sympathetic nervous system.

CLINICAL STUDIES

Hypertension

In an early report, Tam & Yiu (1975) treated a cohort of 28 hypertensive subjects with inner Bladder line and distal points daily for 10 to 40 sessions. Results showed a reduction in symptoms and BP readings in more than half the subjects. The study is flawed, however, because there was only a single baseline measurement of BP. In a study reported briefly by Yin (1992), more stringent inclusion criteria were used to select subjects for acupuncture. The points used were GB-20, ST-36, SP-6, adding PC-6 for hyperlipidaemia, and LR-3 and ST-40 for other indications. Both systolic and diastolic BP fell significantly, but the absence of a control group again limits the value of these findings.

cardiovascular system of 25 healthy subjects. Stimulation of PC-4–6 produced a significant fall in peripheral resistance compared with placebo; there was no change in heart rate or BP, but stroke volume and cardiac output increased. The effect was equivalent to a plasma expander infusion at the rate of 2 ml/kg for 10 minutes. Stimulating LI-4–10 induced a significant increase in radial artery blood flow and vessel diameter 'equivalent to the effect of a stellate ganglion block'. There were no changes in the blood

Huang & Liang (1992) studied the response of 30 hypertensives to auriculotherapy at the Heart point, manipulating the needle to produce a burning sensation, or adding EA if the burning sensation was not achieved. Short-term observations over the following 60 minutes showed a reduction of BP to normal limits in all cases; levels of angiotensin II in seven of the more severe cases were also significantly reduced. As a control procedure, needling the (auricular) Stomach point without stimulation had no such effect. Daily treatment was claimed to produce long-term benefit in over 60% of cases but no data were given.

Gaponjuk, Sherkovina & Leonova (1993) treated 78 hypertensive men by needling a combination of three to six auricular points for 10–12 sessions. A (non-randomized) control group received sham EA to the ear. Systolic and diastolic BP fell significantly by the end of treatment in the active treatment group. There was a decrease in symptoms such as headache and giddiness, and an improvement in work capacity. There were no significant changes in the control group although only limited data were reported.

In a subsequent paper, Gaponjuk & Sherkovina (1994) examined the short-term effects of needling different auricular points in three categories of 104 hypertensive patients. The results suggested that different points can affect BP, cardiac minute volume and peripheral resistance to differing extents. The authors commented that, if true, this may be related to specific innervation of different regions of the auricle. However, the results in various parameters were not compared statistically.

Any treatment that reduces the need for long-term medication in the management of hypertension is potentially very important, so two other techniques that are not strictly acupuncture are discussed here.

First, acupressure was studied by Zhou et al (1991), who randomized a series of 274 patients with grade I or II hypertension to receive either acupressure treatment, or standard Western drug management, or placebo capsule only. The acupressure consisted of 5 or 6 *Vaccaria* seeds placed on appropriate auricular acupuncture points, renewed every 3 days for a period of 3 months. There was no difference between the effects of acupressure and Western drugs, both of which were significantly more effective than the placebo capsule. The methodological rigour of the study was questionable, however, since there were 135 subjects in the acupressure group but only 68 and 71 in the other two groups, without any explanation offered.

Secondly, the effect of TENS on BP was studied by Williams, Mueller & Cornwall (1991) who randomized 12 subjects with essential hypertension to receive electrical stimulation at 10 000 Hz to either genuine points (LR-3, ST-36, LI-11 and auricular Groove for lowering BP) or nearby non-acupuncture points. Blood pressure was measured immediately before and after treatment, and after 5 minutes. There was a significant reduction in BP immediately after treatment but this effect was transient since the difference became insignificant within 5 minutes.

Clearly studies do suggest that acupuncture may reduce hypertension, at least in the short term, and this is encouraging for further studies for this indication.

Ischaemic heart disease

Tang (1987) reviewed the Chinese literature on the value of acupuncture in myocardial infarction. The overall consensus was that acupuncture may improve cardiac function, relieve some symptoms (particularly pain, dyspnoea and palpitations), and reduce arrhythmias and sudden death. The points most commonly used in the Chinese reports were PC-6, BL-14 and 15, Huachuo points at the same levels (T4, 5) and CV-17. Less commonly, PC-4, ST-36 and SP-6 were added. We shall now discuss some quantitative studies that have tested the above hypotheses.

Angina pectoris

Angina is known to respond well to placebo, as discussed in detail by Benson & McCallie (1979).

These authors cited the classic research by Dimond (Dimond, Kittle & Crockett 1960) comparing internal mammary artery ligation with sham operation (i.e. thoracotomy followed by immediate closure). Among the sham-operated group, 100% reduced their use of glyceryl trinitrate and reported increased exercise tolerance. Among the group that received mammary artery ligation, only 76% had similar improvement. Sham-controlled studies are crucial in research into angina.

There are several uncontrolled studies of acupuncture that suggest it may have an effect in angina. Sternfield et al (1987) treated a series of 15 cases of angina with HT-7, PC-6 and CV-17 for 39 sessions. Thirteen achieved significant pain relief and a decrease in drug consumption. Yin & Jia (1991) reported qualitatively on ECG improvements in 70 out of 86 angina patients. Radzievsky, Fisenko & Dmitriev (1988) stopped all medication except glyceryl trinitrate in 48 angina patients and gave them between 20 and 30 treatments with segmental points. This permitted a reduction in glyceryl trinitrate consumption (self-reported) and anxiety (Spielberger index), and improved exercise performance on a bicycle ergometer. Hypertensive subjects also showed improvements in BP, inotropic pumping function and myocardial relaxation function. Similarly, Hansson & Mannheimer (1991) published a small series of three cases in which response to needling the Heart ear point was proportional to the tenderness of that point. Clearly, the need for carefully controlled studies is well justified by these reports.

Richter, Herlitz & Hjalmarson (1991) performed a crossover study of 21 patients with stable angina, comparing 12 sessions of individualized acupuncture (mainly PC-6, HT-5, BL-15 and 20 and ST-36) over 4 weeks with placebo tablet for 4 weeks. The average number of attacks per 4 weeks fell from an average of 12.0 during the run-in period to 6.1 during the acupuncture treatment and to 10.6 during the placebo period. On exercise testing, performance before the onset of pain improved with acupuncture, but not maximal performance. There was a reduction in the mean chest pain score at maximal performance, and ST-segment depression was significantly reduced. Heart rate and BP did not alter.

Ballegaard et al (1986) randomized 28 stable but severe and drug-resistant angina sufferers to receive either 10 genuine treatments at PC-6, ST-36 and BL-14, or 10 sessions of needling of non-acupuncture points within the same segments over the course of 3 weeks. Neither group showed significant changes in the primary outcome measures (i.e. the number of attacks, use of glyceryl trinitrate and exercise tolerance), although there was a significant increase in cardiac work capacity in the genuine treatment group. The study was repeated (Ballegaard et al 1990) with a sample of 49 patients with moderate stable angina. In this study, both active and sham groups showed a median 50% fall in glyceryl trinitrate consumption and angina attack rate, with no difference between groups. There were no significant changes in the exercise test variables in either group.

The lack of difference between the groups can be explained in one of two ways: either there are only non-specific (placebo) effects from both real and placebo treatments, or both interventions have a genuine effect but this is not point specific. In order to distinguish between these alternatives, the authors studied the skin temperature changes in 33 of the original 49 subjects, during and after a session of EA to LI-4 (Ballegaard, Meyer & Trojaborg 1991). Analysis of individual responses showed that the patients whose angina had been helped by acupuncture were significantly more likely to show a rise in skin temperature with acupuncture. Skin temperature changes were significantly correlated with the improvements in exercise tolerance, angina attack rate and nitroglycerine consumption in the earlier study. These results are compatible with the hypothesis that acupuncture reduces sympathetic tone, leading to coronary and skin vasodilatation, although they do not exclude the possibilities either that a vasodilator is released by acupuncture or that acupuncture relieves the pain and this in turn leads to reduced sympathetic tone.

The study was repeated in 43 subjects under rigorously controlled and blinded conditions

(Ballegaard et al 1995) with positive effects on exercise tolerance, cardiac work capacity and decreased glyceryl trinitrate consumption; in this last study expectation, personality and psychosocial factors were found not to be correlated with the response to acupuncture.

It is interesting to note that TENS has also been shown to increase the tolerance to angina induced by atrial pacing, significantly improve lactate metabolism and increase skin temperature (Mannheimer et al 1989). These effects were not reversed by i.v. naloxone.

In summary, there is some evidence that acupuncture has an effect on angina pectoris, at least in the short term, at a segmental level but the value of this in clinical practice is not yet known.

Myocardial infarction

Li et al (1986) randomized 32 patients with acute myocardial infarction to receive standard care plus acupuncture or standard care only. The acupuncture group were treated alternately with (1) CV-14 and Xinping, and (2) CV-17, PC-6 and SP-6. Needles were stimulated to achieve De Qi and then left for 20 minutes. Treatment was given daily for 24 sessions. Circulatory performance was assessed by measuring left ventricular function and stroke volume; the treatment group showed significant improvements. Small blood vessel diameter was assessed by fundoscopy, and again there were significant changes in the acupuncture group but not in the patients who received standard treatment. All changes were more prominent after 24 than after 12 treatments, suggesting that the effects of acupuncture were cumulative.

Arrhythmias

Several authors have commented that pulse and BP remain surprisingly stable during surgery under EA analgesia (e.g. Hollinger, Pongratz & Baum 1979, Kho et al 1991). Li (1985) provided experimental support for an antiarrhythmic effect of acupuncture by showing that EA to ST-36 or PC-6 in anaesthetized rabbits increased the threshold to cardiac arrhythmias that were

artificially induced by electrical stimulation of the hypothalamus through deep implanted electrodes. This effect was dependent on opioid transmitters.

Gao et al (1987) described a series of 54 patients with sinus bradycardia who had been unresponsive to previous medication. They received traditional acupuncture according to syndrome diagnosis together with lifestyle advice (to avoid cold, nicotine, alcohol, greasy foods and emotional disturbances, and to ensure sufficient sleep). Thirty-five subjects noted an improvement of symptoms and a rise in pulse rate to over 60 b.p.m., or by more than 20%. This study is worth repeating under more strictly controlled conditions to examine the acupuncture effects separately from the lifestyle changes.

Cardiomyopathy

Eight patients with stable chronic dilated myopathy were recruited for a study by Huang et al (1985). The subjects were given electroacupuncture to PC-6 on one occasion, and to a sham control point on a second occasion. There was reported to be a significant rise in both end-diastolic volume and stroke volume 1 hour after treatment to the genuine acupuncture point compared with that to the sham point.

Cardiovascular fitness in athletes

Yim (1987) described a study in which junior swimmers in the Japanese team preparing for the 1988 Olympic Games were divided into an experimental group ($n = 13$) and a no-treatment control group ($n = 5$). The experimental group were given daily acupuncture according to the Korean Su-Zi method of multiple needling of the hands. Training continued as normal for both groups, and fitness was assessed by bicycle ergometer. The maximum heart rate of the experimental group decreased, and there was also a 13% increase in maximum oxygen consumption, which was statistically significant. There were no changes in the control group. A test for fatigue after exercise showed no difference between the two groups. While the authors admit that no firm conclusions could be drawn about acupuncture in training of athletes, the study suggests this could be a fruitful area for research.

Peripheral vascular disease

Kaada (1982) reported that TENS at 2 Hz produced marked vasodilatation in six patients with Raynaud's phenomenon or diabetic poly-neuropathy. The TENS pads were applied at LI-4 and SI-3 in all cases including leg ischaemia. A rise in skin temperature was seen after about 20 minutes and lasted for 4–6 hours. Patients with a previous sympathectomy showed the best responses, somewhat surprisingly. High-frequency (100 Hz) TENS showed a similar but smaller effect. In the following year, the same author reported on the use of TENS in 10 cases of chronic ulcers of various causes in leg and sacrum (Kaada 1983). All 10 cases showed either complete healing or marked improvement, and selected photographs were presented.

The author discusses two possible mechan-isms of action, i.e. sympathetic inhibition and the release of a vasodilator substance. Sympa-thetic responses to TENS have been discussed above; Kaada (1982) found that vasodilatation was not reversible by naloxone, atropine, pro-pranolol or a variety of other chemical block-ades, and concluded that vasointestinal active peptide was a candidate for the mechanism. Lundeberg (1993) reviewed other research supporting the value of TENS in chronic diabetic ulcers, and concluded that 40–60 minutes of daily treatment 5–7 days weekly for 12 weeks was probably the minimum needed to produce a clinical response.

A randomized controlled trial of the effect of acupuncture in Raynaud's syndrome was undertaken by Moehrle et al (1995). Forty-one subjects suffering from primary and secondary Raynaud's syndrome were given weekly treat-ment for 8 weeks with either genuine or sham acupuncture. Symptoms were measured by patient diaries, and blood flow during cold stress was assessed by red blood cell velocity in the nailfold capillaries measured with Doppler flowmeter and capillaroscopy. Subjects with primary Raynaud's syndrome who received active treatment recorded significant reduction in the attack rate and increase in blood flow. There was a trend towards a positive effect in the secondary Raynaud's group, but there were no significant changes in any of the subjects who received sham treatment.

Indirect evidence of the effect of acupuncture in improving blood flow can be seen in improved rate of tissue healing. Jansen et al (1989) raised skin flaps in experimental animals and resutured them, giving different modes of acupuncture through two needles at the base of the flap. The flaps survived significantly better after EA (90%) than after manual acupuncture or in control animals (50%). The effects were strongest with daily treatment, and higher intensity was more important than whether the frequency was 2 Hz or 80 Hz. Lundeberg, Kjartansson & Samuelson (1988) applied TENS at 80 Hz to the base of the flap in 14 women who had undergone breast reconstructive surgery for mammary carcinoma. Capillary blood flow and flap survival rate were significantly improved in comparison with 10 controls who received sham TENS. On the other hand, Ekblom et al (1991) found a significantly higher incidence of 'dry socket' (a complication of wound healing) in patients undergoing dental extractions with manual acupuncture analgesia compared with standard anaesthetic.

CONCLUSION

In summary, there are several areas in which acupuncture's ability to reduce sympathetic tone may be of clinical value, for example in the management of angina and myocardial infarc-tion, during surgery and in delayed skin heal-ing. Its place in the management of chronic hypertension appears less certain, but further studies are certainly justified and likely to produce interesting results. Electroacupuncture or TENS may have a role in peripheral ischaemia. It seems clear that acupuncture should be used in support of conventional medical management and not as a substitute.

CENTRAL NERVOUS SYSTEM CONDITIONS

Acupuncture has been used for many conditions of the central nervous system, but largely empirically. Selected scientific and empirical data are now presented.

STROKE

Stroke is the most common cause of severe physical handicap in the adult population and about half the survivors are left with residual neurological impairment and physical disability (Johansson 1993). Yet, despite 'permanent' tissue damage, most surviving stroke patients improve with time. Much debate surrounds the effectiveness of rehabilitation programmes and, even though patients perform better on focused rehabilitation (Ottenbacher & Jannell 1993), there is a relative lack of positive impact on activities of daily living (ADL) (Wagenaar & Meijer 1991).

Johansson et al (1993) performed a randomized study on 78 patients with severe hemiparesis within 10 days of stroke onset. Forty patients in the control group received daily physiotherapy and occupational therapy and 38 had acupuncture in addition (termed sensory stimulation to get around any publication bias!) twice a week for 10 weeks. Motor function, balance and activities of daily living were assessed at baseline levels pretreatment and at 1 and 3 months after stroke onset. Quality of life was measured using the Nottingham Health Profile at 3, 6 and 12 months after the stroke. Patients given acupuncture recovered both faster and to a greater extent than did the control group and had significant differences in improvement of balance, mobility, activities of daily living, quality of life and admission times in hospital/nursing homes. The acupuncture points used were ST-40 and 36, GB-34, LI-4 and 11, TE-5, GV-20 and three extra points. In addition to manual stimulation, electroacupuncture at 2–5 Hz was given to four needles on the paralysed side. Although the study was randomized, the control group did not receive any placebo treatment and the possibility that patient expectation could influence the outcome has been suggested, but partly discounted in the light of previous studies on stroke rehabilitation. Depressed stroke victims are less likely to recover, and any enhancing effects of acupuncture on mental well-being should be considered, as well as its effects on blood flow (Johansson 1993). Furthermore, the mean rehabilitation costs of hospital and nursing home care were estimated at $30 000 US for the patients in the acupuncture group, compared with $56 000 US for a control patient. The impact of this on healthcare budgets could be considerable, although not all countries spend as much on rehabilitation as Sweden. Nevertheless, quality of life benefits cannot be costed. A further study by Magnusson, Johansson & Johansson (1994) on the survivors of this stroke trial on postural function, 2 years' postinjury, showed enhancement of postural function in the acupuncture group; significantly more patients maintained stance during perturbation than the control patients. Barbro Johansson's group has published further reports on brain plasticity (Johansson & Grabowski 1994) and environmental influences (Ohlsson & Johansson 1995), and are currently studying the effects of acupuncture and TENS on stroke patients. Their results are eagerly awaited.

A further randomized controlled study has been performed in the subacute stage of stroke in 45 patients by Sallstrom et al (1995). The median time from stroke onset to inclusion in the study was 40 days and all had hemiparesis following a first-ever stroke. All patients had individually adapted rehabilitation therapy and the 24 randomized to acupuncture had 20–30-minute classical acupuncture treatments three or four times per week for 6 weeks. Both groups improved significantly in motor function and activities of daily living but the improvement was significantly greater among the acupuncture group than in the controls. The acupuncture group additionally rated a significantly improved quality of life following treatment. They concluded that acupuncture gives added benefit to stroke patients' rehabilitation in the subacute phase. Further empirical data are now described.

Chen (1993a) reviewed the historical background and treatment of thousands of cerebrovascular accidents by body and scalp acupuncture and summarized ancient acupuncture prescriptions, especially using GV-20 and GB-20. A formidable attempt was made to promote traditional theory and practice; the text includes clear diagrams of relevant points and merits further study. Her second article (Chen 1993b) concentrated on scalp and eye (orbit) acupuncture and a third (Chen 1993c) outlined preventative methods. Zhao (1990), in a TCM description of treatment of acute cerebrovascular diseases, outlined a detailed group of points for treatment of contractures in various groups of muscles, emotional lability, drooling and chronic disease. Body needling, scalp acupuncture and auricular acupuncture points were described but no patient details were given.

Wei (1977) and Chiao (1977) gave earlier descriptions of scalp acupuncture for various neurological conditions. Yamamoto (1989) has developed a detailed system of scalp acupuncture for a wide variety of conditions including stroke, as has Lu (1991a). Yamamoto & Ishiko (1992) demonstrated that scalp needling improved strength of ankle dorsiflexion and weight-lifting capacity in a small group of patients with paralysed legs. Wang, Ye & Lin (1992) treated 20 patients with hemiplegia of mixed aetiology with scalp acupuncture at points in the region of GV-20 and 21. Fifteen were seen 3 months post onset of stroke. Improvement in muscle strength was experienced by them all and also improvement of other symptoms such as drooling and speech impairment. Ten were deemed 'cured', seven 'markedly improved' and three 'somewhat improved'. Five to 18 treatments were given on average, either daily or on alternate days. However, the contribution of Qigong, psychological influences and natural history were not assessed.

Du (1990) described a series of 200 cases of hemiplegia treated with stroke from 1 month to over 1 year post-insult. The TCM selection of points included GB-20, LI-11 and 4, ST-36, SP-6

and LR-3 bilaterally as principal points. End points were not clearly defined, but 48% were reported to have 'recovered', 20% improved markedly and 29% slightly improved.

Chen & Fang (1990) reported a retrospective analysis of 108 cases of patients with hemiplegia. The degree of paralysis had been graded pretreatment and 24 half-hour acupuncture treatments were given in 1 month to scalp and body points. Scalp points were chosen using Western knowledge on the contralateral side to the paralysis over motor and sensory areas. Larger or multiple loci and multisystem problems or complications such as pneumonia gave unfavourable prognostic indices. Treatment within the first 3 weeks postcerebrovascular accident was statistically superior to treatment more than 3 weeks after the event. Chen raised the interesting question about the puzzle of why lesions of a similar size and aetiology respond differently to acupuncture. He used CT scanning to locate the pathological area and in a similar publication (Fang, Chen & Zhang 1990) reported again on much of the original work.

Qi et al (1990) performed a non-randomized study on 322 cases of cerebral infarction and scored their pretreatment condition out of 100 points based on mental state, speech, cranial nerve function, motor power, sensation and locomotor ability. Scores above 80 were considered mild, 40–79 as moderate damage and 9–40 as severe. 215 were treated within the first month. The four treatment groups were acupuncture alone, acupuncture plus herbal medicine, acupuncture plus i.v. infusion, and acupuncture point injection with root extracts. Up to 36 daily treatments were given and the collective results showed no difference between groups. 48.1% had post-treatment scores above 90 points and 94% showed improvement to a degree that was 'good' or 'fair'. The main points used were GV-20, EX-4, LI-15, TE-5, ST-36 and GB-39, plus or minus GB-20, EX-6, LI-11 and 14, GB-30 and 34, ST-41, LR-3, KI-23, HT-5, ST-2, 4 and 6, depending on the TCM diagnosis. They concluded that acupuncture played a major role in regulating general function and restoring paralysed extremities.

Zhang (1989), described acupuncture treatment for poststroke aphasia, which is notoriously refractory to conventional treatment. One hundred and fifty patients were randomly divided into two groups; 75 had acupuncture and 75 had vasodilators and other symptomatic treatment but details of the drugs were not specified. Vigorous needling deep in the tongue was employed on the side of paralysis in the acupuncture group and 24 treatments were given as a maximum. Although a rather unpleasant-sounding treatment, results were apparently significantly superior in the acupuncture group.

Batlivala (1986) reported a dramatic recovery in a case report of a patient with pseudobulbar palsy treated with EA.

Wong (1988) recommended a series of acupuncture points based not on any meridian theory, but on a functional and detailed Western anatomical point of view that was slightly reminiscent of Chan Gunn's strongly anatomical approach. He successfully treated 30 patients with EA for stroke, polio or paralysis below T12. His charming final sentence that 'we should let a hundred flowers blossom and a hundred schools of thought contend, but in a scientific manner' should encourage us all in further prospective study of these conditions. High- and low-frequency TENS was tried on 15 patients with central poststroke pain and three patients benefitted with ipsilateral high- and low-frequency TENS. Long-term analgesia was also obtained in three patients 23–30 months later (Leijon & Boivie 1989).

HEADACHE

Acupuncture for headache of mixed aetiology, musculoskeletal, tension, migraine and facial neuralgia, is frequently successful and the reader is referred to Chapter 16 for details and results of controlled clinical trials.

CEREBRAL PALSY

No controlled studies of this condition were found. One series of 117 children with mixed aetiology were treated with 'hydroacupuncture therapy' or point injection of various solutions and herbs at three groups of points: (1) GV-15 and BL-23, (2) GB-20 and ST-36 and (3) GV-14 and PC-6 (Shi, Bu & Lin 1992). As all points were injected and insufficient patient details were given, no meaningful conclusions can be drawn, from this study.

In another study, (Sanner & Sundequist 1981), four children aged 11–18 years with dystonic features and hyperkinetic cerebral palsy were reported to have been helped by direct needling to areas of muscle spasm, with long-lasting results even after a short course of treatment.

EPILEPSY

Lai & Lai (1991) described a part of the fascinating history of epilepsy in Chinese traditional medicine. Shi et al (1987) gave acupuncture to 98 patients with poorly controlled epilepsy on a variety of medication, with electroencephalogram (EEG) confirmation in 81 patients. Scalp acupuncture was used in the motor and sensory areas of the scalp and the 'psychic' area, which they describe as being anterior to the motor area. EA for 30 minutes was used at a frequency of 2.5–3 Hz for courses of 15 treatments. Sixty-six per cent had a marked reduction in the frequency of attacks and the worst responders had the least treatments.

A further communication by Petty (unpublished work, 1992) also confirmed a reduction in the number of seizures in a small series of patients who were given a course of acupuncture for drug-resistant epilepsy.

Auricular press needles were used in ear Shenmen points in a group of five epileptic dogs poorly controlled on medication. One animal did not respond, one showed a partial response and three were improved (Panzer & Chrisman 1994).

Chen & Huang (1984) studied the effect of acupuncture on electric shock-induced epilepsy on mice and cats with epilepsy that had been experimentally induced by intracortical or massive intravenous penicillin injections. In this series of experiments on focal and generalized epilepsy, acupuncture did not reduce epileptiform activity and, indeed, in some cases provoked it. Further work by Chen, Huang & How (1986) on rats or cats given intraperitoneal injections of penicillin showed a provoking effect of manual or electroacupuncture at the chosen points. However, in contrast, Wang, Yang & Cheng (1994) have shown an inhibitory effect of EA on microinjection of penicillin into the hippocampus and in the amygdala (Zhang, Yu & Zhang 1992), which was reversed by intraperitoneal microinjection of naloxone.

The most interesting experimental work to date comes from Professor Han's department in Beijing and is described by Oei et al (1992). Cholecystokinin (CCK-8), is a neuropeptide with potent anti-opioid activity. It also possesses anti-epileptic activity (Bajorek, Lee & Lomax 1986, Kadar et al 1984, Zetler 1980). Cholecystokinin is released by EA as well as endogenous opioids and the amount of analgesia obtained is dependent on the balance between the two in the central nervous system (Han, Ding & Fan 1986). Oei et al (1992) demonstrated in a series of elegant experiments that high-frequency EA is more likely to increase the release of CCK-8 in the CNS than is low-frequency EA. Also, rats bred with accoustically evoked epileptic seizures have a functional deficit of CCK-8 and demon-strate prolonged analgesia after EA at 100 Hz, which is similar to the effect in normal Wistar rats given EA at 100 Hz following an injection of a CCK-8 antagonist. This implies that in the treatment of epilepsy the frequency of the EA stimulation is of critical importance and that 100 Hz is more likely than other frequencies to increase CCK-8 with endogenous anti-epileptic activity. This could also go part of the way towards explaining the contradictory results of previous experiments. Further research on these topics is eagerly awaited.

Although not strictly acupuncture, it is interesting to note that chronic electrostimulation of the left vagus has been used in drug resistant epileptics for up to 2 years with no adverse effects on cardiac, gastrointestinal or neurological function (Tougas et al 1992b, Upton et al 1991). Acupuncture by more peripheral and less invasive vagal afferent stimulation may have a contributory effect.

SPINAL CORD INJURY

An established model of spinal cord injury was used in rats at T8 at open laminectomy using a standard-weight contusion device (Politis & Korchinski 1990). The animals were randomized at operation to acupuncture 15 minutes post-injury, acupuncture 24 hours postsurgery, or control animals with no acupuncture. Chosen points were manually and then electrically stimulated at GV-3 and between T2 and T3, BL-60 and BL-54 bilaterally. When assessed at 3 days, rats treated 15 minutes postcontusion showed combined behavioural improvement and morphological sparing caudal to the lesion compared with the 24-hour acupuncture and control groups. The post-traumatic cortisol rise was also reduced in the acupuncture-treated group 15 minutes post-trauma. These results point to the potential usefulness of acupuncture as an adjunctive treatment, but possibly only during the early stages following spinal cord injury.

MULTIPLE SCLEROSIS

Increased irritability and an exaggerated De Qi response was noted in a group of 28 patients with multiple sclerosis (Steinberger 1986); any claims of success are not based on clinical trials to date.

PSYCHOLOGICAL PROBLEMS

In TCM, the heart was considered to be the principal organ that governed mental activities. Indeed, cerebral function would be non-existent without an intact blood supply! The brain is not directly represented in the 12 paired organs and meridians, but the Governor Vessel meridian is the closest equivalent and overlies the brain and the spinal cord. Historically, patients with psychiatric illness were thought of as innocent and defenceless victims in the games and plays of whimsical and wrathful supernatural beings (Cheng 1970). Psychological problems can be broadly caused by endogenous or exogenous factors and in many cases overlap. Acupuncture is more likely to act on neurotransmitters than social circumstances, although any shift in neurotransmitters may conceivably lead a patient to change his or her circumstances. Acupuncture given to a patient with no interaction with the acupuncturist may alter biochemical function, but the contribution of patient's expectations on the outcome could be considerable. Remarkable skill is required therefore in devising clinical trial methodology in this area when the acupuncturist can bias the outcome, for example with empathy. On account of this, it is not so surprising perhaps that such a paucity of clinical papers are available for review in this section.

DEPRESSION

Three studies have been published between 1985 and 1994 from a group in the Institute of Mental Health in Beijing on acupuncture for depression. The first, by Luo, Jia & Zhan (1985), was a series of 47 patients with depression of mixed aetiology who were grouped 'at random' (but probably not formally randomized) into 27 who were treated by EA and 20 treated by amitriptyline. The acupuncture group were electrically stimulated at 80–90 Hz at GV-20 and EX-1 (Yintang) for 30 1-hour sessions over 5 weeks. The amitriptyline group took 100–200 mg per day for 5 weeks. Two psychiatrists assessed patients before and after the trial and the Hamilton depression-rating scale, 'clinical global impression scale' and the antidepressant side-effect rating scales were used. Both treatment groups obtained a statistically significant improvement in all parameters following treatment, with the additional benefit of reduced side-effects in the acupuncture group. Increased serotonin output and noradrenaline turnover were hypothesized to cause relief, as was the regulation and balance of Yin and Yang.

Lou et al (1990), in a further collaborative prospective randomized trial on 241 patients from nine provinces in China, compared EA with amitriptyline for depressive psychosis. Patients were recruited who were depressed or in the depressive phase of manic depression as judged by multiple ratings including the standardized assessment of patients with depressive disorders (SADD) and Hamilton depression-rating scale. One hundred and thirty-three patients had daily EA at GV-20 and Yintang (EX-1) for 6 weeks plus a placebo capsule, and 108 had amitriptyline at doses of 125–300 mg (average 161.4 mg). One hundred and forty-eight patients in total were followed up and both treatments significantly improved the depressive illnesses with no difference in long-term recurrence rates.

Yang (1994), in the third randomized study of 41 cases, treated 21 cases with amitriptyline and 20 cases with acupuncture at GV-12, 14 and 24, CV-14 and 17, GB-20 and PC-6, plus adjuvant points depending on the TCM diagnosis. GV-20 and 24 and GB-20 were electrically stimulated at 80–100 Hz and the rest manually, and six treatments per week were given for 6 weeks. The dose of amitriptyline worked up from 25 mg to between 150 and 300 mg for 6 weeks. As with the previous 2 studies, the results showed that both helped the patients significantly with no significant difference between groups. They also demonstrated that after 4 weeks the acupuncture group arrived at a stable state.

Han (1986) noted the impairment of functioning of monoamine neurotransmitters in the CNS as a major aetiological factor in the development of depression. He included an overview of extensive investigations performed over a decade in his own laboratory on acupuncture and EA stimulation that demonstrate accelerated synthesis and release of serotonin and noradrenaline in the CNS in experimental animals. He suggested a mechanism for how acupuncture could be effective in treatment of depression, based on the changes it could induce.

Faust (1991) described a simplified, very successful form of treatment based on two needles inserted at each base of the nail beds of the third, fourth and fifth digits bilaterally for treatment of reactive depression. He also recommended it to hasten recovery following operations, strokes, myocardial infarction, postpartum and in debilitated patients.

Tao (1993) measured HAD (Hospital Anxiety and Depression scales) in 68 cases with chronic conditions before and after 1 month of acupuncture treatment. All had anxiety, depression or both in the proportions of 11, 8 and 49 respectively pretreatment. Forty-two out of 60 anxiety scores and 45 out of 50 depression scores returned to normal. Lack of details about the chronic illnesses and the natural history of the conditions is, however, a major weakness of this simple study. Nevertheless, the authors recommended that the widespread use of acupuncture could lead to a decrease in psychoemotional problems in patients.

SEDATIVE EFFECT OF ACUPUNCTURE

Following Wen & Cheung's (1973) description of acupuncture for drug addicts to improve well-being, relaxation and alertness, an attempt was made to use it on eight patients from psychological medicine outpatients with anxiety by Lo & Chung (1979). Eight 20-minute treatments were given over 3 weeks by one psychiatrist to LI-4, PC-6 and ST-36. An independent psychiatrist assessed progress using a five-point scale for 10 parameters twice weekly for 3 weeks. Six patients showed moderate to good improvement and two had no benefit. The authors noted a similarity of response to benzodiazepine drugs in a further group of five patients. Faust (1991) described the use of CV-12 and 15, ST-36, LI-4, LR-3 and GV-20 for reactive anxiety, but cautioned against the use of GV-20 in patients suspected of also being depressed.

SCHIZOPHRENIA

Kane & Di Scipio (1979) conducted a 9-week study on three schizophrenics. The patients acted as their own controls with baseline measures of the Psychotic Reaction Profile before and after acupuncture, after washout, after pseudoacupuncture (acupuncture without De Qi in non-traditional points) and after a further no-treatment period. The entire study period was 9 weeks and observers were blinded to the sequence of active and 'inactive' treatment. Two of the patients responded positively to the true acupuncture treatment and negatively to the sham treatment and a third patient showed no significant response to treatment.

Shi & Tan (1986), in a traditional paper on 500 cases of schizophrenics classified into mania, depressive and paranoid groups, gave TCM prescriptions for each type and obtained 'cure' in 275 patients, no help in 58 patients and varying improvement in the rest. In a follow-up of 194 patients, 63 relapsed within 2 years. Patients with a history of less than 1 year showed a more favourable response, but even a 10-year history did not prevent nine patients from responding well. A further anecdotal paper was of 296 cases with hallucinations were treated with acupuncture, 292 of whom had schizophrenia (Zhang, 1988). The major points chosen were GV-19 and 20 plus various auxiliary points. Ten daily sessions with the needles retained between 1 and 3 hours resulted in a 70% 'cure' rate after 10–20 treatments.

MISCELLANEOUS CONDITIONS

Fifty patients with assorted psychosomatic conditions and an asymptomatic control group of 20 patients were given auriculotherapy for 4 weeks. Both groups improved in symptom rating testing, with significantly more pronounced improvement in the stress group than the controls (Romoli & Giommi 1993).

Chein & Zakaria (1974) hypothesized that the rise in L-5 hydroxytryptophan demonstrated in rabbits following acupuncture could be a good reason to use acupuncture in manic-depressive states.

CONCLUSION

Acupuncture has been described for depression, anxiety and schizophrenia with varying success. Very recent research has suggested that oxytocin may play a significant role in sedation. Clearly, the projects reviewed could be regarded as an 'appetizer' before further studies in this field.

GENITOURINARY PROBLEMS

Acupuncture has been used for a variety of

genitourinary problems, although studied most to date in irritative bladder symptoms. Selected empirical and clinical trial data are presented in this section.

RENAL COLIC

A prospective randomized controlled study was performed to compare the effect of acupuncture with that of intramuscular 'Avafortan' on renal colic with radiographic confirmation of stones (Lee et al 1992). Twenty-two patients were randomized to receive acupuncture at bilateral bladder points BL-21–25, and BL-45–47 plus two further bilateral segmental points and two extra points on the hand. Electrical stimulation at 3 Hz was added for the 15 patients who did not obtain analgesia within 1 minute of treatment. Sixteen patients were randomized to 5 ml injections of 'Avafortan' (camylofin, an antispasmodic, and noramidopyrine, an anti-inflammatory). The results showed that acupuncture was as effective at relieving renal colic as the drug, but had a significantly more rapid onset of analgesia and no side-effects. Neither treatment promoted stone passage in the 2-hour study period. The choice of drug was a little unusual for this study and is not widely recommended as the noramidopyrine component can cause agranulocytosis.

A further series of 408 cases of urinary calculi treated by auriculopressure was described by Chen (1991). One hundred and forty-eight patients had stones in the kidney, 162 in the ureter and 98 in the bladder; most were said to be refractory to medication and some to surgical and ultrasonic therapy. Grains of 'semen vacarriae' were placed with adhesive on Kidney, Endocrine, Bladder and Sympathetic otopoints plus auxiliary points in the ear. Treatment was by manual pressure by the patient for 20–30 minutes three times per day and patients were advised to drink liberal quantities of fluids. Two hundred and forty-eight patients' pain subsided after 5–30 minutes' auriculopressure and pain recurred in 16 on the same day. No attempt was made to differentiate between the results of the different sites of stones in stone expulsion data.

Acupuncture has been used successfully for severe pain of the postnephrectomy syndrome but it was given in combination with local anaesthetic (Dewar & El Rakshy 1993).

Uraemic pruritis has been treated by EA in eight patients using SP-6 and 10, ST-36 and LI-11 at 80–100 Hz for 20 minutes (Shapiro, Stockard & Schank 1988). All patients experienced partial or complete relief of itching and improvement in their skin condition. The effects were dramatic in several and the treatment warrants further study.

PROSTATITIS

Acupuncture has been used in two descriptive series of 102 and 350 cases of chronic prostatitis (Ge, Meng & Xu 1988, Ge & Meng 1991). In the first study, on 102 patients, BL-23 and 35 were stimulated daily or on alternate days for 10 treatments; 46% were reported 'cured' and 15.7% had no effect after one course of treatment. In their second study (which coincidentally includes the former study period) patients were divided into two groups; group A had acupuncture to CV-3 and 4, SP-6 and 9, and group B had it to BL-23 and 35. Only 13.4% of 60 patients in group A were 'cured' as opposed to 48.9% of 290 patients in group B. The proximity of group B points to the innervating pelvic plexus was postulated to enhance the neuroregulatory function, improve local blood supply and promote absorption of inflammation. This paper lends further support to a segmental approach to acupuncture.

Combined needle and laser therapy was tried on 122 cases of chronic prostatitis either using BL-30 and 32 as principal points plus a variety of others based on a traditional diagnosis, or including needling adjacent to the prostate, daily or on alternate days for 10 treatments in a course. Chen, Gao & Ling (1990). The addition of the laser stimulation to the needle therapy improved the 'cure' rates from 22 and 26% respectively to 40 and 48% respectively in the patient groups above.

INFERTILITY

One mixed descriptive series of 248 cases was described by Zhang (1987); 153 were impotent,

45 had non-ejaculation and 50 had abnormal or absent sperm. Treatment was given on alternate days for 20 treatments, which could be repeated up to four times. The main points chosen were BL-23 and 32, CV-4 and ST-30 and the following extra points added: ST-36 and KI-3, for impotence, SP-6 and 9 and LR-3 for non-ejaculation and ST-36, KI-3, LR-3, GV-4 and Jiaji (EX-21) for abnormal sperm. The results showed, with impotence, 27.5% cured with 31.4% failures, with non-ejaculation, 76% cured and 24% failures, and, with abnormal or absent sperms, 26% cured with 52% failure, but separate details for abnormal or absent sperm were not supplied.

A further 70 cases with non-ejaculation were treated using a traditional approach by Chen (1993). The principal points selected were CV-3 and 4, SP-6, BL-23, 32 and 65, GV-3, KI-3 and ST-28 for the first three to five treatments, with auxiliary points added subsequently. Ten treatments constituted one course; 65 were 'cured' after one course, with five failures. The authors' success rate is almost unbelievable, as was the further data that 90% of the spouses became pregnant within 3 months of treatment; they suggested that it was a functional disorder.

A paper by Fischl et al (1984) in Germany noted a statistically significant improvement in sperm quality in 28 subfertile males given 10 treatments over 3 weeks using points CV-3 and 6, GV-20, BL-31, ST-30 and 36, SP-6 and LR-8.

NOCTURNAL ENURESIS

Minni et al (1990) studied 22 children aged 5–12 years with enuresis who underwent urodynamic testing prior to acupuncture in which 20 showed bladder instability, but two did not. Three types of treatment were given: group A: SP-6 and 10 and CV-4, group B: SP-6 and 10, CV-4 and ST-44 (electrically stimulated) and group C: SP-6 and 10, CV-4, BL-23 and 28, KI-3 (plus electrical stimulation). The children were treated weekly for 8–10 weeks. Urodynamics were repeated at 30 minutes, 60 minutes and 24 hours after acupuncture. At 30 minutes postacupuncture, an increase in uninhibited bladder contractions was noted, but 1 hour postacupuncture there was a

considerable decrease and less again at the 24-hour testing. Bladder instability disappeared in four out of eight, four out of five, and three out of seven in the respective groups, with a further three, one and three also being improved out of 20 cases tested. Though the long-term results were not described and formal randomization was not applied, these preliminary urodynamic results are of interest.

Tuzuner et al (1989) gave electroacupuncture at between 125 Hz and 259 Hz in 10 daily sessions to 162 children with nocturnal enuresis. The needles were placed in CV-4, SP-6, ST-36, BL-23, 27 and 28 and stimulated for 20 minutes. Ten sessions were given plus fluid restriction 4 hours before bed. All of the 35 7–8 year olds were 'cured' after the first course of treatment. Thirty-eight out of 41 9–10 year olds, all of the 28 11–12 year olds, 27 out of 34 13–14 year olds and 14 out of 24 over 15 years of age were improved after one course of treatment. The term 'cure' was used only in the 7–8 year olds and no real definitions for 'improvement' were given.

Xu (1991) gave acupuncture to CV-3 and 6, LU-9 and SP-6 daily for 10 days for up to four or more courses of treatment, with 221 out of 302 children with enuresis being reported 'cured'. A further descriptive report of 135 cases under 25 years of age with enuresis who were given courses of treatment to 'Shuangxia', above the medial malleolus, gave a figure of 80 'cured' after 1 year and 111 in the short term (Song & Wang 1985). In another study, vigorous scalp acupuncture at GV-20 was used in 100 children with enuresis but only 59 accepted a course of this on account of the pain experienced. There was a 'cure' at 3 months in nine cases and marked improvement in 27 (Chen & Chen 1991).

GYNAECOLOGICAL UROLOGICAL PROBLEMS

Several trials have been performed on the use of acupuncture for irritative bladder problems (frequency, nocturia, urgency and urge incontinence) associated with detrusor instability. Many have been reviewed recently by Kelleher et al (1994). Pigne et al (1985) treated 16 women with detrusor instability using acupuncture at BL-23, 28, 64 and 65, SP-6 and 9 and CV-3. Cystometry revealed a significant improvement in the first desire to void, bladder capacity and bladder compliance. In addition, patients experienced a significant decrease in the frequency of micturition and improvement in urge incontinence following treatment.

Philp, Shah & Worth (1988) performed acupuncture on 20 patients with irritative bladder symptoms of frequency, nocturia, urgency and urge incontinence. Urodynamic testing was performed on all cases and frequency/volume charts were completed for 1 week prior to 10 to 12 weekly acupuncture treatments to BL-23, 28, GV-4 or CV-4 and 6 plus SP-6. Sixteen of the patients had idiopathic detrusor instability and three had sensory urgency. All patients had tried anticholinergic drugs prior to the study. Ten out of 13 patients with detrusor instability and clinical symptoms noted significant symptomatic improvement (77%). Of three patients with enuresis, one was cured for at least 9 months but the others were unchanged. None of the patients with sensory urgency improved. The cystometry results, however, did reflect the objective improvements in one case who was clinically depressed and failed to show symptomatic improvement.

Chang (1988) performed urodynamic testing before and after acupuncture in 52 women with irritative bladder symptoms of frequency, urgency and dysuria. They measured cystometry, anal sphincter electromyography, urethral pressure profilometry and uroflowmetry. Urodynamics were performed before, during and after acupuncture at SP-6 on 26 women and before and after acupuncture at ST-36 on a control group of 26 women. Acupuncture at both points increased cystometric bladder capacity and first sensation to void, but by slightly more in the SP-6 group. Only 14 out of the 52 patients had abnormal cystometry prior to treatment and six out of eight of these improved after SP-6 acupuncture, but only one out of six after ST-36 acupuncture. Subjectively, 22 (84.6%) women had improvement after SP-6 but only six (23.1%) after ST-36

stimulation. Further courses of treatment were required to maintain the beneficial effects in 12 patients in the SP-6 group.

Gibson, Pardey & Neville (1988) used low-power laser therapy on 28 women with detrusor instability with a 6-month to 10-year history. Urodynamics were performed before and 3 months after therapy to BL-23, 28, 64 and 65, SP-6 and 9, CV-2 and 3, which was given twice weekly for 5 weeks. Urgency, frequency and nocturia improved significantly, as did the first desire to void, bladder capacity, detrusor compliance and volume at detrusor instability. Fourteen (50%) of the women were cured and seven (25%) improved at 3 months follow-up, but at 6 months a total of 16 had relapsed and were successfully retreated.

Kelleher & Filshie (1994) compared acupuncture with conventional treatment using oxybutynin in a prospective randomized controlled trial of 39 women with idiopathic low compliance with urgency, urge incontinence, frequency and nocturia. All patients completed a detailed urinary symptom diary, a symptom visual analogue scale (VAS) and a urinary diary prior to videourodynamic investigations. All patients had a diagnosis of low compliance (a tonic detrusor pressure rise of > 15 cm H_2O for < 500 ml during cystometry). Minimal stimulation by acupuncture was given at SP-6, ST-36, CV-3 or 4, BL-23 and 28, plus two further lumbar paravertebral plus four sacral segmental points for possible autonomic effects. Six weekly treatments were given with minimal interaction between patient and acupuncturist; six weekly visits were also given to the oxybutynin group (5 mg b.d.). Symptoms of urgency and frequency were significantly improved by both treatments and nocturia was significantly improved by acupuncture. Greater benefit was found at the 6-week than at the 3-week assessment. Neither group showed improved urge incontinence. Both groups experienced increased first sensation to void and bladder capacity and reduced pressure rise on filling. There were no statistically significant subjective or objective differences between the treatments, but the side-effect profile was considerably better in the acupuncture group, with three women in the oxybutynin group withdrawing from the study owing to side-effects. At 3 months, eight out of 20 in the acupuncture group were symptom free and four had slight urgency but did not require treatment, while seven out of 19 were symptom free on oxybutynin. Thus, in the only comparative study with conventional treatment, acupuncture was found to be comparable in effectiveness but with significantly fewer side-effects. Mechanisms of action need further elucidation but enkephalinergic nerves have been demonstrated in smooth muscle strips by Alm et al (1981). Human detrusor muscle has been shown to be sensitive to methionine and leucine enkephalins *in vitro* by inhibiting evoked detrusor contractions (Klarskov 1987). This suggests a presynaptic inhibitory activity of enkephalins on the bladder. Opioid antagonism with naloxone enhances detrusor activity in cats (Roppolo, Booth & De Groot 1983), rats (Dray et al 1984) and humans (Murray 1983, Murray & Feneley 1982). This lends support to the endogenous opioid theory of acupuncture but it seems possible that normalization of autonomic factors by acupuncture could also contribute to the effects.

TENS to the back at S3 resulted in stabilization of cystometric assessment in 11 out of 24 patients, with reduction of daytime frequency and urgency and also improvement in urge incontinence in 13 patients (Webb & Powell 1992).

Perhaps acupuncture could become a first-line treatment rather than a last resort in patients with irritative bladder symptoms, though this will need further good quality clinical trials measuring endpoints both subjectively and objectively.

URINARY INCONTINENCE

Zhao (1987) described a traditional approach to treatment of patients with postmenopausal urinary incontinence using CV-3 and 4, BL-23 and 28 and SP-6 acupuncture, plus or minus GV-20, ST-36 and Ciliao (BL-32). Sadly, no patient details were provided.

Ellis, Briggs & Dowson (1990) used acupuncture on 20 geriatric patients with nocturia and incontinence. Eleven were given treatment to SP-6 bilaterally and ST-36, and nine were given mock TENS on the medial part of the ankle. Both groups were given daily treatments for 2 weeks. Nine in the acupuncture group showed reduced frequency after 2 weeks and one in the placebo group. These significant short-term results could have a significant cost-reducing potential. Ellis (1993) in a further similar study again showed a significant reduction in nocturia in the acupuncture group.

CONCLUSION

In the areas in which scientific method has been applied to acupuncture for urological problems, promising results have been found. Further study is strongly recommended.

RESPIRATORY DISEASES

ASTHMA

The prevalence of asthma and its morbidity are increasing in several countries at present and some anxiety has been expressed, by Barnes & Chung (1989) amongst others, as to whether current treatment is contributing to the increase in morbidity and mortality of the disease. Naturally an effective non-drug method of control becomes very appealing in this context. The international classification of asthma identifies several sub-groups according to strict criteria (World Health Organization 1995). A stepwise approach to medication is recommended and some asthma remains particularly difficult to treat (Chung 1994).

There is often a discrepancy between the subjective and objective measurements of airways obstruction as shown by Rubinfield & Pain (1976). In this study, 15% of patients studied with methacholine-induced asthma were unable to sense marked airways obstruction, thus emphasizing the need for objective measurements of lung function in the management of asthma. Finally, the placebo effect in asthmatics can be very powerful, as illustrated by Butler & Steptoe (1986) who induced asthma with a sham bronchoconstrictor and then demonstrated prevention of it by pretreatment with a placebo that had been described as a powerful new drug!

These facts lead to extremely difficult dilemmas when devising suitable protocols for acupuncture studies to treat asthmatics.

Scientific approach

Several workers have reviewed evidence for the effects of acupuncture on asthma patients, notably Aldridge & Pietroni (1987), Jobst (1995), Kleijnen, ter Riet & Knipschild (1991), Lane & Lane (1991), Vincent & Richardson (1987). Selected aspects of the more recent reviews will be summarized and discussed.

The meta-analysis by Kleijnen, ter Riet & Knipschild (1991), a group of Dutch epidemiologists, was critical but revealing. Using extensive library search facilities from orthodox and complementary medicine sources, they found 13 controlled trials of acupuncture using the key words acupuncture, clinical trials, asthma and therapy. They included only studies in which needles were used (not TENS or laser therapy) and a reference group was included– some form of 'sham acupuncture'. They outlined the importance of obtaining uniform criteria for patients entering studies, including type of asthma, its severity, current treatment details and objective studies of lung function e.g. FEV1 (forced expiratory volume in 1 second), FVC (forced vital capacity) and peak expiratory flow rate.

They scored methodological criteria, the adequacy of intervention and the adequacy of measurement of effects. A summary of their findings is shown in Table 14.1. The overall quality of each study was scored out of 100, points being awarded for each of the 18 criteria studied (shown in brackets in the table). There was wide variation in the total marks from 16 to 72. Only 8 out of 13 had marks above 50 and the overall quality of the papers was described as mediocre. It is definitely far easier to criticize a study than to complete a good one! Only 8 of the

eight papers that scored above 50 demonstrated a positive effect of acupuncture over sham points and five out of five of the low-scoring papers demonstrated positive results. As the groups were heterogeneous, the authors chose not to pool the results, stating that it made no sense to pool data from good research with data from bad research. They acknowledged the fact that sham acupuncture could be an active placebo. They then qualified this with the assumption that, according to acupuncture theory, therapeutic results are produced only by needle insertions at very specific point locations. This theory has been challenged by Mann (1992) amongst others and lies at the crux of the dilemma of clinician's choice of placebo. This issue is described in greater detail in Jobst's later review (1995). The problem remains as to the choice of a needleless placebo, which is also a credible alternative to acupuncture using a needle.

Kleijnan, ter Riet & Knipschild (1991) concluded that the data were contradictory and that claims that acupuncture was effective were not based on the results of well-performed clinical trials. It is of interest to note that none of the reviewers was an acupuncturist, which may or may not remove bias!

What do we learn from this? Well, unfortunately, the results give more guidance for prospective research workers than for clinical and potential acupuncturists! It is necessary to examine details of these studies in greater depth to try and begin to unravel any useful clinical facts. The authors recommended future experts to study homogeneous populations of patients, larger numbers of patients, longer follow-up periods with more attention to assessment of subjective symptoms, and use of medication and better presentation of the data. This is sound advice.

Scientific curiosity and consumer demand led to the review by Lane & Lane (1991) on acupuncture treatments for asthma. Several other complementary treatments were reviewed. Acupuncture is rarely used as a complete alternative to conventional treatment but more often as an adjunct in both East and the West. Methodological

Table 14.1 Criteria used to assess the trials of acupuncture in asthma reviewed, with scores assigned (maximum possible score 100)*

Criteria	Berger & Nolte 1975	Takishima et al 1982	Virsik et al 1980	Luu et al 1985	Yu & Lee 1976	Christensen et al 1984	Chow et al 1983	Tandon & Soh 1989	Jobst et al 1986	Dias Subramaniam & Lionel 1982	Tashkin et al 1977	Fung, Chow & So 1986	Tashkin et al 1985
Methodological criteria													
Adequate study population													
Homogeneity† (3)	—	—	—	—	—	—	3	3	2	—	—	3	3
Prestratification‡ (3)	—	—	—	—	—	—	—	—	3	—	—	—	—
Random allocation (12)	—	—	—	12	—	12	12	12	12	12	12	12	12
Similarity in relevant respects at baseline (2)	—	1	1	1	2	2	2	—	2	2	—	2	2
At least 50 patients/group (10)	—	—	—	—	—	—	—	—	—	—	—	—	—
No more than 20% lost to follow-up (5)	5	3	5	5	5	5	5	5	5	5	5	5	5
Adequate intervention													
Diffuse noxious inhibitory control avoided§ (2)	—	—	—	—	—	—	—	—	—	—	—	—	—
Acupuncture procedure adequately described‖ (10)	5	10	10	10	10	10	10	10	—	5	10	10	10
Good quality of acupuncture mentioned** (15)	—	—	—	—	8	—	—	5	15	15	15	15	15
Existing treatment modality used in control group†† (3)	—	—	—	—	—	—	—	—	—	—	3	—	—
Adequate measurement of effects													
Patients blinded (10)	5	10	5	—	10	10	10	10	5	5	10	10	10
Evaluator blinded (5)	—	—	—	5	—	5	—	5	5	5	5	—	5
Follow-up after treatment at least 3 months‡‡ (5)	—	—	—	—	—	—	—	—	—	—	—	—	—
Subjective symptoms and frequency of attacks recorded (3)	—	1	—	—	3	3	—	—	3	3	—	—	3
Use of medication noted (2)	—	—	—	—	—	2	—	—	—	2	—	—	2

Table 14.1 (Cont'd)

Criteria	Berger & Nolte 1975	Takishima et al 1982	Virsik et al 1980	Luu et al 1985	Yu & Lee 1976	Christensen et al 1984	Chow et al 1983	Tandon & Soh 1989	Jobst et al 1986	Dias Subra-maniam & Lionel 1982	Tashkin et al 1977	Fung, Chow & So 1986	Tashkin et al 1985
Lung function values given (3)	1	1	3	3	3	2	3	3	3	2	3	3	3
Side-effects mentioned (2)	—	—	2	—	2	—	2	2	—	—	1	2	3
Reader able to do inferential statistics (5)	—	—	5	—	—	—	5	—	5	5	—	5	5
Type of asthma	—	Inf/mix	Mod	Mod	—	St	Ex, atopic	Mod/ sev, atopic	Br	Ch	Mild/ mod	Mild/ mod	Mod/ sev
Control treatment	Irr	Plac	Plac	Plac	Plac	Plac	Irr	Irr	Plac	Irr	Plac	Irr	Plac
Score	16	26	31	36	43	51	52	55	60	61	64	67	72
Outcome of trial	Pos	Pos	Pos	Pos	Pos	Neg	Neg	Neg	Pos	Neg	Pos	Pos	Neg

*Half of the maximum score (rounded up) for any criterion was given if the reviewers agreed that the report was not clear on the particular criterion or the criterion was only partly met.

†This criterion was scored with great caution because it requires considerable knowledge about which factors are prognostically relevant and opinions in this respect vary widely.

‡This was always scored if the authors mentioned it, irrespective of prognostic relevance.

§The phenomenon of extrasegmental counterirritation that could cause sham acupuncture procedures (not at acupoints) to be active placebos.

‖This was scored only if the acupoints used, the number of minutes per treatment, the interval between treatments, and total duration of treatment were mentioned.

**This is difficult but important to assess; if no positive results are found proponents of acupuncture might claim that treatment was administered by inexperienced or badly educated acupuncturists.

††Before a new treatment is implemented its efficacy must be compared with that of other existing treatments.

‡‡Defined as the time from the last treatment to the last measurement of effects.

Inf/mix = infectious or mixed; mod = moderate; st = stable; ex = exercise induced; br = breathlessness (patients had chronic obstructive pulmonary disease and only four had features of asthma); ch = chronic; sev = severe; irr = irrelevant acupuncture points; plac = placebo acupuncture points; pos = positive; neg = negative.

Reproduced from Kleijnen, ter Riet & Knipschild (1991) with permission.

difficulties are discussed, such as the impossibility of blinding the acupuncturist and choice of 'dead' placebo acupuncture points. The authors recommended that relevant methods of assessment should include objective measures of lung function, as recommended by Kleijnen, and daily diary cards. The diary cards should include use of relief medication and questions on quality of life. They reviewed eight of the controlled trials described by Kleijnen, ter Riet & Knipschild (1991) in some depth.

As far as clinical acupuncturists are concerned, the review by Jobst (1995) probably summarizes the trials in a more useful way, based on the type of asthma and choice of acupuncture points. Sixteen studies are summarized in Table 14.2. In his review Jobst has an introductory section on criteria for therapeutic efficacy and shows that acupuncture can be efficacious to the patient, with an acceptable side-effect profile, and can facilitate reduction of pharmacological medication. He attempts to view parallels and similarities between orthodox Western medicine and TCM, but also firmly warns that 'asthma may be fatal and abandoning orthodox Western medicine treatment may be dangerous since it controls asthma and chronic bronchitis very effectively'.

Jobst (1995) reviewed eight blinded studies (in which both patients and evaluators were blind to treatment): Christensen et al (1984), Dias, Subramanian & Lionel (1982), Fung, Chow & So (1986), Jobst et al (1986), Mitchell & Wells (1989), Tandon & Soh (1989) and Tashkin et al (1977, 1985). He also reviewed five single-blind studies in which only the patient was blind to the treatment protocol: Berger & Nolte (1975); Chow et al (1983); Takishima et al (1982); Virsik et al (1980), Yu & Lee (1976), and he listed three unblinded studies by Choudhury & Ffoulkes-Crabbe (1989), Sliwinski & Matusiewicz (1984), and Wen & Chau (1973). Acupuncture was effective in four out of eight of the double-blind, three out of five of the single-blind and three out of three of the unblinded studies (i.e. 10 out of 16 in all). The only trial in which acupuncture points were individually chosen was by Jobst et al (1986) and the others used either incorrect

points or sham points. He discussed the potential contribution of the non-specific effects of needling and made the valid comment that many studies were really comparing two different acupuncture treatments rather than one treatment against a placebo. He elegantly discussed some of the dilemmas, ethical and practical, that confound acupuncture trial methodology. The studies tabulated included acupuncture for acute asthma (Takishima et al 1982, Virsik et al 1980, Yu & Lee 1976), chronic asthma (Choudhury & Ffoulkes-Crabbe 1989, Christensen et al 1984, Dias, Subramaniam & Lionel 1982, Mitchell & Wells 1989, Tashkin et al 1985, Wen & Chau 1973), histamine-induced asthma (Tandon & Soh 1989, Yu & Lee 1976), methacholine-induced asthma (Tashkin et al 1977), exercise-induced asthma (Chow et al 1983, Fung, Chow & So 1986), and chronic disabling breathlessness (Jobst et al 1986). Regrettably, space does not permit the discussion of each clinical trial in detail, but sufficient facts are available in Table 14.2 to permit interested investigators to obtain the literature for themselves and give clinical practitioners some possible useful recipe points for specific conditions.

Jobst (1995) discussed the results in some detail and he also clearly identified the confounding variable in most of the studies—the choice of 'sham' points. Although sham points are supposed to be inactive, many were in fact active in pulmonary disease. He reappraised the studies accordingly and, when both real and sham points had unequivocally shown positive results in comparison with the baseline readings, he concluded that 14 out of 16 studies of acupuncture led to significant improvement. He highlighted the paucity of studies that described subjective improvement and quality of life issues as well as the low incidence of side-effects (7%) experienced by the 320 cases described in the 16 studies.

The review and its results contain much interesting material but the conclusions have been thought by some to be slightly over-generous in favour of acupuncture and traditional acupuncture in particular. Interested

Table 14.2 Acupuncture in pulmonary disease: studies reviewed

Study	Subject	Outcome	Design	No. patients	Acupuncture type	Problems
Christensen et al 1984 MEDC[n]: only at least 4 puffs β-2, never steroids or cromoglycate	Chronic bronchial asthma	Positive: both showed changes but Ac > sham DSA, WSA, PEFR, Puffs β-2, IgE all ↓ $P < 0.05 + P < 0.01$ Medc[n]: clear puffs β-2 Very interesting results	DB: S(NP) vs SA + Electro	17	SA formula 4 points: LI-4 × 2 EX-17 × 2 BI-13 × 2 CV-17	Blinding: only real acupuncture patients had electrostimulation, controls did not. Different needle depths for real + sham. Real worse than sham pre Rx. Incomplete data; no baseline values given
Dias, Subramaniam & Lionel 1982 MEDC[n]: ↓ β-2, franol, ephedrine. Steroids not mentioned; amounts not given	Chronic bronchial asthma	Pos/neg: Sham > Real $P < 0.01$; PEFR Subjective ↑ + both groups; (Medc[n]: ↓ in 13/20, ↑ 4/20, no change in 3/20)	DB: S(TP) vs SA	20	SA formula 3 points: EX-17 × 2 LU-7 × 2 CV-22	Breathing exercises included in some and not controlled for or described. Compliance Methods poorly reported: not repeatable Homogeneity poor (age, duration of Rx + symptoms etc). Stats: should have used non-parametric. Inconsistent number of Rx for the different patients. 'Sham' = active in TCM
Fung, Chow & So 1986 MEDC[n]: on β-2 p.o. + aerosol only. No steroids	Exercise-induced asthma	Positive: β2 > real > sham > none FEV_1, PEFR: $P < 0.01$ Rigorous study Excellent discussion	DB: S(TP) vs SA	19	SA formula 3 points RA: EX-17 × 2 LU-6 × 2 KI-3 × 2 S(TP): SI-14 × 2 PC-4 × 2 GB-39 × 2	'Sham' points can be used in used in TCM Rx. Demographic data missing. 1 × Rx only

Table 14.2 (Cont'd)

Study	Subject	Outcome	Design	No. patients	Acupuncture type	Problems
Jobst et al 1986 (see also Jobst 1987) MEDC[n]: all medication maintained but which medication given not listed	COPD: Chronic disabling breathlessness (COPD + some reversible airways disease)	Positive: Walking distance and subjective $P < 0.01$. Spirometry NS but trend to improvement + trend in blood gases Only study with true TCM Rigorous study Excellent discussion	DB: S(NP) vs TCM	26	TCM Individualized 2–12 points	Points not given
Mitchell, Wells 1989 MEDC[n]: β-2, p.o. aerosol, xanthines, cromoglycate, 6 on steroid aerosol	Chronic bronchial asthma	Pos/neg: both real and sham ↑ ie [SA + S(TP)] > baseline $P < 0.0003$ Real = sham = ↑ but no attacks in real Ac group, × 4 in sham PEFR ↑: $P < 0.0003$, ↓ medc[n] $P < 0.04$, ↓ symptoms $P < 0.04$, ↑ PEFR variation $P < 0.0005$ Very important study Rigorous	DB: (TP) vs SA	31 entered 2 withdrew	SA: formula 4 points SA: CV-17 EX-17 × 2 LR-3 × 2 BI-13 × 2	'Sham' points active in asthma. Homogeneity poor. Raw data for inferential statistics lacking. Some missing data. S(TP): SP-8 × 2, GB-37 × 2, KI-9 × 2
Tandon, Soh 1989 MEDC[n]: β-2, xanthines, cromoglycate, 15/16 on aerosol steroid	Histamine challenge	Negative: NS + No change in all indices ie FVC, FEV_1, histamine challenge, DCO = NS	DB: S(TP) vs SA crossover	16	SA formula 4 points: SA: CV-17 EX-17 × 2 LU-6 × 2 LU-7 × 2	Blinding: no response in either group is suspicious i.e. ?? blinding. Sham points 'active' according to TCM. Placement of EX-17 incorrect. Histamine challenge too soon post Rx. S(TP)-GB-24 × 2, ST-25 × 2, TE-5 × 2

Table 14.2 (*Cont'd*)

Study	Subject	Design	Outcome	No. patients	Acupuncture type	Problems
Tashkin et al 1977 MEDCⁿ: incomplete data; 3 on steroids	Methacholine-induced asthma	DB: S(NP) vs SA vs β-2 + x-over	Positive: Isopren > Ac > saline > sham. Objective: SGaw, Raw, Vt, FEV, 14% MMFR: all $P < 0.05$. No change autonomics: BP, heart rate, respiratory rate	12	SA formula 6 points: LI-4 × 2 EX-17 × 2 ST-36 × 2 LU-7 × 2 GV-14 *Waiting Chuan*	Wide age range. Wide range age of onset of symptoms. Statistics: should have used non-parametric methods. Inclusion/exclusion criteria not given. No stats on β-2 vs SA given. No De Qi at S(NP) sites.
Tashkin et al 1985 MEDCⁿ: steroids; β-2, xanthines, cromoglycate, 19 on oral steroids	Bronchial asthma	DB: S(NP) vs SA crossover	Negative: but trend in subjective, objective and *Meds* to improvement A rigorous study	25	SA formula 6 points: LI-4 × 2 ST-36 × 2 GV-14 LU-7 × 2 EX-17 × 2 *Waiting Chuan*	Blinding: no placebo response is improbable. Insufficient data on diary use. Stats: should also have analysed individual changes with non-parametric stats. Insufficient power
Berger, Nolte 1977 (MEDCⁿ: not given)	Asthma	SB: S(TP): vs SA	Positive: SGaw: 9/12 > 30% Subjective improvement significant in SA + S(TP) Changes last at least 2 h Data indicates should wait at least 10 min for spirometry	12	SA formula ? what 9 points: ? BL-13 BL-15 BL-17 EX-17 LU-1 CV-17	Blinding questionable. Inadequate information given. Raw data not given. No controls. Points used not given (inferred from diagram)
Chow et al 1983 MEDCⁿ: β-2, cromoglycate, steroids not mentioned	Exercise-induced asthma	SB: Ear S(TP) vs SA	Post/neg: NS diff between sham + real *but* both confer significant protection over baseline; >50% improvement in 1/3 points	16	SA Single ear point bilaterally	Data interpretation: both types of ear acupuncture confer protection. Specificity of points dubious. Needs further study. Sham points possibly better than 'real'
Takishima et al 1982 MEDCⁿ: not given	Acute asthma	SB: S(TP/NP) vs SA vs β-2	Positive: Rrs $P < 0.01$ and correlates with significant subjective improvement (20/26 Rx and 5/10 patients) very interesting objective changes	10	SA Single point: ST-10	Blinding dubious. Complex protocol. 'Sham' procedure active according to TCM. 1 × Rx only. Confuse patients with Rx in analysis

Table 14.2 (*Cont'd*)

Study	Subject	Outcome	Design	No. patients	Acupuncture type	Problems
Virsik et al 1980 MEDC[n]: not given	Bronchial asthma	Positive: Subjective: Ac > sham $P < 0.05$ Objective: SGaw, FEV_1, PEFR, RV, VC: all $P < 0.05$	SB: S(NP) vs SA	20	SA formula 6 points: LU-1 × 2 LU-7 × 2 BL-13 × 2 CV-17 LI-4 × 2 Ear × 2	Patients, methods, data insufficient for repeating or inferential stats. Stats: non-parametric should have been used. 1 × Rx only. Impressive results but very poorly reported
Yu & Lee 1976 MEDC[n]: incomplete data, 12 on steroids	Bronchial asthma: 20 pts Histamine challenge: 4 pts	Positive: Isopren > Ac > sham: FEV_1, FVC; $0.05 > P < 0.025$ BP ↓; $P > 0.05$ Heart rate ↑; $P < 0.05$ $PaCO_2$ ↓ $P < 0.05$ Histamine = NS	SB: S(TP + NP) vs SA vs β-2 agonist	20	SA formula 2 points: ST-36 × 1 EX-17 × 2	Blinding (improbable), 'sham' point often indicated for asthma in TCM. Large data overlap for 2 groups. Poor description of point selection. Positioning of needles dubious. 1 × Rx only
Choudhury & Ffoulkes Crabbe 1989 MEDC[n]: not detailed but steroids used	Bronchial asthma	Positive: Spirometry: FEV % 7/10 significant ↑, PEFR ↑ 14% in 9/10 Subjective: significant improvement Medc[n]: 8/10 stopped all Rx	Uncontrolled Unblinded Cohort EA	10	SA formula 7 points: GV-20 CV-17 CV-22 CV-12 LI-4 LI-11 BL-13	Open, non-blinded study. No controls. No statistics on lung function indices
Sliwinski, Matusiewicz 1984 MEDC[n]: steroids p.o. + im, mucolytics antibiotics, β-2, xanthines, sedatives	Chronic bronchitis 3 years Rx	Positive: ↓ Meds particularly steroids ↓: 63.8% stopped, steroids. Stop all drugs, 19.5% 16.7% ↓ steroids, 13.9% ↓ in dose > 60%. spirometry changes reported significant but no data given	Cohort	57 entered 36 completed	SA formula 9 points: GV-14 GV-9 EX-17 × 2 BL-17 × 2 TE-15 × 2 LI-4 × 2 GV-12 CV-17 BL-13 × 2	Uncontrolled evaluation. Raw data missing. No reasons for 15 drop-out given. Data not analysed on intention to Rx

Table 14.2 (Cont'd)

Study	Subject	Outcome	Design	No. patients	Acupuncture type	Problems
Wen & Chan 1973 $MEDC^n$: not clear; probably β-2 + steroids	Status asthmaticus	Positive: Spirometry: FEV_1 ↑ 45%, FVC ↑ 12.5%, FEV_1/FVC ↑ 30%, PEFR ↑ 49.7% Subjective: significant improvement within 4 h Attack rate: ↓ ≤ 50%, sleep: improved $Medc^n$: ↓ > 30% Excellent study Data + patient reports support TCM theory (e.g. warmth, energy etc.)	Uncontrolled ear points only EA	6	SA 2 ear points: Ear 'Lung' × 2	Unblinded. Would have benefitted from more analysis of data

Abbreviations: Beta-2, beta-2 sympathomimetic bronchodilators; BP, blood pressure; DSA, daily severity of asthma score; GH, growth hormone; GWB, general wellbeing; LAI, leukocyte adherence inhibition; $MEDC^n$, medication; MOD BORG, modified Borg score; NP, nonacupuncture point; NS, not statistically significant; O_2 Cost, oxygen cost score; RA, real acupuncture; Rx, treatment; S, sham acupuncture; SA, symptomatic acupuncture formula; SOB, shortness of breath score; $SUBJ^{VE}$, subjective symptoms/wellbeing; TP, true acupuncture point; UNB, unblinded; Vtg, thoracic volume at functional residual capacity; WSA, weekly severity of asthma score; × 1, one side only; × 2, both left and right sides; Rrs, respiratory resistance; DCO, carbon monoxide transfer; Bl, Bladder meridian; LI, Large intestine meridian; CV, conception vessel meridian; Ex, Extra meridian; GB, Gall bladder meridian; GV, Governor meridian; Ki, Kidney meridian; Li, Liver meridian; Lu, Lung meridian; PC, Pericardium or Heart constrictor meridian; SP, Spleen meridian; SI, Small intestine meridian; PEFR, Peak expiratory flow rate; FEV_1, forced expiratory volume in one second; subjve, subjective symptomatic improvement; RV, residual volume; VC, vital capacity; FVC, forced vital capacity; $PaCO_2$, arterial carbon dioxide pressure; SGaw, specific airway conductance; IgE, Immunoglobulin E level; MMFR, maximum mid expiratory flow rate; Raw, airway resistance; PaO_2, arterial oxygen pressure.
Reproduced from Jobst K A (1996) with permission.

readers should draw their own conclusions from all the available data.

Traditional approaches

Asthma or 'xiao/chuan' in TCM texts is apparently derived from 'xiao' meaning wheeze and 'chuan' meaning dyspnoea (Clavey 1993). Choudhury & Ffoulkes Crabbe (1989) discussed a combined approach for both improving immunity and treating precipitating features in 10 subjects by electrically stimulating the points GV-20, CV-12, 17 and 22, LI-4 and 11 and BL-13. Batra, Chari & Singh (1986) demonstrated that steroid reduction was possible in 10 out of 12 patients after treatment using LI-4, LU-7, ST-36, CV-22, BL-13, EX-17 and GV-14.

Traditional Chinese medical descriptions of 'turbid Phlegm secondary to Spleen weakness' or expressions like 'defeated Qi' can be rather lost on a modern medical mind. Sadly, descriptive series such as one written by He et al (1988) reviewing 60 cases are rather typical, in which the patients were classified as 'Cold, Hot or Intermediate'. Acupuncture was given using points GV-14, BL-12 and 13 plus moxibustion plus cupping therapy. The overall effective rate was concluded to be 93.3%. No attempt at classification of asthma was made and three forms of treatment were given together, making it impossible to know what contribution, if any, acupuncture made to the short-term effects.

Zang (1990) recommended needling of LU-6 and LU-10 directing the Qi towards the ipsilateral side of the chest. A further paper by Guorui (1987) gave a summary of the TCM approach to treatment of bronchial asthma. Unfortunately he concluded with a small section on skin pricking and injection of placental tissue fluid! After reading articles like the last two, it is not too surprising perhaps that even two of the best studies on acupuncture for asthma, by Jobst et al (1986) and Fung, Chow & So (1986), came in for some criticism by the late Peter Skrabanek (1987).

TENS

In an interesting study on 20 patients by Sovijarvi & Poppius (1977) the effect of a sequence of adaptation, dummy TENS, active TENS (50 Hz) and isoprenaline was studied by measuring peak flow. Eleven patients' peak flow rates increased significantly following placebo TENS and then did not improve further when true TENS was added. All patients showed an increase in peak expiratory flow rate after isoprenaline. The authors concluded that the bronchodilatory effect of TENS was psychogenic. However, they did not discuss the possibility that the mode of active stimulation may not have been optimal and if an inappropriate active mode was used one could not have expected further improvement. If all modes of stimulation were to be tested then conclusions would be interesting.

Laser therapy

Tandon, Soh & Wood (1991) carried out a double-blind placebo-controlled crossover study in patients with chronic asthma using points SP-6, ST-36, LU-9, LI-11, CV-17 and 22 and BL-13 plus ear points as active, and GB-34, LR-8 and 14, SI-3 and 6, BL-18 and 25 as placebo points with a washout period in between. They failed to show any significant difference between therapies in subjective and objective testing or in the need for additional medication.

Morton, Fazio & Miller (1993) gave 13 subjects laser therapy, placebo laser, salbutamol or no treatment in random order prior to an exercise test. The treatment was given to points CV-17, BL-13, GV-14, LU-7 and KI-3, at 1.5 mW for 20 seconds and patients were blinded to laser or placebo therapy. The authors concluded that the laser treatment showed no difference from placebo in all measures. However, they did not vary the mode of stimulus and therefore it remains to be tested whether different modes of stimulation would give the same results.

CANCER-RELATED BREATHLESSNESS

An open pilot study was conducted on 20 patients with breathlessness at rest that was directly attributable to primary or secondary malignancy

(Filshie et al 1996). Two upper sternal needles and LI-4 bilaterally were used. Outcome measures included respiratory rate, oxygen saturation, pulse rate, patient-rated VAS of breathlessness, anxiety and relaxation. Fourteen out of 20 reported marked symptomatic benefit from treatment and there was a statistically significant improvement in breathlessness scores, relaxation, anxiety and respiratory rate in the short term. The benefits compared favourably with current treatment and further evaluation of long-term effects is under way.

MECHANISMS OF ACTION

The mechanisms underlying the symptoms of breathlessness are complicated and ill understood. The use of naturally occurring opioid peptides in modulating ventilation is unclear and conflicting (Haddad et al 1983). Both δ- and μ-enkephalin agonists directly applied to the medulla depress tidal volume and CO_2 responsivity (Florez, Hurle & Mediavilla 1982). Much further basic scientific research is necessary in the areas of endogenous opioid, steroid, autonomic, sedative and immune effects of acupuncture in respiratory conditions.

CONCLUSION

As with acupuncture in many internal diseases, much of the data on acupuncture for asthma remain conflicting. The accessibility of the respiratory system for objective and subjective testing affords the opportunity for further study so that firm conclusions can be made.

EAR, NOSE AND THROAT PROBLEMS

In 1974 Mann reviewed his own clinical experience of acupuncture and ENT conditions. He maintained that acupuncture was of definite benefit in motion sickness, and of moderate benefit in rhinitis, recurrent tonsillitis and some cases of vertigo; it was useful in a small per-

centage of patients with tinnitus, but had nothing to offer for deafness. That review was remarkably perceptive and these clinical impressions have been largely supported by the (limited) research that has been performed since that time.

DEAFNESS

It should have been self-evident that acupuncture cannot hope to affect a structural problem such as sensorineural deafness. However, in the early 1970s a large number of deaf patients in the USA wasted their money in desperate hope of cure, and the reputation of acupuncture was seriously compromised. Rosen visited China in 1971 and discovered that acupuncture had recently been introduced in many centres as 'treatment' for deaf children (Rosen 1974). It may have been promoted under the banner of Communist achievements, but it seems that no proper evaluation was carried out. Some Western doctors were seduced by the enthusiastic confidence of the Chinese doctors and the enormous potential benefit of this simple therapy for a distressing condition. Reports soon circulated in the American press that acupuncture was being used for deafness, and quick profits were made in 'acupuncture centres' (editorial, JAMA 1974). Both this editorial and an article from Mann (1974), stressed how implausible acupuncture was as a treatment for deafness. It was a hard lesson for the West to learn, but a fundamental one: the fact that acupuncture is used in China for a particular condition does not necessarily mean that it is effective.

Carefully conducted trials, for example by Eisenburg, Taub & DiCarlo (1974), Madell (1975), Taub (1975) and Yarnell, Waylonis & Rink (1976), soon confirmed that acupuncture had absolutely no effect on sensorineural deafness. Any small subjective changes that some patients had reported were simply the result of desperate hope; minor variations in audiometric measurements that had been reported were due to either natural variation or the lack of skill among technicians (Liu et al 1982). The JAMA editorial (1974) reminded the medical profession of its duty to maintain a high standard of critical awareness to protect the public. It is therefore disconcerting that an article appeared in the Chinese literature as recently as 1993, still claiming that 'the treatment of deaf-mutism by acupuncture ... shows a total effective rate of 83.9–94%' (Jia 1993).

TINNITUS

Marks, Emery & Onisiphorou (1984) emphasized the similarities between tinnitus and chronic pain: both are maintained by feedback loops; afferent signals can be inhibited centrally, so that both may respond to counterirritation ('masking' in the case of tinnitus); lignocaine may produce an improvement that outlasts its anaesthetic effect; and there are certain similarities in the personalities of the sufferers of the two conditions.

However, it has not been possible to show that acupuncture is as effective in tinnitus as it is in chronic pain. One of the problems is that there is still no reliable way of measuring tinnitus objectively (Podoshin et al 1989). Hansen, Hansen & Bentzen (1982) performed a randomized controlled trial of acupuncture in unilateral tinnitus, using a crossover design. Eight patients received six sessions of genuine acupuncture over 3 weeks. All patients were treated with the basic points TE-17 and 21, GB-2 and TE-3; for continuous ringing unrelieved by pressure LR-2 was added, and for intermittent symptoms relieved by pressure KI-3 was added. Treatment was followed by a 3-week washout period, followed in turn by six sessions of sham acupuncture (i.e. subcutaneous needles to nearby non-acupuncture points). A second group received the same treatments but in the reverse order. Neither genuine nor placebo treatment had any significant effect on the daily tinnitus ratings recorded by patients.

Axelsson, Andersson & Gu (1994) reported a crossover study on 20 patients randomly selected from a large group with noise-induced tinnitus. Acupuncture was compared with mock TENS, and neither produced any changes in subjective assessment of the annoyance at, awareness of or loudness of the tinnitus. Many patients preferred the acupuncture, however, because of beneficial effects on their sleep pattern and muscle tension.

Marks, Emery & Onisophorou (1984) also used a double-blind crossover design, giving two treatments to LI-4 and 5, SI-4, 5 and 19, KI-6, PC-9, GB-11 and 12 and TE-1 together with the auricular point for vertigo. Patients received EA at 8/100 Hz. The control intervention was two sessions of sham needling. Fourteen patients received the treatments in one or other order, and their tinnitus was rated on a VAS. Five patients noticed an improvement after genuine but not placebo treatment. Mean VAS scores for the two groups were not significantly different, but the results do justify repeating the trial with larger numbers and more treatment sessions.

A four-arm study compared acupuncture with behaviour therapy and cinnarizine, and sham versions of each (Podoshin et al 1989). Subjects assessed the degree to which tinnitus interfered with their daily activities on a five-point scale. Three out of 10 of the acupuncture patients showed an improvement with acupuncture, and seven were unchanged; this result was not statistically significant. Genuine behaviour therapy was the most effective intervention in this study.

Thomas, Laurell & Lundeberg (1988) treated 12 chronic tinnitus sufferers with local and distal points according to traditional diagnosis. A series of 10 treatments was given, and EA was added from the fifth session onwards if there had been no response. Six subjects reported varying degrees of noise reduction during the course of treatment, but there was no long-term benefit. A case series such as this cannot exclude placebo effects. One patient was made temporarily worse.

Nilsson, Axelsson & De (1992) also conducted an uncontrolled study of acupuncture, using TE-3, 17, 19 and 21, GB-20, ST-36, LI-4, and KI-3. As many as a quarter of the 56 patients noticed a worsening of their tinnitus, and one patient withdrew for this reason. Twenty per cent of the subjects improved, and three patients still described themselves as 'better' at the follow-up 10 days later.

It is worth comparing this with the study by Kaada, Hognestad & Haustad (1989) in which low-frequency TENS given to the hand in the LI-4 region (as well as near the ear in some patients) reduced tinnitus in nine out of 20 cases. The nine responders continued using the TENS for the next 3 months, and six reported continuing relief.

Travell & Simons (1983) described unilateral tinnitus associated with myofascial trigger points in masseter muscle, without any impairment of hearing. Controlled trials of acupuncture in the treatment of this condition are awaited with interest.

The balance of this evidence is that acupuncture does not have a specific effect in treating tinnitus, although some people receive some temporary improvement. Trials have recruited only chronic sufferers who have already proved resistant to other forms of treatments and may have associated psychological disturbances. A certain proportion of sufferers feel they benefit from acupuncture, at least during the course of treatment; EA may be more effective than manual acupuncture. Acupuncture may have a supportive role in a therapeutic programme for tinnitus alongside cognitive and relaxation techniques, but it may be necessary to continue therapy in the long term for a sustained effect.

VERTIGO

Zhang, Luo & Bo (1991) reported 65 cases of vertigo of various origins that were treated with a single needle to the 'Vertigo' point above the ear. The needle was inserted into the subcutaneous space and vigorously rotated. One or two courses of 10 daily treatments were reported to have cured 40 of the 65 patients, but this conclusion needs to be verified in a prospective and controlled trial.

Some patients who complain of 'vertigo' turn out to have normal function of the vestibular apparatus and cerebellum. In some of these cases, the symptom may be caused by a reflex response to increased neck muscle tension.

Carlsson & Rosenhall (1990) showed that acupuncture to the neck muscles may relieve these cases (see Eye muscles, p 266).

In the absence of controlled trials we are left with clinical impressions: Mann (1974) suggested that older patients with mild vertigo may be helped, and this view is supported by Campbell (1987) who suggested that periosteal treatment of the cervical vertebrae may reduce the symptoms in moderate cases.

MOTION SICKNESS

Once it was recognized that acupuncture significantly reduced the nausea and vomiting of pregnancy, chemotherapy and general anaesthesia (Dundee & Macmillan, 1991), it was logical to see whether needling PC-6 had any effect on motion sickness since the symptoms are somewhat similar. Warwick-Evans, Masters & Redstone (1991) conducted a well-designed double-blind trial. Matched pairs of healthy volunteer students were treated with either acupressure at PC-6 with Sea Bands, or placebo acupressure with Sea Bands placed 5 cm higher than PC-6 and deactivated by removing the stud. Vertigo was assessed after the subjects had been rotated in a chair at eight rotations per minute while tilting their heads to either side in a standardized way. The acupressure had no effect on their symptoms and signs of motion sickness, although it should be pointed out that acupressure may not be an adequate stimulus.

On the other hand, Hu, Stern & Koch (1992) studied the effect of electrical stimulation across PC-6, delivered through metal plates on flexor and extensor surfaces of one wrist. Motion sickness was induced by sitting the subjects inside a standardized rotating optokinetic drum. Both the symptoms of motion sickness and measurements of gastric contraction were significantly reduced by electrical stimulation of PC-6 when compared with inactive placebo stimulation.

Hu et al (1995) repeated the above study with 64 undergraduate students who were randomized to four groups: they received either finger pressure on PC-6, or finger pressure on a dummy point, or light finger contact without

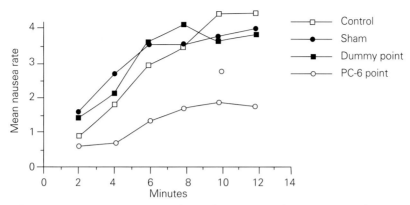

Figure 14.3 Mean nausea ratings for the four groups during drum rotation (From Hu et al 1995, with permission of the Aerospace Medical Association.)

pressure at PC-6 ('sham'), or no intervention. The finger pressure or contact was repeated at 1-minute intervals throughout the time the subject sat in an optokinetic drum (24 minutes). The mean nausea ratings are shown in Figure 14.3 and clearly indicate that PC-6 acupressure has a statistically significant effect. Simultaneous recordings of gastric activity and tachyarrhythmia support these findings.

MENIERE'S DISEASE

The WHO list of diseases for which acupuncture is commonly used includes Menière's disease (WHO 1980) but no controlled studies of the acupuncture treatment of Menière's were found in the Western literature. The clinical impression is that it is of little help. Xu & Shuhan (1987) reported the daily treatment of 75 patients with the points Yintang (EX-2), PC-6 and Anmian (situated between TE-17 and GB-20) together with the adjuvant points GB-20 and SI-19. The report states that 29 were 'cured' and another 25 'markedly improved'.

ALLERGIC RHINITIS

The WHO list also states that acupuncture is commonly used for acute rhinitis, and the clinical impression is that rhinitis is particularly likely to respond when the allergic component is prominent (i.e. in hayfever). The points most commonly used include LI-20 and Yintang locally, together with LI-4 distally. Points BL-2 or ST-2 may be added if allergic conjunctivitis is also present. Other points mentioned in the literature include the local points GV-14, 20 and 23, GB-20, BL-7 and the distal points LI-11, ST-36, 40, and LU-7. Campbell (1987) recommended periosteal pecking over the frontal or maxillary sinuses for chronic rhinitis. The rationale behind using acupuncture for this indication is that local needling may produce immediate reflex vasoconstriction, which reduces the rhinorrhoea and the symptoms of sneezing, blockage and irritation, and it is claimed that distal points may influence the immune system and thereby reduce the allergic response.

Bu & Nakano (1990) elegantly demonstrated the local reflex effect of needling LI-20, measuring the resistance to airflow through the nasal passages by means of a rhinomanometer. Ten hayfever sufferers were given acupuncture at different points and seven showed a 50% increase in nasal airflow after needling at LI-20 (Table 14.3). The results are impressive, although strictly speaking not statistically significant.

Clinical trials in rhinitis include an uncontrolled study by Lau, Wong & Slater (1975) in which 22 patients who suffered from perennial rhinitis were treated at eight acupuncture points bilaterally on six occasions; treatment was with

Table 14.3 Response of nasal airflow to acupuncture at different points

Acupuncture point	n =	Effective*	Ineffective*
LI-20	10	7	3
BL-2	10	1	9
Yintang (EX-2)	10	0	10
ST-2	10	0	10
LI-4	10	2	8
GV-23	10	0	10

*Effective = greater than 50% fall, ineffective = less than 50% fall in nasal airway resistance measured with rhinomanometer. (Data from Bu & Nakano 1990.)

either needles or ultrasound ('sonopuncture'). Symptoms such as congestion, nasal discharge, sneezing and itch were rated at each treatment; there were significant reductions in all symptoms ($P < 0.01$). Half the subjects became symptom free. These changes were accompanied by significant falls in the number of eosinophils and immunoglobulin E levels in blood and in nasal secretions. The timing of the treatment in relation to the allergy season was not stated and natural remission may have contributed to the changes. One-third of the patients recorded a recurrence of some of their symptoms at the 2-month follow-up.

Chari et al (1988) compared the effect of 21 sessions of acupuncture over 7 weeks to thrice-daily chlorpheniramine for the same duration. The points used were LI-4, LU-7, ST-3, Dingchuan (EX-19) and LI-20. The authors reported that there was improvement in both groups, which was significantly superior in the acupuncture group, but the actual data presented do not appear to bear this interpretation.

Lee (1976) argued that the plethora of points that were recommended for rhinitis could confuse the clinical picture and so used a simplified protocol with just LI-4 and LI-20. Deqi was obtained at LI-4 in all cases; LI-20 was needled to a depth of about 2 cm, obliquely upwards along the nasolabial fold; the needle in LI-20 was only manipulated if the patient had shown no improvement with previous treatment. The needles remained in situ for 30 minutes, and treatment was repeated three times a week for an average of seven sessions. Eleven out of 12

patients obtained total or great relief, but as the trial was uncontrolled a placebo response may have accounted for the changes.

Williamson (1994) conducted a pilot study of acupuncture in hayfever in which 31 subjects were randomized to receive either acupuncture to LR-3 on three occasions or standard medication. Subjects assessed their symptoms compared with their usual experience. Four of the 15 who received acupuncture, but none in the control group of 16, reported an excellent response. The mean overall symptom score was significantly lower in the acupuncture group than in the controls.

In the main study (Williamson et al 1996) 102 subjects were randomized to receive either genuine acupuncture to BL-2, LI-20 and 4, or sham acupuncture subcutaneously over the patella. Both interventions were given weekly for 3 or 4 weeks. The endpoints were symptom-rating scores, global rating and use of medication. In the 4-week period following the first treatment, remission of symptoms was reported by 39% of the active treatment group and 45% of the controls. A third of each group felt the treatment had had an excellent or very good effect. There was no significant difference between the two groups for any of the endpoints.

Luo (1992) treated 155 cases of allergic rhinitis by selecting two or three auricular points according to 'pathogenic factors'. When the points had been located with a battery point-locator, two small seeds (*Vaccaria segetalis*) were fixed and held in place with adhesive tape. Patients were instructed to press them for at least 3 minutes until they felt aching or distension, and to repeat this between three and five times daily. Sixty-seven were reported 'cured' and 59 'improved' but no more details were given.

CHRONIC SINUSITIS

Chinese literature has suggested that acupuncture can help chronic sinusitis, using local points over the affected sinus together with LI-4. In acute sinusitis, by contrast, needling over inflamed sinuses is contraindicated, and antibiotics should be prescribed (Outline of Chinese Acupuncture, 1975)

Pothman & Yeh (1982) treated a group of 18 patients aged between 4 and 42 years with acupuncture to GV-20, Yintang (EX-2), LI-20, SI-18 and LI-4. Control groups received either antibiotics or laser therapy. After an average of six sessions, symptoms were relieved for at least 3 months in 13 out of the 18 who received acupuncture (72%), seven of the 19 who had antibiotics (37%) and three of the eight who were treated with laser (37%). Acupuncture was thus significantly superior to the controls.

Lundeberg et al (1988) treated 16 patients suffering from chronic sinus pain with five sessions of deep needling with De Qi and five of superficial needling, the initial intervention being chosen at random. The points used were GB-14, BL-2, GV-23, SI-18, LI-20 and Yintang (EX-2). Assessment of pain was made by VAS pain score, verbal rating and continuous graphic rating. Deep needling produced pain relief in 10 subjects whereas only five were relieved after superficial needling.

FACIAL PAIN

There are several reports of uncontrolled studies of acupuncture for facial pain of various origins. For instance, Silva (1989) treated 42 patients suffering from trigeminal neuralgia with daily 20 Hz electroacupuncture to points in the appropriate area (contralateral if treatment to the affected area was too painful or caused a reaction). Thirty-six patients achieved complete relief.

Johansson et al (1991) randomly allocated 45 individuals with long-standing facial pain to three groups. Six treatments with deep needling of local points and LI-4 were compared with standard occlusal splint treatment and untreated controls. The subjects were assessed by a standard clinical dysfunction score. There was no difference between the two treatment groups, both of which were significantly better than no treatment.

Hansen & Hansen (1983) studied 16 patients who had complained of facial pain (mainly labelled as 'atypical facial pain') for more than a

Table 14.4   Mean index scores for facial pain over periods of 28 days

Order of interventions	Pre-treatment index*	Index* after first intervention	Index* after second intervention
Acupuncture/placebo	47.9	36.6	41.0
Placebo/acupuncture	54.9	53.3	50.2

*Index: 2 points per day if no change in pain; 1 point if improved, 3 points if worse. Improvement after acupuncture significantly greater than after placebo ($P < 0.05$, Wilcoxon test). (Data from Hansen & Hansen 1983.)

year, in a crossover trial. Points appropriate to the affected division of the trigeminal nerve were selected: in the case of the first division, GB-14, Taiyang (EX-5) and TE-5; for the second division ST-2 and 3 and LI-4; and for the third division ST-6, 7 and 45. Genuine treatment consisted of deep needling with De Qi, and sham needling was performed by superficial insertion a short distance away from the correct points. Treatments were given for daily for 10 days with a washout period of 4 weeks between courses. Intensity of facial pain was scored by subjects in comparison with their usual level. Table 14.4 shows that the reduction in pain scores after acupuncture was significantly greater than that after placebo.

Lundeberg et al (1988) compared the effects of different choice of points in the pain clinic report discussed above. Thirty subjects with secondary trigeminal neuralgia following dental extractions or facial trauma received three sessions with segmental stimulation to ST-2, 3, 5, 6 and 7, together with GB-14; three sessions with extra-segmental stimulation to LI-4, ST-36 and 44, TE-5, PC-6 and GB-34; and three sessions with a mixture including ST-3, 5 and 7, LI-4, ST-36 and 44. Treatments were given on the painful side only, in random order. Seventeen patients recorded pain relief after segmental needling, 10 after extrasegmental needling, and 15 after the combination.

THROAT PROBLEMS

Acupuncture is frequently recommended in Chinese texts (e.g. Jia 1993) for throat symptoms such as tonsillitis, pharyngitis, hoarseness and recurrent soreness, particularly in actors and teachers. No controlled studies have been found.

Yang (1990) treated 300 cases of voice disorder from a wide variety of causes, using local points ST-9 and 10, and a number of distal points including LI-4 and 11, LU-11, ST-36 and KI-3. The local points were needled using a 'sparrow-pecking' technique of rapid lift and thrust, after which the needle was advanced deeply 'until a sensation of stuck fishbone was produced'. The author reported 'cure' rates of 100% of acute cases and 58% of chronic cases.

XEROSTOMIA

An uncontrolled study by Goidenko, Pierminova & Sitiel (1985) reported that acupuncture treatment of 32 patients with Sjögren's syndrome reduced salivary flow rates.

Blom, Dawidson & Angmar-Mansson (1992) recruited 21 patients with severe xerostomia into a controlled trial studying acupuncture using points chosen by traditional Chinese principles. The control group received superficial needling 1–2 cm away from genuine points. Both groups received two courses of 12 treatments twice weekly. Salivary flow rates both resting and after paraffin stimulation were measured accurately by a standardized method at five time-points during treatment and for 12 months follow-up (a total of 10 measurements). There were significant increases in the salivary flow rates of the treated group at all time-points compared with baseline, and four subjects still had normal flow rates after 1 year. There was significant improvement in the control group's flow rates at only one time-point. Differences between the two groups were significant in six comparisons. These important findings certainly justify further research into the use of acupuncture for this distressing complaint.

CONCLUSION

In summary, the balance of evidence suggests that acupuncture may be effective in the treatment of chronic sinusitis, chronic facial pain from various causes, motion sickness and xerostomia. It appears to be helpful in treating dizziness associated with neck muscle tension. It is not certain whether acupuncture has a role as an adjunct in the management of tinnitus; the strong clinical impression that acupuncture is of benefit for hayfever is not supported by the existing evidence. Its place in managing Menière's disease does not seem to have been investigated, but there is conclusive evidence that it cannot alleviate sensorineural deafness.

EYE DISEASES

Techniques for the accurate diagnosis of chronic eye disease are now available but treatment for serious conditions has not advanced in parallel; desperate patients may be tempted to try acupuncture. Western physicians would be forgiven for thinking that ophthalmic disease is not a promising area for acupuncture. Infections of the eye are the commonest problem seen and need to be treated with antibiotics; chronic diseases that reduce visual acuity are mainly degenerative and irreversible. It may be surprising therefore to find in the WHO report (WHO 1980) that four eye conditions are frequently treated with acupuncture, viz. acute conjunctivitis, myopia, central retinitis and cataract (without complications). This section looks at the evidence for this rather hopeful statement. Conditions will be discussed in groups according to anatomical structure.

CONJUNCTIVA AND EYELIDS

Deng (1985) reported a series of patients with epidemic fulminating conjunctivitis with systemic upset who were admitted to hospital. In 60 cases, tender points on the ear-lobes were located, and treated with needling and blood letting. Chinese herbs were given to a control group of 30, and both groups received Chloromycetin. All the acupuncture-treated group had recovered after 1 week, but only 80% of the group that were treated with herbs.

Rogvi-Hansen et al (1991) used points for conjunctivitis (BL-1, ST-1, LI-4, ST-36 and LR-2) in their study of Graves' disease (see below). There was a trend towards improvement in conjunctival irritation in six out of eight of the treatment group, but in only two of nine untreated controls. It appears worth investigating the use of acupuncture for persistent conjunctival irritation or blepharitis but it would be negligent to omit the appropriate antibiotic if infection is present.

Five cases of habitual blepharospasm were treated by Story (1989) using local points (EA to the two Eyebrow points directly above centre of pupil in Frontalis muscle, TE-17 and 23, ST-1,2 and 7 and GB-1 and 2) and distal points (manual stimulation to LR-3, LU-7 and LI-4). One patient had an excellent response, two improved somewhat and two, who had a long history of the problem and had undergone surgery, failed to respond. It may be worth using acupuncture in the early stages of blepharospasm, but botulinum toxin is probably the treatment of choice in established cases.

Patients with a variety of periorbital symptoms including blepharospasm, migraine, trigeminal neuralgia and post-traumatic pain were included in a controlled trial (Sold-Darseff & Leydecker 1986, English abstract). Sixty-two subjects had classical acupuncture, and in the control group of 83 only the 'local nerve points' were stimulated. The proportions of patients who were completely free of symptoms after seven sessions were 34% and 38% respectively (no significant difference), but the inclusion of such a mixture of diseases prevents firm conclusions being drawn.

EYE MUSCLES

A feeling of distance or disorientation is quite common among people who are tense. They sometimes say they are 'dizzy', although no abnormality can be found on testing the function of the cerebellum or the vestibular apparatus. Macdonald (1992) described the successful treatment of such cases by needling points in the neck. It now seems clear that the

eye muscles can be affected by tension in neck muscles. Information from proprioceptors in the neck muscles can influence certain central pathways including the occipital and frontal cortices, the cerebellum and brainstem nuclei. The result is that the eyes move more jerkily than normally. This can be tested by measuring the 'smooth pursuit' (i.e. how closely the subject's gaze follows the movement of a light). Carlsson & Rosenhall (1990) studied 48 patients with tension headache, 28 of whom also complained of dizziness. The subjects received either acupuncture (to LI-4 and tender areas around GB-20 and 21), or intensive physiotherapy. Mean scores for smooth pursuit were below normal on entry to the trial, but significantly improved after treatment with acupuncture or physiotherapy. There was a clear association between the complaint of dizziness, the presence of tenderness in the trapezius muscles, and the intensity of headaches. In this trial, the intensive form of physiotherapy used was more effective than acupuncture in improving the smooth pursuit, muscle tenderness and headache severity.

Children in China are often instructed to do '1-minute acupressure exercises' to local points around the eye in an attempt to prevent squint, myopia and other sorts of eye ailments that they believe can be caused by close work (Dale 1988). Östberg, Horie & Feng (1992) discussed the use of similar exercises in factories in the USA and Japan, and conducted a small pilot study into the effects of acupressure on eyestrain. There appeared to be no benefit, but the authors admit that the tests used may not have been entirely appropriate.

ORBITAL CONTENTS

Wu, Jin & Zheng (1985) treated 40 cases of bilateral Graves' ophthalmopathy, who all had at least 18 mm of proptosis together with lid retraction and other eye signs, and had shown no response to treatment including immunosuppressives and local radiotherapy. The main points used were Tianzhu (just above BL-10) and GB-20. TB-23, BL-2 and GB-14 were added for lid retraction, and LIV-3 and EX-2 for conjunctivitis. All points were treated vigorously, and the upper eyelids were lightly percussed with a seven-star needle. Treatments were given every day to a total of 45. The main outcome measure was the degree of proptosis before and after treatment: 70% showed some reduction. In addition, lid retraction was present in 41 eyes before the acupuncture and was reduced in all but four cases. The trial is flawed for several reasons, particularly because the acupuncturist made the clinical measurements.

A controlled trial of the effect of acupuncture on Graves' ophthalmopathy was conducted by Rogvi-Hansen et al (1991); 17 patients who had been euthyroid for a year were treated 10 to 12 times with the points BL-1, ST-1, LI-4, ST-36 and LR-2. The endpoints were eye-muscle volume (estimated by CAT scan), Hertel measure, Hess chart, palpebral fissure and intraocular pressure. There was no difference between the groups in any of the parameters after treatment. However, points on only one side of the body were treated in each patient in order to use the untreated eye as a control. It could be argued that unilateral treatment is less than optimal, and this appears to be an example of the demands of orthodox rigour having unnecessarily compromised an important principle of acupuncture therapy.

MYOPIA

The WHO list of conditions for which acupuncture is commonly used includes myopia. Both French and Chinese writers report on the treatment of myopia in children. Ribaute (1987) treated 10 individuals aged between 6 and 14 years; two of the younger age group were stable for up to 2 years, as were two of the 13 year olds, although of course the natural history of myopia is to stabilize at puberty. Follow-up on the other cases was not sufficient to draw any conclusions. Li, Li & Chen (1993) treated 992 myopic eyes with between 10 and 30 sessions, using LI-4, LR-3, ST-5 and GB-37 bilaterally. All needles were stimulated to produce propagated sensation towards the eye. The trial was uncontrolled. The original report is in Chinese, and only an abstract is available in English. It suggests that objective measurements were made, for the results claimed: 'The vision of 868 eyes was improved . . . the vision completely recovered in 131 eyes and the diopter decreased –0.75 to –1.0 DS in 13 eyes'. Follow-up for 2 years showed that the effects remained stable. This work should be repeated in a controlled trial before firm conclusions can be made, but in any case the strength of treatment described in this study would be unacceptable to children in the West.

GLAUCOMA

Wu, Yue & Zhuang (1990) measured changes in the intraocular pressure during an experimental study of 23 patients (32 eyes) with glaucoma. All glaucoma drugs were stopped 3 days before the trial, which consisted of needling seven ear points. Intraocular pressure was measured during the following 120 minutes. There were statistically significant falls in the pressure during the first hour, and about three-quarters of the patients responded (Table 14.5). The changes were not clinically significant except in one individual who showed a drop of over 20 mmHg. The results at 120 minutes were not stated in the report, although no reason was given, and therefore there is some doubt about longer-term effects.

A detailed case history is given of successful treatment of acute glaucoma (Ralston 1977). The patient presented with acute onset of pain, complete clouding over of one eye and fixed pupillary dilatation of both. Treatment was first given to LI-4 and 11 for about 12 minutes, then fine needles were inserted into BL-2, GB-1 and 14 and ST-1 bilaterally for 15 minutes. The eyes

Table 14.5 Intraocular pressure (mmHg) in glaucoma eyes before and after auricular needling (Wu, Yue & Zhuang 1990)

$n =$	32	25	20
Before treatment	33.53	34.53	32.12
15 min after	28.58		
30 min after		29.84	
60 min after			27.27
P value	< 0.01	< 0.01	< 0.01

had recovered within 36 hours, and the pupillary response was normal and remained so for 8 weeks. The patient was a Chihuahua dog!

PERMANENT VISUAL LOSS

Wong & Ching (1980) performed a prospective case series of acupuncture for 546 patients with permanent visual loss who were attending an ophthalmology outpatients' department in Hong Kong. Diagnoses included retinitis pigmentosa, high myopia with retinal degeneration, optic atrophy, optic neuritis, macular degeneration, choroid retinitis, cataract, detached retina and glaucoma. All had already received every available orthodox therapy, and visual acuity had been constant for months or years. The author started treating these cases with a variety of points according to the diagnosis and the individual, but ended up with a standard procedure with just three needles, twice weekly: GB-14 and the retrobulbar points Hsianchingming and Chiuhou (Extra points just below the inner and outer canthus). The report includes the reassuring statement that 'there is no danger in eye acupuncture when performed by an ophthalmologist' and recommended that doctors who are intending to use this treatment should try it on themselves first so that they can experience De Qi in the eye!

The report gives details of acuity before the intervention, after 12 sessions, and at the end of treatment (which ranged from 12 to 108 sessions) in all 546 cases. Thus the original data can be scrutinized, but there was no statistical analysis. A number of individual records show sustained improvements of two lines on the Snellen chart, but this is probably within the normal margin of error of the test. There were no changes in fields or night vision. Subjects with macular degeneration responded less well than those with other diagnoses. The authors surmised that the major effect of treatment was on the macula itself, improving visual acuity. It is possible that acupuncture has a non-specific effect in optimizing the function of the whole visual pathway.

Dabov et al (1985) reported 50 cases with severe visual deficit resulting from similar diagnoses to those in Wong & Ching's (1980) report; the points used were EX-2, GB-14, LI-4, BL-2 and ST-1, with EA to the last two points. No data were given, but the authors concluded that acupuncture produced its best effect in retinitis pigmentosa. They disagreed with Wong & Ching in finding that the visual fields were enlarged and that there was an improvement in dark adaptation. There was no change in colour vision or night blindness, and the overall conclusion was that acupuncture's effect is modest, calling the results 'more hopeful in younger patients', and overall much less effective than acupuncture for pain control.

RETINITIS PIGMENTOSA

Tian (1991) treated 40 cases of retinitis pigmentosa with needles to EX-2, BL-1, GB-20, ST-36 and KI-3, and added moxibustion of the eye. In order to protect the eye from direct heat, walnuts were collected and carefully halved, sterilized and fixed into specially adapted spectacle frames so that they covered the eyes; the moxa cigar was mounted in a special holder attached to the front of the spectacles! Five out of 40 patients were reported to be 'markedly improved', defined as improved visual acuity with enlargement of the visual field, but no actual figures were given for the changes and therefore claims of success should be treated with caution.

DETACHED RETINA

An ophthalmologist from Pittsburgh, visiting Hang-Zhou in China, performed a prospective cohort study of acupuncture for newly diagnosed retinal detachment in 624 eyes (Lu & Friberg 1987). The diagnosis was made clinically. The standard treatment in Hang-Zhou was conservative, since fluorescein angiography and laser photocoagulation were unavailable. A single point was used, Xiang-yang (near LI-17) needled upwards and inwards until the patient feels De Qi spreading over the jaw and up into the orbit; the author suggests this might stimulate the cervical sympathetic plexus. Treatment courses of 10 days were repeated until the patient was improved; 86% had resolved within

3 months and five to six courses. However, this rate of improvement is the same as the spontaneous resolution rate in untreated cases in epidemiological studies.

OPTIC ATROPHY

Wei (1992) collected 12 papers describing the results of acupuncture treatment for a total of 2647 patients suffering from varying degrees of optic atrophy from different causes. The 'effective rate' was 68% but no data for diagnosis or changes in visual acuity were given, nor details of other treatment such as bed-rest. The 'best results' were obtained in young patients with trauma-induced atrophy of recent onset, which was more likely to resolve spontaneously. Reddy & Fouzdar (1983) from Hyderabad give visual acuity figures before and after treatment of optic atrophy with nine local (including two retrobulbar) and distal points; four out of 12 patients showed a modest improvement. Wu & Ye (1989) studied the treatment of optic atrophy with points GV-20, LI-4, ST-36, LR-3, BL-17 and 18 and EX-4. They claim excellent results after two series of 20 treatments, but the actual figures are extremely difficult to interpret as details and units of measurements are not given. These uncontrolled studies throw little light on whether acupuncture can really affect optic atrophy, which must be regarded as highly unlikely, considering the pathology.

An experimental study of the effects of acupuncture on visual evoked potentials was conducted by Poletti et al (1989). They recruited 12 subjects who had suffered embolism of the visual cortex or the deep visual pathways that had caused a homonymous hemianopia. The outcome measure consisted of cortical potentials evoked by an illuminated chequered pattern shone at the appropriate visual field. These potentials were depressed before treatment, compared with normal controls, but after needling around the eye at EX-1, BL-2, GB-1 and ST-2 there was a significant increase in the strength of the potentials on the same side as the embolus.

CONCLUSION

In summary, there is no firm evidence that acupuncture is indicated as primary therapy for any ophthalmic condition. It may help conjunctival irritation (though it is not a substitute for adequate antibiotic therapy) and it may alleviate the 'dizziness' caused by neck muscle tension. Further research is necessary before it is possible to say whether acupuncture has any effect on chronic visual problems. Retrobulbar needling should be performed only by those who have both a thorough knowledge of anatomy and considerable experience and skill in needling.

IMMUNE SYSTEM CONDITIONS

The Chinese described health as a balance of Yin and Yang, but nowadays clinicians are more familiar with the concept of homeostasis. Acupuncture was believed to create harmony by correcting an 'imbalance in the Yin and Yang', and it is tempting to see a parallel case in its ability to 'modulate the immune system' in either direction as necessary (e.g. Cui 1992). So it is claimed that acupuncture can both stimulate the immune mechanism (e.g. to help treat AIDS) (Chen et al 1992) and suppress the immune system (e.g. in the management of rhinitis, asthma or eczema). A sceptic would argue that this is a convenient way of explaining the contradictory findings in different studies!

As yet, there is no rigorous proof that the immune system responds to needling in different ways under different conditions. The immune system is highly complex, its components interdependent, and specialist knowledge is often required to interpret tests of immunological function. Furthermore, the available evidence consists mostly of piecemeal experiments on isolated parts of the immune system, often published in conference abstracts only. The subject has been reviewed by Bossy (1994), Cui (1992) and Nagano (1991), but these reports by enthusiasts are not systematic surveys of the literature that permit the reader to make an objective assessment of the quality of the evidence. It has to be said that the evidence for acupuncture's action on the immune system, although potentially so important, is both confused and unconvincing.

Bossy (1990) pointed out that the onset of a response to acupuncture is often delayed by 12 to 24 hours and lasts for 5 to 7 days. This time scale appears to be more like that of an immune response than that of neurotransmitter release. In this and a later paper (Bossy 1994), correlations between a modern understanding of acupuncture and the concepts of traditional Chinese acupuncture are pointed out.

PSYCHONEUROIMMUNOLOGY (PNI)

It is now clear that the immune system may be affected by behaviour and is interdependent with both the CNS and the endocrine system. One outstanding example of this link is the way a conditioned (Pavlovian) response can be induced in the immune system: for example, if a distinctly flavoured drink is given to an animal several times together with an immunosuppressant drug, subsequently the drink is able to suppress the immune system in the absence of the drug (Ader et al 1995). Evidence is accumulating that stressful events such as bereavement and depression affect the immune system, mainly the activity of natural killer (NK) cells but also of T lymphocytes (Herbert & Cohen 1993). The mechanisms for this effect include:

1. the release of opioid peptide from the anterior pituitary; most types of immune cell have receptors for a wide variety of peptide transmitters including opioid peptides, thyroid-stimulating hormone, growth hormone, substance P and VIP; β-endorphin has been shown specifically to enhance NK cell activity (McDaniel 1992)
2. the stimulation of lymphoid tissue by the sympathetic nervous system, whose fibres have been found in spleen, thymus and lymph nodes; adrenergic receptor blockade impairs the immune response.

The immune system in turn can influence the CNS by producing lymphokines as part of a feedback loop that regulates immune activity.

A summary of the immune system is presented in Table 14.6 to help identify the roles claimed for acupuncture, but it should be recognized that functions are frequently interdependent (such as the production of lymphokines by T helper lymphocytes, which stimulates the transformation of B lymphocytes into plasma cells). The most accurate tests for the state of the immune system are measurements of function. Changes in cell counts or levels of immunoglobulins are not an accurate measure of short-term responses, although they may be clinically relevant in monitoring changes over longer periods (e.g. in HIV). Examples of reliable in-vitro tests of immune function are the proliferation of lymphocytes in response to various stimulants, and the release of ^{51}chromium from labelled target cells by cytotoxic effect of NK cells.

Acupuncture appears to have the potential to modulate the immune system: it releases β-endorphin from the pituitary in association with ACTH, and has been shown to modulate the sympathetic nervous system via the hypothalamus and at various other levels (see Ch 6). These possibilities are exciting but we should remember that non-specific effects of the acupuncture consultation, including empathy, touch, listening and relaxation, are themselves likely to have marked effects on the immune system.

The theoretical basis of action via endorphin release and autonomic activity suggests a logical approach to point selection (Bossy 1994) in three ways: (1) points around the affected organ, (2) points at the segmental level of the spleen (i.e. LR-13 and BL-18–20), (3) general points that are most likely to have a powerful effect on opioid release, such as LI-4 and ST-36 and possibly the auricular points. GV-14 also appears frequently in formulae for immune activity, although the logic is not clear.

In practice, the points that have been described as having a particularly strong effect on the immune system include LI-4 and 11, ST-25 and 36, BL-18 and 23, GV-14 and 16, and CV-4, 6, 8

Table 14.6 Summary of immune mechanisms and relevant acupuncture studies

Cell	Subdivision/ derivative	Functions	Tests of function	Acupuncture effect	Acupuncture no effect
A. Non-specific immune mechanisms					
Monocyte Leukocyte	Macrophage Eosinophil Neutrophil	Allergic response Phagocytosis	Phagocytic activity Migration phagocytic activity	Sin (1983) Sliwinsky & Kulej (1989) Zhou et al (1988)	Kho et al (1991b)
	Basophil	Immediate allergy, anaphylaxis			
B. Specific immune mechanisms					
a) Humoral B lymphocyte	> Plasma cell	IgG also IgA, D, E, M; bacteria and toxins	Antigen–antibody reaction	Iliev, Popov & Nicolov (1995) Yang et al (1989)	Iliev, Nicolov & Todorova (1990) Kho et al (1991b) Liu, Sun & Xiao (1993)
b) cell-mediated T lymphocyte	T helper	Tumours, viral and fungal infections, delayed-type hypersensitivity (DTH) and PNI	Lymphocyte: proliferation, transformation E-rosetting, plaque formation, DTH	Bianchi et al (1991) Ding, Roath & Lewith (1983) Fujiwara et al (1991) Kasahara et al (1992, 1993) Lundeberg, Eriksson & Theodorsson (1991) Ouyang (1992) Sakic et al (1989) Tohya et al (1989) Wu, Chai & Wang (1985) Xia et al (1986) Zhao & Liu (1988a,b)	Ding, Roath & Lewith (1983) Liu, Sun & Xiao (1993)
	T suppressor	Regulation of immune system			
	Cytotoxic T NK cell	Target Ag-cells Tumour and virus-affected cells, PNI	Cytotoxic activity		Liu (1993)

and 10. Moxibustion is regularly part of a traditional prescription.

STUDIES OF ACUPUNCTURE AND IMMUNITY

Non-specific immune mechanisms

Sliwinski & Kulej (1989) treated 36 patients who suffered severe chronic bronchitis and had been taking either oral or injectable corticosteroids for up to 24 years; leukocyte migration was impaired as a result of the combination of the disease and the steroids. They received formula acupuncture at various chest and back points together with LI-4. Needle insertions were deep, 3.5 to 4 cm in the spinal and paraspinal points, but no additional stimulation was given. The steroids were stopped when the trial began, but in some cases they had to be reintroduced briefly. The results clearly showed that the leukocyte migration returned towards normal in most patients during the course of 42 treatments. No details of the clinical condition of the patients were given, either short or long term, but the authors concluded that the results warrant further studies.

Simple cell counts and immunoglobulin levels have been reported by several authors, although the limitations of these measurements in assessing the immune status have been noted above. Kho et al (1991a) used acupuncture analgesia with low-dose fentanyl in 12 patients undergoing major abdominal surgery; a further 12 patients served as a control group receiving standard-dose fentanyl anaesthesia. Acupuncture did not protect the patients from the usual fall in white cell counts after major surgery; the changes were no different from those of the control group. The author stated that he had previously found that classical acupuncture analgesia (without low-dose anaesthetic drug) in minor surgery did partially prevent this fall in the immune measurements. He surmised that an effect on the immune system might depend on continuing acupuncture stimulation after surgery and choosing points for immune rather than analgesic effects.

Zhou et al (1988) appeared to support this hypothesis with a controlled study of postoperative patients who received strong stimulation to ST-36 and either PC-6 or SP-6 (for surgery above or below the diaphragm respectively) daily for 3 days. There was a significant increase in the phagocytic activity of the neutrophils in the patients who were given acupuncture compared with the no-treatment controls.

Animal studies by Sin (1983) also appear to lend support to the ability of acupuncture or moxibustion to stimulate phagocytosis. Daily treatment to the upper spine increased the uptake of labelled carbon in the reticuloendothelial system of the liver and spleen.

Specific immune mechanisms

Humoral immunity

Iliev, Nicolov & Todorova (1990) found that EA produced no significant changes in immunoglobulin or complement levels among 34 patients with alopecia areata, although there were negative trends. A later study (Iliev, Popov & Nicolov 1995) with 35 patients with lichen ruber planus was reported to show a tendency to regulate immunoglobulin (IgG) and complement levels towards normal values in some subjects, but detailed data were not given and it is not possible to draw conclusions.

In an experimental study with 70 healthy human subjects, Yang et al (1989) measured immunoglobulin levels in serum and saliva before and after acupuncture. Their results appear to indicate that acupuncture regulated the level of salivary IgA in the short term by increasing levels that were low and reducing those that were raised. After repeating acupuncture daily for 14 days there was a significant rise in both IgA and IgG.

In the study already mentioned above, Kho et al (1991a) found that acupuncture given to patients undergoing surgery did not affect the usual postoperative fall in immunoglobulin levels.

Cell-mediated immunity

T lymphocytes The activity of lymphocytes can be measured by their rate of proliferation either spontaneously or when stimulated by incubation with a mitogen. Ding, Roath & Lewith (1983) measured various parameters of the immune system before and after 30 minutes' acupuncture at LI-4 and ST-36. The only consistent and significant change was an increase in spontaneous lymphocyte proliferation during the hours following the needling. One patient showed a reduction, but on further questioning it appeared that he was in the recovery stage of a virus infection.

Bianchi et al (1991) analysed the levels of opioid peptides within white cells and correlated them with immune activity. The levels of β-endorphin in the immune cells of patients with chronic low back pain were reduced before treatment; normal levels were restored after a course of seven treatments with acupuncture, although a single treatment was not sufficient. Changes in T lymphocyte proliferation in the same patients were precisely parallel (i.e. depressed before treatment but returning to normal afterwards).

Moxibustion was tested in a controlled trial of 69 patients with lung cancer (Ouyang, Cao &

Cao 1992). Thirty-six received intensive moxibustion on a bed of salt at the umbilicus, whereas the controls received no intervention. The treatment group showed a significant increase in CD4 and CD11 cells as well as a reduction in digestive, respiratory and mental symptoms.

Liu, Sun & Xiao (1993) studied the effect of warm needling for rheumatoid arthritis, giving intensive treatment to 29 points on 30 occasions. There were no significant changes in numbers of T lymphocytes, NK cells or levels of immunoglobulin after treatment.

Zhao & Liu (1988, 1989) found that the rate of transformation of lymphocytes in rabbits was significantly increased by EA compared with a control group. But when the EA was given after the injection of a neurotoxic agent (6-OHDA), which blocks adrenergic mechanisms of the brain, this increase was no longer seen. This suggests that the immune effects of acupuncture are at least partly dependent on central catecholamines. In a companion paper the same authors studied the effect of morphine and naloxone on the function of lymphocytes, but the results are much less clear cut.

One measure of the immune system that specifically tests the function of T lymphocytes is the tendency of the blood to form plaques when exposed to sheep red cells. Sakic et al (1989) gave either manual or electroacupuncture at 200 Hz to different points in rats for 2 days before and 4 days after the injection of sheep red cells. Control groups were given either no treatment or sham stimulation. The animals treated at LR-8 (but not those treated at SP-5 or KI-2) produced lower levels of plaque-forming cells and anti-sheep red cell antibody than the controls. When the animals were sacrificed, those treated at LR-8 had significantly lighter spleens and heavier adrenal glands than the controls, indicating suppression of the immune response to the injected antigen.

Lundeberg, Eriksson & Theodorsson (1991) used strong manual acupuncture at six points (GB-25, KI-6 and BL-11 bilaterally) in mice, again measuring the activity of T lymphocytes by the rate of plaque formation with sheep red blood cells. Three groups of mice were treated

over 3 days, and two control groups received superficial acupuncture or no treatment. The strong acupuncture produced a doubling of T helper lymphocytes, which was not seen in the other groups; the change was statistically significant. Phentolamine, when administered before acupuncture, increased the effect but propranolol, hexamethonium and lidocaine prevented the response. This is compatible with the hypothesis that these effects of acupuncture involve stimulation of the sympathetic nervous system and release of adrenaline.

These results were confirmed and extended by Fujiwara et al (1991), using ST-36 in mice. They confirmed the nerve pathways involved by showing that the response was prevented by either cutting the sciatic nerve or pretreating with naloxone.

Wu, Chai & Wang (1985) demonstrated increased rosette formation by T lymphocytes 20 minutes after acupuncture in humans, using points LI-4 and ST-36. Subpopulations of lymphocytes stain differentially with α-naphthyl-acetate esterase, and the authors detected a significant increase in those with focal-staining pattern but not other subsets.

Xia et al (1986) conducted a randomized controlled trial on 76 patients with lung, oesophagus or stomach cancer. All patients received radiotherapy or chemotherapy and one group received treatment to a variety of acupuncture points, while the remainder served as a no-treatment control. The acupuncture group had significantly smaller weight loss, improvement of symptoms and increase in lymphocyte rosette formation.

Delayed-type hypersensitivity

Kasahara et al (1992, 1993) investigated the role of acupuncture in modifying delayed-type hypersensitivity in mice. Low-frequency electroacupuncture given to GV-4 suppressed the ear swelling induced by a challenge with trinitrochlorobenzine in animals that had been presensitized to this chemical. The swelling was reduced by 45–73%, a similar figure to the suppression produced by steroids. This effect did not occur with needling non-specific points in the femoral muscle. The mechanism was shown to be dependent on the release of opioid peptides as well as an intact pituitary.

Tohya et al (1989) examined the effect of moxibustion in mice, and showed that daily treatment of BL-20 or LI-15 regions reduced the inflammatory reaction to picryl chloride. When cells from the spleens of the treated animals were transfused into naive mice, they too showed a similar reduction in delayed-type hypersensitivity.

CONCLUSION

Many of the above studies have methodological weaknesses and are reported only sketchily. In summary they do not add up to a body of evidence that is clinically relevant at present. However, they do suggest that acupuncture might have a useful role in modifying immunological processes and further clinical studies are justified and the results awaited with interest.

SKIN DISEASES

Acupuncture would appear to have the potential to influence skin disease at several different levels. It could have local and general effects on the disease processes including possibly the immune response, it may reduce symptoms such as itch, and it might produce generalized effects such as reduced anxiety. However, the quality of research on the subject, as so often in acupuncture, does not allow us to draw any confident conclusions about its precise role. The literature mainly consists of case reports and the only controlled studies are in experimentally induced itch.

Rosted (1994) described three approaches that were commonly combined for treating skin conditions: body acupuncture with strong manual or electrical stimulation, auricular points such as Lung and Adrenal, and a particular technique called 'surrounding the dragon' for specific lesions. In this method, isolated lesions are surrounded by needles, usually about 1 cm from the border of the lesion, placed obliquely to the surface, directed towards the centre of the lesion. Liao & Liao (1992) described a variation in which the needles are inserted tangential to the edge of the lesions in the case of psoriasis. Traditionally the needles would have been placed about 1 Chinese inch apart from each other.

The body points most commonly used for skin disease in the published literature include LI-11, SP-10, GV-14, ST-36, and LI-4. Rosted (1994) pointed out that, although the skin is regarded as part of Lung–Large Intestine complex in Chinese medicine, Chinese doctors do not appear to use Lung points at all. Spinal and paraspinal points commonly appear in the Chinese prescriptions. Rosted (1992a) recommended a standard protocol for skin conditions: points GV-20, EX-HN1 (Sishencong), LR-3, LU-7 and LI-4, subsequently adding the auricular points Lung and Adrenal if there is no response. Lu (1992a,b,c) published a series of papers with recommendations for individual conditions.

Treatment in China is generally given either daily or on alternate days for courses of 10 sessions, repeated as necessary after an interval of a few weeks. In the West treatment is usually given weekly over an extended period: Rosted (1992a) states that the usual course is 4 to 8 months, and that even more prolonged therapy may be necessary, up to 30 sessions.

Since spontaneous remission is quite likely during long courses of treatment, carefully controlled studies are crucial. However, we have been unable to find any such long-term controlled trials.

EXPERIMENTAL ITCH

There are similarities between the neurophysiology of itch and pain. Both sensations depend on the stimulation of C fibres (e.g. by histamine or prostaglandins). Precisely whether this is felt as itch or pain does not seem to depend on the intensity of stimulation, and so it is possible that there are different populations of

C fibres serving each sensation (Lundeberg, Bondesson & Thomas 1987). As is the case with pain, counterstimulation can reduce itch (Belgrade, Solomon & Lichter 1984).

There are two studies into the effect of acupuncture on experimental itch induced by the intradermal injection of histamine. Belgrade, Solomon & Lichter (1984) gave 25 healthy volunteers acupuncture at LI-11 and EA between SP-6 and 10 for 15 minutes before histamine injection. Control groups received sham treatment to nearby non-acupuncture points. The mean duration and intensity of itch were compared with that produced by histamine injection alone. Sham acupuncture reduced both measures significantly ($P < 0.02$), but there was a greater reduction after needling correct acupuncture points ($P < 0.005$), suggesting a point-specific effect as well. In addition, genuine acupuncture produced a greater reduction in the maximal flare area than did sham acupuncture. The authors concluded that acupuncture appears to be an effective inhibitor of histamine-induced itch and flare.

Lundeberg, Bondesson & Thomas (1987) recruited 10 volunteers for a similar test of acupuncture for itch induced by histamine injection in the arm. Three different acupuncture sites were tested, viz. two points in the injection area of the upper arm, two points proximally in the same segment, and two extrasegmental points (LR-5 and 6 in the leg). Manual acupuncture and EA at 2 and 80 Hz were compared with no treatment and with superficial needling of the local points. The results showed a clear reduction of itch intensity after needling locally or in the same segment, but not after needling extrasegmentally. The effect was greatest with stimulation at 80 Hz. The response depended on timing of the acupuncture in relation to the injection: interestingly, when acupuncture was given before the injection, 5 minutes' stimulation had more effect than did 20 minutes. Acupuncture had a greater effect when given after the injection. A dose–response curve was noted, the effect being weakest with superficial needling, stronger with manual acupuncture and with 2 Hz EA, and maximal with 80 Hz EA.

The above studies in healthy volunteers indicate that acupuncture may be of some value in controlling the symptom of itch.

PRURITUS

Shapiro, Stockard & Schank (1988) reported anecdotally eight cases of severe uraemic pruritus, all of whom were treated with EA (80–100 Hz) to SP-6 and 10, ST-36 and LI-11. Seven out of eight achieved virtually total relief of itch within the first four treatments, but the eighth required 10 sessions. The relief lasted over 4 months in all cases.

Liu JD (1987) selected six patients with end-stage renal failure and severe uraemic pruritus, and gave them EA (frequency 0.5–50 Hz) to LI-11 and ST-36 thrice weekly for 26 sessions. Severity and frequency of itch and disturbance to sleep were measured with a points system and compared before and after treatment. All patients showed significant improvement and in two-thirds the benefit lasted more than a month.

Huang et al (1987) described similar excellent results in the treatment of 56 patients with chronic pruritus vulvae, where infection had been excluded and other treatments had failed. The follow-ups were between 3 and 19 months.

Gao (1991) reported a series of 65 patients with chronic urticaria treated with acupuncture at GV-20, 14 and 12, GB-20, LI-11, BL-17 and ST-36, including letting blood from selected points. He claimed that 61 had lasting benefit from 10–20 treatments. These figures should be treated with caution as no detailed breakdown of the results is given.

ECZEMA AND DERMATITIS

Eczema is referred to as neurodermatitis in Chinese texts. Liu J (1987) and Yang (1993) reported acupuncture treatment in 86 and 139 patients respectively with chronic neurodermatitis, using either needles surrounding isolated lesions, or distal points in widespread cases. They both reported success rates of nearly 90% but since details were very sparse this result must be open to some doubt.

Pothmann (1992) reported a prospective case series of 10 patients with dermatitis solaris, all of whom responded to 2 consecutive days' brief stimulation of SP-10 and LI-11. In four cases the benefit lasted through the summer.

Liao (1988) reported four cases of poison ivy contact dermatitis. The plant's resin causes a vesicular rash that is intensely itchy, and usually lasts 2 to 3 weeks. The points used included LI-11, SP-10 and ST-36. In three cases the itch subsided within hours, and in the fourth case within 2 days, that is, considerably sooner than expected. No follow-up data were presented.

PSORIASIS

Rosted (1992b) made the observation that psoriasis is the skin disease that responds best to acupuncture. Liao & Liao (1992) described a series of 61 patients in the USA who requested acupuncture because their chronic psoriasis had not responded to conventional management. The authors discussed the traditional Chinese approach to skin lesions, but used a standard prescription of LI-11, SP-10 and ST-36—that is, the same points that they had used for poison ivy contact dermatitis (Liao 1988) and herpes simplex (Liao & Liao 1991). The average age of the group was 52 and the overall duration of psoriasis was over 16 years. Thirty-seven cases were classified as severe before treatment. The patients received an average of nine sessions of acupuncture. Thirty-one of the patients were reported as having excellent improvement that was defined as 'complete or almost complete clearance of all the skin lesions with no recurrence'. There was a clear correlation between the number of sessions of acupuncture and the effectiveness of the treatment. Seven patients withdrew when they noticed no improvement after two or three sessions, and nine patients persisted with treatment but did not benefit ultimately.

Zhao, Wang & Hua (1991) reported a case series of 600 patients with psoriasis whom they treated with blood letting, cupping, paraspinal long subcutaneous needling, and EA on alternate days for 30 sessions. The authors reported a marked improvement in 86% of patients.

WARTS

Su & Tu (1987) described their method of treatment of 119 patients with warts that had been present more than 2 months. They inserted the needle perpendicularly into the centre of the largest (or earliest) wart. At the same time the base of the wart was pinched with the other hand to try to reduce the pain. The needle was advanced to the base of the wart then 'fast and heavy twirling with lift-thrusting' performed 30 times. Then the needle was withdrawn slightly and forced round in a circle inside the wart, at the level of the border between normal skin and wart. This technique was disarmingly called the 'open door' method. It was repeated four times (in those who returned—the percentage of drop-outs was not recorded!) once after 4 days and then twice after intervals of 15 days. Ninety cases were followed up for 3 months: in 87 cases the warts had disappeared completely. The authors discuss possible mechanisms of the treatment, concluding finally that it probably works by the simple disruption of the blood supply to the wart.

Lu (1992b) recommended a special point between first and second phalanges of thumb or hallux, with TE-3, LI-4 and auricular points for warts.

MISCELLANEOUS CONDITIONS

Alopecia areata was treated by Ge (1990) with two different techniques: one consisted of needling GB-20 together with two standard needles placed horizontally in the margin of the bald area, manipulated to achieve De Qi and left for 20 minutes; the other involved plum-blossom needling over the whole bald area in a spiral pattern, followed by plum-blossom needling to the lumbar region (centrally and paravertebrally). It was claimed that eight out of the nine cases responded satisfactorily.

Liao & Liao (1991) described a series of five cases of chronic relapsing herpes simplex treated with acupuncture in a standard formula: LI-11, SP-10 and ST-36. The authors report that the lesions cleared during the 2 or 3 weeks' course of acupuncture. They gained the impression from two of the cases with longer follow-up that there might be some reduction in the frequency of relapse, but clearly some caution is required in interpreting these data.

Iliev, Popov & Nicolov (1995) reported good results in 14 out of 35 patients with lichen ruber planus who received 15 treatments at GV-20, BL-13, 17 and 20, LI-4 and 11, ST-36 and SP-6 and 10. Immunological parameters also improved but no data are given.

No case series have been found of acupuncture for acute herpes zoster. Lu (1992b) recommended the use of GV-12, GB-34, LI-11 and SP-6 for this condition plus relevant local points and points 'surrounding the dragon'.

Successful treatment of a case of mycosis fungoides with acupuncture was reported by Lao (1988).

SCARS

There appears to be a lack of even published case series of the treatment of scars by acupuncture. Problems can arise from scars from the formation of either neuromata or soft tissue trigger points. Sometimes the whole scar appears to be involved. Symptoms may be restricted to local pain, although scars have been blamed for widespread reflex effects (e.g. on the abdominal organs). Acupuncture offers a variety of techniques that may be useful as an alternative to local anaesthetic injection (Peck 1989). Tender points should be carefully identified by lifting the scar off the underlying structures and rolling it between the fingertips and thumb. Treatment can range from local superficial needling to produce erythema, to deep needling directly into the tender point, or EA applied to needles either side of the tender area. The latter techniques can be applied to whole scars by threading the needles subcutaneously along either side (Peck 1989).

FACIAL CONDITIONS

Xu (1989) treated acne with several ear points,

including Lung and Kidney, twisting the needles then leaving them for 30 minutes; 16 treatments on alternate days were reported to be effective in over 90% of cases, though the author suggested continuing treatment on a monthly basis. In the following year, Xu (1990) reported on the treatment of facial acne together with acne rosacea and chloasma, using local and distant points. He claimed a 90% success rate in 15 sessions.

Chen & Hu (1985) used auricular acupuncture in a similar way to treat the butterfly rash of lupus erythematosus. Feng et al (1985) treated 10 patients who had suffered systemic lupus (skin, joint and haemopoietic system affected, but without renal involvement) for an average of 3.2 years. Using the main distal points as well as the Huatuojiaji points, they reported that a variety of symptoms, signs and laboratory findings were improved. Abnormal appearances of capillaries in the nailfold and associated stasis of blood flow were improved after treatment.

A series of 34 cases of progressive systemic sclerosis was described by Maeda et al (1988). They received low-frequency (1–10 Hz) EA connected from interdigital points to the elbow or knee respectively. Treatment was repeated between one and five times a week for long periods, up to 9 years in one case. Ulcerations of tips of digits, arthralgia, cutaneous sclerosis and morning stiffness improved, and photographs are provided of six cases that responded. Immune parameters showed no response, however, and the patients' overall clinical condition was not improved. This is a realistic retrospective study from Japan with positive clinical findings that are worth pursuing in controlled trials.

Wang (1991) used ST-36, KI-3, LI-4 and GB-20 together with points 'surrounding the dragon' in a series of 11 cases of local scleroderma. Two patients were 'cured', one 'markedly improved' and the remainder 'improved'.

CONCLUSION

In summary, there are optimistic case series of the use of acupuncture in a variety of skin conditions. However, controlled clinical trials are required before acupuncture can claim definitely to be effective in treating skin diseases. Two controlled studies strongly suggest that acupuncture has an antihistaminic effect in healthy volunteers.

GYNAECOLOGICAL AND OBSTETRIC COMPLAINTS

Many acupuncturists, both medical and lay, say anecdotally how satisfying it is to treat a variety of gynaecological complaints. One could expect a plethora of good clinical trials to back up these widely held claims. Sadly this is not the case at present. An attempt has been made to present this topic in some sort of order with gynaecological problems preceding the obstetrics section.

PREMENSTRUAL SYNDROME

The only article on this subject by Flaws (1985) was rather amusing, listing the threat of nuclear wars, a background music of discordant jazz and TV news as three of the many predisposing factors. Acupuncture was only part of the treatment, three times per week, advocated by the TCM paper, which included herbs, relaxation and diet.

DYSMENORRHOEA

Table 14.7 represents a summary of some of the literature on dysmenorrhoea. There is quite a variation in technique—the TCM papers being mostly labour intensive with treatments on alternate days, premenstrually and occasionally daily of 20–30 minutes duration. The pretreatment classification of primary or secondary dysmenorrhoea and investigations are often minimal, the scoring systems crude and follow-up often inadequate. Nevertheless good success rates are claimed. One form of dysmenorrhoea apparently often occurred in patients who had been wading across rivers, exposed to rain, swimming, sitting, lying on damp ground or eating raw and cold food, according to Lu

(1991b). A modern acupuncturist may have considerable conceptual difficulties with this type of information. Wang (1987) and Zhao (1988) further illustrate a TCM approach to treatment. Helms in 1987 performed a randomized controlled prospective study on 43 patients. They were followed up for 1 year. He studied four groups; (1) a group treated with real acupuncture at SP-4, KI-3, ST-30 and 36, CV-2 and 4 and PC-6 which he stimulated for 30 minutes; (2) a placebo acupuncture group who were given needles in the lateral arm and thighs and similar stimulation; (3) a standard control group had no treatment and (4) a 'visitation' control group who had monthly non-acupuncture visits to try to compensate for the extra attention that the acupuncture groups were receiving. The treatment groups were given one treatment per week for 12 weeks, apart from the weeks in which they were menstruating. Improvement was defined as an average post-treatment score of less than half of the pre-treatment pain score. The results were: (1) real acupuncture, 10 out of 11 improved; (2) placebo acupuncture, four out of 11 improved; (3) standard control group, two out of 11 improved; (4) visitation group, one out of 10 improved. While not statistically significant, a trend towards improvement was seen in the real and placebo acupuncture groups, with the real acupuncture showing the more dramatic drop in reported pain. Analgesic consumption was reduced by the greatest amount in the acupuncture group and dropped by 54% during treatment and by 41% after treatment.

Thomas et al (1995) has recently reported an interesting placebo-controlled trial on the comparative effectiveness of four different modes of acupuncture and three different modes of TENS prior to the onset of recurrent pain of primary dysmenorrhoea. Twenty-nine patients were treated at 7 and 3 days before their expected periods. Seventeen patients were given acupuncture premenstrually by different methods (manual, low-frequency 2 Hz or high-frequency 100 Hz EA at BL-32, CV-4, SP-6 and 9 or periosteal stimulation at SP-6 and 9). Each of these four modes was used sequentially for 4

Table 14.7 Dysmenorrhoea

Author date	Study type	TCM or modern	No. of patients	Length of follow-up	Type of treatments	Success	Points
Zhang 1984	Descriptive	TCM	49	3/12	EA + Moxa + ear	42—cure 6—marked improvement 1—failure	Several TCM groups
Steinberger 1981	Descriptive	TCM	48	6 — 12/12	Manual acupuncture + moxa	28—good 12—improved 4—failure 4—lost to follow-up	ST-36 SP-6 LI-14 CV-4
Wang 1987	Descriptive	TCM	100	6/12	Manual acupuncture	54—cure 27—marked improvement 13—some improvement 6—failure	TCM
Zhan 1990	Descriptive	TCM	32	6/12	Manual acupuncture + moxa	20—cure 11—effective 1—failure	LI-4 SP-6 CV-4 and 6
Helms 1987	Randomized controlled 4 groups: (1) acupuncture (2) placebo acupuncture (3) control (4) visitation alone	Modern diagnosis first. Pain scores	43	1 year	Manual acupuncture	Group 1—10/11 improved 2—4/11 improved 3—2/11 improved 4—1/10 improved	SP-4 KI-3 ST-30 ST-36 CV-2 CV-4 PC-6
Neighbors 1987	Controlled acupuncture vs sugar pill	Modern	20		Acupuncture-like TENS	Group 1—7/10 improved 2—1/10 improved	BL-21 BL-29 ST-30 SP-6
Lewers 1989	Controlled acupuncture vs sugar pill	Modern	21	24 hrs	Acupuncture-like TENS	Both groups improved	BL-21 BL-29 ST-30 SP-6
Thomas 1995	Controlled 4 groups acupuncture 3 groups TENS	Modern diagnosis first. Good scoring system	29	3/12	Manual acupuncture 2 Hz EA 100 Hz EA periosteal	Significant improvement	BL-32 CV-4 SP-6 SP-9
					TENS 2 Hz 100 Hz	Significant improvement	SP-6 SP-9
					Inactive TENS	no improvement	

consecutive months and entry to the initial mode was randomized. The 5th month's treatment was then repeated in the mode of the patient's choice. Twelve patients in another group were treated with two active modes of TENS 2 Hz or 100 Hz and one inactive mode for each of 3 months and then the patient's choice of mode was repeated on the 4th month. Pain, blood loss, nausea and vomiting, hours of work lost, daily analgesic consumption and subjective assessments were made. Although two of the acupuncture group did not complete the treatment schedule, all modes of acupuncture gave improvement in outcome measures and were significant for pain, analgesic intake and subjective assessment, except that low-frequency EA did not result in decreased analgesic consumption. Low-frequency TENS also gave a significant reduction in pain, analgesic consumption and subjective assessment. High-frequency TENS and placebo TENS did not result in significant improvement. At 3 months' follow-up, significant improvement continued with pain and subjective assessment in the acupuncture group and in subjective assessment in the low-frequency TENS group. They concluded that a reduction in pain and discomfort in primary dysmenorrhoea was obtained by the pre-emptive use of different modes of acupuncture or low-frequency TENS, but not high-frequency or placebo TENS.

One paper on TENS by Neighbors et al (1987) studied 20 patients using a single treatment with acupuncture-like TENS on BL-21 and 29, ST-36 and SP-6 or a sugar pill (placebo) and showed that seven out of 10 had a statistically significant drop in pain beyond the one out of 10 placebo group using validated pain scores. Another paper trying to replicate this (Lewers et al 1989), despite getting better analgesia, failed to show a statistical difference between the control and the acupuncture group. They attributed this to the fact that the patients had had auricular pressure testing prior to their treatment and that this in itself had induced analgesia in both groups.

PELVIC PAIN

The bulk of the literature is on dysmenorrhoea.

One descriptive study used injection of local anaesthetic into trigger points (Slocumb, 1984). Xia et al (1987) claimed excellent results (80%) in 55 patients with Kraurosis vulvae using CV-1 and 2 and distant points using a thermoelectric acupuncture device to normalize skin pigmentation following treatment. Heated needles were used and 30–60 daily treatments were recommended. However the treatment was even recommended for early stages of squamous carcinoma but on the basis of only three cases. This advice should be regarded with extreme caution.

DYSFUNCTIONAL UTERINE BLEEDING

Hallberg et al (1966) found a definite decrease in haemoglobin concentration and plasma iron concentrations when the menstrual loss exceeded 80 ml and this value is now taken as the upper limit of normal. To date, no study has been performed comparing any reduction of menstrual loss in patients taking conventional therapy with acupuncture.

The bulk of the literature is traditional and descriptive with substandard reporting of gynaecological work-up pretreatment and relatively short post-treatment follow-up.

Some TCM papers describe acupuncture as second-line treatment to herbal therapy. Liu et al (1988), in a descriptive series of 30 patients, aimed to (1) stop the bleeding using CV-4 and 6, SP-6 and BL-20 and 23 and (2) improve the general condition using ST-36, BL-20 and 23 and CV-4. Only 20 patients had a 3-monthly follow up. One traditional paper on endometriosis by Lyttleton (1988) after an interesting introduction gave only two unclear case histories. Another case report by Sternfield et al (1993) in a patient with a 12–14-week size fibroid uterus showed that it began to shrink to 7–8-week size after 30 treatments and enabled an in-vitro fertilization pregnancy. The points used were ST-29 and 36, CV-1 and 4, SP-6 and 11, KI-3, LR-3 and GB-34 for 25 weeks. Wu et al (1987) recommended laser therapy for chronic pelvic inflammation at the following points; CV-3 and 6, BL-23 and SP-6 and 10. Unfortunately, gynaecological work-up pretreatment was extremely poor, rendering the cure and markedly improved rate of 61% and the 87% totally effective rate uninterpretable.

AMENORRHOEA

Amenorrhoea is either primary or secondary. Primary amenorrhoea is most commonly due to reproductive failure or an anomaly of the reproductive tract and would not be helped by acupuncture. Secondary amenorrhoea is most commonly due to anovulation and could be helped by acupuncture. One descriptive series of 225 cases of presumed secondary amenorrhoea is described by Liu, Liu & Liu (1992) in cases with 3–16-month histories. A TCM diagnosis was made and treatment was more successful in patients with a shorter history of amenorrhoea. Two groups of patients apparently fared better than two others based on TCM diagnosis; the points chosen were KI-6, BL-20 and 23, SP-6 and 10 and ST-36, or SP-6, 8 and 10, KI-6, PC-6, LR-3 and TE-6. The patients were neither matched nor randomized in any way and so this conclusion may well be inaccurate or merely reflect that the points chosen in the good groups were better than the other groups. Out of all TCM groups, 162 were 'cured', 59 'effective' and four failed after five to 10 treatments of 20–30 minutes' duration. A further descriptive series by Yu (1990) of 20 cases showed a 70% success rate using CV-4, ST-36, SP-6 and two points lateral to the second lumbar vertebra bilaterally.

INFERTILITY

Takeshi et al (1976) gave women who ovulated normally acupuncture stimulation and the effect on plasma levels of luteinizing hormone, follicle-stimulating hormone, progesterone and oestradiol were measured. As tests were performed in the same cycle as the acupuncture and would be expected to change during the cycle, the validity of the results could be questioned. The timing of tests in relation to the cycle is also not clearly stated. Nevertheless, they did see a noticeable increase in luteinizing hormone response to luteinizing hormone-releasing hormone test

under acupuncture stimulation, this trend being more obvious around the time of ovulation and in the luteal phase.

Gerhard & Postneek 1992 used auricular acupuncture according to Nogier on a group of 45 women with infertility and compared them with matched patients undergoing active infertility treatment. The patients all had at least one patent fallopian tube and positive postcoital sperm test. The results were not statistically significantly different. Side-effects were observed only in the hormone treatment group, which would give an advantage to acupuncture. Further study is recommended.

A further paper by Deng & Han (1990) showed the effect of laser therapy on 50 patients with tubal infertility. The entry criteria did not clearly include an HSG or laparoscopy so cautious interpretation of the results should be made. 26 patients conceived within 12 months after infertility of 2–12 years, which was not insignificant. The treatment was given over four sacral foramina bilaterally and three low abdominal points and the patients were given a course of 25 treatments. Ten out of 24 patients who did not conceive had significant pelvic pathology.

Lin et al (1988) has shown acupuncture to render anoestrous sows oestrous after acupuncture to back points compared with treatment in the foreleg or in a third group receiving gonadotropin-releasing hormone (GnRH):

group 1   four sows – EA back, three oestrous
group 2   three sows – EA foreleg and hindleg, one oestrous
group 3   four sows – GnRH, one oestrous

This paper appears to reinforce the fact that acupuncture can decrease luteinizing hormone in anovulatory sows and in group 1 this was associated with an increase in progesterone, continuing ovulation and subsequent pregnancy in three of four sows. Although the numbers were low, the acupuncture results showed promise.

PREVENTION OF MISCARRIAGE

The only articles that mention acupuncture for prevention of miscarriage are anecdotal and not validated. If there is a history of threatened miscarriage, Staebler (1985) recommends treatment at CV-4, ST-36, BL-23, SP-6, KI-3 and LR-3 preconception. CV-3 and KI-9 have been suggested to help decrease contractions and stop a threatened abortion (Rempp & Bigler 1991). Zharkin (1990) recommends KI-3, KI-7 as primary points and PC-6, HT-5 and CV-6 as secondary points mainly for early threatened abortion, and PC-6, SP-4 and 6, HT-5 and GV-20 for late threatened miscarriage.

TERMINATION OF PREGNANCY

Although not recommended per se to induce abortion, Ying, Lin & Robins (1985) have recommended strong electrical low-intensity, high-frequency stimulation at SP-6 and manual stimulation at LI-4 to aid cervical dilatation prior to termination of pregnancy in 20 patients and a cervical dilatation to 7 mm was found in the acupuncture group compared with controls. It may be useful to help to prevent tearing of the cervix prior to therapeutic termination of pregnancy.

GYNAECOLOGICAL UROLOGICAL PROBLEMS

Table 14.8 summarizes the data from 4 trials. Kelleher et al (1994) have performed the only prospective randomized trial of acupuncture versus conventional treatment, oxybutynin, studying urodynamics, diaries and quality of life. In a minimal-stimulating technique, acupuncture was found to be as effective as conventional anticholinergic therapy, with a statistically significant reduction in nocturia and also minimal side-effects. There was a high degree of patient acceptability and compliance. Interestingly, the benefit often occurred between the 3rd and 6th weekly 10-minute acupuncture treatments in this group. One paper by Chang (1988) is slightly difficult to interpret as only 14 of the 52 patients had abnormal urodynamics prior to treatment.

Two further descriptive series included male patients (Ellis 1993, Philp et al 1988) Auriculo-therapy plus body acupuncture has also been described (Zhao 1987).

MENOPAUSE

Only one descriptive TCM study exists. It is in French, by De Giacomo (1989) who recommends the use of Bl-23, CV-3, LR-3, GB-20 and 34 and ST-40. Wyon et al (1995) have shown a significant reduction in hot flushes after a course of acupuncture and decreased excretion of the potent vasodilating neuropeptide calcitonin gene-related peptide after acupuncture.

MISCELLANEOUS CONDITIONS

Radiation rectitis following radiation therapy for carcinoma of the cervix can be very debilitating. One study on 44 patients by Zhang (1987) using LI-4, ST-25, 36 and 37 plus additional points 'cured' 73% and helped or improved a further 27%. Further formal study is recommended.

OBSTETRICS

Zharkin (1990) states that traditional Chinese texts hardly discuss obstetrics but that acupuncture is useful for inducing and augmenting labour and treating endometritis and mastitis. He states that there are no absolute contraindications in pregnancy but some restrictions such as moxibustion, although it is used for breech pregnancy. It is not advisable to needle parts below the umbilicus or on the anterior abdominal wall or to stimulate strongly BL-31–34 or LI-4 or ST-36, SP-2 or 3 within the first trimester, but treatment later in pregnancy is thought to carry a very much lower risk of abortion or premature labour. Treatment should not be more than 30 minutes in length and the report recommends that the patient should ideally be treated by an obstetrician. No prospective randomized controlled trials are available to date on acupuncture for their indications.

Table 14.9 summarizes some of the literature for inducing labour and some postpartum problems.

NB. It is advisable for anyone contemplating using acupuncture for labour or during pregnancy to read the relevant literature immensely carefully and not to take any unnecessary chances.

Table 14.8 Irritative bladder problems

Author	No.	Randomized	Control	Urodynamics	Rx details pre	Results post	Follow-up
Chang 1988	51	—	✓	✓ ✓ (only 14/52 abnormal pre-Rx however)	SP-6 true, ST-36 placebo	Both helped but 22/26 helped 6/26 helped	2–14/12
Pigne 1985 (abstract)	16	—	—	✓ ✓	BL-23, BL-28, BL-64, BL65, SP-6, SP-9, CV3	Frequency ↓ urgency ↓ bl. capac. ↑ improved 1st desire to void	—
Gibson 1988 (abstract)	28	—	—	✓ ✓	Laser therapy BL-23, BL-28, BL-64, BL-65, SP-6, SP-9, CV-3	Frequency ↓ urgency ↓ nocturia ↓ bl. capac. ↑	3/12
Kelleher et al 1994	39	✓	✓	✓ ✓	Minimal Rx BL-23, BL-28, SP-6, ST-36, CV-3 or 4 2 lumbar 4 sacral points vs oxybutynin	Frequency ↓ urgency ↓ nocturia ↓ bl. capac. ↑ both Rx's effective nocturia sig. ↓ with acup. side-effects sig. ↓ with acup.	3/12

Table 14.9 Obstetrics

Induction	Labour	Post partum
Remp 1991 Treat apprehension HT-5, HT-7 Prepare cervix & perineum CV-4, TE-6, LR-3, CV-4 1000 patients	Remp 1991 BL-32, BL-33 & BL-34 Skelton 1988 83 patients ST-36, SP-6, etc +1 or 2 ear points	Remp 1991 Post partum pain CV-2, CV-4, KI-14, ST-29, ST-30, BL-31, BL-32 Perineal pain GV-20, SP-4, SP-6, ST-30 Sphincter problems LR-2, CV-3, BL-23 28 and 67 Lactation CV-17 Depression SI-1
Kubista 1975 EA 2 hrs 8HZ K-18, ST-36, CV-6 31/35 induced	Martoudis 1990 EA 20–30 mnts Ear Shenmen LI-4 168 patients	Yang 1985 Post partum urine retention 49 patients SP-6 ST-36
Dunn 1989 TENS SP-6, LR-3	Staebler 1995 Selected points for several different obstetric problems	Li 1993 Post partum urine retention 56 patients CV-2, CV-4, SP-6, SP-8 +/-CV-6, BL-22 & 23
	Yagudin 1987 LI-4 Ear Shenmen 20 mnts EA 29 patients	Hou 1989 Post partum dysuria 30 patients CV-3, CV-4, SP-6

Breech presentation

Moxibustion to BL-67 appears to be the favourite treatment of breech presentation (Cardini et al 1991, Rempp & Bigler 1991, Zharkin 1990). One large descriptive series recommends the use of auricular plaster therapy for abnormal foetal positions (Qin & Tang 1989). The results are better before the 36th week of pregnancy (Cardini et al 1991).

Several other aspects of acupuncture during pregnancy are covered by Rempp & Bigler

(1991) in one series of 1000 patients and by Staebler (1985).

There is one controlled trial comparing TENS to dummy TENS at SP-6 and LR-3 for induction of labour by Dunn, Rogers & Halford (1989); it demonstrates a significant increase in higher-intensity contractions during labour with TENS than with dummy TENS.

CONCLUSION

Clearly, there is considerable potential for further trials of acupuncture for gynaecological and obstetric conditions.

REFERENCES

Ader R, Cohen N, Felten D 1995 Psychoneuroimmunology: interactions between the nervous system and the immune system. Lancet 345:99–103

Aldridge D, Pietroni P C 1987 Clinical assessment of acupuncture in asthma therapy: discussion paper. Journal of the Royal Society of Medicine 80:222–224

Alm P, Alumets J, Hakanson R et al 1981 Enkephalin immunoreactive nerve fibres in the feline genitourinary tract. Histochemistry 72:351–355

Axelsson A, Andersson S, Gu L-D 1994 Acupuncture in the management of tinnitus: a placebo-controlled study. Audiology 33:351–360

Bajorek J G, Lee R J, Lomax P 1986 Neuropeptides: anticonvulsant and convulsant mechanisms in epileptic model systems and in humans. Advances in Neurology 44:489–500

Ballegaard S, Christophersen S J, Dawids S G, Hesse J, Olsen N V 1985 Acupuncture and transcutaneous electric nerve stimulation in the treatment of pain associated with chronic pancreatitis. A randomised study. Scandinavian Journal of Gastroenterology 20:1249–1254

Ballegaard S, Jensen G, Pedersen F, Nissen V H 1986 Acupuncture in severe, stable angina pectoris: a randomized trial. Acta Physiologica Scandinavica 220:307–313

Ballegaard S, Pedersen F, Pietersen A, Nissen V H, Olsen N V 1990 Effects of acupuncture in moderate, stable angina pectoris: a controlled study. Journal of Internal Medicine 227:25–30

Ballegaard S, Meyer C N, Trojaborg W 1991 Acupuncture in angina pectoris: does acupuncture have a specific effect? Journal of Internal Medicine 229:357–362

Ballegaard S, Muteki T, Harada H, Ueda N, Tsuda H, Tayama F 1993 Modulatory effects of acupuncture on the cardiovascular system: a cross-over study. Acupuncture and Electro-therapeutics Research 18:103–115

Ballegaard S, Karpatschoff B, Holck J, Meyer C, Trojaborg W 1995 Acupuncture in angina pectoris: do psycho-social and neurophysiological factors relate to the effect? Acupuncture and Electro-therapeutics Research 20: 101–116

Bannerman R H 1979 Acupuncture: the WHO view. World Health, 27/28 December

Barnes P J, Chung K F 1989 Difficult asthma. British Medical Journal 299:695–698

Batlivala S 1986 Acupuncture acts dramatically in dysphagia to acute pseudo-bulbar palsy. British Journal of Acupuncture 9:12–13

Batra Y K, Chari P, Singh H 1986 Acupuncture in corticosteroid-dependant asthmatics. American Journal of Acupuncture 14:261–264

Belgrade M J, Solomon L M, Lichter E A 1984 Effect of acupuncture on experimentally induced itch. Acta Dermatologica Venereologica (Stockholm) 64:129–133

Benson H, McCallie DP 1979 Angina pectoris and the placebo effect. New England Journal of Medicine 300:1424–1429

Berger D, Nolte D 1975 Hat Akupunktur einen nachweisbaren brocho-spasmolytischen Effekt beim Asthma bronchiale? Medizinische Klinik (München) 70:1827–1830

Bianchi M, Jotti E, Sacerdote P, Panerai A E 1991 Traditional acupuncture increases the content of beta-endorphin in immune cells and influences mitogen induced proliferation. American Journal of Chinese Medicine 19(2):101–104

Blom M, Dawidson I, Angmar-Mansson B 1992 The effect of acupuncture on salivary flow rates in patients with xerostomia. Oral Surgery, Oral Medicine, Oral Pathology 73(3):293–298

Bondi N, Bettelli A 1981 Trattamento del singhiozzo con agopuntura in soggetti anestetizzati ed in soggetti coscienti. Minerva Medica (Torino) 72: 2231–2234

Bossy J 1990 Immune systems, defense mechanisms and acupuncture: fundamental and practical aspects. American Journal of Acupuncture 18(3):219–232

Bossy J 1994 Acupuncture and immunity: basic and clinical aspects. Acupuncture in Medicine 12(1):60–62

Bu G, Nakano T 1990 Clinical application of rhinomanometer. Chinese Medical Journal 103(11):956–958

Butler C, Steptoe A 1986 Placebo responses: an experimental study of psychophysiological processes in asthmatic volunteers. British Journal of Clinical Psychology 25:173–183

Cahn A M, Carayon P, Hill C, Flamant R 1978 Acupuncture in gastroscopy. Lancet 1:182–183

Campbell A 1987 Acupuncture: the modern scientific approach. Faber & Faber, London

Campbell A 1992 Acupuncture treatment of gastrointestinal disorders. Acupuncture in Medicine 10:70–71

Cao X-D, Xu S-F, Ly W-X 1983 Inhibition of sympathetic nervous system by acupuncture. Acupuncture and Electro-therapeutics Research 8:25–35

Cardini F, Basevi V, Valentini A, Martellato A 1991 Moxibustion and breech presentation: preliminary results. American Journal of Chinese Medicine XIX:105–114

Carlsson J, Rosenhall U 1990 Oculomotor disturbances in patients with tension headache treated with acupuncture or physiotherapy. Cephalalgia 10:123–129

Chang P L 1988 Urodynamic studies in acupuncture for women with frequency, urgency and dysuria. Journal of Urology 140:563–566

Chari P, Biwas S, Mann S B S, Sehgal S, Mehra Y N 1988 American Journal of Acupuncture 16(2):143–147

Chein E Y M, Zakaria S 1974 Acupuncture for psychiatric disorders. Journal of the American Medical Association 229:639

Chen A 1993a Effective acupuncture therapy for stroke and cerebrovascular diseases: part 1. American Journal of Acupuncture 21:105–122

Chen A 1993b Effective acupuncture therapy for stroke and cerebrovascular diseases. Part 2. American Journal of Acupuncture 21:205–218

Chen A 1993c Effective acupuncture therapy for stroke and cerebrovascular disease. Part 3 (Prescription for prevention). American Journal of Acupuncture 21:305–318

Chen C, Gao Z, Ling P 1990 Clinical research on He-Ne laser acupuncture in treating 122 cases of chronic prostatitis. International Journal of Clinical Acupuncture 1:345–350

Chen H, Cai D, Zhai D, Zhao C 1992 Investigation on the feasibility of treating AIDS with acupuncture and moxibustion. International Journal of Clinical Acupuncture 3(1):13–17

Chen L 1991 408 cases of urinary calculus treated by auriculoacupoint pressure. Journal of Traditional Chinese Medicine 11:193–195

Chen R, Huang Y 1984 Acupuncture on experimental epilepsies. Proceedings of the National Science Council 8:72–77

Chen R, Huang Y, How S 1986 Systemic penicillin as an experimental model of epilepsy. Experimental Neurology 92:533–540

Chen Y 1993 Acupuncture treatment of functional non-ejaculation: a report of 7 cases. Journal of Traditional Chinese Medicine 13:10–12

Chen Y, Fang Y 1990 108 cases of hemiplegia caused by stroke: the relationship between CT scan results, clinical findings and the effect of acupuncture treatment. Acupuncture and Electro-therapeutics Research 15:9–17

Chen Y, Hu X 1985 Auriculo-acupuncture in 15 cases of discoid lupus erythematosus. Journal of Traditional Chinese Medicine 5(4):261–262

Chen Z, Chen L 1991 The treatment of enuresis with scalp acupuncture. Journal of Traditional Chinese Medicine 11:29–30

Cheng J C C 1970 Psychiatry in traditional Chinese medicine. Canadian Psychiatric Association Journal 15:399–401

Cheng Z C, Shi P F, Ji S H et al 1979 The clinical observation on the acupuncture treatment of acute bacillary dysentery. People's Medical Publishing House 39

Chiao S 1977 Scalp acupuncture in brain diseases. Chinese Medical Journal 3:325–328

Choudhury K J, Ffoulkes Crabbe DJO 1989 Acupuncture for bronchial asthma. Alternative Medicine 3:127–132

Chow O K W, So S Y, Lam W K, Yu D Y C, Yeung C Y 1983 Effect of acupuncture on exercise-induced asthma. Lung 161:321–326

Christensen P A, Laursen L C, Taudorf E, Sorensen S C, Weeke B 1984 Acupuncture and bronchial asthma. Allergy 39:379–385

Chu H, Zhao S, Huang Y 1987 Application of acupuncture to gastroscopy using a fibreoptic endoscope. Journal of Traditional Chinese Medicine 7:279

Chung K F 1994 Management of difficult asthma. British Journal of Hospital Medicine 51:80–81

Clavey S 1993 Asthma. The standard TCM approach. Pacific Journal of Oriental Medicine 1:9–21

Cui M 1992 Present status of research abroad concerning the effect of acupuncture and moxibustion on immunologic functions. Journal of Traditional Chinese Medicine 12(3):211–219

Dabov S, Goutoranov G, Ivanova R, Petkova N 1985 Clinical application of acupuncture in ophthalmology. Acupuncture and Electro-therapeutics Research 10:79–93

Dai J-L, Ren Z J, Fu Z M, Zhu Y H, Xu S F 1993 Electroacupuncture reversed the inhibition of intestinal peristalsis induced by intrathecal injection of morphine in rabbits. Chinese Medical Journal 106:220–224

Dale R A 1988 The Chinese acupressure eye exercises. American Journal of Acupuncture 16(4):366–367

De Giacomo E 1989 Céphalée et syndrome climatérique. La Revue Française de Médicine Traditionnelle Chinoise 133:60–61

Deng Q, Han Z 1990 Therapy of female tubal infertility under defocused CO_2 and He-Ne laser acupoint irradiation. Laser Therapy 2:117–118

Deng S 1985 Treatment and prevention of fulminant red-eye by acupuncture and blood-letting. Journal of Traditional Chinese Medicine 5(4):263–264

Dewar J, El Rakshy M 1993 Interpleural analgesia compared with acupuncture for post-nephrectomy syndrome. Acupuncture in Medicine 11:47–48

Dias P L R, Subramaniam S, Lionel N D W 1982 Effects of acupuncture in bronchial asthma preliminary communication. Journal of the Royal Society of Medicine 75: 245–248

Dill S G 1992 Acupuncture for gastrointestinal disorders. Problems in Veterinary Medicine 4:144–154

Dimond E G, Kittle C F, Crockett J E 1960 Evaluation of internal mammary artery ligation and sham procedure in angina pectoris. American Journal of Cardiology 5:483–486

Ding V, Roath S, Lewith G T 1983 Effect of acupuncture on lymphocyte behaviour. American Journal of Acupuncture 11(1):51–54

Dong S, Zhang Y, Yang K et al 1988 Clinical analysis of therapeutic efficacy in 365 cases of cholelithiasis treated by pressure over ear points. Journal of Traditional Chinese Medicine 6:1–5

Dong S, Zhang Y, Yang K et al 1988 Clinical analysis of therapeutic efficacy in 365 cases of cholelithiasis treated by pressure over ear points. Journal of Chinese Medicine 28:3–5

Dray A, Metsch R, Davis T P 1984 Endorphins and the central inhibition of urinary bladder motility. Peptides 5:645–647

Du X 1990 Clinical observation on acupuncture treatment of 200 cases of hemiplegia. International Journal of Clinical Acupuncture 1:229–233

Dundee J W, McMillan C 1991 Positive evidence for P6 acupuncture antiemesis. Postgraduate Medical Journal 67:417–422

Dunn P A, Rogers D, Halford K 1989 Transcutaneous electrical nerve stimulation at acupuncture points in the induction of uterine contractions. Obstetrics and Gynecology 73:286–290

Editorial 1974 Ear specialists doubt acupuncture has any effect in nerve deafness. Journal of the American Medical Association 228(12):1505–1514

Eisenberg L, Taub H A, DiCarlo L 1974 Acupuncture therapy of sensorineural deafness. New York State Journal of Medicine October:1942–1949

Ekblom A, Hansson P, Thomsson M, Thomas M 1991 Increased postoperative pain and consumption of analgesics following acupuncture. Pain 44:241–247

Ellis N 1993 A pilot study to evaluate the effect of acupuncture on nocturia in the elderly. Complementary Therapies in Medicine 1:164–167

Ellis N, Briggs R, Dowson D 1990 The effect of acupuncture on nocturnal urinary frequency and incontinence in the elderly. Complementary Medical Research 4:16–17

Ernst M, Lee M H M 1986 Sympathetic effects of manual and electrical acupuncture of the Tsusanli knee point: comparison with the Hoku hand point sympathetic effect. Experimental Neurology 94:1–10

Fang Y, Chen Y, Zhang Q 1990 CT scanning and therapeutic effects of acupuncture on 108 cases of hemiplegia due to apoplexy. International Journal of Clinical Acupuncture 1:1–6

Faust S 1991 Acupuncture for psychological problems. Acupuncture in Medicine 9:80–82

Feng R 1984 Relief of oesophageal carcinomatous obstruction by acupuncture. Journal of Traditional Chinese Medicine 4:3–4

Feng S, Fang L, Bao G et al 1985 Treatment of systemic lupus erythematosus by acupuncture. Chinese Medical Journal 98(3):171–176

Feng W 1989 Acupuncture treatment for 30 cases of infantile chronic diarrhea. Journal of Traditional Chinese Medicine 9:106–107

Filshie J, Penn K, Ashley S, Davis C L 1996 Acupuncture for the relief of cancer-related breathlessness. Palliative Medicine 10:145–150

Fischl F, Riegler R, Bieglmayer C, Nasr F, Neumark J 1984 Die beeinflußbarkeit der samenqualitat durch akupunktur bei subfertilen mannern. Geburtshilfe Frauenheilkunde 44:510–512

Flaws B 1985 Premenstrual syndrome (PMS): its differential diagnosis and treatment. American Journal of Acupuncture 13:205–222

Florez J, Hurle M A, Mediavilla A 1982 Respiratory responses to opiates applied to the medullary ventral surface. Life Sciences 31:2189–2192

Fu W 1991 Clinical practice of eye acupuncture. American Journal of Acupuncture 19(3):229–236

Fujiwara R, Zhou G T, Matsuoka H, Shibata H, Iwamoto M, Yokoyama M M 1991 Effects of acupuncture on immune response in mice. International Journal of Neuroscience 57:141–150

Fung K P, Chow O K W, So S Y 1986 Attenuation of exercise-induced asthma by acupuncture. Lancet 2: 1419–1422

Gao H 1991 Clinical observation of 65 cases of chronic urticaria treated with acupuncture. International Journal of Clinical Acupuncture 2(4):415–417

Gao Z, Yu X, Shen A, et al 1987 Acupuncture treatment of 54 cases of sinus bradycardia. Journal of Traditional Chinese Medicine 7(3):183–189

Gaponjuk P J, Sherkovina T J 1994 The clinical and physiological foundation of auricular acupuncture therapy in patients with hypertensive disease.

Acupuncture in Medicine 12(1):2–5

Gaponjuk P J, Sherkovina T J, Leonova M V 1993 Clinical effectiveness of auricular acupuncture treatment of patients with hypertensive disease. Acupuncture in Medicine 11(1):29–31

Ge S 1990 Treatment of alopecia areata with acupuncture. Journal of Traditional Chinese Medicine 10(3):199–200

Ge S, Meng F 1991 Acupuncture in the treatment of chronic prostatitis: a report of 350 cases. International Journal of Clinical Acupuncture 2:19–23

Ge S, Meng F, Xu B 1988 Acupuncture treatment in 102 cases of chronic prostatitis. Journal of Traditional Chinese Medicine 8:99–100

Gerhard I, Postneek F 1992 Auricular acupuncture in the treatment of female infertility. Gynecological Endocrinology 6:171–181

Gibson J S, Pardey J, Neville J 1988 Infrared low power laser therapy on acupuncture points for the treatment of detrusor instability. Proceedings of the International Continence Society: 146–147

Goidenko V S, Pierminova I S, Sitiel A B 1985 Use of auricular acupuncture reflexotherapy in treating Sjögren's disease. Stomatologia 64:47–48

Gu Y 1992 Treatment of acute abdomen by electro-acupuncture. A report of 245 cases. Journal of Traditional Chinese Medicine 12:110–113

Guorui J 1987 Lectures on formulating acupuncture prescriptions—selection and matching of acupoints. British Journal of Acupuncture 10:8–10

Gwee K A, Read N W 1994 Rolling review: disorders of gastrointestinal motility—therapeutic potentials and limitations. Alimentary Pharmacology and Therapeutics 8:105–118

Haddad G G, Gandhi M R, Hochwald G M, Lai T L 1983 Enkephalin-induced changes in ventilation and ventilatory pattern in adult dogs. Journal of Applied Physiology 55:1311–1320

Hallberg L, Hogdahl A, Nilsson L, Rybo G 1966 Menstrual blood loss—a population study. Acta Obstetricia et Gynaecologica Scandinavica 45:320–351

Han J S 1986 Electroacupuncture: an alternative to antidepressants for treating affective diseases? International Journal of Neuroscience 29:79–92

Han J S, Ding X Z, Fan S G 1986 Cholecystokinin octapeptide (CCK-8): Antagonism to electroacupuncture analgesia and a possible role in electroacupuncture tolerance. Pain 5:101–115

Hansen P E, Hansen J H 1983 Acupuncture treatment of chronic facial pain—a controlled cross-over trial. Headache 23(2):66–69

Hansen P E, Hansen J H, Bentzen O 1982 Acupuncture treatment of chronic unilateral tinnitus—a double-blind cross-over trial. Clinical Otolaryngology 7:325–329

Hansson S O, Mannheimer C 1991 Treatment with ear acupuncture in patients with severe angina pectoris. Pain Clinic 4:53–56

He J, Ma R, Zhu L, Wang Z 1988 Immediate relief and improved pulmonary functional changes in asthma symptom-complex treated by needle warming moxibustion. Journal of Traditional Chinese Medicine 8:164–166

He Z, Yie X, Gong H 1986 Acupuncture can influence the motive function of the stomach and intestine. Chen Tzu Yen Chiu 282–283

He-Jz 1989 The clinical application of helium-neon laser in paediatric ailments: a report of 1420 cases treated with low level laser therapy. Laser Therapy 1:75–78

Heinzl M W R 1986 When there is gallbladder trouble. American Journal of Acupuncture 14:83–84

Helms J M 1987 Acupuncture for the management of primary dysmenorrhea. Obstetrics and Gynecology 69:51–56

Herbert T B, Cohen S 1993 Depression and immunity: a meta-analytic review. Psychology Bulletin 113:472–486

Hollinger J A, I R, Pongratz W, Baum M 1979 Acupuncture anesthesia for open heart surgery: a report of 800 cases. American Journal of Chinese Medicine 7(1):77–90

Hou X 1989 30 Cases of postpartum dysuria treated with acupuncture. Journal of Traditional Chinese Medicine 9(2): 186

Hsu G S, Chen R X, Shen P K 1987 Protective effect of acupuncture on gastric mucosa in rats. Chen Tsu Yen Chiu 214–217

Hu S, Stern R M, Koch K L 1992 Electrical acustimulation relieves vection-induced motion sickness. Gastroenterology 102(6):1854–1858

Hu S, Stritzel R, Chandler A, Stern R M 1995 P6 acupressure reduces symptoms of vection-induced motion sickness. Aviation, Space, and Environmental Medicine 66:631–634

Huang D, Cheng D T, Das S K, Buda A J, Pitt B 1985 Effect of acupuncture on left ventricular size and function assessed by echocardiography in patients with stable dilated cardiomyopathy. Journal of Traditional Chinese Medicine 5(4):243–245

Huang H, Liang S 1992 Acupuncture at otopoint heart for treatment of vascular hypertension. Journal of Traditional Chinese Medicine 12(2):133–136

Huang W, Guo Z, Yu J, Hu X 1987 56 cases of chronic pruritus vulvae treated with acupuncture. Journal of Traditional Chinese Medicine 7(1):1–3

Hwang Y C, Jenkins E M 1988 Effect of acupuncture on young pigs with induced enteropathogenic Escherichia coli diarrhea. American Journal of Veterinary Research 49:1641–1643

Iliev E, Nicolov K, Todorova I 1990 The effects of psychological factors and the influence of electroacupuncture on immunological parameters in patients with alopecia areata. Acupuncture in Medicine 8(2):56–58

Iliev E, Popov J, Nicolov K 1995 Evaluation of clinical and immunological parameters in patients with lichen ruber planus treated with acupuncture. Acupuncture in Medicine 13(2):91–92

Iwa M, Sakita M 1994 Effects of acupuncture and moxibustion on intestinal motility in mice. American Journal of Chinese Medicine 22:119–125

Jansen G, Lundeberg T, Samuelson U E, Thomas M 1989 Increased survival of ischaemic musculocutaneous flaps in rats after acupuncture. Acta Physiologica Scandinavica 135:555–558

Jia D 1993 Current applications of acupuncture by otorhinolaryngologists. Journal of Traditional Chinese Medicine 13(1):59–64

Jiang R 1990 Analgesic effect of acupuncture on acute intestinal colic in 190 cases. Journal of Traditional Chinese Medicine 10:20–21

Jiao G 1986 Lectures on formulating acupuncture prescriptions—selection and matching of acupoints.

Journal of Traditional Chinese Medicine 6:128–130

Jin A 1987 Acupuncture therapy in 67 cases of asthenic childhood prolapse of rectum. Journal of Traditional Chinese Medicine 7:141–142

Jobst K A 1995 A critical analysis of acupuncture in pulmonary disease: efficacy and safety of the acupuncture needle. Journal of Alternative and Complementary Medicine 1:57–85

Jobst K, Chen J H, McPherson K et al 1986 Controlled trial of acupuncture for disabling breathlessness. Lancet 2:1416–1419

Johansson A, Wenneberg B, Wagersten C, Haraldson T 1991 Acupuncture in treatment of facial muscular pain. Acta Odontologica Scandinavica 49:153–158

Johansson B B 1993 Has sensory stimulation a role in stroke rehabilitation? Scandinavian Journal of Rehabilitation Medicine Suppl 29:87–96

Johansson B B, Grabowski M 1994 Functional recovery after brain infarction: plasticity and neural transplantation. Brain Pathology 4:85–95

Johansson K, Lindgren I, Widner H, Wiklund I, Johansson B B 1993 Can sensory stimulation improve the functional outcome in stroke patients? Neurology 43:2189–2192

Kaada B 1982 Vasodilatation induced by transcutaneous nerve stimulation in peripheral ischaemia (Raynaud's phenomenon and diabetic polyneuropathy). European Heart Journal 3:303–314

Kaada B 1983 Promoted healing of chronic ulceration by transcutaneous nerve stimulation (TNS). VASA 12:262–269

Kaada B, Hognestad S, Haustad J 1989 Transcutaneous nerve stimulation (TNS) in tinnitus. Scandinavian Audiology 18:211–217

Kadar T, Pesti A, Penke B, Telegdy G 1984 Inhibition of seizures induced by picrotoxin and electroshock by cholecystokinin octapeptides and their fragments in rats after intracerebroventricular administration. Neuropharmacology 23:955–961

Kane J, Di Scipio W J 1979 Acupuncture treatment of schizophrenia: report on three cases. American Journal of Psychiatry 136:297–302

Kasahara T, Wu Y, Sakurai Y, Oguchi K 1992 Suppressive effect of acupuncture on delayed type hypersensitivity to trinitrochlorobenzene and involvement of opiate receptors. International Journal of Immunopharmacy 14(4):661–665

Kasahara T, Amemiya M, Wu Y, Oguchi K 1993 Involvement of central opioidergic and nonopioidergic neuroendocrine systems in the suppressive effect of acupuncture on delayed type hypersensitivity in mice. International Journal of Immunopharmacy 15(4):501–508

Kelleher C J, Filshie J, Burton G, Khullar V, Cardozo L D 1994 Acupuncture and the treatment of irritative bladder symptoms. Acupuncture in Medicine 12:9–12

Kho H G, Eijk R J R, Kapteijns W M M J, van Egmond J 1991a Forum. Acupuncture and transcutaneous stimulation analgesia in comparison with moderate-dose fentanyl anaesthesia in major surgery. Clinical efficacy and influence on recovery and morbidity. Anaesthesia 46:129–135

Kho H G, Van Egmond J, Eijk R J R, Kapteyns W M M J 1991b Lack of influence of acupuncture and transcutaneous stimulation on the immunoglobulin levels and leucocyte counts following upper-abdominal surgery. European Journal of Anaesthesiology 8:39–45

Khoe W H 1975 Chronic ulcerative and spastic colitis treated with acupuncture and nutrition. American Journal of Acupuncture 3:211–214

Klarskov P 1987 Enkephalin inhibits presynaptically the contractility of urinary tract smooth muscle. British Journal of Urology 59:31–35

Klauser A G, Rubach A, Bertsche O, Muller-Lissner S A 1993 Body acupuncture: effect on colonic function in chronic constipation. Zeitschrift für Gastroenterologie 31:605–608

Kleijnen J, Ter Riet G, Knipschild P 1991 Acupuncture and asthma: a review of controlled trials. Thorax 46:799–802

Kubista E, Kucera H, Muller-Tyl E 1975 Initiating contractions of the gravid uterus through electro-acupuncture. American Journal of Chinese Medicine 3:343–346

Lai C, Lai Y C 1991 History of epilepsy in Chinese Traditional Medicine. Epilepsia 32:299–302

Lane D J, Lane T V 1991 Alternative and complementary medicine for asthma. Thorax 46:787–797

Lao H H 1988 Acupuncture treatment of mycosis fungoides. American Journal of Acupuncture 16(3):221–224

Lau B H S, Wong D S, Slater J M 1975 Effect of acupuncture on allergic rhinitis: clinical and laboratory evaluations. American Journal of Chinese Medicine 3(3):263–270

Lee G T C 1974 A study of electrical stimulation of acupuncture locus susanli (ST-36) on mesenteric microcirculation. American Journal of Chinese Medicine 2:53–66

Lee T-N 1976 Treatment of rhinitis with acupuncture. American Journal of Acupuncture 4(4):357–361

Lee Y, Lee W, Chen M, Huang J, Chung C, Chang L S 1992 Acupuncture in the treatment of renal colic. Journal of Urology 147:16–18

Leijon G, Boivie J 1989 Central post-stroke pain—the effect of high and low frequency TENS. Pain 38:187–191

Lewers D, Clelland J A, Jackson J R, Varner R E, Bergman J 1989 Transcutaneous electrical nerve stimulation in the relief of primary dysmenorrhea. Physical Therapy 69:3–9

Lewis P J 1992 Irritable bowel syndrome. Emotional factors and acupuncture treatment. Journal of Chinese Medicine 40:9–11

Li B, Li L L, Chen J 1993 Observation on the relation between propagated sensation along meridians and the therapeutic effect of acupuncture on myopia of youngsters. Chen Tzu Yen Chiu 18(2):154–158 [Chinese]

Li C, Bi L, Zhu B et al 1986 Effects of acupuncture on left ventricular function, microcirculation, cAMP and cGMP of acute myocardial infarction patients. Journal of Traditional Chinese Medicine 6:157–161

Li F, Wang D, Ma X 1991 Treatment of hiccoughs with auriculoacupuncture. Journal of Traditional Chinese Medicine 11:14–16

Li P 1985 Modulatory effect of electroacupuncture on cardiovascular functions. Journal of Traditional Chinese Medicine 5(3):211–214

Li P, Sun F, Zhang A-Z 1983 The effect of acupuncture on blood pressure: the interrelation of sympathetic activity and endogenous opioid peptides. Acupuncture and Electro-therapeutics Research 8:45–46

Li W, Chen H, Mao Z 1993 Therapeutic effects of acupuncture in 56 cases of postpartum retention of urine. International Journal of Clinical Acupuncture 4 (1):101–103

Li X, Yi J, Qi B 1990 Treatment of hiccough with auriculo-acupuncture and auriculo-pressure. A report of 85 cases. Journal of Traditional Chinese Medicine 10:257–259

Li Y, Tougas G, Chiverton S G, Hunt R H 1992 The effect of acupuncture on gastrointestinal function and disorders. American Journal of Gastroenterology 87:1372–1381

Li Z 1987 Observation of curative effects of emergency acupuncture treatment in 172 cases of infantile toxic intestinal paralysis. Journal of Traditional Chinese Medicine 7:209–210

Liao S J 1988 Acupuncture for poison ivy contact dermatitis, a clinical case report. Acupuncture and Electro-therapeutics Research 13:31–39

Liao S J, Liao T A 1991 Acupuncture treatment for herpes simplex infections. Acupuncture and Electro-therapeutics Research 16:135–142

Liao S J, Liao T A 1992 Acupuncture treatment for psoriasis: a retrospective case report. Acupuncture and Electro-therapeutics Research 17: 195–208

Lin J H, Liu S H, Chan W W, Wu L S, Pi W P 1988 Effects of electroacupuncture and gonadotropin-releasing hormone treatments on hormonal changes in anoestrous sows. American Journal of Chinese Medicine XVI: 117–126

Lin Y 1987 Observation of therapeutic effects of acupuncture treatment in 170 cases of infantile diarrhea. Journal of Traditional Chinese Medicine 7:203–204

Liu G, Liu J, Liu S 1992 A clinical report of 255 cases of amenorrhea treated by acupuncture and moxibustion. International Journal of Clinical Acupuncture 3:419–421

Liu J 1987 Treatment of 86 cases of local neurodermatitis by electro-acupuncture (with needles inserted around diseased areas). Journal of Traditional Chinese Medicine 7(1):67

Liu J D 1987 Electrical needle therapy of uremic pruritus. Nephron 47:179–183

Liu Q, Deng Y, Li L, Lin G 1982 Evaluation of acupuncture treatment for sensorineural deafness and deafmutism based on 20 years' experience. Chinese Medical Journal 95(1):21–24

Liu W, Zhang J, Zhang Y, Pei T 1988 Acupuncture treatment of functional uterine bleeding—a clinical observation of 30 cases. Journal of Traditional Chinese Medicine 8:31–33

Liu X, Sun L, Xiao J I 1993 Effect of acupuncture and point-function in rheumatoid arthritis. Journal of Traditional Chinese Medicine 13(3):174–178

Lo C W, Chung Q Y 1979 The sedative effect of acupuncture. American Journal of Chinese Medicine VII:253–258

Lou H, Jia Y, Wu X, Dai W 1990 Electro-acupuncture in the treatment of depressive psychosis. A controlled prospective randomised trial using electro-acupuncture and amitriptyline in 241 patients. International Journal of Clinical Acupuncture 1:7–13

Lu J-G, Friberg T 1987 Idiopathic central serous retinopathy in China: a report of 600 cases (624 eyes) treated by acupuncture. Ophthalmic Surgery 18(8):608–611

Lu S 1990 Stomachache treated with acupuncture and moxibustion. International Journal of Clinical Acupuncture 1:283–288

Lu S 1991a Scalp acupuncture therapy and its clinical application. Journal of Traditional Chinese Medicine 11:272–280

Lu S 1991b Acupuncture therapy in the treatment of dysmenorrhea. International Journal of Clinical Acupuncture 2:283–291

Lu S Acupuncture therapy in skin diseases (1) 1992a

International Journal of Clinical Acupuncture 3(2):67–72

Lu S Acupuncture therapy in skin diseases (2) 1992b International Journal of Clinical Acupuncture 3(2):159–164

Lu S Acupuncture therapy in skin diseases (3) 1992c International Journal of Clinical Acupuncture 3(2):289–295

Lundeberg T 1993 Peripheral effects of sensory nerve stimulation (acupuncture) in inflammation and ischemia. Scandinavian Journal of Rehabilitation Medicine 29(suppl): 61–86

Lundeberg T, Bondesson L, Thomas M 1987 Effect of acupuncture on experimentally induced itch. British Journal of Dermatology 117:771–777

Lundeberg T, Hurtig T, Lundeberg S, Thomas M 1988 Long-term results of acupuncture in chronic head and neck pain. Pain Clinic 2(1):15–31

Lundeberg T, Kjartansson J, Samuelson U 1988 Effect of electrical nerve stimulation on healing of ischaemic skin flaps. Lancet 2:712–715

Lundeberg T, Eriksson S V, Theodorsson E 1991 Neuroimmunomodulatory effects of acupuncture in mice. Neuroscience Letters 128:161–164

Luo F 1992 Auricular-plaster therapy for treating 155 cases of allergic rhinitis. International Journal of Clinical Acupuncture 3(2):205–207

Luo H C, Jia Y K, Li Z 1985 Electroacupuncture vs amitriptyline in the treatment of depressive states. Journal of Traditional Chinese Medicine 5:3–8

Luu M, Maillard D, Pradalier A, Boureau F 1985 Controle spirometrique dans la maladie asthmatique des effets de la puncture de points douloureux thoraciques. Respiration 48:340–345

Lux G, Hagel J, Backer P et al 1994 Acupuncture inhibits vagal gastric acid secretion stimulated by sham feeding in healthy subjects. Gut 35:1026–1029

Lyttleton J 1988 The treatment of endometriosis. Journal of Chinese Medicine 26:3–7

McDaniel J S 1992 Psychoimmunology: implications for future research. Southern Medical Journal 85(4):388–396

Macdonald M 1992 Acupuncture in ophthalmology. Acupuncture in Medicine 10(1):18–21

Madell J R 1975 Acupuncture for sensorineural hearing loss. Archives of Otolaryngol 101:441–445

Maeda M, Ichiki Y, Sumi A, Mori S 1988 A trial of acupuncture for progressive systemic sclerosis. Journal of Dermatology 15:133–140

Magnusson M, Johansson K, Johansson B B 1994 Sensory stimulation promotes normalization of postural control after stroke. Stroke 25:1176–1180

Mann F 1974 Acupuncture in auditory and related disorders. British Journal of Audiology 8:23–25

Mann F 1992 Reinventing acupuncture: a new concept of ancient medicine. Butterworth Heinemann, Oxford

Mannheimer C, Emanuelsson H, Waagstein F, Wilhelmsson C 1989 Influence of naloxone on the effects of high frequency transcutaneous electrical nerve stimulation in angina pectoris induced by atrial pacing. British Heart Journal 62:36–42

Marks N J, Emery P, Onisiphorou C 1984 A controlled trial of acupuncture in tinnitus. Journal of Laryngology and Otology 98:1103–1109

Martoudis S G, Christofides K 1990 Electroacupuncture for pain relief in labour. Acupunct Med 7:51–53

Minni B, Capozza N, Creti G, De Gennaro M, Caione P, Bischko J 1990 Bladder instability and enuresis treated by acupuncture and electrotherapeutics: early urodynamic observations. Acupuncture and Electro-therapeutics Research 15:19–25

Mitchell P, Wells J E 1989 Acupuncture for chronic asthma: a controlled trial with six months follow-up. American Journal of Acupuncture 17:5–13

Moehrle M, Blum A, Lorenz F, Roesch G, Steins A, Juenger M, Hahn M 1995 Proceedings of the 2nd Asian Congress for Microcirculation, Beijing, p 10

Morton A R, Fazio S M, Miller D 1993 Efficacy of laser-acupuncture in the prevention of exercise-induced asthma. Annals of Allergy 70:295–298

Murray K H A 1983 Effect of naloxone induced opioid blockade on idiopathic detrusor instability. Urology 22: 329–331

Murray K H A, Feneley R C A 1982 Endorphins. A role in lower urinary tract function? The effect of opioid blockade on the detrusor and urethral sphincter mechanisms. British Journal of Urology 54:638–640

Nagano K 1991 Immune enhancement through acupuncture and moxibustion: specific treatment for allergic disorders, mild infectious disease and secondary infections. American Journal of Acupuncture 19(4):329–338

Neighbors L E, Clelland J, Jackson J R, Bergman J, Orr J 1987 Transcutaneous electrical nerve stimulation for pain relief in primary dysmenorrhea. Clinical Journal of Pain 3:17–22

Nilsson S, Axelsson A, De G L 1992 Acupuncture for tinnitus management. Scandinavian Audiology 21:245–251

Oei L T, Chen X H, Van Ree J, Han J S 1992 Potentiation of electroacupuncture-induced analgesia by CCK-8 antagonist L-365, 260 in Wistar rats but not in acoustically-evoked epileptic rats. Acupuncture in Medicine X:47–52

Ohlsson A L, Johansson B B 1995 Environment influences functional outcome of cerebral infarction in rats. Stroke 26:644–649

Östberg O, Horie Y, Feng Y 1992 On the merits of ancient Chinese eye acupressure practices. Applied Ergonomics 23(5):343–348

Ottenbacher K J, Jannell S 1993 The results of clinical trials in stroke rehabilitation research. Archives of Neurology 50:37–44

Outline of Chinese acupuncture 1975 Foreign Language Press, Peking

Ouyang J Y, Ding X J, Fan Le 1984 Electroacupuncture protects gastric mucosa from chemical injury. Abstract. Abstracts of National Symposuim of Acupuncture, Beijing, p 381

Ouyang Q, Cao M, Cao Q 1992 An observation on the effect of moxibustion on the immunological functions in 69 cases of lung cancer. International Journal of Clinical Acupuncture 3(4):369–373

Ouyang Z R, Fan L, Gong Q H 1987 Comparison of the effect of stimulating the femoral nerve, artery and lymphatic vessels with acupuncture at Zusanli on intestinal motility in rabbits. Shanghai Journal of Acupuncture 4:14–16

Panzer R B, Chrisman C L 1994 An auricular acupuncture treatment for idiopathic canine epilepsy: A preliminary report. American Journal of Chinese Medicine 22:11–17

Peck G 1989 The treatment of scars by acupuncture. Journal of Chinese Medicine (May) 30:23–24

Philp T, Shah P J R, Worth P H L 1988 Acupuncture in the treatment of bladder instability. British Journal of Urology 61:490–493

Pigne A, de Goursac C, Nyssen C, Barrat J 1985 Acupuncture

and Unstable Bladder. Abstracts of the 15th Meeting of the International Continence Society pp 186–187

Podoshin L, Ben-David Y, Fradis M, Gerstel R, Felner H 1989 Idiopathic subjective tinnitus treated by biofeedback, acupuncture and drug therapy. Ear, Nose and Throat Journal 70(5): 284–289

Poletti J, Poletti A, Franzini S, Durand F 1989 Etude des potentiels evoqués visuels par renversement de pattern en hémichamp sous acupuncture au cours d'hémianopsies latérales homonymes. Bulletin de la Société Ophthalmologique de France 11(89):1339–1342

Politis M J, Korchinski M A 1990 Beneficial effects of acupuncture treatment following experimental spinal cord injury: a behavioral, morphological, and biochemical study. Acupuncture and Electro-therapeutics Research 15:37–49

Pothmann R 1992 Brief acupuncture treatment for dermatitis solaris: a multicentre pilot study. Acupuncture in Medicine 10(2):64–65

Pothman R, Yeh H L 1982 The effects of treatment with antibiotics, laser and acupuncture upon chronic maxillary sinusitis in children. American Journal of Chinese Medicine 10(1–4):55–58

Qi L Y, Zhang Z H, Ye C G, Li J B, Hu J K 1990 Observation on acupuncture treatment of 322 cases of cerebral infarction and changes in serum HDL-C, fibrinogen, FDP, hemorrheological indices etc. during treatment. International Journal of Clinical Acupuncture 1:39–46

Qin G, Tang H 1989 413 cases of abnormal fetal position corrected by auricular plaster therapy. Journal of Traditional Chinese Medicine 9:235–237

Qiu M L, Sheng C R, Li N Y 1979 Researches on treatment of acute bacillary dysentery by acupuncture. Abstracts of 1st National Symposium of Acupuncture, Beijing, pp 2–5

Radzievsky S A, Fisenko L A, Dmitriev V K 1988 Possible mechanisms of acupuncture as an independent method for treating ischaemic heart disease. American Journal of Acupuncture 16(4):323–328

Ralston N C 1977 Successful treatment and management of acute glaucoma using acupuncture. American Journal of Acupuncture 5(3):283

Reddy N S, Fouzdar N M 1983 Role of acupuncture in the treatment of 'incurable' retinal diseases. Indian Journal of Ophthalmology 31 (suppl 31):1043–1046

Rempp C, Bigler A 1991 Pregnancy and acupuncture from conception to postpartum. American Journal of Acupuncture 19:305–313

Requena Y 1981 Ulcerative colitis treated by traditional Chinese acupuncture. American Journal of Acupuncture 9:341–346

Ribaute A 1987 Stabilisation de la myopie évolutive, par acupuncture, chez des enfants prépubères. La Revue Française de Médicine Traditionelle Chinoise 125:309–311

Richter A, Herlitz J, Hjalmarson A 1991 Effect of acupuncture in patients with angina pectoris. European Heart Journal 12:175–178

Rogvi-Hansen B, Perrild H, Christensen T, Detmar S E, Siersbæk-Nielsen K, Hansen J E M 1991 Acupuncture in the treatment of Graves' ophthalmopathy. A blinded randomized study. Acta Endocrinologica (Copenhagen) 124:143–145

Romoli M, Giommi A 1993 Ear acupuncture in psychosomatic medicine: the importance of the sanjiao (triple heater) area. Acupuncture and Electro-therapeutics Research 18:185–194

Roppolo J R, Booth A M, De Groot W C 1983 The effects of naloxone on the neural control of the urinary bladder of the cat. Brain Research 264:355–358

Rosen S 1974 Acupuncture and Chinese medical practices. Volta Review 76:340–350

Rosted P 1992a A protocol for successful treatment of chronic skin diseases with acupuncture. American Journal of Acupuncture 20(4):321–326

Rosted P 1992b The treatment of skin disease by acupuncture. Acupuncture in Medicine 10(2):66–68

Rosted P 1994 Survey of recent clinical studies on the treatment of skin diseases with acupuncture. American Journal of Acupuncture 22(4):357–361

Rubinfeld A R, Pain M C F 1976 Perception of asthma. Lancet 882–884

Sakic B, Kojic L, Jankovic B D, Skokljev A 1989 Electroacupuncture modifies humoral immune response in the rat. Acupuncture and Electro-therapeutics Research 14: 115–120

Sallstrom S, Kjendahl A, Osten P E, Stanghelle J K, Borchgrevink C F 1996 Acupuncture in the treatment of stroke patients in the subacute stage: a randomised controlled study. Complementary Therapies in Medicine 4: 193–197

Salvi E, Pistilli A, Romiti P, Bedogni G, Pedrazzoli C 1983 Ulcera duodenale. Aspetti gastroscopici prima e dopo trattamento agopunturale. Minerva Medica 74(42):2541–2546

Sanner G, Sundequist U 1981 Acupuncture for the relief of painful muscle spasms in dystonic cerebral palsy. Developmental Medicine and Child Neurology 23:544–545

Shapiro R S, Stockard H E, Schank A 1988 Uremic pruritus successfully controlled with acupuncture. Dialysis and Transplantation 17(4):180–183, 189

Shi B, Bu H, Lin L 1992 A clinical study on acupuncture treatment of pediatric cerebral palsy. Journal of Traditional Chinese Medicine 12:45–51

Shi Z, Gong B, Jia Y, Huo Z 1987 The efficacy of electro-acupuncture on 98 cases of epilepsy. Journal of Traditional Chinese Medicine 7:21–22

Shi Z, Tan M 1986 An analysis of the therapeutic effect of acupuncture treatment in 500 cases of schizophrenia. Journal of Traditional Chinese Medicine 6:99–104

Silva S A 1989 Acupuncture for the relief of pain of facial and dental origin. Anesthesia Progress 36(4–5):244–245

Sin Y M 1983 Effect of electric acupuncture and moxibustion on phagocytic activity of the reticulo-endothelial system of mice. American Journal of Acupuncture 11(3):237–241

Skelton I F, Flowerdew M W 1988 Acupuncture and labour—a summary of results. Midwives Chronicle and Nursing Notes 101:134–137

Skrabanek P 1987 Acupuncture and asthma. Lancet 1:1082–1083

Sliwinski J, Kulej M 1989 Acupuncture induced immunoregulatory influence on the clinical state of patients suffering from chronic spastic bronchitis and undergoing long-term treatment with corticosteroids. Acupuncture and Electro-therapeutics Research 14:227–234

Sliwinski J, Matusiewicz R 1984 The effect of acupuncture on the clinical state of patients suffering from chronic spastic bronchitis and undergoing long term treatment with corticosteroids. Acupuncture and Electro-therapeutics Research 9:203–215

Slocumb J C 1984 Neurologic factors in chronic pelvic pain. Trigger points and the abdominal pelvic pain syndrome. American Journal of Obstetrics and Gynecology 149:536–543

Sodipo J O A, Falaiye J M 1979 Acupuncture and gastric acid studies. American Journal of Chinese Medicine 7:356–361

Sold-Darseff J, Leydecker W 1986 Acupuncture for pain in the cranial region and for blepharospasm without organic cause. Klinische Monatsblätter für Augenheilkunde 189(2):167–169 [German]

Song B, Wang X 1985 Short-term effect in 135 cases of enuresis treated by wrist-ankle needling. Journal of Traditional Chinese Medicine 5:27–28

Sovijarvi A, Poppius H 1977 Acute bronchodilating effect of transcutaneous nerve stimulation in asthma. A peripheral reflex or psychogenic response. Scandinavian Journal of Respiratory Diseases 58:164–169

Staebler F E 1985 Acupuncture in childbirth. British Journal of Acupuncture 8:3–12

Steinberger A 1981 The treatment of dysmenorrhea by acupuncture. American Journal of Chinese Medicine IX: 57–60

Steinberger A 1986 Specific irritability of acupuncture points as an early symptom of multiple sclerosis. American Journal of Chinese Medicine 14:175–178

Sternfield M, Shalev Y, Eliraz A, Kauli N, Hod I, Bentwich Z 1987 Effect of acupuncture on symptomatology and objective cardiac parameters in angina pectoris. American Journal of Acupuncture 15(2):149–152

Sternfeld M, Finkelstein Y, Segal Y, Katz Z, Eliraz A, Hod I 1993 The effect of acupuncture on functional and anatomic uterine disturbances: case report—secondary infertility and myomas. American Journal of Acupuncture 21:5–7

Story R T 1989 Acupuncture and blepharospasm: a five case study. American Journal of Acupuncture 17(4):321–324

Su J, Tu J 1987 Experience with treatment of warts by acupuncture and its evaluation. Journal of Traditional Chinese Medicine 7(3):199–202

Su X 1987a The treatment of haemorrhoids by acupuncture. Journal of Chinese Medicine 25:23–24

Su X 1987b The treatment of acute pancreatitis by acupuncture. Journal of Chinese Medicine 25:24–25

Su Z 1992 Acupuncture treatment of infantile diarrhea: a report of 1050 cases. Journal of Traditional Chinese Medicine 12:120–121

Sun X-Y, Yu J, Yao T 1983 Pressor effect produced by stimulation of somatic nerve on hemorrhagic hypotension in conscious rats. Acta Physiologica Sinica 35(3):264–270

Takeshi A, Toru M, Masayoshi M, Toshio N, Kaname K, Seiya K 1976 The influence of acupuncture stimulation on plasma levels of LH, FSH, progesterone and estradiol in normally ovulating women. American Journal of Chinese Medicine 4: 391–401

Takishima T, Mue S, Tamura G, Ishihara T, Watanabe K 1982 The bronchodilating effect of acupuncture in patients with acute asthma. Annals of Allergy 48:44–49

Tam K-C, Yiu H-H 1975 The effect of acupuncture on essential hypertension. American Journal of Chinese Medicine 3(4):369–375

Tandon M K, Soh P F T 1989 Comparison of real and placebo acupuncture in histamine-induced asthma. A double-blind crossover study. Chest 96:102–105

Tandon M K, Soh P F T, Wood A T 1991 Acupuncture for bronchial asthma? A double-blind crossover study. Medical Journal of Australia 154:409–412

Tang Z 1987 Assessment of acupuncture in the prevention of sudden death from coronary heart disease. Journal of Traditional Chinese Medicine 7(2):142–146

Tao D J 1993 Research on the reduction of anxiety and depression with acupuncture. American Journal of Acupuncture 21:327–330

Tashkin D P, Bresler D E, Kroening R J, Kerschner H, Katz R L, Coulson A H 1977 Comparison of real and simulated acupuncture and isoproterenol in methacholine-induced asthma. Annals of Allergy 39:379–387

Tashkin D P, Kroening R J, Bresler D E, Simmons M, Coulson A, Kerschner H 1985 A controlled trial of real and simulated acupuncture in the management of chronic asthma. Journal of Allergy and Clinical Immunology 76:855–864

Taub H A 1975 Acupuncture and sensorineural hearing loss: a review. Journal of Speech and Hearing Disorders 40:427–433

Tayama F, Muteki T, Bekki S et al 1984 Cardiovascular effects of electro-acupuncture. Kurume Medical Journal 31:37–46

Thomas M, Laurell G, Lundeberg T 1988 Acupuncture for the alleviation of tinnitus. Laryngoscope 98:664–667

Thomas M, Lundeberg T, Bjork G, Lundstrom-Lindstedt V 1995 Pain and discomfort in primary dysmenorrhea is reduced by preemptive acupuncture or low frequency TENS. European Journal of Physical Medicine and Rehabilitation 5:71–76

Tian C 1991 Moxibustion on walnut shells in the frames of spectacles in treating pigmentary degeneration of the retina. International Journal of Clinical Acupuncture 2(1):45–49

Tohya K, Mastrogiovanni F, Sugata R et al 1989 Suppression of the DTH reaction in mice by means of moxibustion at electro-permeable points. American Journal of Chinese Medicine 17(3–4): 139–144

Tougas G, Yuan L Y, Radamaker J W, Chiverton S G, Hunt R H 1992a Effect of acupuncture on gastric acid secretion in healthy male volunteers. Digestive Diseases and Sciences 37:1576–1582

Tougas G, Fitzpatrick D, Hudoba P et al 1992b Effects of chronic left vagal stimulation on visceral vagal function in man. PACE 15: 1588–1596

Travell J G, Simons D G 1983 Myofascial pain and dysfunction. Williams & Wilkins, Baltimore

Tuzuner F, Kecik Y, Ozdemir S, Canakci N 1989 Electro-acupuncture in the treatment of enuresis nocturna. Acupuncture and Electro-therapeutics Research 14:211–215

Upton A R M, Tougas G, Talalla A et al 1991 Neurophysiological effects of left vagal stimulation in man. PACE 14:70–76

Vincent C A, Richardson P H 1987 Acupuncture for some common disorders: a review of evaluative research. Journal of the Royal College of General Practitioners 37:77–81

Virsik K, Kiristufek P, Bangha O, Urban S 1980 The effect of acupuncture on pulmonary function in bronchial asthma. Progress in Respiratory Research 14:271–275

Wagenaar R C, Meijer O G 1991 Effects of stroke rehabilitation (1). A critical review of the literature. Journal of Rehabilitation Sciences 4:61–73

Wan Y, Yu L 1981 Volvulus of the stomach successfully treated with acupuncture. Report of 9 cases. Journal of Traditional Chinese Medicine 1:39–42

Wang B E, Yang R, Cheng J S 1994 Effect of electroacupuncture on the level of preproenkephalin mRNA in rat during penicillin-induced epilepsy. Acupuncture and Electro-therapeutics Research 19:129–140

Wang G, Zhang S, Lin H et al 1987 Nonoperative treatment of Hirschsprung's disease: a new approach. Journal of Pediatric Surgery 22:439–442

Wang H, Ye D, Lin Q 1992 Scalp acupuncture in treating 20 cases of hemiplegia. International Journal of Clinical Acupuncture 3:307–309

Wang M 1991 Treatment of local scleroderma of progressive systemic sclerosis by acupuncture. International Journal of Clinical Acupuncture 2(2):207–209

Wang X 1987 Observations of the therapeutic effects of acupuncture and moxibustion in 100 cases of dysmenorrhea. Journal of Traditional Chinese Medicine 7:15–17

Warwick-Evans L A, Masters I J, Redstone S B 1991 A double-blind placebo controlled evaluation of acupressure in the treatment of motion sickness. Aviation, Space, and Environmental Medicine August 1991:776–778

Webb R J, Powell P H 1992 Transcutaneous electrical nerve stimulation in patients with idiopathic detrusor instability. Neurourology and Urodynamics 11:327–328

Wei Q 1992 Treatment of optic atrophy with acupuncture. Journal of Traditional Chinese Medicine 12(2): 142–146

Wei W 1977 Scalp acupuncture in China. American Journal of Chinese Medicine 5: 101–104

Wen H L, Chau K 1973 Status asthmaticus treated by acupuncture and electro-stimulation. Asian Journal of Medicine (January) 9:191–195

Wen H L, Cheung S Y C 1973 Treatment of drug addiction by acupuncture and electrical stimulation. Asian Journal of Medicine 9:138–141

WHO 1980 Use of acupuncture in modern health care. WHO Chronicle 34:294–301

Williams T, Mueller K, Cornwall M W 1991 Effect of acupuncture-point stimulation on diastolic blood pressure in hypertensive subjects: a preliminary study. Physical Therapy 71:523–529

Williamson L 1994 Hay fever prophylaxis using single point acupuncture: a pilot study. Acupuncture in Medicine 12(2):84–87

Williamson L, Yudkin P, Livingstone R, Prasad K, Fuller A, Lawrence M 1996 Hay fever treatment in general practice—randomised controlled trial comparing standardised Western acupuncture with sham acupuncture. Acupuncture in Medicine 14(1):6–10

Wong L P 1988 Successful treatment of paralysis of the lower extremity with acupuncture. American Journal of Acupuncture 16:329–344

Wong S, Ching R 1980 The use of acupuncture in ophthalmology American Journal of Chinese Medicine 8(2):104–153

Wong S K A 1983 Treatment of hiccough by acupuncture—a report of two cases. Medical Journal of Malaysia 38:80–81

World Health Organization 1995 International Statistical Classification of Disease and Related Health Problems, 10th revision

Wu B, Yue Y, Zhuang X 1990 A primary study on the effect of ear needling to reduce intraocular pressure in glaucoma patients. International Journal of Clinical Acupuncture 1(4):409–412

Wu J-L, Chai X-M, Wang Y-L 1985 Acupuncture effects upon alpha-naphthyl-acetate esterase staining patterns of circulating lymphocytes and e-rosette forming cells.

Chinese Medical Journal 98(10):753–758

Wu, X, Cui Y, Yang B, Zhou Q 1987 Observations on the effect of He-Ne laser acupoint radiation in chronic pelvic inflammation. Journal of Traditional Chinese Medicine 7: 263–265

Wu Z, Jin S, Zheng Z 1985 The effect of acupuncture in 40 cases of endocrine ophthalmopathy. Journal of Traditional Chinese Medicine 5(1):19–21

Wu Z, Ye X 1989 Optic atrophy teated with acupuncture. Journal of Traditional Chinese Medicine 9(4):249–250

Wyon Y, Lindgren R, Lundeberg T, Hammar M 1995 Effects of acupuncture on climacteric vasomotor symptoms, quality of life and urinary-excretion of neuropeptides among postmenopausal women. Menopause Journal of the North American Menopause Society 2(1): 3–12

Xia L, Huang S 1991 Acupuncture treatment in 8 cases of dysphagia. International Journal of Clinical Acupuncture 2:427–428

Xia Y, Qi R, Xu H, Li L 1987 On the therapeutic efficacy of thermoelectric acupuncture in 55 cases of kraurosis vulvae. Journal of Traditional Chinese Medicine 7:161–164

Xia Y Q, Zhang D, Yang J C, Xu H, Li Y, Ma L 1986 An approach to the effect on tumours of acupuncture in combination with radiotherapy or chemotherapy. Journal of Traditional Chinese Medicine 6(1):23–26

Xiao J, Xie G, Dong J 1992 Study on the effect of acupuncture analgesia for postoperative pain of anal disease. International Journal of Clinical Acupuncture 3:183–185

Xu B 1991 302 cases of enuresis treated with acupuncture. Journal of Traditional Chinese Medicine 11:121–122

Xu B, Shuhan G 1987 Treatment of Meniere's disease by acupuncture: report of 75 cases. Journal of Traditional Chinese Medicine 7(1):69–70

Xu Y 1989 Treatment of acne with ear acupuncture—a clinical observation of 80 cases. Journal of Traditional Chinese Medicine 9(4):238–239

Xu Y 1990 Treatment of facial skin diseases with acupuncture. Journal of Traditional Chinese Medicine 10(1):22–25

Yagudin E 1987 Electroacupuncture during labour. Acupuncture in Medicine 4:20

Yamamoto T 1989 New scalp acupuncture. Acupuncture in Medicine 6:46–48

Yamamoto T, Ishiko N 1992 The effect of scalp acupuncture on the weight-lifting capacity of the healthy and paralyzed lower limb. American Journal of Acupuncture 20:47–54

Yan L 1988 Treatment of persistent hiccupping with electro-acupuncture at 'hiccup-relieving' point. Journal of Traditional Chinese Medicine 8: 29–30

Yan R 1988 The research on the acupuncture treatment of acute bacillary dysentery. Ancient Science of Life VII:166–171

Yang C 1990 Acupuncture treatment of 300 cases of voice disorders. International Journal of Clinical Acupuncture 1(4):333–337

Yang D 1985 Acupuncture therapy in 49 cases of postpartum urinary retention. Journal of Traditional Chinese Medicine 5(1):26

Yang M M P, Ng K K W, Zeng H L, Kwok J S L 1989 Effect of acupuncture on immunoglobulins of serum, saliva and gingival sulcus fluid. American Journal of Chinese Medicine 17(1–2):89–94

Yang Q 1993 Acupuncture treatment of 139 cases of neurodermatitis. Journal of Traditional Chinese Medicine 13(1):3–4

Yang W B, Kong F W 1987 Acupuncture for anal fissures. American Journal of Acupuncture 15:384–385

Yang X 1994 Clinical observation on needling extrachannel points in treating mental depression. Journal of Traditional Chinese Medicine 14:14–18

Yao T 1993 Acupuncture and somatic nerve stimulation: mechanism underlying effects on cardiovascular and renal activities. Scandinavian Journal of Rehabilitation Medicine 29 (suppl):7–18

Yarnell S K, Waylonis G W, Rink T L 1976 Acupuncture effect on neurosensory deafness. Archives of Physical Medicine and Rehabilitation 57(4):166–168

Yim M-J 1987 Acupuncture: preliminary report of its role as a stimulus for cardiorespiratory enhancement in swimmers. Medicine and Sport Science 24:23–29

Yin K, Jia C 1991 Treatment of chronic coronary insufficiency with acupuncture on Ximeni point. Journal of Traditional Chinese Medicine 11(2):99–100

Yin Z 1992 Acupuncture treatment of hypertension and hyperlipidaemia. International Journal of Clinical Acupuncture 3(2):191–192

Ying Y K, Lin J T, Robins J 1985 Acupuncture for the induction of cervical dilatation in preparation for first-trimester abortion and its influence on HCG. Journal of Reproductive Medicine 30:530–534

Yu D Y C, Lee S P 1976 Effect of acupuncture on bronchial asthma. Clinical Science and Molecular Medicine 51: 503–509

Yu X 1990 Experiences in the treatment of amenorrhoea with acupuncture together with syndrome differentiation. International Journal of Clinical Acupuncture 1:155–158

Yuan C, Li R, Zhu J, Jin N, Zhang D, Yan C 1986 The curative effect and mechanism of action of the acupoints pishu and weishu. Journal of Traditional Chinese Medicine 6: 249–252

Yuan C X, Zhu J, Zhing L Xe 1985 Gastroscopic observation of the effect of acupuncture on gastric motility. Jiangxi Journal of Chinese Traditional Medicine 3:33–44

Zang J 1990 Immediate antiasthmatic effect of acupuncture in 192 cases of bronchial asthma. Journal of Traditional Chinese Medicine 10:89–93

Zetler G 1980 Anticonvulsant effects of caerulein and cholecystokinin octapeptide compared with those of diazepam. European Journal of Pharmacology 65:297–300

Zhan C 1990 Treatment of 32 cases of dysmenorrhea by puncturing hegu and sanyinjiao acupoints. Journal of Traditional Chinese Medicine 10:33–35

Zhang J 1987 The acupuncture treatment of 248 cases of male infertility. Journal of Chinese Medicine 25:28–30

Zhang J 1992 Treatment with acupuncture at zusanli (St 36) for epigastric pain in the elderly. Journal of Traditional Chinese Medicine 12:178–179

Zhang M 1988 Treatment of 296 cases of hallucination with scalp-acupuncture. Journal of Traditional Chinese Medicine 8:193–194

Zhang S, Luo Y, Bo M 1991 Vertigo treated with scalp acupuncture. Journal of Traditional Chinese Medicine 11(1):26–28

Zhang T Q, Jin A D, Li S Se 1979 The curative effect of acupuncture on bacillary dysentery in Rhesus monkey

and the experimental study of its mechanisms. Abstracts of 1st National Symposium of Acupuncture, Beijing, pp 40–41

Zhang Y 1984 A report of 49 cases of dysmenorrhea treated by acupuncture. Journal of Traditional Chinese Medicine 4:101–102

Zhang Z 1987 Effect of acupuncture on 44 cases of radiation rectitis following radiation therapy for carcinoma of the cervix uteri. Journal of Traditional Chinese Medicine 7:139–140

Zhang Z 1989 Efficacy of acupuncture in the treatment of post-stroke aphasia. Journal of Traditional Chinese Medicine 9:87–89

Zhang Z, Yu Z, Zhang H 1992 Inhibitory effect of electro-acupuncture on penicillin-induced amygdala epileptiform discharges. Chen Tzu Yen Chiu 17:96–98

Zhao C 1987 Postmenopausal urinary incontinence. Journal of Traditional Chinese Medicine 7:305–306

Zhao C 1988 Acupuncture treatment of menstrual pain. Journal of Traditional Chinese Medicine 8:73–74

Zhao C 1989 Acupuncture and moxibustion treatment of hiccup. Journal of Traditional Chinese Medicine 9:182–183

Zhao C 1990 Treatment of acute cerebro-vascular diseases and sequelae with acupuncture. Journal of Traditional Chinese Medicine 10:70–73

Zhao F, Wang P, Hua S 1991 Treatment of psoriasis with acupuncture: retrospective case report. Acupuncture and Electro-Therapeutics Research, International Journal 17:195–208

Zhao J 1991 Acupuncture at huatuojiaji (extra 21) points for treatment of acute epigastric pain. Journal of Traditional Chinese Medicine V:258

Zhao J, Liu W 1988 Relationship between acupuncture-induced immunity and the regulation of central neurotransmitters in the rabbit: I Effect of central catecholaminergic neurons in regulating acupuncture-induced immune function. Acupuncture and Electro-therapeutics Research 13:79–85

Zhao J, Liu W 1989 Relationship between acupuncture-induced immunity and the regulation of central neurotransmitter system in rabbits: II Effect of the endogenous opioid peptides on the regulation of acupuncture-induced immune reaction. Acupuncture and Electro-therapeutics Research 14:1–7

Zharkin N A 1990 Acupuncture in obstetrics. Journal of Chinese Medicine 33:10–13

Zhongxin X 1989 Clinical observation of 500 cases with pediatric diarrhea treated by acupuncture. Chinese Acupuncture and Moxibustion 9:3–10

Zhou R, Huang F, Jiang S, Jiang J 1988 The effect of acupuncture on the phagocytic activity of human leukocytes. Journal of Traditional Chinese Medicine 8(2):83–84

Zhou R, Zhang Y, Wang J et al 1991 Anti-hypertensive effect of auriculo-acupoint pressing therapy. Journal of Traditional Chinese Medicine 11(3):189–192

Zhu J, Huang X, Zhang S 1984 A clinical study of acupuncture treatment of gastric and duodenal ulcer. 2nd National Symposium of Acupuncture and Moxibustion, Beijing, pp 54–55

15

Acupuncture for nausea and vomiting

Christine M. McMillan

INTRODUCTION

Since the mid 1980s reports have suggested a growing use of non-orthodox therapies as a supplement to conventional health care (Thomas et al 1991). One aspect of this has been a renewed interest in the use of acupuncture for the symptomatic relief of nausea and vomiting in a variety of clinical situations.

Chinese doctors have used acupuncture, based mainly on meridian theory, for the treatment of nausea and vomiting for at least 2000 years (Chiang et al 1973, Foster & Sweeney 1987, Heine 1988). Traditionally, acupuncture has been used in the treatment of gastrointestinal disorders, in which nausea and vomiting often present as symptoms, and also for sickness of early pregnancy (Beijing College of Traditional Chinese Medicine et al 1980). Western textbooks describe the acupuncture treatment of these conditions in terms of Western diagnosis, considered in relation to the traditional Chinese diagnostic categories of Excess and Deficiency disturbances (Stux & Pomeranz 1987). Despite far-reaching claims for its efficacy in alleviating nausea and vomiting associated with these conditions, however, reports from China are for the most part anecdotal in nature and its use largely remains empirical.

The traditional, theoretical concept of acupuncture is difficult to deal with in modern, scientific terms in the light of our knowledge of anatomy and physiology and for this reason acupuncture has stimulated limited scientific interest in the

Western world. It has become apparent, however, that if acupuncture is to become an accepted treatment, objective studies are needed to evaluate its effectiveness for the relief of pain and other symptoms, including nausea and vomiting (Prance et al 1988, Richardson & Vincent 1986, Vincent & Richardson 1986).

It is as a result of this recognition that a number of studies on the use of acupuncture in the treatment of nausea and vomiting are now appearing in medical publications. The main objective of these has been to see if acupuncture, or a modification of the technique, has indeed any antiemetic action, rather than attempt to explain how it works.

Much of this research has been in areas in which nausea and vomiting present as a specific clinical problem, rather than in conditions where they coexist with other symptoms of gastrointestinal disease. While nausea and vomiting, of non-obstructive origin, can be a problem in early pregnancy (Fagan & Chadwick 1983), it may also require therapeutic intervention after some operations (Watcha & White 1992) and following the use of some drugs. The latter include morphine and related compounds, and most of the cytotoxic drugs used in the treatment of cancer (Priestman 1989).

Although a wide range of antiemetic drugs is now available, these may not be totally effective and may cause unpleasant extrapyramidal effects or drowsiness (Bateman 1991, Cunningham 1990). Furthermore, to be effective they have to be administered before the emetic stimulus (Watcha & White 1992, Williams et al 1989). Since there is an individual variation in the susceptibility to sickness, their routine use results in some patients being given drugs that they do not actually require.

Undoubtedly, however, the multiplicity of factors that predispose to nausea and vomiting make reliable evaluation of antiemetic treatments very difficult. Furthermore, antiemetic treatment is only one component of a very complex care system and should remain, if at all possible, secondary in importance to the correct treatment of the disease (Clarke, Dundee & Loan 1970, Soukop & Cunningham 1987). Indeed, on

reviewing individual antiemetic drugs in a variety of clinical situations, it becomes apparent that there are few well-controlled trials in this area. Despite these difficulties, practitioners have responded to the challenge of scientifically evaluating the antiemetic effects of acupuncture.

ACUPUNCTURE POINTS

The therapeutic value of acupuncture in the symptomatic relief of nausea and vomiting is referred to in both traditional Chinese and Western acupuncture textbooks, and a number of points are identified for their antiemetic action (Beijing College of Traditional Chinese Medicine et al 1980, Chang 1976, Lewith & Lewith 1983, Mann 1987, Stux & Pomeranz 1987, 1991).

Generally speaking within these books, in addition to a description of the location of the points and indications for their specific use, there is a classification of the most important points in relation to different diagnoses. It is common practice for the treatment of nausea and vomiting to be described in relation to symptoms of gastrointestinal disorders and pregnancy.

The PC-6 acupuncture point

Neiguan ('Inner Pass', PC-6) is the point most commonly described for its antiemetic effect (Fig. 15.1). It is located on the pericardial 'meridian' 2 'Cun' or Chinese inches proximal to the distal wrist crease between the tendons of palmaris longus and flexor carpi radialis muscles of the forearm.

A 'Cun' is equivalent to the distance between the creases of the flexed index finger, or approximately the width of the thumb across the interphalangeal joint. The exact depth of location is not clear, but textbooks refer to the use of a 2.5 cm needle. Insertion to a depth of 1 cm has been found to elicit De Qi, a non-anatomically distributed sensation of heaviness, numbness or tingling radiating into the fingers and up the arm.

While PC-6 is described as having a specific effect on the upper digestive tract (Stux &

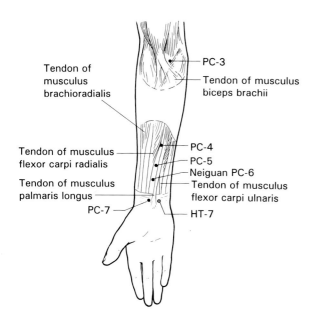

Tendon of
musculus
brachioradialis

PC-3

Tendon of musculus
biceps brachii

Tendon of musculus
flexor carpi radialis

Tendon of musculus
palmaris longus

PC-4

PC-5

Neiguan PC-6

Tendon of musculus
flexor carpi ulnaris

PC-7

HT-7

Figure 15.1 Location of the PC-6 Neiguan point.

Pomeranz 1987), there is little scientific evidence to support this. Its antiemetic action, however, has been demonstrated in a number of well-designed, controlled clinical studies.

Other points for antiemesis

A number of other points are referred to in textbooks in relation to the treatment of nausea and vomiting, although the clinical efficacy of these has not been scientifically evaluated.

Zusanli (ST-36) is situated one finger breadth lateral to the lower border of the tibial tuberosity, 3 Cun below the knee joint. In addition to its being regarded as a very important point in the treatment of a wide range of gastrointestinal disorders, it is considered to be useful in the alleviation of nausea and vomiting of non-specific aetiology.

Recent studies carried out observing gastric peristalsis during gastroscopy, concluded that stimulation of ST-36 altered peristalsis in a significant number of patients. The effect was related to initial motility, with a promoting effect of acupuncture in patients with low initial gastric motility, and a suppressing effect in patients with active initial motility (Yuan, Zhu & Zhing 1985).

Although the importance of these findings in understanding the possible effect stimulation has on the alleviation of nausea and vomiting is unclear, the observations are consistent with the traditional Chinese hypothesis that acupuncture exerts a differential effect on internal organs to restore the homeostatic balance. It is, however, difficult to provide a physiological basis for this hypothesis (Li et al 1992).

Similar results to these have been reported with stimulation of the Pishu and Weishu points, which are also considered to have an antiemetic action (Beijing College of Traditional Chinese Acupuncture et al 1980, Yuan, Li & Zhu 1985). Furthermore, in animal studies, a suppression of gastric acid output has been demonstrated with stimulation of these points (Department of Physiology Guangsi Medical University 1961). Pishu (Transport point to the spleen, BL-20) is situated 1.5 Cun lateral to the lower border of the spinous process of the 11th thoracic vertebra. Weishu (Transport point to the stomach, BL-21) is situated 1.5 Cun lateral to the lower border of the spinous process of the 12th thoracic vertebra.

Some other points referred to for their anti-emetic effect (Stux & Pomeranz 1991) include:

- Zhongwan (in the middle of the stomach pit), influential point for the Fu (hollow) organs, Mu point of the stomach (CV-12), which lies on the midline, midway between the xiphoid process and the umbilicus.
- Liangmen (Beam Gate, ST-21) which is located 2 Cun lateral to the midline, 4 Cun above the umbilicus. As this point lies lateral to CV-12 the two are often stimulated together.
- Tianshu ('Celestial Pivot', Mu point of large intestine, ST-25) which is located 2 Cun lateral to the umbilicus.

Taichong ('Large Impulse', LR-3) located between the first and second metatarsal bones, 2 Cun proximal to the margin of the web, and HoKu ('Closed Valley', LI-4) situated at the highest point of the muscle adductor pollicis with the thumb and index finger adducted, have been noted for their effect on nausea and vomiting (Deng, Tan & Han 1986, Mann 1987).

These two points are also indicated in the reduction of states of anxiety and mental agitation (Stux & Pomeranz 1987) and this effect may indirectly play a part in the alleviation of nausea and vomiting symptoms.

Although nausea and vomiting are frequently referred to as symptoms that can be alleviated by stimulation of any of the above points, the textbooks do not generally distinguish between different causes of sickness.

In clinical practice it is not uncommon for a number of points to be used for a combined effect in treating specific diagnoses. One such example of this is in the case of morning sickness. A 'prescription' for treatment could include stimulation of two antiemetic points, PC-6 and ST-36, with Gongsun (SP-4), which is indicated in the treatment of dyspepsia and gastritis (Lewith & Lewith 1983) or with Shangwan (CV-13), a local point for treating 'fullness' in the epigastric region (Beijing College of Traditional Chinese Medicine et al 1980).

Furthermore, in severe cases of morning sickness (hyperemesis gravidarum), Stux & Pomeranz (1987) suggest, in addition to stimulation of three antiemetic points, namely PC-6, ST-36 and CV-12, the use of Shenmen (HT-7), for its effect on anxiety and Baihui (GV-20), which is considered to have a general sedative effect.

EAR ACUPUNCTURE

While ear acupuncture is used in China mainly for the treatment of acutely painful conditions, it can be used for any condition that will respond to acupuncture (Lewith & Lewith 1983). Auricular points can be selected directly for the areas they represent, or on the basis of TCM. The main ear points indicated, for example, in the treatment of morning sickness are Liver, Stomach, Ear-Shenmen and Sympathetic Nerve (Beijing College of Traditional Chinese Medicine et al 1980).

Methods of stimulation

Different methods, including traditional needling acupuncture, are available for stimulation and these can be grouped as follows. The methods are described with reference to PC-6 as the non-invasive techniques have been developed specifically for stimulation of this particular point (Choy, personal communication, 1990, Dundee, Yang & McMillan 1991):

- invasive: acupuncture with manual rotation of needle (ACP)
  acupuncture with electrical stimulation of the needle (electro-ACP)
- non-invasive: transcutaneous electrical stimulation (TCES) (Fig. 15.2)
  acupressure– pressure over the point (see Fig. 15.3).

Electroacupuncture involves a current applied to the needle from a battery-operated, direct current, rectangular wave stimulator, with a variable current output adjusted until the patient is aware of the stimulation. The same apparatus is used for TCES via surface electrodes with the frequency of output set at 10–15 Hz, a technique developed by Professor John Dundee and his colleagues (McMillan & Dundee 1991a). With both these applications the opposite polarity electrode is placed somewhere on the same limb. While this technique is similar to transcutaneous electrical nerve stimulation (TENS), used for pain relief, the term 'TCES' is considered to be more appropriate in this application.

In addition to this technique there are now a number of commercially available hand-held

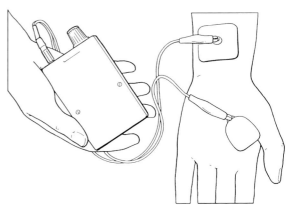

Figure 15.2   TCES via surface electrodes.

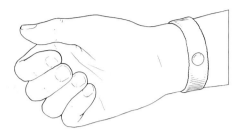

Figure 15.3 Acupressure applied by commercially available Sea Bands.

stimulators available for administering non-invasive electroacupuncture (Dickinson 1991).

Acupressure can be applied manually or by the use of an elasticized band with a large plastic stud that is easily positioned over PC-6. Originally devised by Daniel Choy from New York and commonly known as 'Choy bands' or 'Choy straps' these are now available commercially under the name of 'Sea Bands' (Fig. 15.3).

DEVELOPMENT OF THE NON-INVASIVE TECHNIQUE FOR STIMULATION OF PC-6

Professor Dundee was one of the first medical practitioners to become involved in the scientific evaluation of the antiemetic effects of acupuncture. During a visit to the People's Republic of China in 1983 he observed pregnant girls at an antenatal clinic at the Peking Maternity Hospital using acupressure (at the Neiguan point) as a prevention for morning sickness. This stimulated his interest in this ancient Chinese treatment, which he pursued up until his death in 1991. He initiated a series of studies that considered the antiemetic effect of acupuncture in a number of clinical situations and this work led to the development and evaluation of the non-invasive technique using TCES.

Scientific basis

Initial studies carried out by Professor Dundee in Belfast were concerned with perioperative nausea and vomiting. The Department of Anaesthetics, The Queens University of Belfast, had previous experience of studying antiemetics under clinical conditions using 'opioid premedication–postoperative sickness' as a model (Clarke, Dundee & Loan 1970). In well-controlled, randomized, single-blind studies of perioperative sickness following a standardized premedication–anaesthetic sequence, Professor Dundee and his co-workers convincingly demonstrated the antiemetic action of PC-6 stimulation (Dundee et al 1989a).

Fry (1986) had briefly described the antiemetic effect of acupuncture in postoperative vomiting and many of the early findings of the Belfast workers were confirmed by Barsoum, Perry & Fraser (1990) and Ho et al (1990).

The British Medical Association (1986) published a report on alternative therapy in which it pointed out that 'new and unconventional techniques should be evaluated with the same scientific methods as have been applied to therapeutic methods now known'. While this was possible in the perioperative studies, the same scientific approach could not be adopted in the case of cancer chemotherapy sickness.

Nausea and vomiting are among the most common and distressing side-effects of chemotherapy (Coates et al 1983) and if left unchecked can result in possible rejection of potentially useful treatment (Frytek & Moertel 1981, Wilcox et al 1982). Until recently, emesis was poorly controlled by standard antiemetic drugs, even in high doses or in combination. In particular, antiemetic activity was unsatisfactory against strongly emetic stimuli such as cisplatin (Gralla, Itri & Pisko 1981, Kris et al 1985).

The serious nature of the condition thus dictated that the dosage and the choice of cytotoxic drugs should not be affected by the antiemetic regimen. Until the efficacy of acupuncture antiemesis was established it was not justifiable to stop the currently prescribed, though not totally effective, antiemetics.

Following the findings of the perioperative studies, but with a modified approach, Dundee et al (1989b) demonstrated a synergistic effect of PC-6 acupuncture antiemesis with tolerable doses of standard antiemetics in the relief of nausea and vomiting associated with cancer chemotherapy. Aglietti, Roila & Tonato (1990) later confirmed these findings.

The efficacy of a single acupuncture stimulation was limited to about 8 hours and this brevity of action indicated a limited place in clinical practice, particularly in patients treated on an outpatient basis. The use of acupressure, using commercially available Sea Bands, while alone relatively ineffective with perioperative sickness (Bill & Dundee 1988), was shown to prolong the effect of invasive acupuncture in patients having cancer chemotherapy (Dundee & Yang 1990).

The studies at this stage had shown PC-6 acupuncture to be effective in the control of emesis induced by cancer chemotherapy, with no major side-effects identifed. In the studies by Dundee and others the median nerve was touched by the needle in only one patient and Barsoum, Perry & Fraser (1990) describe one patient experiencing symptoms like those of the carpal tunnel syndrome when using acupressure bands.

However, for the technique to be adopted in clinical practice for chemotherapy-induced emesis, certain factors had to be considered. Invasive acupuncture, while effective, required some technical skill and not unexpectedly many patients would have preferred a non-invasive approach. Dundee, Yang & McMillan (1991) reported limited benefit from the use of acupressure on its own with chemotherapy-induced emesis, however, the antiemetic effect of a technique involving TCES via surface electrodes was marked. The findings indicated that, while TCES, similarly non-toxic and inexpensive, did not produce the degree of benefit derived from invasive acupuncture, it could be considered as a useful alternative.

The only possible contraindication to the use of TCES is with patients with cardiac pacemakers (Rasmussen et al 1988). Skin rashes, although reported by others using large self-adhesive electrodes (Mannheimer & Lampe 1984), were not a major problem, a transient rash occurring in only two patients.

The non-invasive technique (TCES) that evolved is described as being most effective as an antiemetic when:

- administered prior to the emetic stimulus and for several days after
- used as an adjunct to standard antiemetics
- applied for 5 minutes duration at 2-hourly intervals during waking hours with stimulus frequency of 10–15 Hz.

Non-invasive TCES is clearly a compromise between the highly effective needle acupuncture and what can be adopted as a routine adjunct to treatment. The feasibility of modifying this technique to enable self-administration of the stimulus at regular intervals by the patient in order to sustain the effect was then considered (McMillan & Dundee 1991b).

Dundee and colleagues completed a series of randomized, crossover studies to evaluate the relative efficacy of some commercially available equipment as a preliminary to the development of a self-administered technique (Dundee, Yang & McMillan 1991). Replacement of the large multichannel acupuncture machine by a small, easy to operate, single-output stimulator, with a fixed frequency of 15 Hz, reduced errors in the use of the devices. The use of large, diffuse surface electrodes rather than conventional small copper or rare-earth cobalt stud electrodes removed the need for exact accuracy of placement over PC-6. Furthermore, the current necessary for skin penetration was less with the larger electrodes, thus increasing battery life. Identical results were obtained with self-adhesive ECG-type and black carbonized rubber electrodes, which were both more robust than the studs and could be worn for 4–5 days with low incidence of side-effects to the skin. Patient preference, however, was for the self-adhesive ECG type as these were easier to apply to the skin and connect to the leads of the stimulator with a crocodile clip attachment (Fig. 15.2).

The adoption of these modifications increased acceptability by both patients and medical staff and made self-administration feasible. Indeed this method of self-administered transcutaneous electrical stimulation of PC-6 later proved to be invaluable as a treatment option for antiemesis at the Northern Ireland Centre for Clinical Oncology in Belfast. Furthermore, a consideration with the use of any treatment is its cost and this technique was considered to be extremely cost effective in comparison with other antiemetic regimens (Warrington 1991)

The concurrent introduction of ondansetron and other 5-HT receptor antagonist antiemetics somewhat revolutionized the treatment of nausea and vomiting associated with cancer chemotherapy. However, there remain some patients for whom this group of drugs offers only a partial alleviation of symptoms, particularly on the third and fourth day of treatment. Even when there is no vomiting, a percentage of patients still remain nauseated. Observations by Kris, Gralla & Tyson (1988), and Cubeddu et al (1990) have confirmed this clinical impression. Smith et al (1990, 1991) and Jones et al (1991), aware of these limitations, supplemented the use of ondansetron with dexamethasone and demonstrated synergistic activity by the steroid. In a comparable randomized, crossover study monitoring the degree of sickness over a 5-day period, McMillan, Dundee & Abram (1991) subsequently demonstrated that self-administered TCES of PC-6 can be used to enhance significantly the antiemetic action of ondansetron.

The use of this technique of self-administered transcutaneous electrical stimulation of PC-6 has also been evaluated in the alleviation of emetic sequelae following opioid analgesia in major orthopaedic surgery (McMillan 1994).

A REVIEW OF THE EFFICACY OF ACUPUNCTURE ANTIEMESIS

Much of the evidence for the efficacy of the aforementioned acupuncture points, in terms of their antiemetic effect, remains anecdotal and still requires scientific evaluation. There is now, however, a considerable body of scientific evidence confirming that stimulation of PC-6 results in a significant antiemetic effect. Concurrent with the studies initiated by Dundee et al (1986), others have carried out similar investigations.

Initially, manual acupuncture at the PC-6 point was used, but later studies have involved other methods of stimulation. These modified methods have already been described in detail.

PC-6 antiemesis has been used in the following fields:

1. postoperative sickness
2. morning sickness
3. sickness from cancer chemotherapy
4. travel sickness.

The findings will be reviewed in the above order.

It will become apparent that most of the reliable scientific data were obtained in the first group. There have been comparatively few studies in sickness of early pregnancy or in travel sickness, while with cytotoxic drug therapy the medical condition of the patients has often restricted the use of randomization and control (no-treatment) groups.

While some workers refer only to antinausea effect, the majority include both nausea and vomiting. Objections to including nausea, which is a subjective sensation, are minimized by simply noting its presence and not attempting to quantify it, although methods of quantifying it have been described (Del Favero et al 1990). Some researchers attempt to quantify the severity of vomiting, based on the number of episodes, while others simply note its occurrence in a given time period. In the cancer chemotherapy field, while some quantify the severity of sickness, the majority look at the reduction in sickness with different forms of therapy.

Very recently a systematic review by Vickers (1996) found that 27 out of 33 controlled trials of acupuncture for nausea and vomiting were positive.

Postoperative sickness

The most complete study in this field is by Dundee et al (1989a). This involved over 500 female patients having short (8–12 minute) gynaecological operations (cervical dilatation and uterine curettage) under a standard methohexitone–nitrous oxide anaesthetic. Premedication was with 10 mg nalbuphine given intramuscularly. Except in one series, PC-6 was stimulated before administration of the opioid. No drugs were given that are known to reduce the incidence of sickness. All four methods of stimulation of PC-6 were used in random order and a control (no-treatment) group was included. In addition, a small group had needling of a point near the right elbow that is not on a traditionally described acupuncture meridian (sham acupuncture).

Initially all treatments were applied to the right forearm, but later this was changed to the dominant side. Patients were visited at the end of the first and sixth postoperative hours by a person who was unaware of the treatment given, and the occurrence of nausea alone or vomiting (including retching) with or without nausea was noted. All were told that the study was designed to reduce side-effects and improve the efficacy of the premedication; nausea and vomiting were not mentioned at this stage, but a full description of the study objectives was given at the time of the last postoperative visit. There was a minimum of 31 patients in each group.

The incidence of sickness was reduced to a significant degree ($P < 0.001$) by both invasive and non-invasive stimulation of PC-6, but not by stimulation of the 'dummy point'. The non-invasive approach was not as effective ($P < 0.01$) as the invasive, the difference being in the duration of action; both were equieffective in the first postoperative hour, but the benefit of both TCES and acupressure was less in the 1–6-hour period. With electrical stimulation of the acupuncture needle and TCES, best results were obtained with a frequency of 10–15 Hz applied for a 5-minute duration.

In a subsequent investigation using the same study model, it was found that infiltration of the acupuncture site with lignocaine abolished the antiemetic action of PE-6 stimulation, compared with subjects in whom the injection was with saline (Dundee & Ghaly 1991).

Contemporaneously with the first Belfast study, Fry (1986) reported an antiemetic action from acupressure applied just before induction

of general anaesthesia and in the immediate postanaesthetic period and commented on its brevity of action. At the same time, in a small but well-designed study in patients having eye surgery, Masuda et al (1986) noted a reduction in postoperative sickness in those having acupuncture carried out at the time of induction of neuroleptanaesthesia compared with untreated controls.

A more recent study by Barsoum, Perry & Fraser (1990) investigated the benefit of acupressure (Sea Bands) at the PC-6 point in relieving sickness following 162 major operations. Patients received a variety of premedicants and anaesthetics but postoperative analgesia was standardized (papaveretum). Adjuvant therapy, (acupressure, 'dummy' Sea Bands and prochlorperazine) was given in random order and one group received no treatment. Nausea scores (as assessed on a linear analogue scale) were significantly lower in the first two postoperative days in those patients treated by acupressure when compared with the other groups. Vomiting was recorded in fewer patients amongst the acupressure groups than in the control or drug group, but the difference was not statistically significant.

Sacco et al (1990) later confirmed these findings in a study involving 225 female patients undergoing laparoscopy and laser gynaecology surgery. In this study a standardized anaesthetic regimen was used for all the patients. The incidence of nausea and vomiting was compared with the use of bilateral PC-6 acupressure (Sea Bands), placebo bands without studs and a control 'non-treatment' group.

While Dundee et al (1989a) suggested that PC-6 acupuncture was effective only when administered before the emetic stimulus, in a well-controlled, prospective study of female patients with a standard operation that involved four anaesthetic techniques, Ho et al (1990) demonstrated a significant antiemetic action from PC-6 acupuncture administered postoperatively in patients whose anaesthesia included an opioid. The reduction in incidence was similar to that produced by 5 mg prochlorperazine intravenously. These workers did not, however, include nausea in their study, but they did find acupuncture more effective than TCES.

Two studies in which acupuncture was given intraoperatively during an opioid-containing anaesthetic failed to demonstrate any antiemetic action (Dundee, Milligan & McKay 1988, Weightman, Zacharias & Herbison 1987), suggesting that there may be a strong psychological element in acupuncture antiemesis; however, this is refuted by the comparative ineffectiveness of 'dummy' acupuncture demonstrated in many of the aforementioned studies. It is possible that it is not the timing of the acupuncture in relation to the administration of the emetic stimulus that is the important factor, but rather that the general anaesthesia may have a suppressing effect on its antiemetic action. If this is indeed the case, and acupuncture antiemesis requires patients to be awake in order to produce an effect, this may limit its acceptability as a therapy in certain groups of patients, for example young children.

To complete this discussion an alternative approach adopted by Yang et al (1993) is worthy of mention. They considered that the instrumentation involved in electroacupuncture may limit its clinical applicability and investigated a simpler alternative method. The effect of PC-6 acupoint injection with 0.2 ml 50% glucose in water was compared prospectively with intravenous injection of $20 \mu g/kg$ droperidol in 120 consecutive outpatients undergoing gynaecological laparoscopy. They concluded that PC-6 injection with 50% glucose in water provided a simple and effective method for reducing the incidence of postoperative emesis in this type of outpatient surgery.

Three studies have considered the efficacy of PC-6 antiemesis following paediatric surgery. Lewis et al (1991), in a double-blind study, compared the effect of pressure at the PC-6 point with placebo in children undergoing strabismus correction. Children participating in the study were allocated randomly to either an acupressure or a placebo group. The acupressure group wore Sea-Bands and the placebo group wore bands with no studs. The bands were positioned 1 hour before the operation and were worn continuously until discharge from hospital the same day. They found no significant difference in the incidence of vomiting recorded in the two groups.

Yentis & Bissonnette (1992) evaluated the antiemetic effects and side-effects of PC-6 acupuncture and droperidol following strabismus repair in 90 children. The invasive acupuncture was administered immediately following induction of the anaesthesia. They found no difference in the incidence of postoperative vomiting after acupuncture, droperidol or both treatments. In all the groups the incidence of emetic sequelae was high and compares with previously reported control group incidences (Broadman et al 1990, Hardy et al 1986, Lerman, Eustis & Smith 1986). Postoperative restlessness was, however, more frequent in children who received droperidol than those who received acupuncture alone. They conclude that acupuncture is as effective, or ineffective, as droperidol and comment that the value of droperidol in anaesthesia for strabismus surgery requires reassessment.

Concurrent with this study, Yentis & Bissonnette (1991) also found no antiemetic effect of acupuncture administered during anaesthesia on postoperative vomiting after tonsillectomy in children.

Although these three studies failed to demonstrate any antiemetic effect of PC-6 stimulation, the results should be considered in relation to previous studies investigating vomiting in children following these particular surgical procedures, and the antiemetic effect of PC-6 stimulation in adults. Both strabismus correction and tonsillectomy are associated with a high incidence of postoperative vomiting, which is likely to be multifactorial. Factors including, in the former case, manipulation of the eye with stretching of the muscles and visual sensory disturbance and, in the latter case, pharyngeal stimulation and swallowing of blood may be important in the aetiology of vomiting, but the administration of opioid analgesia and early ambulation may also play a part. Interestingly, Veroli & Astier (1992) attempt to explain the negative result in the study by Lewis et al (1991) in terms of the physiopathological basis of TCM. In TCM the treatment of the symptom depends on the aetiology and in this situation the frequency of vomiting is particularly great probably because of the perioperative manipulation of the eye and its muscles. They conclude therefore that the stimulation of PC-6 may not be very effective as it does not act on the eye.

While non-invasive acupressure was considered by Lewis et al (1991) to be more clinically acceptable to children, it has been suggested that it is less effective than an invasive technique and therefore following these particular surgical procedures its effect may be limited. In the studies by Yentis & Bissonnette (1991, 1992) the acupuncture was administered during anaesthesia, while evidence from previous studies would suggest that PC-6 stimulation to be effective should be administered before (Dundee et al 1989a), after (Ho 1990), but not during anaesthesia (Weightman, Zacharias & Herbison 1987).

To summarize, the use of acupuncture in the prevention of postoperative nausea and vomiting has stimulated considerable debate. It seems clear that there is some positive evidence of an antiemetic effect in postoperative sickness in adults from stimulation of PC-6 with acupuncture and related techniques. Furthermore, compared with conventional pharmacological therapies, this approach is free from side-effects. However, a number of recent studies would suggest that PC-6 acupressure and PC-6 acupuncture, when administered after induction of anaesthesia, are ineffective in reducing postoperative vomiting in children following certain surgical procedures. It would seem, therefore, that further studies are required in this area to define more clearly the relative importance of factors such as age, gender, timing of stimulation, type of surgery or emetic stimulus and anaesthetic technique.

To conclude, in recent years, a more serious problem with emetic sequelae has evolved from the development of techniques adopting opioid administration for pain relief following major surgery (Robinson & Fell 1991). It is now widely recognized that the use of patient-controlled analgesia systems (PCA), extradural infusion analgesia (EIA) and the use of intrathecal diamorphine, while providing an enhanced degree of pain relief, is associated with a high incidence of emetic sequelae of sufficient severity to require antiemetic therapy (Wheatley et al 1991). The efficacy of acupuncture and related techniques in this area provides further scope for research and to date a number of studies have been completed. McMillan (1994), in a well-controlled study, demonstrated the efficacy of transcutaneous stimulation of PC-6 in controlling the sickness following opioid analgesia in major orthopaedic surgery. A significant difference in the incidence of sickness in female patients ($n = 137$) in the active treatment group compared with the control/placebo groups was demonstrated. The difference in the incidence of sickness within the different groups was not, however, significant in male patients ($n = 93$). McConaghy, Bland & Swales (1996), using invasive acupuncture, reported a significant reduction in nausea in patients receiving parenteral morphine following surgery via a PCA system. Allen, Kitching & Nagle (1994) found that the use of Sea Bands was of benefit in reducing the severity of nausea, but not the overall incidence of nausea and vomiting, in patients receiving PCA following laparotomy for major gynaecological surgery.

Morning sickness

When acupressure at PC-6 was practised in an obstetric outpatient clinic in Beijing, the mothers were told that 'it always works'. Supporting evidence for this could not be obtained, but the remedy has been used for 4000 years and is quoted in most acupuncture textbooks. Much of the Chinese literature is anecdotal and concentrates mainly on the condition from a TCM point of view. Two recent, inadequately documented Chinese studies claim benefit from needling a number of points including PC-6 in patients with morning sickness, claiming 'fairly satisfactory results' without giving any details (Zhao 1988, Zhao 1987). A Russian paper is likewise lacking in data (Osadchaia & Shabadash 1989), as is one from Czechoslovakia (Jindrak 1980).

With regard to the use of invasive needling acupuncture in the alleviation of symptoms of nausea and vomiting there would appear to be a hesitancy on the part of many Western practitioners to use this technique in the first trimester of pregnancy. A number of textbooks refer to this in general terms, while others mention the contraindication with specific reference to certain points. It may be partly due to this, and also perhaps to the anticipated problems of obtaining ethical approval, that the studies carried out in this field by Western practitioners have been confined to the scientific evaluation of non-invasive techniques.

The beneficial effect of self-administered acupressure has been studied in 350 consecutive women attending an antenatal clinic in Belfast (Dundee et al 1988). A self-reporting system of study was adopted, patients being given either no treatment, told to press PC-6 for 5 minutes every 2 to 3 hours, or to press a dummy point on the right elbow. Although the incidence of returned records (70%) was less than hoped for, the findings demonstrated a benefit from PC-6 acupressure ($P < 0.0005$), with lesser benefit ($P < 0.01$) from pressing the 'dummy' point. Since patients had to have the reason for pressing their elbows explained to them, the latter would appear to be a psychological effect. This study was far from ideal and has been criticized for low incidence of returned records—a factor outside the control of the workers (Root 1989). However, the study is not without some merit as the limitations encountered have clearly been considered in the design of studies by other workers who have attempted to define further the efficacy of this treatment in pregnancy sickness.

A more scientifically controlled clinical trial, limited only by the small numbers involved, has been reported by Hyde (1989). Commercially available wrist bands with a stud pressing on PC-6 were worn for 5 days, followed by a similar band without a stud, the order being reversed in half the patients. Using a VAS, a significant reduction in nausea was demonstrated ($P < 0.05$) from acupressure, with relief of symptoms in 12–16 subjects.

In Italy, De Aloysio & Penacchioni (1992), in a double-blind, crossover, placebo-controlled study demonstrated that acupressure (Sea Bands) at PC-6 resulted in an antiemetic effect twice that induced by placebo therapy. In this study the placebo treatment involved the use of a 'blunted' button in the wristband applied to the PC-6 point. The results were limited only by a population size ($n = 60$) just significant to allow reliable and appreciable statistical analysis, as the inclusion criteria were deliberately severe.

Two more recently published studies also suggest that acupressure may be useful in relieving nausea and vomiting of pregnancy. Stainton & Neff (1994), in an uncontrolled study, demonstrated a 50% reduction in the incidence of nausea and vomiting with the use of Sea Bands. Twenty-seven pregnant women (5–22 weeks' gestation) participated in the study and it was concluded that the Sea Bands were more effective if applied early in the onset of symptoms. Belluomini et al (1994) adopted a well-controlled design to evaluate the effectiveness of acupressure to PC-6 compared with a sham control point located on the palmar aspect of the hand proximal to the head of the fifth metacarpal head. Sixty women completed the study. While there was a significant difference in the incidence of nausea in the treatment group compared with the control group, there was none in the severity of emesis. A significant positive correlation was noted between the maternal age and severity of nausea. Brill (1995) questioned whether the findings of this study could be generalized to other populations, as the referral route for those women participating in the study inferred a group of individuals who had an interest in alternative methods. Furthermore, he commented on the high dropout rate (33%), even in this select group, demonstrating that compliance with acupressure may be problematic.

In conclusion, despite the limitations of these studies, there would appear to be sufficient evidence of the beneficial effects to adopt acupressure as a useful technique for this common problem in clinical practice.

Sickness from cancer chemotherapy

The emetic effect of cisplatin and other potent cytotoxic drugs is well known and until the introduction of the 5-HT antagonists treatment of this was unsatisfactory. This is clearly illustrated by the large number of reported studies in which a wide range of antiemetics and combination therapies have been evaluated (Fetting et al 1982, Gralla, Itri & Pisko 1981, Grunberg 1990). In cancer treatment centres the reported incidence of troublesome vomiting is in the region of 56% (Hoskins & Hanks 1988) to 76% (Dundee et al 1989b). In the latter survey, 96% of patients who were sick with one course of treatment experienced the same on the second occasion.

This was the setting for the studies reported by Professor Dundee on the antiemetic action of PC-6 acupuncture in patients receiving cancer chemotherapy (Dundee et al 1989b, Dundee & Yang 1990). Those who had had troublesome sickness with a previous course of chemotherapy, despite the use of standard antiemetics, had acupuncture before starting the next course, but continuing their antiemetics. At that time these were metoclopramide, cyclizine and some phenothiazines (prochlorperazine, thiethylperazine and chlorpromazine) with lorazepam and steroids as adjuvants.

Before discussing the findings, the limitations of the studies should be outlined. First, patients knew they were being referred for a 'new treatment for sickness' and, even when acupuncture was not mentioned, patients talked among themselves and the subject had good media coverage. Secondly, ethical considerations limited the use of a 'dummy point' technique to a very few patients. Assessment of benefit was based on the opinion of the patient and attendants, all of whom knew the treatment that had been given, and the four-point scale for benefit attributed to acupuncture did not attempt to quantify the degree of nausea or vomiting (Dundee et al 1989b). Both hospitalized and outpatients were studied. Daily visits to the former gave more reliable data than that obtained from outpatients on their next visit to the clinic, which was normally 3–4 weeks later, although these patients were often contacted by phone. The input by the nursing staff on the severity and frequency of sickness also made the inpatient data more reliable.

The initial studies were with manual or electrical acupuncture (Dundee et al 1989b) and these were followed by non-invasive approaches to stimulation of PC-6 (Dundee, Yang & McMillan 1991, McMillan & Dundee 1991a). Best results were obtained with invasive acupuncture, which benefited more than 90% of patients, although the effect often lasted less than 8 hours. The beneficial effects were marginally, but not significantly, less in patients having highly emetic compounds as compared with other forms of chemotherapy. In a small, single-blind, crossover study, only one out of 10 patients benefited from 'dummy acupuncture' as compared with nine from PC-6 stimulation.

Indirect TCES had many practical advantages over an invasive approach, with 85% of patients benefiting from it. By the use of large, diffuse, low-impedance ECG electrodes, it could easily be self-administered by patients (McMillan & Dundee 1990, 1991b).

While 2-hourly acupressure prolonged the beneficial effect of both acupuncture and TCES, better results were obtained when TCES was used every 2 hours. In this series, acupressure alone was not very effective, but in a smaller study Stannard (1989) found that the wearing of Sea Bands reduced nausea.

In Italy, workers (Aglietta, Roila & Tonato 1990) have confirmed Dundee's findings with acupuncture. The study involved 26 female patients receiving highly emetic cisplatin chemotherapy. Both an increase in the incidence of complete protection from nausea and a decrease in the intensity and duration of vomiting were demonstrated when acupuncture was administered in addition to routine standard antiemetic therapy.

Price, Lewith & Williams (1991), in a well-controlled, crossover study, compared the benefit of PC-6 acupressure (Sea Bands) to that of acupressure bands applied to a placebo ankle point. Those patients receiving wrist acupressure had significantly less sickness and nausea, and their overall mood and condition was better than those treated at the placebo ankle point. The benefit appeared to be confined to patients receiving drugs with a high emetic potential.

Price, Lewith & Williams (1991) comment that larger studies are required to see whether there is a similar effect in patients treated with drugs less likely to cause emesis. However, as conventional antiemetics provide comparatively better control of symptoms in this group of patients, it may be difficult to document significant improvements.

To complete the discussion of evidence of an antiemetic effect of stimulation of the PC-6 point after chemotherapy, a study by Liu et al (1991) is worthy of comment. In this study magneto-therapy was applied to the PC-6 point in patients in whom standard antiemetics had not been effective. The control groups consisted of a non-magnetotherapy group and a point compression group. In the magnetotherapy group, a flat piece of magnet was sewn to a cotton band. The magnet piece was a disc of 5 mm thick and 20 mm in diameter, made of strontium and calcium-containing ferrite. The magnetic intensity on the surface of the disc was 60 mT. The cotton band was fastened to the wrist of the side receiving no drip, with the North pole of the magnet exactly on the PC-6 point. In the non-magnetotherapy group, a similar cotton band with a disc of the same size but made of ordinary iron was used and in the point compression group a 0.5 cm diameter steel ball was used instead of a disc. The three types of band were applied in the same way and for the same length of time. Of 161 cases in the magneto-therapy group the treatment was markedly effective in 61.4% of the cases, effective in 28% and ineffective in 10.6%. Comparison of the three groups showed a statistically significant benefit ($P < 0.001$) from the magnetotherapy technique compared with the controls.

Travel sickness

Only acupressure has been used in this field employing either the Choy strap or Sea Bands. The idea arose from the personal experience of Dr Choy in the Newport–Bermuda boat race in 1980. Pressure on PC-6, although effective in relieving his nausea, left him with only one hand to sail his 40-foot sloop (Choy 1990). Most of the supportive evidence is anecdotal, including a strong recommendation in the press (Fishman 1981).

There have been three scientific investigations into the efficacy of these acupressure bands (Bruce et al 1990, Lentz 1982, Warwick-Evans, Masters & Redstone 1991). These have involved laboratory-induced symptoms employing motor challenge tests. Bruce et al (1990) exposed male subjects on four successive weeks to a cross-coupled nauseogenic motion challenge and compared the relative effects of active and placebo drug and acupressure combinations. Warwick-Evans, Masters & Redstone (1991) adopted a matched-pairs design and compared the efficacy of Sea Bands with a 'no-stud' placebo band in response to a Coriolus machine stimulus. None of the studies found acupressure using a Sea Band on PC-6 point, to be effective in preventing laboratory-induced motion sickness.

Table 15.1 summarizes the above data.

Discussion

Acupuncture literature refers to other sites from which an antiemetic action is claimed. However, presumably ease of access and simplicity of technique have led to all studies being limited to stimulation of PC-6.

Under certain circumstances, there is undoubtedly a psychological element in the antiemetic action of acupuncture. This probably played a part in the reported studies of morning sickness where stimulation of a 'dummy' point had some benefit. It may also have been a contributory factor in the cancer chemotherapy studies where patients knew what to expect. However, in both postoperative and cancer chemotherapy studies, stimulation of a 'dummy acupuncture point' or 'sham acupuncture' had no antiemetic action. The ability to 'block' the antiemetic action by injection of PC-6 with local anaesthesia (Dundee & Ghaly 1991) also points to a non-psychological action. Similar observation has been made in respect to acupuncture analgesia (Chiang et al 1975, Lu et al 1979).

Table 15.1 Summary of the efficacy of acupuncture antiemesis

Postoperative sickness	Good experimental and clinical evidence of efficacy. Acupuncture and TCES equieffective, but acupuncture benefit lasts longer Timing of administration may be important in relation to emetic stimulus General anaesthesia appears to suppress the antiemetic action Local anaesthesia blocks the antiemetic effect
Morning sickness	Acupressure only studied. Some benefit claimed Psychological factors may play a part
Cancer chemotherapy	PC-6 stimulation used adjunct to standard antiemetic drug therapy Good clinical evidence of efficacy Acupuncture more effective than TCES. Acupressure alone has some benefit but also is useful in prolonging the action of acupuncture and TCES
Travel sickness	Acupressure only studied Scientific evaluation limited to laboratory induced motion sickness Much anecdotal evidence of efficacy

While there is an increasing amount of evidence indicating the possible mode of action of acupuncture analgesia, the mechanism of acupuncture antiemesis remains unknown. The role of endogenous opioids in acupuncture analgesia has been investigated with some contradictory results. Some report antagonism of analgesia by naloxone (Hosobuchi, Adams & Linchitz 1977, Mayer, Price & Rafii 1977), while others found no antagonism (Chapman et al 1980, Lindblom & Tegner 1979). The consensus of opinion appears to favour the view that endogenous opioids are released by acupuncture, but this is unlikely to apply to its antiemetic action. Nash (1992) suggests that acupuncture antiemesis requires an intact nervous system, as it has been shown to reduce vomiting when administered before (Dundee et al 1989a) and after (Ho et al 1990) but not during (Weightman, Zacharias & Herbison 1987) anaesthesia. In addition, Dundee & Ghaly (1991) have reported

that local anaesthetic injection at the PC-6 point prevents the antiemetic effect of stimulation.

In general it appears that a lower frequency of stimulation is required for an antiemetic compared with an analgesic action (Ho et al 1990, Johnson et al 1989), but even this view is not universally accepted (Baldry 1989).

In a study of acupuncture as a prophylaxis for migraine headaches, Lenhard & Waite (1983) found a decrease in sickness without any analgesia. This suggests a different mechanism for the two actions of acupuncture.

A further example of this interesting hypothesis is found in a paper by Kho et al (1991) investigating acupuncture analgesia following major surgery. In this study the effect of fentanyl analgesia is compared with combined acupuncture and TCES analgesia. Of the four body and three ear points stimulated, none is regarded as having a specific antiemetic action. Although specific data on the incidence of nausea and vomiting are not given, the authors comment that their findings suggest that those patients who had the combined acupuncture and TCES analgesia experienced less sickness than those having fentanyl analgesia. While this would not be an unexpected finding in view of the different mean doses of fentanyl in the two groups, it is none the less interesting as it clearly highlights the fact that generalities in reporting studies, while apparently simple, may well be inappropriate and if quoted out of context can be misleading.

Harris (1982) has suggested that vomiting induced by cytotoxic therapy is mediated via enkephalinergic pathways, which would preclude an endorphin-mediated action for acupuncture antiemesis.

It is many years since Borison & Wang (1953) demonstrated the existence of a vomiting centre, which receives stimuli from various sites including the chemoreceptor trigger zone (CTZ), the gastrointestinal tract and the cerebral cortex. The CTZ, located on the floor of the fourth venticle within the area postrema, senses chemical stimuli that can provoke emesis when present in the blood in sufficient concentration. Based on the response to therapy, a number of possible neurotransmitters have been postulated : receptors for dopamine, serotonin, cholinergic and possibly adrenergic and histaminergic drugs may all be involved in the transmission of neurochemical signals (Borison & McCarthy 1983, Peroutka & Synder 1982). This may explain the efficacy of a five-drug regimen in preventing sickness induced by cisplatin combination therapy (Kessler, Alberts & Plezia 1986, Editorial Lancet 1987). The synergistic effect of PC-6 stimulation with standard antiemetics suggests that it may be acting on another, as yet unknown, transmitter.

PROBLEMS ENCOUNTERED IN THE EVALUATION OF ACUPUNCTURE ANTIEMESIS

If acupuncture is to become accepted as a valued treatment in the Western world, scientific evaluation by experienced research teams and perseverance in gaining publication for the results are vital. Although few would disagree with this, there is still a paucity of scientific data and only a few 'orthodox practitioners' with experience in scientific studies have shown an interest in complementary techniques. Those who have, however, can attempt to identify some prejudices and present some of the specific problems encountered in a scientific evaluation of acupuncture antiemesis. This experience may be of benefit to others who wish to evaluate different aspects of acupuncture or to try and explain its effects.

The studies carried out by Professor Dundee and his colleagues are of particular importance, as they encompass not only a variety of techniques of stimulation but also a range of different clinical situations. In an attempt to describe and emphasize some of the problems inherent in the scientific evaluation of acupuncture antiemesis, specific reference will be made to the work of these researchers (Dundee & McMillan 1992).

Preliminary considerations

When designing any study, consideration of some of the reported pitfalls is helpful. While acupuncture is used in a wide range of clinical situations, despite claims for its efficacy, its use remains largely empirical. This may be owing to the hesitation of Western practitioners to attempt to apply scientific method to the assessment of treatment techniques that derive from an unfamiliar system of medicine that, by their standards, is not in itself scientifically based. Indeed Prance et al (1988) clearly define problems encountered in the reporting of acupuncture research arising from existing differences in the underlying concepts and methodology.

A problem with much of the literature, particularly that originating in China, is the fundamental, totally uncritical acceptance of the effectiveness of the technique, with emphasis being placed mainly on descriptive reporting in the form of case histories or studies with too-small samples. Further discrepancies arise from the lack of clear definition of the exact technique and method of stimulation adopted. While the term acupuncture means simply 'piercing the skin with a sharp instrument', it is often used in broader terms to include both invasive needling with manual or electrical stimulation and the non-invasive transcutaneous application of an electical current via surface electrodes. Recently there have been some studies reporting specifically the effects of the non-invasive acupressure technique (Barsoum, Perry & Fraser 1990, Fry 1986, Lewis et al 1991, Price, Lewith & Williams 1991). It is essential in reporting findings to differentiate between invasive and non-invasive stimulation of acupuncture points as it is becoming clear that the clinical effect may vary according to how the technique is applied.

Criteria for the ideal clinical trial

Box 15.1 outlines the generally acceptable criteria for scientific clinical evaluations in any field (Dundee 1974, Mirakhur 1988). While some of these are unachievable in acupuncture studies, others can be considered in the light of experience of previously reported studies.

Having considered the criteria and identified an adequate source of suitable patients, it is necessary to write a protocol that defines the object of the study and details the procedure involved. On occasion a preliminary protocol

---

Box 15.1 Criteria for the ideal clinical trial

1. A proposed study must be acceptable to the regional ethical committee or other responsible review body.
2. The method under study should be compared with a recognized 'standard' technique, where this exists.
3. If ethically acceptable a 'dummy treatment' (placebo) should be included in the study.
4. All three forms of treatment (new, standard, dummy) should be given in random order.
5. Patients should be typical of a larger population in whom the condition to be treated presents a real clinical problem.
6. Informed verbal/written consent should be obtained from the patients.
7. Explanation of the procedure to the patients should not be suggestive of one particular outcome.
8. Patient variables must be reduced to a minimum where possible e.g. sex, age group, severity of illness. Surroundings and attendants may be important in some studies.
9. Concomitant medication should be standardized as far as possible.
10. There should be a limited number of observers, with at least one participating throughout the study.
11. A specific end point for the particular trial and exclusion criteria for subjects must be defined.
12. An acceptable method is needed for quantifying and recording data.
13. Assessment of benefit should be on a 'single-blind' or 'double-blind' basis.

---

may be necessary, followed by a feasibility (pilot) study, which would also look at consistency of results, after which a final version can be prepared. This is often an acceptable compromise of what the researcher would like to do and what can actually be achieved (Dundee 1974).

In some instances it may be that only those patients who have already failed to derive benefit from all the relevant Western treatment methods are allowed to join in an acupuncture study. There may also be the insistence that these patients should continue their existing orthodox treatment during the study: since these trials are carried out on a 'difficult' group of patients the question may be raised, if any success is achieved, as to which form of treatment is the effective one.

Ethical permission

The function of a medical ethical research committee is to examine the scientific validity of the study and oversee the ethical considerations. No research should be detrimental to the patients' well-being with disadvantages or side-effects outweighing any potential benefit. Furthermore, a procedure should not be administered unless there are reasonable grounds to believe it to be of some therapeutic value.

When, in 1984, Professor Dundee submitted the protocol that initiated the study of acupuncture for its antiemetic action in the postoperative field it was only after considerable amendment that approval was granted (Chestnutt & Dundee 1985). Fewer difficulties were encountered in subsequent studies and, indeed, it is unlikely that problems would exist to the same extent today, which is attributable mainly to the extent of work that has now been completed in the area of acupuncture antiemesis. If there exists some scepticism of the use of complementary techniques among individuals involved in ethical committees, submission of a carefully prepared, detailed protocol should help to minimize the effect this will have on gaining approval.

Uncontrolled and controlled clinical trials

Uncontrolled trials can be useful only in giving preliminary indications of the general effectiveness of a particular treatment. The presence of a control group enables a comparison to be made and subsequently a judgement may be drawn as to which particular method reported findings can be attributed.

Three different types of control can be adopted: no treatment, an alternative established treatment or a placebo. In many of the reported studies the alternative treatment consisted of using standard, acceptable antiemetic drugs whose efficacy in the particular clinical situation, had previously been assessed.

Acupuncture might well be expected in itself to have a powerful placebo effect. Beecher (1955) found, in a series of studies, that a number of subjective symptoms including nausea can be temporarily relieved in about 35% of patients by placebo effect alone. Other psychological mechanisms, as described by Lu (1983), including anxiety reduction, patient motivation and distraction, may also be involved in its efficacy.

Possible placebos for use in acupuncture trials include the use of non-acupuncture sites or sham points (Lewith & Machin 1983) and the application of mock TCES in which no current actually reaches the patient (McMillan 1994). An interesting finding reported by Vincent et al (1989) is that elicitation of De Qi (needling sensation), which was considered to be a favourable prerequisite to successful treatment, does not occur any more frequently at classical acupuncture sites than at sham points.

In acupressure studies, using the commercially available Sea Bands, the placebo treatment can consist of stimulation of a sham point at the ankle (Price, Lewith & Williams 1991) or alternatively 'stimulation' of the PC-6 point using a band without a stud or incorporating a 'blunted' button (De Aloysio & Penacchioni 1992).

Randomization

Theoretically this should be easy, but problems have been encountered. In one of the morning sickness studies involving acupressure (Dundee et al 1988), patients were given a card with full instructions as to which point to press (or not to press any) and how to complete the record of sickness. When attending the antenatal clinic the women talked freely to each other and compared experiences, so a number of them then asked why they were to use different points from others. True randomization became impossible as it was necessary to change the system of allocation so that one treatment was given to all patients attending in the same week.

Patient explanation and consent

These can be a problem for which there is no universal solution as each situation requires an individual approach. In many of the postoperative sickness studies there was no specific mention of sickness, but patients were told that the aim was to establish whether the acupuncture technique would improve the 'quality of recovery'. It has been considered necessary in antenatal studies to inform the patients that the incidence and severity of morning sickness is being assessed.

In the oncology studies carried out by Professor Dundee and his colleagues (Dundee et al 1989b, 1991), the chemotherapy patients referred for acupuncture initially were those who had been sick after a previous dose of medication, and nursing staff and oncologists freely referred to 'reducing or stopping sickness'. Details of the technique spread quickly among the patients and reports of the findings by the media left no one in any doubt as to the aim of the study. As assessment was dependent on the patient's detailed description of their symptoms, prior knowledge of the trial's intentions was not found to be a problem in studying acupuncture antiemesis in this group of patients. It was felt that the use of a written record in the form of a diary was not appropriate for these patients, as a personal approach by a familiar member of staff was more acceptable.

Reducing variables

In any evaluation study, for the purposes of replication or use in clinical practice it is important to use as standardized an approach as possible—not only as regards the patient variables, but also the regimen of acupuncture treatment implemented and concomitant medication administered.

In postoperative studies it is possible to adhere strictly to these criteria. The effective emetic stimulus, for example a moderately emetic opioid premedication, is given prior to a standardized surgical procedure with all other factors held constant. The standardized anaesthetic technique, adopted by Dundee et al (1989a) using nalbuphine premedication in women patients undergoing minor gynaecological surgery, was successfully evaluated in over 500 cases.

Interestingly, however, when he returned to this area of study in 1990 to evaluate modifications in the technique of electrical stimulation of PC-6, although access to the same type of patient was freely available, anaesthetic practice had changed considerably. Minor gynaecological operations were now mainly done on an out-patient basis, requiring a much more rapid recovery than previously, and the introduction of the intravenous anaesthetic propofol with its known antiemetic action (Gunawardene & White 1988, McCollum, Milligan & Dundee 1988, Mehernoor et al 1991) had reduced post-operative sickness to negligible levels. An alternative technique, using i.v. alfentanil as the opioid, produced a slightly higher incidence of emetic sequelae but recovery was still too prolonged to be acceptable (McMillan, Moore & Dundee 1992). Needless to say, as a result of this changing pattern in medical practice the proposed follow-up study could not materialize.

In the oncology setting it is not possible to follow the criteria for standardization so closely. There is considerable variability in the emetic potential of the various chemotherapy drugs and combinations, and in these patients other factors, such as concomitant medication and site of tumour, may indirectly affect the nature and severity of symptoms. It is therefore necessary to subdivide the patients according to likely emetic outcomes associated with type and dose of chemotherapeutic agents and also consider male and female patients separately, as it is well recognized that women patients are more susceptible to sickness (Dundee et al 1991, Marty 1989).

The introduction of the new, highly effective antiemetic, ondansetron, a 5-HT antagonist (Smith et al 1990, 1991) had a dramatic effect on the standardization of the ongoing studies by Dundee and his colleagues at that time. Indeed, initially it was thought that the acupuncture antiemesis studies might have to come to a premature close because of a reduction in patient numbers; however, it soon transpired that the drug still left some patients with an unacceptable level of sickness (Dundee et al 1992), so they used this opportunity to evaluate the concomitant use of the new drug with TCES and successfully demonstrated a reduction in

incidence of sickness with this combination (McMillan, Dundee & Abram 1991).

The attitude of medical, nursing and ancillary staff can influence the outcome of a study involving subjective findings and this is obviously important with acupuncture antiemetic studies. Not all of the staff may view studies evaluating complementary techniques with equal enthusiasm, and in the presence of frank scepticism by some it is difficult to see how a good clinical trial could be carried out.

Completion and exclusion criteria

Factors to be considered in estimating the total number of patients needed for a satisfactory completion of the trial include the anticipated clinical differences between the efficacy of the techniques being evaluated, the degree of statistical significance considered to be appropriate to the area of study and the possibility of detecting that difference. Each of the different clinical situations that have been studied clearly indicated the need for this decision to be 'tailor made' for each particular set of circumstances. Specific contraindications should be defined. There is some anecdotal comment on avoiding acupuncture in early pregnancy and the use of electrical acupuncture when a pacemaker is in situ should be avoided (Rasmussen et al 1988).

Assessing benefit

How does one quantify the benefit of acupuncture? There is no clear answer to this (Lewith 1984), but before seeking statistical advice the clinician must have some idea of the degree of benefit considered necessary to recommend a specific treatment. Is a 10% reduction in emetic sequelae adequate, or should one look for complete relief of symptoms? Many factors have to be considered including the severity and likely duration of the symptoms, the prognosis regarding any coexisting condition and the effect the symptoms are having on patients' quality of life. It is therefore necessary to consider the implications of each clinical situation in such an evaluation.

Furthermore, the experience of the research coordinator must override the enthusiasm of the research worker and a clinically important finding is preferable to a statistically significant one.

Ideally, assessment of outcome should include both subjective and objective elements. Nausea is a purely subjective symptom and the reports by patients and the judgements of the observer can therefore be subject to bias. Unlike trials involving chronic pain, where methods such as the VAS and the McGill Pain Questionnaire have been developed, no comparable means of measuring nausea has yet been established although Del Favero et al (1990) have attempted to define a reliable measurement of nausea in conducting clinical trials on antiemetic treatments. In contrast, vomiting can be more clearly defined in objective terms—usually with a differentiation being made between a retch and a vomit.

In the majority of studies reported to date, a number of comparable schemes of assessment have been employed in which presence/absence, severity of sickness or a combination of the two have been used to evaluate the symptoms. These schemes usually assess nausea and vomiting separately and the subjective nature of the former has not been found a problem, with reliable and reproducible findings being reported.

Single blind or double blind?

While the double-blind approach is the ideal, a number of studies by different workers have indicated that a single-blind or even an open assessment can be acceptable. Ultimately the number of available staff will often determine the method to be used.

For example in the early postoperative studies Dundee employed both single- and double-blind methods but even here he recorded that a number of patients proudly showed the 'blinded' assessor the spot where the needle was inserted, remarking that the insertion of the needle was painless and did not cause bleeding.

Vincent & Richardson (1986) indeed question whether a double-blind approach can be applied adequately in the evaluation of any therapeutic effects of acupuncture. They argue that for a truly blind procedure the technique must be administered by a naive and inexperienced practitioner who may not produce an adequate standard of treatment; they therefore advocate single-blind studies with independent outcome assessment.

Discussion

Despite the inherent problems associated with the evaluation of a technique such as acupuncture, it would appear that a scientific approach to this aspect is possible and that a properly designed trial can conform for the most part to the generally accepted criteria of conventional studies. The experience of Professor Dundee and his colleagues has been highlighted because this work considers different methods of stimulation and their application to a number of clinical situations. The reported problems give a clear illustration of the likely pitfalls that may be encountered and it is hoped that this will be helpful to other workers who may consider further evaluating this technique.

The studies reported to date on acupuncture antiemesis have involved controlled study experimentation, as in the clinical situations studied the emetic sequelae were expected to persist for a limited duration. In situations where sickness is likely to present over a more extended period of time, evaluation of the efficacy of acupuncture could be carried out satisfactorily by adopting single-case experiment designs, which can also be considered in scientific terms (Hersen & Barlow 1976).

It is normal practice to get the opinion of one's peers on research work and in the past decade there has been a gradual increase in the number of presentations at conferences all over the world and also publications on the topic of acupuncture antiemesis. It is important that even negative findings should be presented at some forum and published, even if only as an abstract. Data that remain unanalysed and findings that are not communicated to colleagues are a betrayal of the trust that the participating patients and colleagues place in the investigator.

In the future, perseverance and properly designed trials will further improve the acceptance of publications and it is vital that papers are submitted to and published in journals associated with the speciality related to the clinical condition in which the acupuncture techniques have been evaluated, rather than only in complementary medicine journals.

CONCLUSION

Traditional Chinese explanations of how acupuncture works remain difficult to understand in the light of current knowledge of anatomy and physiology. Nevertheless it is possible to apply Western methods of evaluation in terms of properly controlled, scientific trials. In China acupuncture has been established in the treatment of nausea and vomiting for several thousand years but only in the past decade has it been subjected to objective scientific study.

While the mechanisms involved in nausea and vomiting are complex and the aetiology multifactorial, nevertheless there is a growing body of evidence to support a limited clinical efficacy of acupuncture. To date much of the evidence has come from evaluation of PC-6 stimulation in certain well-defined clinical situations (Dundee & McMillan 1991). The findings, however, demand further study and it may be necessary to broaden investigations to include other antiemetic acupuncture points, initially singly, but with a possible view to evaluation of combined points in order to maximize therapeutic outcome.

Current knowledge offers no understanding of how acupuncture works in controlling nausea and vomiting, but this should not limit the use of a technique that may enhance patient care. Ignorance of how a treatment works has not previously been a hindrance to its use in the practice of modern medicine. For practitioners involved in the treatment of patients, the pursuit of scientific goals may have to take second place to the achievement of clinical goals. It is more important to establish, using scientific methodology, that a treatment is safe and that it works. Patients cannot always wait for the scientists and practitioners to have the luxury of knowing how and why.

REFERENCES

Aglietti L, Roila F, Tonato M 1990 A pilot study of metoclopramide, dexamethasone, diphenhydramine and acupuncture in women treated with cisplatin. Cancer Chemotherapy Pharmacology 26:239–240

Allen D L, Kitching A J, Nagle C 1994 P6 acupressure and nausea and vomiting after gynaecological surgery. Anaesthesia and Intensive Care 22:691–693

Baldry P E 1989 Acupuncture: Trigger points and musculoskeletal pain. Churchill Livingstone, New York

Barsoum G, Perry E P, Fraser I A 1990 Postoperative nausea is relieved by acupressure. Journal of the Royal Society of Medicine 83:86–89

Bateman N 1991 Selected side-effect: 4. Metoclopramide and acute movement disorders. Prescribers Journal 31:212–215

Beecher H K 1955 The powerful placebo. Journal of the American Medical Association 159:1602–1606

Beijing College of Traditional Chinese Medicine, Shanghai College of Traditional Chinese Medicine, Nanjing College of Traditional Chinese Medicine, The Acupuncture Institute of the Academy of Traditional Chinese Medicine 1980 Essentials of Chinese acupuncture. Foreign Languages Press, Beijing

Belluomini J, Litt R C, Lee K A, Katz M 1994 Acupuncture for nausea and vomiting of pregnancy: a randomized, blinded study. Obstetrics and Gynecology 84:245–248

Bill K M, Dundee J W 1988 Acupressure for postoperative nausea and vomiting. British Journal of Clinical Pharmacology 26:225 p

Brill J R 1995 Acupuncture for nausea and vomiting of pregnancy: a randomized, blinded study [letter]. Obstetrics and Gynecology 85:159–160

British Medical Association Board of Science and Education 1986 Alternative Therapies. British Medical Association, London

Borison H L, McCarthy L E 1983 Neuropharmacology of chemotherapy-induced emesis. Drugs 25:8–17 (Suppl. 1)

Borison H L, Wang S G 1953 Physiology and pharmacology of vomiting. Pharmacological Reviews 5:193–230

Broadman L M, Ceruzzi W, Patane P S, Hannallah R S, Ruttimann U, Friendly D 1990 Metoclopramide reduces the incidence of vomiting following strabismus surgery in children. Anesthesiology 72:245–248

Bruce D G, Golding J F, Hockenhull J, Pethybridge R J 1990 Acupressure and motion sickness. Aviation Space Environmental Medicine 61:361–365

Chang S T 1976 The complete book of acupuncture. Celestial Arts, Berkeley, CA

Chapman C R, Colpitts Y M, Benedetti C, Kitaeff R, Gehrig J D 1980 Evoked potential assessment of acupuncture analgesia; attempted reversal with naloxone. Pain 9:183–197

Chestnutt W N, Dundee J W 1986 Acupuncture for the relief of meptazinol-induced vomiting. British Journal of Anaesthesia 57:825P–826P

Chiang C Y, Zhang Q C, Khu X L, Yang L F 1973 Peripheral afferent pathways for acupuncture analgesia. Scientia Sinica 16:210–217

Chiang C Y, Liu J Y, Chu T H, Pai Y H, Chang S C 1975 Studies on spinal ascending pathway for effect of acupuncture analgesia in rabbits. Scientia Sinica 18:651–658

Clarke R S J, Dundee J W, Loan W B 1970 The use of postoperative vomiting as a means of evaluating antiemetics. British Journal of Pharmacology 40:568–569

Coates A, Abraham S, Kaye S B, Sowerbutts S T, Frewin C, Fox R M, Tattersall M H N 1983 On the receiving end—patient perception of the side effects of cancer chemotherapy. European Journal of Cancer Clinical Oncology 19:203–208

Cubeddu L X, Hoffmann I S, Fuenmayor N T, Finn A L 1990 Efficacy of ondansetron (GR38032F) and the role of serotonin in cisplatin-induced nausea and vomiting. New England Journal of Medicine 322:810–815

Cunningham D 1990 Treatment of emesis induced by cytotoxic drugs. Hospital Update 16:104

De Aloysio D, Penacchioni P 1992 Morning sickness control in early pregnancy by Neiguan point acupressure. Obstetrics and Gynecology 80:852–854

Del Favero A, Roila F, Basurto C, Minotti V, Ballatori E, Patoia L, Tonato M, Tognoni G 1990 Assessment of nausea. European Journal of Clinical Pharmacology 38:115–120

Deng D H, Tan O L, Han J S 1986 Observations on combatting nausea by finger pressure on the Hegu point. Journal of Traditional Chinese Medicine 6:111–112

Department of Physiology, Guangsi Medical University 1961 The mechanisms of acupuncture for gastric acid secretion. Guangdong Traditional Chinese Medicine 2:55–58

Dickinson D 1991 Acupuncture without needles. Which? Way to Health 12:188–190

Dundee J W 1974 Introduction of new drugs symposium—clinical trials in anaesthesia. Proceedings of the Royal Society of Medicine 67:586–588

Dundee J W, Chestnutt W N, Ghaly R G, Lynas A G A 1986 Traditional Chinese acupuncture: a potentially useful antiemetic? British Medical Journal 293:583–584

Dundee J W, Ghaly R G 1991 Local anaesthesia blocks the antiemetic action of P6 acupuncture. Clinical Pharmacology and Therapeutics 50:78–80

Dundee J W, McMillan C 1991 Positive evidence for P6 acupuncture antiemesis. Postgraduate Medical Journal 67:417–422

Dundee J, McMillan C 1992 Some problems encountered in the scientific evaluation of acupuncture antiemesis. Acupuncture in Medicine 10:2–8

Dundee J W, Yang J 1990 Prolongation of the antiemetic action of P6 acupuncture by acupressure in patients having cancer chemotherapy. Journal of the Royal Society of Medicine 83:360–362

Dundee J W, Milligan K R, McKay A C 1988 The influence of intraoperative acupuncture and droperidol on postoperative emesis. British Journal of Anaesthesia 61:116–117

Dundee J W, Sourial F B R, Ghaly R G, Bell P F 1988 P6 acupressure reduces morning sickness. Journal of Royal Society of Medicine 81:456–457

Dundee J W, Ghaly R G, Bill K M, Chestnutt W N, Fitzpatrick K T J, Lynas A G A 1989 Effect of stimulation of the P6 antiemetic point on postoperative nausea and vomiting. British Journal of Anaesthesia 63:612–618

Dundee J W, Ghaly R G, Fitzpatrick K T J, Abram W P, Lynch G A 1989 Acupuncture prophylaxis of cancer chemotherapy-induced sickness. Journal of the Royal Society of Medicine 82:268–271

Dundee J W, Yang J, McMillan C 1991 Non-invasive stimulation of P6 (Neiguan) antiemetic acupuncture point in cancer chemotherapy. Journal of the Royal Society of Medicine 84:210–212

Dundee J W, Yang J, McMillan C M, Mahdi A 1991 Some factors influencing cancer chemotherapy sickness. British Journal of Clinical Pharmacology 31:601p

Dundee J W, McMillan C M, Yang J, Wright P M C 1992 Is ondansetron a less effective antiemetic against moderately emetic as compared with highly emetic chemotherapy? British Journal of Clinical Pharmacology 33:200–201

Editorial 1987 The chemoreceptor trigger zone revisited. Lancet i:144

Fagan E A, Chadwick V S 1983 Drug treatment of gastrointestinal disorders in pregnancy. In: Lewis P (ed) Clinical pharmacology in obstetrics. Wright, Bristol, pp 114–137

Fetting J H, Grochow L B, Folstein M F, Ettinger D S, Colvin M 1982 The course of nausea and vomiting after high dose cyclophosphamide. Cancer Treatment Reports 66:1487–1493

Fishman J A 1981 Seasickness cure: it's all in the wrists. New York Times March 15

Foster J M G, Sweeney B P 1987 The mechanisms of acupuncture analgesia. British Journal of Hospital Medicine 38:308–312

Fry E N S 1986 Acupressure and postoperative vomiting. Anaesthesia 41:661–662

Frytak S, Moertel C G 1981 Management of nausea and vomiting in the cancer patient. Journal of the American Medical Association 245:393–396

Gralla R J, Itri L M, Pisko S E 1981 Antiemetic efficacy of high dose metoclopramide; randomised trials with placebo and prochlorperazine in patients with chemotherapy-induced nausea and vomiting. New England Journal of Medicine 305:905–909

Grunberg S M 1990 Making chemotherapy easier. New England Journal of Medicine 322:846–848

Gunawardene R D, White D C 1988 Propofol and emesis. Anaesthesia 43 (Suppl.):65–67

Hardy J F, Charest J, Girouard G, Lepage Y 1986 Nausea and vomiting after strabismus surgery in preschool children. Canadian Anaesthetic Society Journal 33:57–62

Harris A L 1982 Cytotoxic-therapy induced vomiting is mediated via enkephalic pathways. Lancet i:714–716

Heine H 1988 Anatomische Struktur der Akupunkturpunkie. Deutshe Zeitschrift Akupunktur 31:26–30

Hersen M, Barlow D H 1976 Single case experimental designs: strategies for studying behavioural change. Pergamon, Oxford

Ho R T, Jawan B, Fung S T, Cheung H K, Lee J H 1990 Electroacupuncture and postoperative emesis. Anaesthesia 45:327–329

Hoskin P J, Hanks G W 1988 The management of symptoms in advanced cancer: experience in a hospital-based continuing care unit. Journal of the Royal Society of Medicine 81:341–344

Hosobuchi Y, Adams J E, Linchitz R 1977 Pain relief by electrical stimulation of the central gray matter in humans and its reversal by naloxone. Science 197:183–186

Hyde E 1989 Acupressure therapy for morning sickness. A controlled clinical trial. Journal of Nurse-Midwifery 34:171–178

Jindrak M 1980 (Treatment of vomitus matutinus and emesis gravidarum by acupuncture in clinical practice.) Ceska Gynekologie 45:303–304 (In Czech)

Johnson M I, Ashton C H, Bousfield D R, Thompson J W 1989 Analgesic effects of different frequencies of transcutaneous electrical nerve stimulation on cold induced pain in normal subjects. Pain 39:231–236

Jones A L, Hill A S, Soukop M, Hutcheon A W, Cassidy J, Kaye S B, Sikora K, Carney D N, Cunningham D 1991 Comparison of dexamethasone and ondansetron in the prophylaxis of emesis induced by moderately emetogenic chemotherapy. Lancet 338:483–487

Kessler J F, Alberts D S, Plezia P M 1986 An effective five-drug antiemetic combination for prevention of chemotherapy-related nausea and vomiting. Cancer Chemotherapy Pharmacology 16:282–286

Kho H G, Eijk R J R, Kapteijns W M M J, Van Egmond J 1991 Acupuncture and transcutaneous stimulation analgesia in comparison with moderate-dose fentanyl anaesthesia in major surgery. Anaesthesia 46:129–135

Kris M G, Gralla R J, Tyson L B, Clark R A, Kelsen D P, Reilly L K, Groshen S, Bosl G J, Kalman L A 1985 Improved control of cisplatin-induced emesis with high dose metoclopramide and with a combination of metoclopramide, dexamethasone and diphenhydramine. Cancer 55:527–534

Kris M G, Gralla R J, Clark R A, Tyson L B 1988 Dose ranging evaluation of the serotonin antagonist GR38032F when used as an antiemetic in patients receiving anticancer chemotherapy. Journal of Clinical Oncology 6:659–662

Lenhard L, Waite P M E 1983 Acupuncture in the prophylactic treatment of migraine headaches: pilot study. New Zealand Medical Journal 96:663–666

Lentz J M 1982 Two experiments on laboratory induced motion sickness I. acupressure II. repeated exposure. US Naval Aerospace Medical Research Laboratory Report, Pensacola, Florida

Lerman J, Eustis S, Smith D R 1986 Effect of droperidol pretreatment on postanaesthetic vomiting in children undergoing strabismus surgery. Anesthesiology 65:322–325

Lewis I H, Pryn S J, Reynolds P I, Pandit U A, Wilton N C T 1991 Effect of P6 acupressure on postoperative vomiting in children undergoing outpatient strabismus correction. British Journal of Anaesthesia 67:73–78

Lewith G T 1984 Can we assess the effects of acupuncture? British Medical Journal 288:1475–1476

Lewith G T, Lewith N R 1983 Modern Chinese acupuncture. Thorsons, London

Lewith G T, Machin D 1983 On the evaluation of the clinical effects of acupuncture. Pain 16:111–127

Li Y, Tougas G, Chiverton S G, Hunt R H 1992 The effect of acupuncture on gastrointestinal function and disorders. American Journal of Gastroenterology 87:1372–1381

Lindblom U, Tegner R 1979 Are the endorphins active in clinical pain states? Narcotic antagonism in chronic pain patients. Pain 7:65–68

Liu S, Chen Z, Hou J, Wang J, Zhang X 1991 Magnetic disk applied on Neiguan point for prevention and treatment of cisplatin-induced nausea and vomiting. Journal of Traditional Chinese Medicine 11:181–183

Lu G W 1983 Neurobiologic research on acupuncture in China as exemplified by acupuncture analgesia. Anesthesia and Analgesia 62:335–340

Lu G, Liang R, Xie J, Wang Y, He G 1979 Role of peripheral afferent nerve fibers in acupuncture analgesia elicited by needling point Zusanli. Scientia Sinica 22:680–692

McCollum J S C, Milligan K R, Dundee J W 1988 The antiemetic action of propofol. Anaesthesia 43:239–240

McConaghy P M, Bland D G, Swales H A 1996 Acupuncture in the management of postoperative nausea and vomiting in patients receiving morphine via a patient-controlled analgesia system. Acupuncture in Medicine, 14:2–5

McMillan C M 1994 Transcutaneous electrical stimulation of Neiguan antiemetic acupuncture point in controlling sickness following opioid analgesia in major orthopaedic surgery. Physiotherapy 80:5–9

McMillan C, Dundee J W 1990 Problems of self-administration of P6 (Neiguan) antiemesis. British Journal of Clinical Pharmacology 31:236p

McMillan C M, Dundee J W 1991 The role of transcutaneous electrical stimulation of Neiguan antiemetic acupuncture point in controlling sickness after cancer chemotherapy. Physiotherapy 77:499–502

McMillan C, Dundee J W 1991b Is self-stimulation of P6 feasible as an antiemetic in cancer chemotherapy? British Journal of Anaesthesia 66:394p–414p

McMillan C, Dundee J W, Abram W P 1991 Enhancement of the antiemetic action of ondansetron by transcutaneous electrical stimulation of the P6 antiemetic point, in patients having highly emetic cytotoxic drugs. British Journal of Cancer 64:971–972

McMillan C M, Moore J, Dundee J W 1992 Changing clinical anaesthetic practice influences the evaluation of antiemetic therapy. Irish Journal of Medical Sciences 161:20–21

Mann F 1987 Textbook of acupuncture. William Heinemann, London

Mannheimer J S, Lampe G N 1984 Clinical transcutaneous electrical nerve stimulation. Davies, Philadelphia, pp 59–61

Marty M 1989 Ondansetron in the prophylaxis of acute cisplatin-induced nausea and vomiting. European Journal of Cancer Clinical Oncology 25 (Suppl. 1):S41–S45

Masuda A, Miyazaki H, Yamazki M, Pintov S, Ito Y 1986 Acupuncture in the anesthetic management of eye surgery. Acupuncture Electro-Therapeutics Research 11:259–267

Mayer D J, Price D D, Rafii A 1977 Antagonism of acupuncture analgesia in man by narcotic antagonist naloxone. Brain Research 121:368–372

Mirakhur R K 1988 Designing a clinical trial. Bailliere's Clinical Anaesthesiology 2:157–174

Nash T P 1992 Acupuncture and postoperative vomiting in children. British Journal of Anaesthesia 68:633–634

Osadchaia O V, Shabadash V V 1989 Changes of central nervous system function in patients with hyperemesis gravidarum treated by acupuncture. Akusherstvoi Ginerologii (Mosk) 5:55–56

Peroutka S J, Snyder S H 1982 Antiemetics: neurotransmitter

receptor binding predicts therapeutic actions. Lancet
i:658–659

Prance S E, Dresser A, Wood C, Fleming J, Aldridge D,
Pietroni P C 1988 Research on traditional Chinese
acupuncture science or myth: a review. Journal of the
Royal Society of Medicine 81:588–590

Price H, Lewith G, Williams S C 1991 Acupressure as an
antiemetic in cancer chemotherapy. Complementary
Medical Research 5:93–94

Priestman T J 1989 The management of the side effects of
cytotoxic drugs in cancer chemotherapy: an introduction,
3rd edn. Springer-Verlag, Berlin

Rasmussen M J, Hayes D L, Vlietstra R E, Thorsteinsson G
1988 Can transcutaneous electrical nerve stimulation be
safely used in patients with permanent cardiac
pacemakers? Mayo Clinic Proceedings 63:443–445

Richardson P H, Vincent C A 1986 Acupuncture for the
treatment of pain: a review of evaluative research. Pain
24:15–40

Robinson S L, Fell D 1991 Nausea and vomiting with use
of a patient-controlled analgesia system. Anaesthesia
46:580–582

Root D T 1989 P6 acupressure reduces morning sickness.
Journal of the Royal Society of Medicine 82:635

Sacco J J, Grant W D, Luthringer D D, London A, Kamps C A
1990 The reduction of post-surgical nausea and vomiting
in patients receiving NO. Anesthesiology 73:A15

Smith D B, Newlands E S, Spruyt O W, Begent R H J,
Rustin G J S, Mellor B, Bagshawe K D 1990 Ondansetron
(GR 38032F) plus dexamethasone: effective antiemetic
prophylaxis for patients receiving cytotoxic
chemotherapy. British Journal of Cancer 61:323–324

Smith D B, Newlands E S, Rustin G J S, Begent R H J,
Howells N, McQuade B, Bagshawe K D 1991 Comparison
of ondansetron and ondansetron plus dexamethasone as
antiemetic prophylaxis during cisplatin containing
chemotherapy. Lancet 338:487–490

Soukop M, Cunningham D 1987 The treatment of nausea
and vomiting induced by cytotoxic drugs. Baillière's
Clinical Oncology 1:307–326

Stainton M C, Neff E J 1994 The efficacy of Seabands for the
control of nausea and vomiting in pregnancy. Health Care
Woman International 15:563–575

Stannard D 1989 Pressure prevents nausea. Nursing Times
85:33–34

Stux G, Pomeranz G S B 1987 Acupuncture: textbook and
atlas. Springer-Verlag, Berlin

Stux G, Pomeranz B 1991 Basics of acupuncture. Springer-
Verlag, Berlin

Thomas K J, Carr J, Westlake L, Williams B T 1991 Use of
non-orthodox and conventional health care in Great
Britain. British Medical Journal 302:207–210

Veroli P, Astier V 1992 Acupressure and postoperative
vomiting in strabismus correction. British Journal of
Anaethesia 68:634

Vickers A 1996 Can acupuncture have specific effects on
health? A systematic review of acupuncture antiemesis
trials. Journal of the Royal Society of Medicine 89: 303–311

Vincent C A, Richardson P H 1986 The evaluation of
therapeutic acupuncture: concepts and methods. Pain
24:1–13

Vincent C A, Richardson P H, Black J J, Pither C E 1989
Significance of needle placement site in acupuncture.
Journal of Psychosomatic Research 33:489–496

Warrington P 1991 Hidden costs of chemotherapy. Hospital
Doctor 7 February:48

Warwick-Evans L A, Masters I J, Redstone S B 1991 A
double-blind placebo controlled evaluation of acupressure
in the treatment of motion sickness. Aviation, Space and
Environmental Medicine 62:776–778

Watcha M F, Simeon R M, White P F, Stevens J L 1991 Effect
of propofol on the incidence of postoperative vomiting
after strabismus surgery in pediatric outpatients.
Anesthesiology 75:204–209

Watcha M F, White P F 1992 Postoperative nausea and
vomiting. Its etiology, treatment and prevention.
Anesthesiology 77:162–184

Weightman W M, Zacharias M, Herbison P 1987 Traditional
Chinese acupuncture as an antiemetic. British Medical
Journal 295:1379–1380

Wheatley R G, Madej T H, Jackson I J, Hunter D 1991 The
first year's experience of an acute pain service. British
Journal of Anaesthesia 67:353–359

Wilcox P M, Fetting J H, Nettesheim K M, Abeloff M D 1982
Anticipatory vomiting in women receiving
cyclophosphamide, methotrexate and 5FU (CMF)
adjuvant chemotherapy for breast carcinoma. Cancer
Treatment Reports 66:1601–1604

Williams C J, Davies C, Raval M, Middleton J, Luken J,
Stone B 1989 Comparison of starting antiemetic treatment
24 hours before or concurrently with cytotoxic
chemotherapy. British Medical Journal 298:430–431

Yang L C, Jawan B, Chen C N, Ho R T, Chang K A, Lee J H
1993 Comparison of P6 acupoint injection with 50%
glucose in water and intravenous droperidol for
prevention of vomiting after gynecological laparoscopy.
Acta Anaesthesiologica Scandanavica 37:192–194

Yentis S M, Bissonnette B 1991 P6 acupuncture and
postoperative vomiting after tonsillectomy in children.
British Journal of Anaesthesia 67:779–780

Yentis S M, Bissonnette B 1992 Ineffectiveness of
acupuncture and droperidol in preventing vomiting
following strabismus repair in children. Canadian Journal
of Anaesthesia 39:151–154

Yuan C X, Li P M, Zhu J 1985 Clinical value and mechanisms
of the action of the acupuncture points 'Pishu' and
'Weishu'. Chinese Acupuncture 4:5–8

Yuan C X, Zhu J, Zhing L X 1985 Gastroscopic observation of
the effect of acupuncture on gastric motility. Jiangxi
Journal of Chinese Traditional Medicine 3:33–34

Zhao C X 1988 Acupuncture treatment of morning sickness.
Journal of Traditional Chinese Medicine 8:228–229

Zhao R J 1987 39 cases of morning sickness treated with
acupuncture. Journal of Traditional Chinese Medicine
7:25–26

ARCHIVE

16

Acupuncture in the pain clinic

Joan Hester

INTRODUCTION

Pain management clinics have evolved in Britain and throughout the world over the past 20 years as a response to the tremendous challenge of chronic intractable pain. The prevalence of chronic pain is not known, although a survey of 1489 adults in New Zealand (James et al 1991) reported that 82% of subjects had experienced more than one life-disrupting experience of pain. The Office of Population Censuses and Surveys (OPCS) in Great Britain surveyed disabled people between 1985 and 1988. The survey was not widely published, but produced some startling results (Coniam & Diamond 1994); it found that 10% of the population was disabled and, of the 10%, 41% suffered from severe pain, 36% stated that it limited their daily activity, and 28% said that it was excruciating, terrible or distressing pain, severely affecting their normal life.

Such pain not only affects the life of the individual and is costly in terms of human suffering but it is also costly in terms of provision of care, drugs and medical intervention. The late Dr John Bonica of the University of Washington Medical School devoted his life to the understanding of pain and attempted to relieve it using a combination of drugs, local anaesthetic nerve blocks, psychological manipulation and other more sophisticated techniques.

In 1965 Ronald Melzack from McGill University, Montreal, and Patrick Wall of University College, London propounded the 'gate control theory' of pain. This new and original thinking has greatly influenced the attitudes of health care professionals world-wide to the perception and treatment of pain, and has provided a neurophysiological basis for many symptoms previously thought to be 'in the mind' (Melzack & Wall 1965).

Since then there has been much neuro-physiological research that has greatly increased our understanding as to why pain becomes intractable. Finding a solution to the problem is a much more difficult task. Prior to 1965 it was thought that cutting a nerve pathway to the painful area would stop the pain. This is not so; in fact it can lead to much more painful dysaesthesiae after nerve transection, owing to changes of neurotransmission within the spinal cord.

Modern techniques look towards manipulation of drugs that affect pain transmission in the CNS and neurostimulatory techniques such as TENS and acupuncture, which act to increase inhibition of nociceptive impulses.

WHAT IS PAIN?

Pain is defined as an 'unpleasant sensory and emotional experience, associated with actual or potential tissue damage or expressed in terms of such damage' (International Association for the Study of Pain 1994). Chronic pain is defined as a pain that persists past the normal time of healing (Bonica 1953). In practice this may be less than 1 month, but often more than 6 months. With non-malignant pain, 3 months is the most convenient point of division between acute and chronic pain but for research purposes 6 months will often be preferred. (International Association for the Study of Pain 1994).

There are four types of pain:

- nociceptive pain
- neuropathic pain
- sympathetically mediated pain
- psychogenic pain.

In any one chronic pain disorder there can be overlap between these types of pain, for example:

- a stump pain may have a nociceptive component if, say, the prosthesis is rubbing on a specific area, causing localized pain
- there may be also a neuropathic component from neuroma formation at the end of the cut nerve
- there may be a sympathetically mediated component if there is cutaneous coldness, discoloration and evidence of poor skin blood flow and
- a psychogenic component if the patient is depressed or anxious.

THE PAIN CLINIC

The pain clinic, or pain management clinic as it is now usually termed, was instituted as a referral centre for patients with chronic intractable pain. The types of pain referred to such a clinic are shown in Box 16.1.

Such patients usually have a long history of pain and have had multiple referrals to other specialists, frequently with unsuccessful outcomes.

Box 16.1   Major referral patterns of painful disorders

1. *Nociceptive*
   Back pain e.g. — degenerative disease
                   — post surgery
                   — osteoporosis
   Neck pain
   Headaches
   Cancer pain
   Vascular disorders
   Other musculoskeletal pains, including fibromyalgia

2. *Neuropathic*
   e.g. postherpetic neuralgia, malignant neuropathy, post-traumatic neuropathy

3. *Sympathetically mediated*
   Vascular disorders
   Complex regional pain disorder type I — previously reflex sympathetic dystrophy
   Complex regional pain disorder type II — causalgia
   NB These pains are not always sympathetically mediated

4. *Psychogenic*
   Depression
   Somatization disorders
   Hysterical conversion

Hope has been replaced by anger and resentment and there are often unresolved psychosocial problems. The expectation of the general population is that the symptoms will be cured, and the pain physician's role is often to explain carefully that this may not be possible and to find ways to lessen the pain, using psychological strategies to help the patient cope better with symptoms, to improve daily activity and to return to a useful role in life.

A pain management clinic is multidisciplinary. A trained physician, often an anaesthetist, performs the initial assessment and plans the treatment. Many other personnel may be involved, such as specialist nurses trained in pain management, physiotherapists, occupational therapists, social workers, psychologists, other physicians and surgeons.

A detailed history of the pain is taken at the first interview, taking into account psychological aspects, the history of the pain and its subsequent treatment, the patient's past medical history, behavioural patterns, social status, drug intake and former response to therapy. An examination is performed to confirm the diagnosis and to reassure the patient. A more formal psychological assessment may be made, usually by a questionnaire such as the Hospital Anxiety and Depression Scale (Zigmund & Snaith 1983). Twelve simple questions are asked, the patient ticks appropriate boxes and a score is made for depression and anxiety. Alternative questionnaires are listed in Box 16.2.

Results of previous investigations are examined. New investigations may be ordered if necessary, such as isotope bone scans, CT scanning, MRI or nerve conduction studies. A plausible explanation is given to the patient for his pain and its apparent severity. Explanation may be expressed in simple terms with respect to neurophysiological mechanisms that can be understood by the majority of patients and provide instant reassurance that the pain is 'not all in the mind'.

A treatment plan is then devised for that particular patient; this may include counselling, drug therapy, exercises, relaxation techniques or tapes, TENS, acupuncture, nerve blocks or other invasive procedures. A plan is explained to the patient who must then agree to a long-term commitment to try and lessen the pain severity and help him to cope better with the symptoms. Types of therapy offered in pain clinics are listed in Box 16.3.

It is evident that acupuncture is offered as one treatment modality amongst the list of proposed treatments. Acupuncture is used to a variable degree, depending largely on the personal beliefs of the pain clinic physician and also on logistical problems related to delivery of treatment. Acupuncture needs space for frequent patient attendances and requires skilled personnel. Whilst the actual equipment used is simple and cheap, it is not cheap in terms of professional time for each

---

Box 16.2   Psychological assessment scales used in pain clinics

HAD Scale (Hospital Anxiety and Depression Score) (Zigmund & Snaith 1983)
MPQ (McGill Pain Questionnaire) (Melzack 1975)
GHQ (General Health Questionnaire) (Benjamin et al 1991)
BDI (Beck Depression Inventory) (Beck et al 1961)
Illness Behaviour Questionnaire (Pilowsky & Spence 1975)
Sickness Impact Profile (Bergner et al 1981)
Oswestry Low Back Pain Disability Questionnaire (Fairbank et al 1980)
West Haven–Yale Multi-dimension Pain Inventory (Kerns, Turk & Rudy 1985)

Box 16.3   Types of chronic pain therapy (for non-malignant pain)

Drug therapy
Counselling
TENS
Acupuncture
Local anaesthetic/ steroid injections { into scar, trigger point, peripheral nerve block
Intravenous regional blockade
Epidural/caudal injections
Sympathetic ganglion block
Facet joint block
Cryoanalgesia
Radiofrequency lesioning
Spinal drug delivery systems
Spinal cord stimulation
Pain management programme

treatment, frequency of attendance and the number of personnel involved. Trained practitioners in acupuncture may be doctors, physiotherapists, specially trained nurses or non-medical acupuncturists. Pain clinics in Britain are controlled by the National Health Service and the pain clinician involved will decide who performs acupuncture. This subject is controversial. Should a non-medical acupuncturist be employed to treat patients? Do Western doctors undergo sufficient training in the application of acupuncture? The British Medical Acupuncture Society is addressing these problems, and has recently agreed to work closely with physiotherapists who are trained in the use of acupuncture in musculoskeletal disorders. After treatment the patient is reassessed by the pain clinic physician.

APPLICATION OF ACUPUNCTURE

Acupuncture may be performed in a variety of ways, depending on the training and experience of the acupuncturist. Those trained in TCM will use more distal points inserted with reference to the pulse diagnosis, usually deeply placed (1–2 cm) and stimulated manually to elicit a needling sensation ('De Qi'); this is a feeling of dullness, numbness, warmth or tingling around the needle site, sometimes with similar sensation radiating proximally (see Ch 3, p 27). Needles can then be left in situ or continuously stimulated by hand with a thrust–retraction action or a twirling movement. Sometimes the stimulation is applied intermittently every 5–10 minutes, or just at insertion and prior to removal. The length of time the needles are left in situ varies from 2 to 30 minutes. Sometimes the skin is wiped with an alcohol swab prior to insertion of the needles, but there is no bacteriological rationale for this.

Some practitioners (McDonald et al 1983) electively use superficial acupuncture, where fine needles are inserted over acupuncture points to a depth of 4–5 mm. A still more superficial insertion of needles 2–3 mm depth at non-acupuncture points is used in many papers as a method of sham or placebo acupuncture. Distances from traditional acupuncture points vary from 3 to 10 cm; in one study (Mendelson et al 1983) such

areas were anaesthetized with a small quantity of lignocaine prior to acupuncture needle insertion. In sham acupuncture no needling sensation is obtained. 'Western' practitioners of acupuncture tend to use more segmental points, local dermatomal points or trigger points. A trigger point is defined (Kellgren 1939) as an exquisitely tender spot in the muscle, such that palpation makes the patient wince. Melzack, Stillwell & Fox (1977) found that brief intense stimulation of trigger points frequently produced prolonged relief of pain and also found a 71% correspondence between trigger points and acupuncture points.

Acupuncture points may be identified by anatomical landmarks, by descriptive markings from Chinese acupuncture point charts, by measurement of skin electrical resistance, by finger pressure to find trigger points or by using an algometer. Johansson et al (1976) found the measurement of temperature higher at acupuncture points than at false points 3 mm distance from the real points ($P < 0.001$) and electrical resistance was lower at acupuncture points ($P < 0.00001$). However, thermal and electrical measurements on skin are notoriously unreliable.

WESTERN ACUPUNCTURE METHODS

Practitioners of 'Western' acupuncture mostly use manual stimulation, with or without leaving needles in situ, or periosteal acupuncture, where the tip of the needle pricks the periosteum for a few seconds.

Electrical stimulation is often employed for the treatment of painful conditions; a standard acupuncture stimulator is used with a square wave biphasic impulse of variable frequency of 2 up to 200 Hz (see Ch 10). Length of stimulation varies from 1 to 2 minutes up to 30 minutes and the frequency of treatment from one to five times weekly, up to a maximum of 10 sessions; most practitioners stop treatment when the pain is better. Stimulation with a 2 Hz frequency setting has been shown to produce the most satisfactory long-term pain relief in low back pain (Thomas & Lundeberg 1994).

HOW EFFECTIVE IS ACUPUNCTURE IN THE MANAGEMENT OF PAIN?

Lewith & Machin (1983) reviewed randomized trials with particular reference to the definition of placebo, sham acupuncture and real acupuncture. Response rates of 30, 50 and 70% respectively were suggested for these groups of patients studied. The majority of trials had very low power at a conventional 5% level of significance, but the authors emphasized that one cannot necessarily conclude from these trials that acupuncture is ineffective.

Lewith & Kenyon (1984) also reviewed a number of trials and suggested that acupuncture is no more effective than placebo, but again emphasized the poor design of the existing trials and the short-term follow-up. They concluded that acupuncture has an analgesic effect in approximately 60% of patients suffering from chronic pain, that this effect is greater than that of a placebo and probably greater than that of random needling. They also concluded that acupuncture therapy is probably as effective for musculoskeletal pain as are other conventional treatments such as physiotherapy or drugs and is likely to cause fewer adverse reactions than do analgesics and anti-inflammatory medications.

Richardson & Vincent (1986) also reviewed existing studies on the use of acupuncture for the relief of pain. They commented on the paucity of well-written and randomized controlled studies, and noted that the results for headache were equivocal but the role of acupuncture in the treatment of back pain appeared to be better established. They questioned the role of physical and psychological variables in determining an individual's response to treatment and wanted further data on the needling procedures themselves.

There are two meta-analyses at present in the literature. Ter Riet, Kleijnen & Knipschild (1990) in a criteria-based quality review, analysed 51 controlled clinical studies on the effectiveness of acupuncture in chronic pain and reviewed the studies using a list of predefined methodological criteria. The results from the better-constructed studies proved to be highly contradictory; the authors therefore concluded that the efficacy of acupuncture in the treatment of chronic pain remains doubtful. Patel et al (1989) studied the results of 14 randomized controlled trials of acupuncture for chronic pain in a meta-analysis and concluded that, whilst a few individual trials had statistically significant results, there was no one conclusive finding, although most results apparently favoured acupuncture.

In the interpretation of trial results for particular pain categories in the following sections, it is important to remember that any treatment group that involves needling, such as 'minimal acupuncture', whether or not it uses traditional Chinese acupoints, is still acupuncture and cannot, therefore, be considered to be a placebo. Trials that compare two needling variants are thus a comparison between two types of acupuncture, not between acupuncture and a placebo. The results should be interpreted accordingly (see Ch 13).

Headache

The main categories of headache classification include migraine, tension headache or muscle contraction headache, mixed headache, cluster headache and psychogenic headache (Headache Classification Committee of the International Headache Society 1988). There have been anecdotal reports of the successful treatment of migraine headache with acupuncture (Cheng 1975, Kim 1974, Poitinen & Salmela 1977). Bovie & Brattberg (1987) found a 40% reduction in migraine index from baseline after acupuncture treatment followed up for 24 weeks. The above are, however, uncontrolled studies. There is one paper reporting acupuncture for migraine prophylaxis (Laitinen 1975); this noted an initial 92% improvement, but at 6 months 54% of patients had relapsed to the preacupuncture state. There is one case report (Gwan 1977) of a woman treated successfully for cluster headache where medical therapy had failed.

Many papers report a low incidence of side-effects from acupuncture, however, especially compared with medical treatment (Hesse,

Mogelvang & Simonsen 1994, Laitinen 1975, Loh et al 1984).

Headache is known to be a disorder that is particularly responsive to placebo treatment (Hossenloop & Leiber 1976). Controlled clinical trials have proved, with few exceptions, to be inconclusive. Different trials on migraine (Dowson, Lewith & Machin 1985, Hesse, Mogelvang & Simonsen 1994, Vincent 1989b) have used a variety of control groups. Dowson, Lewith & Machin (1985) used mock TENS as placebo and found that acupuncture was 20% more effective in controlling severity and frequency of migraine attacks but this result was not significant. Vincent (1989b), in a single-blind randomized controlled trial, found a significant reduction in pain severity between classic acupuncture and minimal acupuncture. Hesse, Mogelvang & Simonsen (1994) compared trigger point needling and a placebo tablet with sham acupuncture (needle just touching the skin) and metoprolol. Both groups showed a significant reduction in frequency of attacks ($P < 0.01$) but the meto-prolol group showed a significantly greater reduction in global rating than did the acupuncture group ($P < 0.05$) (see Table 16.1).

In the treatment of tension headache, results have been equally disappointing. Hansen & Hansen (1985), in a randomized crossover study, showed a significant effect of real over sham acupuncture ($P < 0.05$) but there was a high drop-out rate of seven out of 25 patients, which may have skewed the results. Vincent (1990) showed a greater than 50% pain reduction in both real and sham acupuncture treatment of tension headache, but without any significant difference between the two groups. Carlsson & Sjölund (1994) compared acupuncture with physiotherapy and found a reduction of pain intensity and muscle tenderness in both groups, with physiotherapy faring better than acupuncture, but no significant difference. Tavola et al (1992) compared real with sham acupuncture for tension headaches with follow-up at 1, 6 and 12 months. Statistical analysis showed a significant reduction in both groups of frequency of headache and of analgesic con-sumption. The trend in favour of acupuncture

was not significant, which the authors attributed to wide variance in the symptoms.

There appears to be a trend in favour of real versus sham acupuncture (Hansen & Hansen 1985, Vincent 1989b, Johansson et al 1976, Borglum Jensen et al 1979) in the treatment of classic migraine or muscle contraction headache, though sham acupuncture also proves to be an effective treatment. Most papers find a greater reduction in frequency of headache and analgesic consumption than reduction in pain severity and duration. EMG studies (Ahonen et al 1983, Borglum Jensen et al 1977) show an average decrease in postural activity of the temporalis or frontalis muscles, although marked individual variations in muscular response are noted. The way in which outcome is quantified in a clinical trial may be of importance.

These results are summarized in Table 16.1.

Facial pain

Lundeberg et al (1988) discussed the long-term treatment of 177 patients with facial and neck pain, the facial pain due to trigeminal neuralgia following tooth extraction, chronic sinus pain, temporomandibular pain or muscle contraction headache. Patients were followed for up to 2 years, although the majority did not continue with treat-ment for longer than 3 months and the group in which acupuncture was most effective was pain associated with muscle tenderness. Johansson et al (1991) studied 45 patients with chronic facial muscular pain in a randomized trial, comparing acupuncture, in a combination of local and distal points, with occlusal splint therapy and an un-treated control group. They measured pain score and subjective dysfunction score and followed patients up for 3 months. Both the acupuncture and the occlusal splint group showed a signifi-cantly reduced subjective dysfunction score, but there was no difference in effectiveness between the two therapies.

These results have been reproduced by List & Helkimo (1987, 1992). The latter, randomized trial studied 80 patients with craniomandibular disorders, comparing acupuncture with occlusal splint therapy and following them up for a year.

Both treatment groups showed a significant benefit compared with untreated controls.

Raustia and colleagues (Raustia & Pohjola 1986, Raustia, Pohjola & Virtanen 1985) studied TMJ dysfunction, comparing acupuncture with conventional stomatognathic therapy such as exercises, splints and counselling. Measurement of the Helkimo dysfunction index at 1 week and 3 months showed that both treatments were equally effective and that conventional treatment was better initially. Raustia and colleagues stated that acupuncture is more effective in patients with functional disorders and that it is less effective in patients with organic changes in the joint; they concluded that acupuncture is a useful, early form of treatment or may be complementary to stomatognathic treatment in temporomandibular dysfunction.

These results are summarized in Table 16.2.

Neck pain

Several authors have studied the effect of acupuncture on chronic cervical pain, usually with underlying cervical spondylosis. Coan, Wong & Coan (1982) randomly selected 30 patients who either received traditional acupuncture three to four times weekly, or no treatment. After 12 weeks, 80% of the treated patients expressed subjective improvement, with a 40% reduction in pain score, 54% reduction in analgesia intake and 32% increase in activity levels. The improvements were clearly much greater than those shown by the waiting-list control group.

Peng, Behar & Yue (1987) studied 37 patients with chronic neck and shoulder pain in an un-controlled study in which over 50% of treated patients attained a significant 'long-term improvement'. Hypnotic profiles were also measured; there was no correlation shown between hypnotic profile and efficacy of acupuncture.

Two controlled studies have compared acupuncture with placebo TENS. Petrie & Langley (1983), in a pilot study of 13 patients, found acupuncture to be better than placebo with a significance level of $P < 0.01$. However, when Petrie repeated the study with Hazelman (Petrie & Hazelman 1986) as a randomized controlled trial

with 26 patients, assessing analgesia intake and with more detailed pain measurements, the results of the pilot study were not repeated and no significant improvement was found in the acupuncture group. However, there were trends towards significance in the measurement of daily pain intensity and pill count.

Loy (1983) compared electroacupuncture with physiotherapy in the form of short-wave therapy or traction. Neck movement was measured with a goniometer and assessments were made at 3 weeks and 6 weeks. Both the electroacupuncture and physiotherapy groups showed a satisfactory improvement at 3 and again at 6 weeks. He commented that acupuncture appeared to be of greater benefit in patients with milder initial symptoms than in those with more severe symptoms.

Lundeberg et al (1988) treated 177 patients with chronic head and neck pain using different types of acupuncture, including extrasegmental points, superficial acupuncture and electro-acupuncture. He found that the most effective sites for acupuncture were located in the painful area and that deep stimulation followed by the 'De Qi' sensation was more effective than intra-dermal placing of the needles. He found that acupuncture worked better when the pain was coming from muscle spasm and that low-frequency electrical stimulation at 2 Hz produced more prolonged alleviation of pain than did either manual stimulation or high-frequency electro-acupuncture. However, manual stimulation, low- and high-frequency electroacupuncture were equally effective in producing immediate pain relief, lasting up to 8 hours. To achieve a maximal duration of pain relief, acupuncture stimulation had to be applied for at least 30 minutes. Thirty-eight out of 177 patients discontinued treatment as they were pain free. Eighty-four continued long-term treatment with acupuncture, seven for more than 2 years.

Thomas, Eriksson & Lundeberg (1991) studied 44 patients with chronic cervical osteoarthritis, comparing the effect of one acupuncture treatment lasting 40 minutes with either sham acupuncture, diazepam 5 mg, or a placebo pill. The patients were randomized to the overlap of treatments

Table 16.1 Trials of acupuncture in headache

Author name(s)	Year	Condition treated	Type of trial	No. of pts.	Type of acu.	Length/no of treatments	Control group	Assessment	Duration	Results	Analysis
Borglum Jensen, Melsen Borglum Jensen	1979	Unspecified headache	Crossover	29	MS 1 needle	1×20 min	Skin touched by needle	Frequency of attacks, analgesia intake	2 months	↓ frequency of headaches in both groups. Acu. ↓ analgesia intake	N/S
Loh et al	1984	Migraine	Crossover	48	MS. Local and distal points	2 min, variable no.	Medical treatment	Frequency, severity, and duration of attacks	3 months	Improvement in 60%	N/A
Dowson, Lewith & Machin	1985	Migraine	RC SB	48	CA body and seg. points	6×10 min	Mock TENS	Pain diary, analgesia intake	2 years	Acupuncture 20% more effective	N/S
Vincent	1989b	Migraine	RC SB	30	CA MS Local and distal pts.	15 min 6×weekly	Sham acupuncture	Severity, frequency of attacks, analgesic intake	6 weeks 4 months 1 years	Pain reduction both groups	N/S
Hesse, Mogelvang & Simonsen	1994	Migraine	RC DB	85	TP needling	6–8×weekly	Point touched with blunt end of needle	Pain dairy, severity and frequency of attacks	17 weeks	Significant ↓ frequency in both groups No difference between groups	$P < 0.01$ N/S
Johansson et al	1976	Tension	SB	33	CA MS	Not stated	Sham acupuncture	Not specified	8 weeks	Acu had a better effect than sham acu.	N/S
Borglum Jensen et al	1977	Myogenic	U/C	21	MS 1 point	1×20 min	None	EMG recordings	1 day 1 month 4 months	60% improved. EMG showed decrease in postural activity	N/S
Ahonen et al	1983	Myogenic, tension	U/C	22	CA	10 min ×4	Physio, U/S	Pain, VAS, EMG recording	2 months	Similar pain relief and alteration EMG in all groups	N/S
Hansen & Hansen	1985	Tension	RC Crossover	18	CA MS	6 needles 2× weekly for 3 weeks	Sham acupuncture	Pain scores, pain index	15 weeks	Significant reduction pain scores	$P < 0.05$
Vincent	1990	Tension	Single case/ time series	14	CA	MS 15 min 8×weekly	Sham acupuncture	Pain scores, pain diaries	8 weeks 4 months	>50% reduction in pain scores both groups	N/S

Table 16.1 (Cont'd)

Author name(s)	Year	Condition treated	Type of trial	No. of pts.	Type of acu.	Length/no of treatments	Control group	Assessment	Duration	Results	Analysis
Carlsson & Sjölund	1994	Tension and neck pain	U/C	62	CA	7–8 times weekly	Physio	Pain intensity, muscle tenderness	17 weeks	Reduction in both groups	N/S
Tavola et al	1992	Tension	RC	30	CA	8 × 20 min	Sham acupuncture	Frequency, severity, duration, headache index, analgesia intake	1 month, 6 months 12 months	Both groups ↓ frequency and analgesia intake	N/S

CA = classical acupuncture; DB = double blind; MS = manual stimulation; N/A = not applicable; N/S = not significant; RC = randomized controlled; SB = single blind; U/C = uncontrolled; U/S = ultrasound; VAS = Visual analogue scale.

Table 16.2   Trials of acupuncture in facial pain

Author name(s)	Year	Condition treated	Type of trial	No. of pts.	Type of acu.	Length/no of treatments	Control group	Assessment	Duration	Results	Analysis
Raustia, Pohjola & Virtanen	1985	TMJ dysfunction	RC	50	Seg. and distal	20 min × 3	Standard stomatognathic treatment	Clinical dysfunction index	1 weeks and 3 months	Both groups improved at 1 month	N/S
Raustia & Pohjola	1986	TMJ dysfunction	RC SB	50	Seg. and distal	20 min × 3	Standard stomatognathic treatment	Painful movement of mandible	1 week and 3 months	Dental treatment better initially, no difference at 3 months	N/S
List & Helkimo	1987	Chronic facial pain, mandibular dysfunction	U/C	10	MS EA	10 min × 8	None	Clinical index dysfunction, VAS, analgesic cons.	3 months and 7 months	Subjective improvement in all	N/A
Johansson et al	1991	Facial muscular pain	R	45	Local and distal	30 min × 6	Occlusal splint or untreated	Pain score, dysfunction score	3 months	Both treatments reduced subjective dysfunction score	N/S
List & Helkimo	1992	Cranio-mandibular disorders	R	80	Local and distal	30 min × 6	Occlusal splint or untreated	ADL/VAS, pain diary, examination	1 year	Both groups significant benefit; no difference between treatment groups	N/S

ADL = Activities of Daily Living; EA = Electroacupuncture; R = randomized; other abbreviations as Table 16.1.

and crossed over to each treatment, with a rest of 3–5 days between the different trials. Assessments were made on a visual analogue scale (VAS) for pain, pain intensity, and an unpleasantness score. There was significant reduction of pain intensity and unpleasantness in the acupuncture group compared with the placebo pill ($P < 0.05$), but compared with the sham acupuncture and diazepam groups there was no significant difference.

These results are summarized in Table 16.3 Figure 16.1 shows an example of needle placement for neck pain.

Back pain

Low back pain, with or without radicular symptoms and signs, often presenting with disability and patterns of illness behaviour, is one of the commonest reasons for referral to a pain clinic. The diagnoses are many and varied. The numbers (and types) of treatment are also diverse and often not of proven efficacy. Figure 16.2 shows an example of needle placement for low back pain, while Figure 16.3 is an example of electroacupuncture for low back pain. There are several controlled studies in the literature comparing the treatment of uncomplicated chronic low back pain by acupuncture or sham acupuncture, TENS or mock TENS.

The only study of these to achieve significant results is that of McDonald et al (1983), who treated 17 patients with either superficial acupuncture or mock TENS. A VAS was used to measure pain and to assess activity, mood, percentage of pain relief and reduction in physical signs; it showed a significant benefit of acupuncture over placebo in four out of five of the outcome measures. The pain score reduction (by VAS) was not significant. The combined average reduction was, however, significant ($P < 0.01$).

Papers comparing acupuncture with sham acupuncture (Edelist, Gross & Langer 1976, Mendelson et al 1983) have not achieved significant results, although there was an overall reduction of pain score in both groups. Mendelson also commented that there were increased depression, neuroticism and hypochondriasis

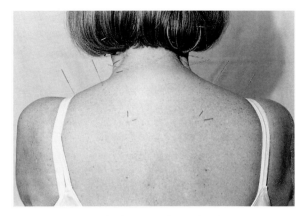

Figure 16.1 Needle placement for neck pain.

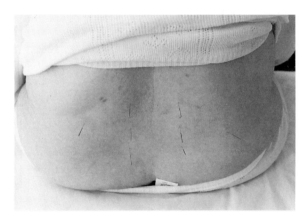

Figure 16.2 Needle placement for low back pain.

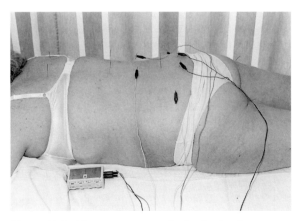

Figure 16.3 Electroacupuncture for low back pain.

Table 16.3 Trials of acupuncture in neck pain

Author name(s)	Year	Condition treated	Type of trial	No. of pts.	Type of acu.	Length/no of treatments	Control group	Assessment	Duration	Results	Analysis
Coan, Wong & Coan	1982	Neck pain	R	37 30	CA	3/week < 10	No treatment	Pain score, analgesia intake, activity levels	12 weeks	80% improved 40% ↓ pain score 54% ↓ analgesia intake, 32% increase activity	N/A
Loy	1983	Cervical spondylosis	R	60	EA	30 min 3 × weekly for 3–6 weeks	Physiother.	Pain score neck movement	6 weeks	EA 87% improvement Physio 54% imp. EA. produced earlier imp.	N/A
Petrie & Langley	1983	Chronic cervical pain	R pilot	13	CA	20 min MS 2 × weekly for 4 weeks	Mock TENS	PRS	1 month	Acupuncture better than placebo	$P < 0.01$
Petrie & Hazelman	1986	Chronic cervical pain	RC	26	CA	20 min MS 2 × weekly for 4 weeks	Mock TENS	VAS, MPQ, analgesia pain diary, neck movement	1 month	No significant improvement in acu. group. Trends in daily activity and pill count	N/S
Peng, Behar & Yue	1987	Neck and shoulder pain	U/C	37	EA tender points	20 min<15 2 × weekly	U/C	Hypnotic profile	Not stated	50% long term improvement	N/A
Lundeberg et al	1988	Chronic head and neck pain	U/C	177	Local and intraseg. points	2/weekly × 10	Superficial acupuncture	Pain scores	2 years	Pain score reduced by acupuncture in 56%	N/A
Thomas, Eriksson & Lundeberg	1991	Chronic cervical OA	R crossover	44	CA MS	1 × 40 min	Sham acu. diazepam, placebo	VAS, intensity and unpleasantness	3 weeks	Significant ↓ pain and unpleasantness in acu. group	$P < 0.05$ compared with placebo

EA = electroacupuncture; MPQ = McGill Pain Questionnaire; OA = osteoarthritis; PRS = pain rating scale; other abbreviations as Table 16.1.

scores in the treated group compared with normal population. Garvey, Marks & Wiesel (1989) compared one single trigger point needling with an injection of lidocaine, lidocaine with steroid, or vapocoolant spray and acupressure. All groups improved. The acupuncture and vapocoolant spray group improved more than the injection groups, but this did not achieve significance. Lehmann et al (1986) compared acupuncture with TENS and mock TENS and found no difference in VAS scores, disability rating or physical measures in the three groups, although there was a trend on the VAS scores towards less pain with acupuncture treatment. Education of the patient was assumed to have a very positive role.

There have also been studies in veterinary journals. Klide & Martin (1989) compared traditional needle acupuncture with laser therapy or injections of saline near acupuncture points in horses. All three types of treatment were equally useful in treating back pain. Thirty-seven out of 45 horses had alleviation of clinical signs of pain and could once again train and compete.

Fox & Melzack (1976) treated 12 patients suffering from chronic low back pain with both acupuncture and TENS. Changes in intensity and quality of pain were measured with the McGill Pain Questionnaire (Melzack 1975). Results showed that pain relief greater than 33% was produced in 75% of patients by acupuncture, and in 66% by TENS. The mean duration of pain relief was 40 hours after acupuncture, and 23 hours after TENS. There was, however, no significant difference between the two methods of treatment.

Thomas & Lundeberg (1994) assessed the importance of different modes of acupuncture in the treatment of chronic nociceptive low back pain. They randomly allocated 30 patients into three trial treatment groups and a control group; one received manual stimulation of needles, the second group had low-frequency electrical stimulation at 2 Hz and the third group had high-frequency electrical stimulation at 80 Hz, while the no-treatment control group consisted of a further 10 patients. Six local and four distal points were stimulated for 30 minutes. Assessments, which took place at 6 weeks and 6 months,

included activity related to pain, mobility, verbal pain ratings and patients' subjective pain assessment. At 6 weeks all treated groups achieved significant improvement, but at 6 months only the low-frequency acupuncture group, suggesting that 2 Hz electrical stimulation is the mode of choice when using acupuncture in the treatment of chronic nociceptive low back pain.

The above studies are summarized in Table 16.4.

Other types of musculoskeletal pain

Godfrey & Morgan (1978) studied 193 patients with musculoskeletal pain in a number of sites. 57% of the patients were self-referred. They were randomized into 'appropriate' (i.e. needles placed relevant to the site of the pain) and 'inappropriate' acupuncture groups. They attempted to make the trial triple-blind in that neither the patients, the assessor, nor the acupuncturist knew if the site of acupuncture was appropriate to the patient's symptoms. After 3 treatments 63% of the acupuncture group had reduced pain but there was no significant difference between this and the inappropriate acupuncture group. Both Moore & Berk (1976) and Gaw et al (1975) have produced similar results.

Christensen et al (1992) performed a randomized, single-blind, crossover study on 29 patients with osteoarthritic knees who were waiting for knee replacement. He compared an acupuncture treatment group with a no-treatment control group and found that range of movement, pain score and analgesic consumption were all improved in the acupuncture-treated group: seven patients took themselves off the waiting list as a result of relief. Another study on osteoarthritis of the knee by Takeda & Wessell (1994) showed that both real and sham acupuncture decreased pain, stiffness and physical difficulty.

Lundeberg (1984) studied 36 patients with chronic myalgia, and found that electroacupuncture, vibratory stimulation and TENS all produced better pain relief than did placebo in the form of a pill.

Molsberger & Hille (1994) treated 48 patients with chronic tennis elbow, using non-segmental

Table 16.4 Trials of acupuncture in back pain

Author name(s)	Year	Condition treated	Type of trial	No. of pts.	Type of acu.	Length/no of treatments	Control group	Assessment	Duration	Results	Analysis
Edelist, Gross & Langer	1976	Low back pain	R SB	30	EA	3 × 30 min	Sham acu.	Pain relief, range of movement, neurological testing	1–3 weeks	40% improvement in sham group, 46% in acu. group	N/S
Fox & Melzack	1976	Low back pain	R crossover	12	MS	3 min 3 × weekly	TENS -	MPQ	4 months	Pain relief >33% in 75% acu. group. 66% TENS group	N/S
McDonald et al	1983	Low back pain	R SB	17	Superficial acu., EA	4–6 × 20 min	Mock TENS	VAS, activity ratings, mood, pain relief	6 weeks 6 months	Significant benefit of acu. in pain relief, activity, & overall severity	P < 0.01
Mendelson et al	1983	Chronic back pain	DB cross-over	95	CA, MS	1 × 30 min	Intradermal injection 2% lidocaine into non-acu. points	Pain score	3 months	↓ pain score 26% acu. group, 22% control group	N/S
Lehmann et al	1986	Low back pain	R	54	EA	2 × weekly for 3 weeks	TENS, mock TENS	VAS, disability rating, physical measures	3 weeks	No difference between 3 groups, trend towards less pain with acu.	N/S
Garvey, Marks & Wiesel	1989	Low back pain	R DB	63	MS, TP	1 treatment	Lidocaine inj, lidocaine with steroid, vapo spray and acupressure	VAS	2 weeks	All groups improved	N/S
Thomas & Lundeberg	1994	Low back pain	R DB	40	MS EA 2 Hz EA 80 Hz	1 × 30 min	No treatment	Activity level, mobility, verbal pain rating	6 weeks 6 months	At 6 weeks all groups significantly improved at 6 months EA 2 Hz group only	N/S

Abbreviations as Tables 16.1, 16.3.

distal points in the true acupuncture treatment group. In the placebo group they used a needle placed on the skin close to the thoracic spine and stimulated it without penetrating the skin for 5 minutes. Significantly better results were reported in the acupuncture-treated group ($P < 0.01$).

Deluze et al (1992) treated fibromyalgia in a group of 70 patients randomized to electro-acupuncture or a sham procedure using non-acupuncture points superficially needled and a weak electric current. Post-treatment values were significantly better after electroacupuncture in five of the eight parameters studied when compared with the control group. Pain threshold at tender sites improved by 70% in the electro-acupuncture group and only 4% in the control group. This difference was significant ($P < 0.03$). However, the use of electroacupuncture instead of manual stimulation of needles in this study was questioned by Lewis (1993) who suggested it led to an unusually high dropout rate of 17% (15% in the control group). Emery & Lythgoe (1986) reporting on the treatment of ankylosing spondylitis in 10 patients, also compared real with sham apcupuncture, and found no significant effect on pain in either group; however, stiffness improved in both groups ($P < 0.01$).

Puett & Griffin (1994) have surveyed the published trials of non-medical and non-invasive therapies for hip and knee osteoarthritis and comment that results of acupuncture trials are inconsistent. Single, well-designed studies suggest that topically applied capsaicin and laser treatment reduce pain better than other therapies, and exercise is consistently better at reducing pain and improving function. However, they comment that more data are needed to evaluate the roles of different therapies.

One study (Moore & Berk 1976) assessed the effect of positive versus negative settings for acupuncture and found no difference, and also tested hypnotic susceptibility in terms of pain reduction, but again found no significant trends. Takeda & Wessell (1994) in the above-mentioned study of acupuncture for pain in osteoarthritic knees, commented that men responded better than women to acupuncture treatment and that subjects experiencing De Qi regularly during treatment responded better to acupuncture than did those not experiencing this sensation. Bulow et al (1992) tried to determine whether it is possible to predict the outcome of acupuncture treatment by evaluating parameters such as age, duration of disease, pain score, range of knee movement, analgesic consumption and knee score. They concluded that it was not possible to predict the outcome and that immediate results were not a guide to long-term results; those who achieved the best immediate results were not necessarily the ones with the best long-term effect.

Berry et al (1980) compared five different treatments for painful stiff shoulder: acupuncture, steroid injections with placebo, and with active tolmetin sodium (a non-steroidal anti-inflammatory drug), physiotherapy in the form of ultrasound, and 'placebo' physiotherapy with placebo tolmetin sodium tablets. Pain was measured by VAS and a four-point scale, and goniometer readings were taken to measure shoulder abduction. With very few exceptions, patients in all groups improved markedly and no differences between treatments were detected. The authors suggested that any beneficial effect may have been due to natural recovery as stiff painful shoulder is a self-limiting condition.

Acupuncture for musculoskeletal pain appears to be equal in effect to more conventional therapies, and may be better where muscle spasm is present. There is also a noticeable lack of side-effects.

The above results are summarized in Table 16.5.

Figure 16.4 shows electroacupuncture for hip pain; Figure 16.5 shows acupuncture for knee pain.

Miscellaneous pain

Non-specific chronic pain

There have been many uncontrolled studies (Carlsson & Sjölund 1994, Fischer, Behr & Reumont 1984, Johnstone et al 1994, Junnila 1987, Lee & Modell 1975, Mann et al 1973, Sodipo 1979, Strauss 1981) on the treatment of chronic pain patients with acupuncture. These studies show that a high proportion of patients, 42–97%, report

Table 16.5 Trials of acupuncture in musculoskeletal pain

Author name(s)	Year	Condition treated	Type of trial	No. of pts.	Type of acu.	Length/no of treatments	Control group	Assessment	Duration	Results	Analysis
Gaw et al	1975	Chronic OA pain	R DB	40	CA	8 × 30 min	Sham acu.	Joint tenderness, VRS, mobility, range of movement	3 weeks	Significant improvement pain and mobility in both groups	N/S
Moore & Berk	1976	Chronic shoulder pain	R SB	42	CA	1 × weekly	Needle strapped to-skin	Pain score, range of movement	3 weeks	Significant improvement in pain in both groups	N/S
Godfrey & Morgan	1978	Musculoskeletal pain	R DB	193	CA	3–5 treatments	Sham acu.	Pain score	3 weeks	↓ pain in 63% of acupuncture group, 54% sham group	N/S
Berry et al	1980	Shoulder cuff lesions	R DB	60	CA	5 × weekly	Steroid inj., physio., NSAID, placebo pill	VAS, movement, comparative assessment	4 weeks	All groups improved, no difference between them	N/S
Lundeberg	1984	Myalgia	R crossover	36	EA	2 × weekly for 3 weeks	TENS, vibratory stimulation, placebo pill	VAS	3 weeks	> 50% pain relief in 40% of treated patients, 20% placebo group	N/A
Emery & Lythgoe	1986	Ankylosing spondylitis	DB crossover	10	EA	3 × 20 min	Sham acu.	Pain score and stiffness	9 weeks	No significant effect on pain, stiffness improved in both groups	N/S
Christensen et al	1992	OA knee	R SB crossover	29	MS	20 min 2 × weekly for 3 weeks, then monthly	No treatment	Range of movement, pain score, analgesia intake	40 weeks	↓ pain score, analgesia intake and ↑ movement	P < 0.01
Deluze et al	1992	Fibromyalgia	R SB	70	EA	6 × 2 weekly	Sham acu.	Pain threshold, analgesia intake, VAS, pain score, sleep quality, morning stiffness	3 weeks	Significant difference for 5 out of 8 outcome measures	P < 0.03
Molsberger & Hille	1994	Chronic tennis elbow	R SB	48	Non-seg. distal points	5 min × 1	Needle placed on skin	Pain relief	72 hours	75% reported 50% pain relief	P < 0.01
Takeda & Wessell	1994	OA knee	R SB	40	MS	3 × weekly for 3 weeks	Sham acu.	PRS, OA index, pain threshold	3 weeks	Reduction of pain, stiffness and physical difficulty in both groups	N/S

VRS = Verbal Rating Scale. NSAID = non-steroidal anti-inflammatory drug; other abbreviations as Tables 16.1, 16.3.

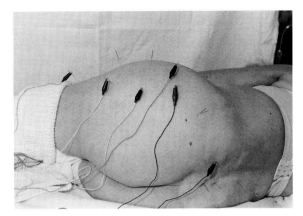

Figure 16.4 Electroacupuncture for hip pain.

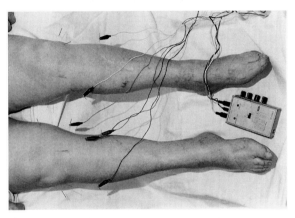

Figure 16.5 Electroacupuncture for knee pain.

immediate pain relief after treatment. A longer-term follow-up shows that this improvement rapidly declines. Lee et al (1975), assessing pain relief after 4 weeks, found 45% of patients still reporting improvement. Junnila (1987a) showed a reduction in pain score persisting for 2 years in 26% of patients. Carlsson & Sjölund (1994) found that at 6 months only 17% of patients report sustained pain relief and these were patients suffering from nociceptive pain; patients with neuropathic pain and psychogenic pain reported a rapid return to baseline. Fischer, Behr & Reumont (1984) found the best results in patients suffering from cephalalgia, sinusitis, cervical spine syndrome, shoulder arm syndrome, ischialgia, back pain, constipation, herpes zoster and allergic rhinitis. Junnila (1987b) found that acupuncture

appeared to be less effective in elderly patients, those with a psychiatric history, those on high doses of analgesics and those with long-standing pain. Response was not influenced by social status or expectation of benefit. Sodipo (1979), in his unselected group of chronic pain patients, also reported benefits in terms of improved appetite, sleep pattern, bowel regulation, an increase of energy and less tension. He found that young patients responded better, as did those with a shorter duration of pain before treatment. A further trial (Ghia et al 1976) compared acupuncture with tender area needling in 40 patients with pain below the waist. There was no statistical difference between the two groups. Both reported significant improvement in pain scores.

Other pain

A variety of other types of pain have been studied in the literature. Filshie & Redman (1985) studied acupuncture in 183 patients suffering from malignant pain of various causes. Gauge 36 needles were used and medication was continued; 52% of patients were significantly helped but multiple treatment proved necessary. Muscle spasm and bladder spasm were also helped and, in one patient, thermography showed a sustained rise in temperature of the affected limb after acupuncture. A poor response after a previous good response often indicated relapse of the malignant disease.

Two studies have been performed on post-traumatic reflex sympathetic dystrophy (RSD). Chan & Chow (1981) found an improvement in terms of pain relief in 70% of patients, with reduction of swelling and tenderness, but observed no difference in range of movement. In a randomized controlled study, Fialka et al (1993) compared classical acupuncture with sham acupuncture, measuring VAS scores at 3 weeks, and found that both groups showed a significant reduction in pain score, but with no significant difference between groups.

Longobardi et al (1989) performed a pilot study on 15 patients with distal extremity pain, comparing auricular acupuncture with a placebo pill and measuring VAS for pain at 30 minutes.

There was no change in the VAS scores but the pain rating index (PRI) showed a significant difference between the two groups.

Lewers et al (1989) studied 21 patients with primary dysmenorrhea, using a single treatment of acupuncture-like TENS versus a placebo pill and measuring VAS and PRI at 24 hours. There was a 50% reduction in scores in both groups but no difference between them.

Lee et al (1992) studied 38 patients with acute renal colic using electroacupuncture or intramuscular analgesia. They measured pain scores and found that significant pain reduction occurred in 86% of the acupuncture group and 62.5% of the analgesia group. There were fewer side-effects in the acupuncture group.

Co et al (1979) studied acupuncture for pain from sickle cell crises in 10 patients, comparing real acupuncture with sham acupuncture and measuring VAS pain scores up to 24 hours. Both groups improved. Ballegaard et al (1985) performed a crossover study in 23 patients with chronic pancreatitis, using electroacupuncture or TENS and measuring VAS and analgesia intake. After 6 weeks, at the end of the crossover time, neither treatment proved effective and there was no reduction in analgesia requirement. Lewith, Field & Machin (1983) studied 62 patients with post-herpetic pain in a randomized single-blind study, comparing auricular or body acupuncture with mock TENS, and measuring VAS scores, pain diary and sleep pattern. Patients were followed up at 4 and 8 weeks after the study; only 30% of the patients in each group improved. Acupuncture was therefore considered an ineffective therapy for post-herpetic neuralgia.

The above results are summarized in Table 16.6. Results of these trials are somewhat inconsistent but acupuncture does appear to have an immediate pain-relieving role and may be a very useful means of treating acute pain. It appears to be much less effective in chronic states, such as chronic pancreatitis, and in neuropathic pain.

PSYCHOLOGICAL FACTORS

Levine, Gormley & Fields (1976) treated 37 patients with either traditional or Western acupuncture with either manual or electrical stimulation for a variety of problems. Of these, 10 patients had nerve damage and did not respond to acupuncture, while 27 patients had other problems such as migraine, neck, back pain, headaches, etc.; in the latter group the response to treatment was very much better. Patients with high initial anxiety and depression scores had significantly more relief of their symptoms than those with low initial scores. Good pain relief also correlated with a positive rapport between the patient and the therapeutic team. Katz, Kaocy Spiegel & Katz (1974) studied normal volunteers receiving needle puncture analgesia and found a positive correlation between analgesia produced and hypnotizability. Kreitler, Kreitler & Carasso (1987) studied cognitive orientation as a predictor of pain relief after acupuncture in 30 chronic pain patients who were assessed by questionnaire. After 4–6 acupuncture sessions, over 50% of patients showed some improvement and the effects persisted for at least 8 months. The patient's positive belief in the therapeutic effect of acupuncture was an important influence in predicting the outcome. Berlin, Bartlett & Black (1975) in a group of 120 patients suffering from long-term chronic pain syndromes, found that patients with a higher level of anxiety attained a greater reduction of pain after treatment. Biederman et al (1986) treated a woman with chronic facial pain with acupuncture before and after the medical treatment of her depression. After prolonged intake of a tricyclic, acupuncture no longer produced analgesia. Thomas, Arner & Lundeberg (1992) used periosteal acupuncture in the treatment of idiopathic pain disorder and found acupuncture ineffective.

It is hard to draw any firm conclusions on the role of psychological factors in predicting the outcome of acupuncture for the treatment of chronic pain. However, it does appear that positive belief in a successful outcome may be important.

The methodology of controlled trials of acupuncture has been very well reviewed by Vincent (1989). Many papers, for example Coan, Wong & Coan (1980), found that acupuncture has highly significant results when compared with no

Table 16.6 Miscellaneous pain trials

Author name(s)	Year	Condition treated	Type of trial	No. of pts.	Type of acu.	Length/no of treatments	Control group	Assessment	Duration	Results	Analysis
Chan & Chow	1981	Post-traumatic RSD	U/C	20	EA	50 Hz for 20–30 min ×5–10	None	Pain relief, swelling, range of movement	3 < 22 months	70% improvement in terms of pain relief	N/A
Fialka et al	1993	Post-traumatic RSD	RC	14	CA	5 × weekly for 3 weeks	Sham acu.	VAS	3 weeks	Both groups ↓ pain scores	N/S
Lewith, Field & Machin	1983	Post-herpetic pain	R SB	62	Auric. or body acu.	1 × 10 min	Mock TENS	VRS, pain diary, sleep pattern	4 weeks 8 weeks	30% patients improved in each group	N/S
Ballegaard et al	1985	Chronic pancreatitis	SB cross-over	23	EA	5 treatments in 2 weeks	TENS	VAS, analgesia intake	6 weeks	Neither treatment effective	N/A
Longobardi et al	1989	Distal extremity pain	Pilot	15	Ear acu.	5 × 10min	Placebo pill	VAS, PRI	0, 10 and 30 min	VAS no change, PRI significant difference	$P < 0.05$
Lewers et al	1989	Primary dysmenorrhoea	RC	21	Acu-like TENS	1 × 30 min	Placebo pill	VAS, PRI	1 day	50% ↓ pain in both groups	N/S
Lee et al	1992	Acute renal colic	RC	38	CA, EA	1 × 10 min	IM, analgesia	Pain score, paralytic ileus	30 min	Acu. group 86% pain relief; analgesia group 62.5% pain relief	N/A

PRI = Pain rating index; other abbreviations as Tables 16.1, 16.3.

treatment. However, it is more important to know whether acupuncture offers any advantage over conventional treatment and many papers show very little difference when acupuncture is compared with other physical treatments such as TENS or steroid injections. A double-blind trial methodology cannot be applied to trials of acupuncture. The great majority of controlled trials in the literature use a form of sham acupuncture that proves to be equally effective as real acupuncture. More appropriate control groups have been developed, such as mock TENS and minimal acupuncture which has a very slight specific effect. Some such trials (Hansen & Hansen 1985, McDonald et al 1983, Vincent 1989) have produced statistically significant results. Vincent & Lewith (1995) suggest that it is important to monitor the adequacy of the control procedure, suggesting assessment of the credibility of the two treatment procedures. (See also Ch 13.)

ACUPUNCTURE AND PLACEBO

The word 'placebo' has been used since 1811 to mean 'a medicine given more to please than to benefit the patient'. Placebos are catalysts for the transformation of expectation to effect (Edmeads 1984). Positive expectations may evoke positive effects; negative expectations evoke no effects or adverse effects. According to Beecher & Boston (1955), placebos are found to have an average effectiveness of $35.2 \pm 2.2\%$. Placebo-induced analgesia can be blocked by naloxone (Levine, Gordon & Fields 1978) and it has been shown that moderate to severe pain is more likely than mild pain to ease with placebo (Levine et al 1979). Pain due to disease or injury responds more readily to placebo than does pain inflicted in the laboratory and a positive expectation of benefit is of great importance (Fields & Levine 1981). Is acupuncture a placebo response? Kenyon, Knight & Wells (1983) found no significant change in pain relief after the injection of naloxone in patients receiving acupuncture. Berlin, Bartlett & Black (1975) studied experimental pain in volunteers and suggested that acupuncture increases the latency of terminating response to a painful stimulus and that this effect is greater than that of placebo alone. Vincent & Lewith (1995) have tackled the difficult subject of an effective placebo-controlled condition used in acupuncture trials and suggest that a credibility rating as conceived by Borkovec & Nau (1972) should be used to assess the credibility of acupuncture and a control group, whether this is mock TENS or minimal acupuncture. Such a procedure has been used by Petrie & Hazelman (1986) and Vincent (1989); they suggest that the credibility measure is a check that both the treatment and control group are equivalent in their psychological impact. This credibility may vary from one study to another, involving different clinicians, a different group of patients, and a different setting, which in turn may influence the patient's perception of treatment or control procedures.

CONCLUSION

Acupuncture is widely offered as a treatment option in pain management clinics. It appears to have a therapeutic role in the treatment of a variety of chronic pain disorders, especially where there is nociceptive pain of musculoskeletal origin associated with muscle spasm and anxiety. It appears to be definitely more effective than dummy treatment; however, many trials have used sham acupuncture, which consistently has a therapeutic effect, as a control group. Acupuncture is also equally as effective as other conventional therapies, the role of which have often not been carefully assessed. It is costly in terms of professional staff involved, but causes very few side-effects or problems. More clinical trials are, however, required to establish further the role of acupuncture in the pain clinic.

REFERENCES

Ahonen E, Hakumaki M, Mahlamaki S, Partanen J, Reikkinen P, Sivenius J 1983 Acupuncture and physiotherapy in the treatment of myogenic headache patients: pain relief and EMG activity. Advances in Pain Research and Therapy 5:571–576

Ballegaard S, Christophersen S J, Dawids S G, Hesse J, Olsen N V 1985 Acupuncture and transcutaneous electric nerve stimulation in the treatment of pain associated with chronic pancreatitis. Scandinavian Journal of Gastroenterology 20:1249–1254

Beck A T, Ward C H, Mendelson M et al 1961 An inventory for measuring depression. Archives of General Psychiatry 4:561–571

Beecher H K, Boston M D 1955 The powerful placebo. Journal of the American Medical Association 159:1602–1605

Benjamin S, Lennon S, Gardner G 1991 The validity of the general health questionnaire for first stage screening for mental illness in pain clinic patients. Pain 47:197–202

Bergner M, Bobitt R A, Carter W B, Gilson B S 1981 The sickness impact profile: development and final revision of a health status measure. Medical Care 19:787–805

Berlin F, Bartlett R, Black J 1975 Acupuncture and placebo. Anesthesiology 42:527–531

Berry H, Fernandes L, Bloom B, Clark R, Hamilton E 1980 Clinical study comparing acupuncture, physiotherapy, injection and oral anti-inflammatory therapy in shoulder-cuff lesions. Current Medical Research and Opinion 7:121–126

Biedermann H J, Lapeer G L, Mauri M, McGhie A 1986 Acupuncture and myofascial pain: treatment failure after administration of tricyclic antidepressants. Medical Hypotheses 19: 397–402

Bonica J J 1953 The management of pain. Lea & Febiger, Philadelphia

Borglum Jensen L, Tallgren A, Troest T, Borglum Jensen S 1977 Effect of acupuncture on myogenic headache. Scandinavian Journal of Dental Research 85:456–470

Borglum Jensen L, Melsen B, Borglum Jensen S 1979 Effect of acupuncture on headache measured by reduction in number of attacks and use of drugs. Scandinavian Journal of Dental Research 87:373–380

Borkovec T D, Nau S D 1972 Credibility of analogue therapy rationales. Journal of Behavioral Therapy and Experimental Psychiatry 3:257–260

Boivie J, Brattberg G 1987 Are there long lasting effects on migraine headache after one series of acupuncture treatment? American Journal of Chinese Medicine 15:69–75

Bulow H, Christensen B, Wilbek H, Iuhl I, Dreijer N, Rasmussen H 1992 Predictive value of subjective and objective evaluation before acupuncture treatment. American Journal of Chinese Medicine 20:17–23

Carlsson C P, Sjölund B H 1994 Acupuncture and subtypes of chronic pain: assessment of long-term results. Clinical Journal of Pain 10:290–295

Chan C S, Chow S P 1981 Electroacupuncture in the treatment of post-traumatic sympathetic dystrophy. (Sudeck's atrophy) British Journal of Anaesthesiology 53:899–902

Cheng A C K 1975 Treatment of headache employing acupuncture. American Journal of Chinese Medicine 3:181–185

Christensen B, Iuhl I, Vilbek H, Bulow H, Dreijer N, Rasmussen H 1992 Acupuncture treatment of severe knee osteoarthrosis. A long-term study. Acta Anaesthesiologica Scandinavica 36:519–525

Co L L, Schmitz T H, Havdala H, Reyes A, Westerman M P 1979 Acupuncture: an evaluation in the painful crises of sickle cell anaemia. Pain 7:181–185

Coan R, Wong G, Coan P 1981 The acupuncture treatment of neck pain: a randomized controlled study. American Journal of Chinese Medicine 9:326–332

Coniam S W, Diamond A W 1994 Practical pain management. Oxford University Press, Oxford

Deluze C, Bosia L, Zirbs A, Chantraine A, Vischer T 1992 Electro-acupuncture in fibromyalgia: results of a controlled trial. British Medical Journal 305:1249–1252

Dowson D, Lewith G, Machin D 1985 The effects of acupuncture versus placebo in the treatment of headache. Pain 21:35–42

Edelist G, Gross A E, Langer F 1976 Treatment of low back pain with acupuncture. Canadian Anaesthesiology Society Journal 23:303–306

Edmeads J 1984 Placebos and the power of negative thinking. Headache: 24(6):342–343

Emery P, Lythgoe S 1986 The effect of acupuncture on ankylosing spondylitis. British Journal of Rheumatology 25:132–133

Fairbank J C T, Couper J, Davies J B, O'Brien J P 1980 The Oswestry low back pain disability questionnaire. Physiotherapy 66:271–273

Fialka V, Resch K L, Ritter-Dietrich D, Alacamlioglu Y, Chen O, Leitha T, Kluger R, Ernst E 1993 Acupuncture for reflex sympathetic dystrophy. Archives of Internal Medicine 153: 661–665

Fields H L, Levine J D 1981 Biology of placebo analgesia. American Journal of Medicine 70:745–746

Filshie J 1988 The non-drug treatment of neuralgic and neuropathic pain of malignancy. Cancer Surveys 7:161–193

Filshie J, Redman D 1985 Acupuncture and malignant pain problems. European Journal of Surgical Oncology 11:389–394

Fischer M V, Behr A, von Reumont J 1984 Acupuncture—a therapeutic concept in the treatment of painful conditions and functional disorders. Report on 971 cases. Acupuncture and Electrotherapeutics Research 9:11–29

Fox E, Melzack R 1976 Transcutaneous electrical stimulation and acupuncture: comparison of treatment for low back pain. Pain 2:141–148

Garvey T, Marks M, Wiesel S 1989 A prospective, randomised, double blind evaluation of trigger-point injection therapy for low back pain. Spine 14:962–964

Gaw A C, Chang L W, Shaw L C 1975 Efficacy of acupuncture in osteoarthritic pain. A controlled double-blind study. New England Journal of Medicine 293:375–378

Ghia J, Mao W, Toomey T, Gregg J 1976 Acupuncture and chronic pain mechanisms. Pain 2:285–299

Godfrey C, Morgan P 1978 A controlled trial of the theory of acupuncture in musculoskeletal pain. Journal of Rheumatology 5:121–124

Gwan K H 1977 Treatment of cluster headache by acupuncture. American Journal of Chinese Medicine 5:91–94

Hansen P E, Hansen J H 1985 Acupuncture treatment of chronic tension headache—a controlled cross-over trial. Cephalalgia 5:137–142

Headache Classification Committee of the International Headache Society 1988 Classification and diagnostic criteria for headache disorders, cranialneuralgias, and facial pain. Cephalalgia 8:(Suppl M)

Hesse J, Mogelvang B, Simonsen H 1994 Acupuncture versus metoprolol in migraine prophylaxis: a randomised trial of trigger point inactivation. Journal of Internal Medicine 235:451–456

Hossenloop C M, Leiber L, Mo B 1976 Psychological factors in the effectiveness of acupuncture for chronic pain. In: Bonica J J (ed) Advances in pain research and therapy, vol 1. Raven Press, New York 41:903–909

International Association for the Study of Pain (Sub-Committee on Taxonomy) 1994 Classification of chronic pain, 2nd edn IASP, Seattle

James F R, Large R G, Bushnell J A, Wells J E 1991 Epidemiology of pain in New Zealand. Pain 44:279–283

Johansson V, Kosic S, Lindahl O, Lindwall L, Tibbling L 1976 Effect of acupuncture in tension headache and brainstem reflexes. Advances in Pain Research and Therapy 1:839–841

Johansson A, Wenneberg B, Wagersten C, Haraldson T 1991 Acupuncture in treatment of facial muscular pain. Acta Odontologica Scandinavica 49:153–158

Johnstone H, Marcinak J, Luckett M, Scott J 1994 An evaluation of treatment effectiveness of the Chicago Health Outreach Acupuncture Clinic. Journal of Holist-Nursing 12:171–183

Junnila S. 1987a Long-term treatment of chronic pain with acupuncture Part I. Acupuncture and Electrotherapeutics Research 12:23–36

Junnila S 1987b Long-term treatment of chronic pain with acupuncture Part II. Acupuncture and Electrotherapeutics Research 12:125–138

Katz R L, Kaocy Spiegel H, Katz G J 1974 Pain, acupuncture, hypnosis. In: Bonica J J (ed) Advances in neurology, vol 4. International Symposum on Pain. Raven Press, New York, pp 749–754

Kellgren H J 1939 The distribution of pain arising from deep somatic structures with charts of segmental pain areas. Clinical Science 4:35–46

Kenyon J, Knight C, Wells C 1983 Randomised double-blind trial on the immediate effects of naloxone on classical Chinese acupuncture therapy for chronic pain. Acupuncture and Electrotherapeutics Research 8:17–24

Kerns R D, Turk D C, Rudy T E 1985 The West Haven-Yale Multidimensional Pain Inventory (WHYMPI). Pain 23:345–356

Kim C K 1974 The effect of acupuncture on migraine headache. American Journal of Chinese Medicine 2:407–411

Klide A, Martin B 1989 Methods of stimulating acupuncture points for treatment of chronic back pain in horses. Journal of the American Veterinary Medical Association 195:1375–1379

Kreitler S, Kreitler H, Carasso R 1987 Cognitive orientation as predictor of pain relief following acupuncture. Pain 28:323–341

Laitinen J 1975 Acupuncture for migraine prophylaxis: a prospective clinical study with six months' follow-up. American Journal of Chinese Medicine 3:271–274

Lee P, Anderson T W, Modell J 1975 Treatment of chronic pain with acupuncture. Journal of the American Medical Association 232:1133–1135

Lee P, Thorkild W, Andersen, Modell J, Saga S 1975 Treatment of chronic pain with acupuncture. Journal of the American Medical Association 232:1133–1135

Lee Y, Lee W, Chen M, Huang J, Chung C, Chang L 1992 Acupuncture in the treatment of renal colic. Journal of Urology 147:16–18

Lehmann T R, Russell D W, Spratt K F et al 1986 Efficacy of electroacupuncture and TENS in the rehabilitation of chronic low back pain patients. Pain 26:277–290

Levine J D, Gormley J, Fields H L 1976 Observations on the analgesic effect of needle puncture (acupuncture). Pain 2:149–159

Levine J D, Gordon N C, Fields H L 1978 The mechanism of placebo analgesia. Lancet 2:654–657

Levine J D, Gordon N C, Bornstein J C, Fields H L 1979 Role of pain in placebo analgesia. Proceedings of the National Academy of Sciences 76:3528–3531

Lewers D, Clelland J A, Jackson J, Varner R E, Bergman J 1989 Transcutaneous electrical nerve stimulation in the relief of primary dysmenorrhea. Physical Therapy 69:3–9

Lewis P J 1993 Electroacupuncture in fibromyalgia. [Letter] British Medical Journal 306:393

Lewith G T 1984 How effective is acupuncture in the management of pain? Journal of the Royal College of General Practitioners 34:275–278

Lewith G T, Kenyon J N 1984 Physiological and psychological explanations for the mechanism of acupuncture as a treatment for chronic pain. Social Science in Medicine 19:1367–1378

Lewith G T, Machin D 1983 On the evaluation of the clinical effects of acupuncture. Pain 16:111–127

Lewith G T, Field J, Machin D 1983 Acupuncture compared with placebo in post-herpetic pain. Pain 17:361–368

List T, Helkimo M 1987 Acupuncture in the treatment of patients with chronic facial pain and mandibular dysfunction. Swedish Dentistry Journal 11:83–92

List T, Helkimo M 1992 Acupuncture and occlusal splint therapy in the treatment of craniomandibular disorders. Acta Odontologica Scandinavica 50:375–385

Loh L, Nathan P W, Schott G D, Zilkha K J 1984 Acupuncture versus medical treatment for migraine and muscle tension headaches. Journal of Neurology, Neurosurgery and Psychiatry 47:333–337

Longobardi A, Clelland J A, Knowles C J, Jackson J 1989 Effects of auricular transcutaneous electrical nerve stimulation on distal extremity pain: a pilot study. Physical Therapy 69:10–17

Loy T 1983 Treatment of cervical spondylosis. Electroacupuncture versus physiotherapy. Medical Journal of Australia 2:32–34

Lundeberg T 1984 A comparative study of the pain alleviating effect of vibratory stimulation, transcutaneous electrical nerve stimulation, electroacupuncture and placebo. American Journal of Chinese Medicine 12:72–79

Lundeberg T, Hurtig T, Lundeberg S, Thomas M 1988 Long-term results of acupuncture in chronic head and neck pain. The Pain Clinic 2:15–31

MacDonald A, Macrae K, Master B, Rubin A 1983 Superficial acupuncture in the relief of chronic low back pain. Annals of the Royal College of Surgeons of England 65:44–46

Mann F, Bowsher D, Mumford J, Lipton S, Miles J 1973 Treatment of intractable pain by acupuncture. Lancet 2:57–60

Martin B, Klide A 1987 Use of acupuncture for treatment of chronic back pain in horses. Journal of the American Veterinary Medical Association 190:1177–1180

Melzack R, Wall P D 1965 Pain mechanisms; a new theory. Science 150:971–979

Melzack R 1975 The McGill Pain Questionnaire; major properties and scoring methods. Pain I:277–299

Melzack R, Stillwell D, Fox E 1977 Trigger points and acupuncture points for pain: correlations and implications. Pain 3:3–23

Mendelson G, Selwood T, Kranz H, Loh T, Kidson M, Scott D 1983 Acupuncture treatment of chronic back pain. A double-blind placebo controlled trial. American Journal of Medicine 74:49–54

Molsberger A, Hille E 1994 The analgesic effect of acupuncture in chronic tennis elbow pain. British Journal of Rheumatology 33:1162–1165

Moore M E, Berk S N 1976 Acupuncture for chronic shoulder pain. Annals of Internal Medicine 84:381–384

Patel M, Gutzwiller F, Paccaud F, Marazzi A 1989 A meta-analysis of acupuncture for chronic pain. International Journal of Epidemiology 18:900–906

Peng A T, Behar S, Yue S J 1987 Long-term therapeutic effects of electroacupuncture for chronic neck and shoulder pain—a double blind study. Acupuncture and Electrotherapeutics Research 12:37–44

Petrie J P, Hazelman B L 1986 A controlled study of acupuncture in neck pain. British Journal of Rheumatology 25:271–275

Petrie J P, Langley G B 1983 Acupuncture in the treatment of chronic cervical pain. A pilot study. Clinical and Experimental Rheumatology 1:333–336

Pilowsky I, Spence N D 1975 Patterns of illness behaviour in patients with intractable pain. Journal of Psychosomatic Research 19:279–287

Poitinen P J, Salmela T M 1977 Acupuncture treatment of migraine In: Sicuteri F (ed) Headache new vistas. Biomedical Press, Florence, pp 251–257

Puett D, Griffin M 1994 Published trials of non-medicinal and non-invasive therapies for hip and knee osteoarthritis. Annals of Internal Medicine 121:133–140

Raustia A M, Pohjola R T 1986 Acupuncture compared with stomatognathic treatment for TMJ dysfunction III. Journal of Prosthetic Dentistry 56:616–623

Raustia A M, Pohjola R T, Virtanen K K 1985 Acupuncture compared with stomatognathic treatment for TMJ dysfunction I. Journal of Prosthetic Dentistry 54:581–585

Reeves J, Jaeger B, Graff-Radford S 1986 Reliability of the pressure algometer as a measure of myofascial trigger point sensitivity. Pain 24:313–321

Richardson P H, Vincent C A 1986 Acupuncture for the treatment of pain: a review of evaluative research. Pain 24:15–40

Sodipo J O 1979 Therapeutic acupuncture for chronic pain. Pain 7:359–365

Strauss S 1981 Acupuncture therapy in conditions of chronic pain. American Journal of Acupuncture 9:73–75

Takeda W, Wessell J 1994 Acupuncture for the treatment of pain of osteoarthritic knees. Arthritic Care and Research 1:118–122

Tavola T, Gala C, Conte G, Invernizzi G 1992 Traditional Chinese acupuncture in tension-type headache; a controlled study. Pain 48:325–329

Ter Riet G, Kleijnen J, Knipschild P 1990 Acupuncture and chronic pain: a criteria-based meta-analysis. Journal of Clinical Epidemiology 43:1191–1199

Thomas M, Lundeberg T 1994 Importance of modes of acupuncture in the treatment of chronic nociceptive low back pain. Acta Anaesthesiologia Scandinavica 38:63–69

Thomas M, Eriksson S V, Lundeberg T 1991 A comparative study of diazepam and acupuncture in patients with osteoarthritis pain—a placebo controlled study. American Journal of Chinese Medicine 19:95–100

Thomas M, Arner S, Lundeberg T 1992 Is acupuncture an alternative in idiopathic pain disorder? Acta Anaesthesiologia Scandinavica 36:637–642

Vincent C A 1989a The methodology of controlled trials of acupuncture. Acupuncture in Medicine VIII:9–13

Vincent C A 1989b A controlled trial of the treatment of migraine by acupuncture. Clinical Journal of Pain 5:305–312

Vincent C A 1990 The treatment of tension headache by acupuncture: a controlled single case design with time series analysis. Journal of Psychosomatic Research 34:553–561

Vincent C A, Lewith G 1995 Placebo controls for acupuncture studies. Journal of the Royal Society of Medicine 88:199–202

Vincent C A, Richardson P H 1986 The evaluation of therapeutic acupuncture: concepts and methods. Pain 24:1–13

Zigmund A S, Snaith R P 1983 The Hospital Anxiety and Depression Scale. Acta Psychiatrica Scandinavica 67:361–371

17

Acupuncture for rheumatological problems

Anne Virginia Camp

The specialty of rheumatology encompasses diseases that vary from the most serious and potentially fatal, such as progressive systemic sclerosis and systemic lupus erythematosus, through to a variety of mild but tiresome and chronically painful disorders, such as soft tissue rheumatism and tenosynovitis. Rheumatologists have, as have all physicians, to maintain a detailed knowledge of all the body systems and the ability to apply a truly holistic approach to the diagnosis and management of rheumatic diseases. This encompasses the classical history, examination and treatment triad as well as the use of the skills of empathy, listening, communication and teaching to assist patients in the management of their problems. The symptoms occurring commonly in this very varied group of patients are pain, stiffness, lack of mobility and actual or perceived swelling. Although rheumatologists are specialists in diseases and problems arising within the connective tissue system of the body, the occurrence of these symptoms, together with the propensity for many serious diseases such as cancer and infections to spread to the system, mean that many rheumatological patients will in fact require referral to other specialists, such as oncologists, surgeons, cardiologists and, very frequently, psychiatrists and psychologists. The diagnosis of a patient presenting with chronic pain requires meticulous history taking and observation, far more than high-powered technological investigations, to arrive at a clear idea of the true problem. It is therefore vitally important that anyone undertaking to treat patients presenting with rheumatological symptoms should have a clear idea of this background to the problems, the ability to diagnose and exclude serious disease and the humility to recognize that individual skills are insufficient alone to treat such a patient.

Rheumatic diseases are mostly chronic, recurring and incurable. Many can be treated adequately by local or systemic drugs, physiotherapy procedures or surgery but for the majority such treatments are in general only suppressive, frequently fail or may not even be available for that particular disease. Rheumatologists recognize their inability to treat many of the diseases adequately and a lot of time is spent in education of patients and explanation of the problems and how to apply reasonable management principles. For all these reasons, patients with rheumatological disorders frequently seek alternative therapy. The percentage of patients with rheumatoid arthritis who made use of alternative methods at least once has been found to be as high as 94% (Higham, Ashcroft & Jayson 1983, Kestin et al 1985, Kronenfield & Wasner 1982, Struthers, Scott & Scott 1983). A study from the Netherlands that looked at attitudes of both patients and rheumatologists to alternative therapists revealed that acupuncture, homeopathy and healing by touch were the three most popular alternative practitioners visited by Dutch patients (Visser, Peters & Rasker 1992). Overall probably some 50% of patients with rheumatic diseases will visit an alternative practitioner at some time or other during the course of their illness. This is not so much a reflection of general practitioner or rheumatological care (Moore et al 1985) as the nature of the condition of chronic pain and unrelieved symptoms (James, Fox & Taheri 1983). Despite the popularity of alternative or complementary therapies and the increasing popularity of acupuncture and homeopathy in particular, rheumatologists remain both sceptical and unaccepting of alternative therapies, although non-judgemental in their attitude to patients (Visser, Peters & Rasker 1992). Scepticism, particularly for a treatment such as acupuncture, which is by no means harmless, is reasonable and well founded. A search of the world literature for published trials of the treatment of osteo-

arthritis of the knee by acupuncture has revealed only two published randomized controlled trials (Puett & Griffin 1994). Such paucity of publications contrasts strongly with the 60 papers per year published on the subject of osteoarthritis, but probably compares well with the lack of randomized controlled trials of surgical intervention for the treatment of many diseases (Brooks & Kirwan 1995). The medical profession is certainly beginning to take complementary therapies seriously and acupuncture in particular is increasingly widely used in the UK National Health Service (British Medical Association 1993). Acupuncture will undoubtedly find its correct place in rheumatological practice so long as practitioners accept the need for and carry out adequate randomized controlled trials (Ernst 1995) but the difficulties and pitfalls in carrying out such studies should not be underestimated (Camp 1995).

INDICATIONS FOR TREATMENT

The potential scope of therapeutic effects of acupuncture in rheumatic diseases is fairly wide (Box 17.1). Acupuncture has been shown to be effective in the treatment of chronic pain in a

---

Box 17.1 Indications for acupuncture treatment in rheumatology

Acute musculoskeletal pain:
- muscle strain
- acute osteoarthritis
- enthesopathy
- shoulder pain
- neck and low back pain.

Chronic musculoskeletal pain:
- osteoarthritis
- shoulder pain
- neck and low back pain
- postlaminectomy pain
- scar pain
- inflammatory polyarthritis
  — where drugs are refused; following systemic control for residual joint pain
  — postjoint replacement pain (particularly following knee arthroplasty)
- fibromyalgia
- soft tissue rheumatism.

number of areas of the musculoskeletal system such as the back (MacDonald et al 1983), the elbow (Molsberger & Hills 1994) and the neck (Coan, Wong & Coan 1980). It can also be used in the short term for acute pain, particularly pain that is frustrating and disabling in everyday life, such as that in the back (Hackett, Seddon & Kaminski 1988). Acupuncture can certainly be used in the relief of stiffness and has been shown to increase significantly the range of movement in knee joints of patients with severe osteoarthritis (Christensen et al 1992). Numerous studies, including those where release of endorphins and enkephalins by acupuncture were originally described (Ho & Wen 1989), have shown that acupuncture can reduce the overall burden of symptoms in painful conditions by improving muscle spasm, sleep pattern, depression, anxiety and restlessness. Despite reports that seemingly indicate that acupuncture has the potential for immunological effects (J L Chou, unpublished work, 1985, Liu et al 1993), there have as yet been no adequate controlled trials in vivo demonstrating that acupuncture has an effect on acute or chronic inflammation by reducing swelling, affecting leukocyte migration or changing the biological markers of disease. Acupuncture cannot be recommended for the treatment of inflammatory arthritis, except perhaps to reduce pain temporarily in patients unable to take anti-inflammatory or analgesic drugs.

Acupuncture is essentially a treatment for symptoms, not diseases. The types of conditions that should therefore be considered for acupuncture management, both early on in the course of the problem or as a last resort, are those for which there are no adequate long-term treatments, where other treatments can be dangerous, with adverse effects on mortality or morbidity, and those where other more comparable symptomatic treatments, such as physiotherapy or osteopathy, have proved ineffective or inadequate. Such conditions therefore include muscle strain, osteoarthritis, shoulder pain, neck and lower back pain, postlaminectomy and scar pain, fibromyalgia and soft tissue rheumatism (Camp 1992). Acupuncture can be used also for many symptoms associated with musculoskeletal disorders. These include sympathetic or parasympathetic symptoms, such as coldness, cramps, anxiety, frequency of micturition, palpitations, muscle spasm, other neurological symptoms such as numbness, paraesthesiae, weakness and hyperaesthesia, smooth muscle abnormalities of the gastrointestinal tract or of the smaller blood vessels and a host of other associated symptoms, such as giddiness, mild tinnitus, nausea, vomiting and visual problems.

DISADVANTAGES AND ADVANTAGES OF ACUPUNCTURE

The dangers of acupuncture treatment in rheumatic patients, although in general mild, should not be disguised. The commonest side-effects encountered are those resulting from the physiological effects of needling, namely bruising and vasovagal attacks. There are particular problems in rheumatic diseases to which a practitioner should pay attention; these are the effects that bleeding from the needle may have on the original condition treated, as well as other systems. Bleeding into a joint can cause an intense inflammatory reaction and act as a nidus for infection. The intensity of the inflammatory reaction may lead to a severe and rapid form of osteoarthritis. Even mild bleeding can lead to considerable and lasting disability in patients who are already disabled by virtue of musculoskeletal symptoms. Bleeding into the soft tissue can lead to swelling, stiffness and worsening of overall pain, which may interrupt a rehabilitation programme (e.g. for fibromyalgia) and lead to abandonment of the correct overall treatment regimen.

There are further inherent difficulties in acupuncture treatment that arise from its very success. Relief of pain and stiffness without relief of inflammation or an effect on the overall progression of the disease can disguise such progression and remove from the patient the ability to observe developing deformity, muscle wasting and weakness or serious complications such as infection. A false sense of security can be given to both the practitioner and the patient that the disease is well under control and that there is no necessity to provide a continuous reassessment of chronic disease. This may mean that surgery is deferred until too late, that patients will refuse the best, albeit inadequate, forms of drug therapy such as immunosuppressive treatment, and may avoid the best medical practice, which is now recognized as the multidisciplinary approach to the overall management of rheumatic problems. The most important disadvantage to the single-minded use of acupuncture for the treatment of rheumatic diseases is the disguise, through the removal of pain, of the development of serious symptoms and diseases such as tumours of bone, vasculitis, inflammatory muscle disease or other serious manifestations of connective tissue disease. It is therefore essential that acupuncture is practised in the context of best medical practice.

Having said this, it is also true that to the patient, as well as the doctor, acupuncture offers many advantages. Patients are always anxious to pursue every avenue of treatment for chronic diseases and it is well recognized that self-efficacy is an important component of a patient's approach to treatment and acceptance of therapy (Lorig et al 1989). Pain remains the main concern for patients with rheumatic conditions (Lorig et al 1984). The use of a treatment that is successful in controlling the pain with fewer side-effects is very acceptable to patients. Self-efficacy and satisfaction with health care have been shown to influence patient behaviour, both in understanding education programmes and in adhering to medical regimens. Patients are more likely to attend regularly for treatment, but nevertheless reduce the frequency of attendance for minor symptoms, if they have some locus of control of their disease (Fitzpatrick & Hopkins 1976, Ley et al 1976, Pryn et al 1985). Clinicians who offer acupuncture treatment as part of an overall treatment for rheumatoid arthritis and include a careful critique of alternative therapies amongst educational programmes for such patients have found that overall patient knowledge, compliance and satisfaction with care can be considerably increased (A Kirk et al, unpublished work, 1991).

TREATMENT MODES

There is no universally accepted nor correct mode of treatment for the use of acupuncture in rheumatological patients. At different times particular types of treatment and forms of needling may be necessary.

The placing of the acupuncture needle, the method of needling and the length of treatment will all be governed initially by the history. Patients who display a great amount of fear and who appear to have a heightened sensitivity to pain (often seen in long-standing back pain, fibromyalgia and nerve pain) should be treated initially with particular care, with gentle needling for a short time and a very careful explanation that the symptoms may initially be made worse.

At the start of each acupuncture treatment, a detailed history of the type of pain, its distribution and referral, its diurnal variation, and features that can make it better or worse should be taken. The site of origin of the pain may often lead to the identification of particular trigger points. The spread of the pain may show secondary trigger points and help to decide which segmental acupuncture points may be used.

Associated symptoms will show whether or not classical Chinese acupuncture points should be used or whether a simple anatomical approach is all that is necessary.

In the examination of the patient, areas of tenderness should be identified. These might include the tendon ends (entheses), joint margins, osteophytes, tender points or trigger points in muscles and areas of increased spasm or sympathetic signs in related dermatomes, myotomes or sclerotomes.

Muscle shortening may be identified by contractures or joint deformity. This should lead to an examination of the shortened muscles for trigger spots or areas of muscle spasm. A patient may complain of pain in an overstretched muscle, whereas the muscle to treat should be the shortened and sometimes asymptomatic one.

Many of the classical acupuncture points, such as those along the Bladder meridian and around the knee and hip joints are exquisitely tender in rheumatological disorders. A knowledge, therefore, of a selection of commonly used classical acupuncture points is important for the treatment of rheumatological conditions. Examination of a few relevant points will help to shorten the treatment time. There are a number of classical peripheral and central acupuncture points that can be used in most rheumatological disorders for their known effects on pain and their anatomical association with spinal nerves. These are: LR-3, SI-3, LI-4, 9 and 11, BL-25, 27, 54 and 57, GB-20 and 21 and ST-36 (Box 17.2)

There are no particular needles that are specially for use in musculoskeletal diseases. Standard 30 or 40 mm needles are sufficient for most patients, although occasionally longer needles may be necessary particularly around the buttock area. Needling may be deep into very superficial muscle, periosteal, or actually into the joint space. (The latter require particular care in patients with rheumatoid arthritis who have a tendency to infection. In these patients, if joints are to be needled then aseptic precautions should be used.)

The different types of needling used in musculoskeletal disease are:

Box 17.2 Acupuncture for the musculoskeletal system

Key points:
LI-4, LR-3, SP-6, SP-9, SP-10,
GB-30, ST-36, LR-11, SI-3,
GB-20, GB-21, BL-54, BL-57
Dominant meridians:
Bladder
Governor Vessel
Large Intestine
Gall Bladder
Miscellaneous:
Muscle cramps—BL-57
Muscle spasm—motor point of nerve—teach stretching
Tinnitus—KI-3, EAR, GB-20 } only in association
Blurred vision—GB-20, BL-2 } with neck pain
'Sciatica'
— Diagnose it first—is it myofascial or nerve root?
— Which is the dominant root?
Select from:
1. BL-50, BL-52, BL-54, BL-57, BL-60, BL-25, BL-27
2. SP-9, SP-10, GB-30
3. Sacral flats
4. SP-6

- **Classical**: The traditional approach where the aim is to elicit needling sensation ('De Qi'). The depth and slope of the needle will depend upon the area and associated structures. The needles are usually left in for 5 to 20 minutes.
- **Superficial**: The needles are flicked under the skin and almost immediately withdrawn.
- **Deep, intramuscular**: Used for trigger point therapy.
- **Periosteal pecking**: The aim is to reach the periosteal plexus of nerves and stimulate them repeatedly for perhaps 10 seconds. This is mainly of use over bony prominences or osteophytes.

There are three particular techniques that may be of special use for musculoskeletal conditions. These are the 'fanning' technique for needling of tendon ends, the use of subcutaneous needles along the passage of nerves and the technique known as 'surrounding the dragon'.

- The needling of tendon ends by 'fanning' is an extension of periosteal pecking (Fig. 17.1). It is the same technique that is used for the injection of hydrocortisone under local anaesthetic for conditions such as tennis elbow. The needle is inserted perhaps 1 to 2 cm away from the tendon end and is advanced to tap the periosteum. It is then moved in different directions around the full extent of the insertion of the tendon and at the end of each movement the periosteum should be touched. This technique is painful and can lead to bruising but

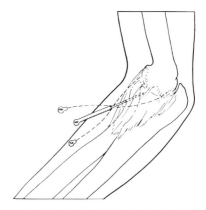

Figure 17.1 'Fanning' technique for the treatment of tendinitis.

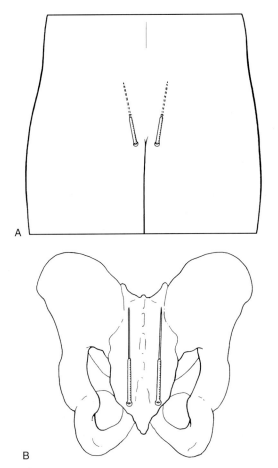

Figure 17.2 A and B: Technique of subcutaneous needling: application of 'sacral flats' for back pain, bladder problems and autonomic symptoms in the lower limbs.

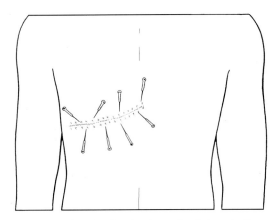

Figure 17.3 'Surrounding the dragon' technique for the treatment of postherpetic neuralgia, scar pain, etc.

may be extremely successful as a substitute for corticosteroid injections, which are unacceptable to many patients and lead to side-effects such as fat atrophy. The technique can be used for lateral epicondylitis, calcaneal spurs, bicipital tendinitis, the various enthesopathies associated with ankylosing spondylitis and as a method of treating chondromalacia patellae, where the needles are inserted into the quadriceps muscle just above the patella.

• The insertion of subcutaneous needles above or along the course of a nerve has long been used by the Chinese for acupuncture analgesia (Fig. 17.2b). It has also been used in childbirth. The placing of a TENS machine over the sacral nerves during labour mimics this form of acupuncture without the use of needles. This may be used for bladder symptoms as well as for low back pain. The technique consists of the insertion of a needle usually over the point of exit of the nerve from the spinal column. In the sacral area, the needle can be inserted just above the third or fourth sacral foramen and then placed so as to lie subcutaneously above the first to third sacral foramina. Electrical stimulation can if necessary be applied through the needles.

• The technique known as 'surrounding the dragon' has been used particularly over denervated or partially denervated areas and in herpes zoster (Fig. 17.3). The needles are placed, in a circular fashion, fairly superficially around the edge or just beyond the area of denervation. They may be stimulated electrically. A TENS machine placed with its electrodes on either side of a painful scar can also be tried.

Whilst many practitioners feel that better results will be achieved by obtaining needling sensation when using traditional Chinese meridian points, this is certainly not necessary for all points or in all conditions. The exact level of stimulation will depend upon which points are used and the condition. It is seldom necessary to maintain stimulation at all times or to use electro-acupuncture at each treatment. It is sometimes important just to use superficial acupuncture (for instance in fibromyalgia initially) and sometimes necessary to use only one or two needles with deep stimulation, such as when treating myofascial syndrome.

It is worthwhile studying a few points in the ear, especially where pain is associated with autonomic symptoms. Points suggested are: Shenmen (HT-7), cervical, thoracic and lumbar areas, the eye point and ACTH point.

NON-NEEDLE 'ACUPUNCTURE'

All types of non-needle 'acupuncture' may be used in rheumatological disorders with benefit. Those patients who have experienced both types of acupuncture usually say that the needles are more successful. Lasers (see Ch 12) may be used over acupuncture points with or without a point finder: TENS (see Ch 11) can also be used over acupuncture points to give an acupuncture type of treatment and electroacupuncture machines can be attached to surface electrodes rather than to the needles themselves (see Ch 10).

Inactive electroacupuncture or TENS machines are frequently used as placebo treatments in randomized controlled trials (Dowson, Lewith & Machin 1985, Hackett, Seddon & Kaminski 1988, MacDonald et al 1983). The use of non-needle acupuncture has had both success and failure in clinical trials (Dowson, Lewith & Machin 1985, Fargas-Babjak, Pomeranz & Rooney 1992, Hackett, Seddon & Kaminski 1988, Lehmann et al 1986, Lisenyuk & Yakupov 1992). The above forms of treatment have the advantage that they are virtually painless and can be used for patients in whom needle acupuncture is relatively contra-indicated, such as those with needle phobia or who are on anticoagulants.

The electrical stimulus can be varied considerably for the different types of pain. This technique effectively replaces the traditional Chinese method of the use of heat or moxa to acupuncture needles or an acupuncture point, providing greater refinement of stimulation and greater safety. Electrical stimulation of acupuncture needles may be used in rheumatology, although this is seldom necessary for straightforward joint or soft tissue pain. It has a particular advantage in relieving stiffness, sensitivity of the skin and some nerve pain and in providing superficial analgesia for areas of hyperaesthesia or scar tenderness. Most electroacupuncture and TENS machines are not accurately calibrated but in practice this seems to make little difference to the success of treatment.

The low-level laser used for rheumatology treatment does not penetrate as deeply as can needles and is probably not of a great deal of use for deep pain, although its well-demonstrated anti-inflammatory effect may well reduce soft tissue pain. Modern lasers can reach a power output of 15 mW but the depth of penetration is not accurately known. More work is required to establish their true place in acupuncture treatment.

TREATMENT SCHEDULE

An individual treatment can last anything from 5 to 20 minutes depending upon the patient, the type of condition and the response to previous treatments. Although it is possible to achieve some pain relief at the first treatment in most patients, this is seldom long lasting and is really only of use in treating acute pain. All patients should plan on having four treatments initially, either once or twice a week, before expecting any lasting benefit. With really chronically painful conditions, particularly where low back pain or intractable joint pain have been present for more than 3 years, six treatments may be necessary for a response. It is important to realize that this response may be delayed for several weeks after the last treatment. It is seldom necessary to plan more than six treatments initially before a gap to assess response. If there has been no effect on pain 10 weeks after starting an acupuncture course, it is not worth while continuing.

The pattern of future treatments, after the initial four to six, depends very much on the response. Rheumatological conditions are chronic and recurrent. An acupuncture response seldom lasts at any reasonable level for longer than 3 months. In some patients, sufficient relief may occur for a course of treatment to be repeated only once a year, but, in the majority, two or three courses a year will usually be required.

The alternative is to give a 'top-up' treatment every 6 or 8 weeks. Acupuncture treatment of rheumatological diseases may need to be continued for many years. Both patient and practitioner must be aware of this before embarking on a trial of treatment.

It is difficult to avoid patients becoming habituated to acupuncture. A considerable therapeutic bias results from the positive benefits of feeling that something is being done for chronic pain and the extra time given by the therapist in personal treatment. The effects of acupuncture recorded by many patients and doctors make a true therapeutic benefit easy to recognize. At the first visit the patient usually feels relaxed, sleeps better that night and has increased energy and mobility. A transient relief of long-standing pain may then be followed by rebound worsening of the pain for 24 hours. At the second visit drowsiness may be less but relaxation is usually achieved. The patient recognizes a sense of well-being, and pain relief may last longer. By the third visit the patient is usually able to recognize that the overall pain level is less, particularly at night, and finds it easier to bear. After the fourth visit a long-term acupuncture response is recognized, the pain is relieved in part or in total for up to 3 months and everyday activities become easier. The duration of the response to acupuncture depends on many factors. Foremost is the length of time that pain has been present and the extent of pathology treated. A good therapeutic response in rheumatological conditions can be expected in 60% of patients overall. Miraculous cure at the first visit is extremely rare and achieved in general only for acute conditions. Even then the effect may be short lasting and the rebound pain doubly difficult to bear.

EVALUATION

It is vitally important that evaluation of the acupuncture response takes place regularly. To the patient, even a slight diminution of chronic disabling pain is worth while and it is tempting to continue treatment on demand. However acupuncture is not without side-effects and is time consuming. Response to acupuncture should not be confused with response to a sympathetic ear. Evaluation of the acupuncture response can be made in a number of ways. The use of visual analogue scales, scales of well-being, scales of night pain and analgesic counts are all well known in therapeutic trials and are quick and easy to use in everyday practice. The addition of a patient diary, kept perhaps once a week, may help to evaluate the treatment on a more long-term basis and sort out a true acupuncture response from normal disease fluctuations. For more detailed audit and outcome measurement, the short-form McGill pain questionnaire has been found useful (Collier et al 1995, Melzack 1987). The best method of evaluation is to obtain a careful clinical record of the patient's symptoms, signs and disability in everyday life, recorded for preference at least 3 months prior to treatment and monthly after the start of treatment. Where specific drugs such as carbamazepine for trigeminal neuralgia are used, records of change of dosage can provide further evidence of the efficacy of acupuncture treatment.

PSYCHOLOGICAL FACTORS

It is well known that psychological factors such as expectations, values, attitudes, personality traits, emotions and social culture affect perception of pain and a person's response to it (Kreitler, Kreitler & Carrassa 1987). Tolerance of high pain levels may be directly related to attitudes that either deny the existence of pain or avoid dealing with it (Weisenberg et al 1975). Research into attitudes that affect a person's recovery from pain after a treatment such as acupuncture is sparse and has been equivocal. A study by Norton et al (1984) looked at the effects of belief on acupuncture analgesia and found that subjects with more positive beliefs in the effectiveness of acupuncture reported significantly lower pain in cold pressure tests than did those who were sceptical. Conversely, earlier work on patients with dental pain (Chapman et al 1982) found that a person's beliefs did not influence the effects of acupuncture. Other studies by Kreitler, Kreitler & Carrassa (1987) and Knox, Handfield Jones & Schum (1979) appeared to show that a positive attitude of the recipient to acupuncture potentiates its effects. A study of acupuncture for chronic shoulder pain, which was specifically designed to test the part that both placebo and hypnotic susceptibility may play in a patient's response to acupuncture, showed no real difference in effect when the acupuncture was given in either a positive or a negative setting, nor any significant effect of susceptibility to hypnosis (Moore & Berk 1976).

A recent study of the influence of attitudes to acupuncture and the outcome of treatment is of particular relevance to practitioners of rheumatological acupuncture because it specifically looked at a group of rheumatological patients who had never previously received acupuncture and studied them both before, during and after a course of acupuncture given on the National Health Service (Collier et al 1995). This study showed that 55% of the subjects respond to acupuncture given for chronic long-standing rheumatological conditions. There was no difference between responders and non-responders either in their attitudes to or knowledge of acupuncture, but there was a negative correlation between acupuncture response and the trait of anxiety. Other interesting findings in the study, which was carried out in the context of a large NHS rheumatological clinic with patients very positive to the idea of acupuncture, were the findings that patients felt very inadequately prepared for acupuncture, had a considerable lack of knowledge, particularly about the side-effects and the amount of pain to be expected and that older patients were more anxious than younger patients.

Combining the result of this study with those on self-efficacy would seem to indicate that preparation of a patient for acupuncture by a careful discussion of its likely outcome, mode of working, side-effects and the placing of the needles would reduce a patient's anxiety, ensure cooperation with the whole of the acupuncture course and with other treatments for the condition and probably increase the efficacy of the acupuncture.

TREATMENT FAILURES

Whilst no treatment can be universally successful there are a number of other reasons why acupuncture for the treatment of musculoskeletal conditions may fail. The first is poor selection. Somatization is very common to the musculoskeletal system and it may take some considerable time to recognize. This does not mean that the autonomic features of some conditions caused by anxiety or post-traumatic stress cannot be treated by acupuncture but that they must be recognized and treated accordingly. In general, patients in whom the pain has a strong non-anatomical element and where features of somatization are present do not respond well to acupuncture.

Point selection may be at fault and it is always worth while trying a further approach using either the classical Chinese diagnostic techniques, contralateral points, electrical stimulation or the ear. It is also useful to examine patients' drug treatment. Poorly controlled or undiagnosed diabetes may well alter pain sensitivity. High doses of corticosteroids can also affect pain and severe rebound pain may occur after withdrawal of corticosteroids or drugs such as diazepam. This may well have altered the pain threshold and pain sensitivity and make acupuncture less effective. Such changes may also alter a previously successful acupuncture response to an unsuccessful one.

Drugs may also be used as an adjunct to acupuncture. Tricyclic antidepressant drugs in small doses can be useful in this way, as can some of the antiepileptic drugs. There is every reason for combining two treatments such as pain modulation by drugs and pain modulation by acupuncture. Overall success in the treatment of pain depends not just on applying acupuncture but on applying all other known methods of successful treatment for the condition. This should include training in relaxation, self-motivation, exercise, lifestyle advice and cognitive therapy.

Finally electrical stimulation or non-needle 'acupuncture' for those in whom the fear of acupuncture produces heightened pain may increase the success rate of acupuncture.

TREATMENT OF SPECIFIC CONDITIONS

Inflammation arthritis

Few attempts have been made to carry out adequate clinical studies of acupuncture for patients with rheumatoid arthritis. Only four controlled trials were discovered by Bhatt-Saunders (1985) in a survey of world literature. Man & Baragar (1974) studied two groups of 10 patients with definite or classical rheumatoid arthritis for 4 years or longer, who had major problems in the knees. These patients were randomly assigned to treatment either with a standard course of acupuncture to one knee and an intra-articular steroid injection (50 mg hydrocortisone acetate) to the other knee or with placebo acupuncture (an inappropriately placed needle) to one knee and intra-articular steroid to the other. Assessment was by a blinded observer and assessments were made at 24 hours, weekly for 4 weeks and monthly for 3 months after treatment. All patients in the active group achieved some reduction of pain, which lasted in some patients for the full 4 months, whilst only one patient in the control group achieved any reduction of pain. This study has been criticized for the type of placebo acupuncture used, on the grounds that it constituted a noxious stimulus, for the paucity of acupuncture treatments, and for the use of standardized acupuncture points. Assessments were made of the intensity of pain and of evidence of inflammation: no effect was seen on inflammation in either group. Further studies in rheumatoid arthritis have been marred either by the use of a crossover design or by lack of control. Conclusions from these and other sources are that acupuncture has a weak effect on inflammation, if any.

Best medical practice in the treatment of inflammatory arthritis should be directed towards suppressive drug therapy and a multidisciplinary approach to the prevention of joint deformity and muscle weakness. If acupuncture is to be used in rheumatoid arthritis it should be only in the context of a single joint that is extremely painful and unresponsive to other measures. The approach to treatment would be that of treatment of the local joint. In late stage rheumatoid arthritis, particularly in patients with gastrointestinal disease, where anti-inflammatory drugs cannot be used, acupuncture may help intractable pain and stiffness prior to orthopaedic surgery. The treatment approach should be as that used for osteoarthritis.

Osteoarthritis

Osteoarthritis, wherever it occurs, is a condition that can respond excellently to acupuncture. The disease leads to a number of symptoms and signs, each of which can be treated differently. There is seldom any systemic upset in osteoarthritis and inflammation is generally mild and localized.

The early symptoms are those of localized, flitting, aching pain, joint margin tenderness and immobility stiffness. These fluctuate considerably from day to day and may cause varying degrees of disability and depression. At this stage, apart from histological changes within the cartilage, the pathological changes are those of joint capsule stiffness and early osteophyte formation. The latter results in stretching of the periosteal nerves, with pain and sometimes inflammation of the skin and localized tenderness. Stiffness and shortening of associated muscles may show as tenderness, trigger points and deformities. There is frequently also tenosynovitis and inflammation of the tendon ends such as lateral epicondylitis.

Primary osteoarthritis presents typically in early middle age but may be confused with other conditions, including fibromyalgia, thyroid deficiency, menopausal symptoms and parathyroid disease. It is important to check for associated systemic disease by examination and baseline blood tests in all patients presenting with these symptoms. X-rays at this stage make no contribution to the diagnosis.

Osteoarthritis is a lifetime but non-life-threatening disease. Apart from major surgery, such as arthroplasty, there are no corrective treatments of adequately proven efficacy. Acupuncture can play a major role in symptom control, but only in the context of other aspects of general treatment, such as weight reduction, exercise, relaxation and pain management strategies. Apart from simple on-demand analgesics, drug therapy plays no part in the management of osteoarthritis in its early stages, as the risk of serious side-effects of anti-inflammatory drugs is too great.

The techniques of acupuncture of particular use in osteoarthritis are:

- periosteal needling of osteophytes
- superficial needling of joint capsule
- superficial needling over tender muscles
- LI-4, Shenmen ear point for pain and sleep disturbance
- stimulation of tendon ends
- electroacupuncture.

Success can often be immediate in early disease and only one or two treatments may be required. A TENS machine can be very helpful for self-management of the unpredictable flares of this disease. Electroacupuncture may be used in some acute flare-ups when a joint becomes 'stuck'. The acupuncture should be used to stimulate the nerves to the joint, to provide analgesia. This will often restore mobility rapidly. Apart from these general principles, the treatment of osteoarthritis should be similar to that used for individual joints.

Knee joint problems

Acupuncture treatment of the knee joint is probably the simplest treatment to learn. There are few general points, the treatment is successful in up to 80% of patients and the condition is common enough for practical knowledge to be acquired rapidly. As in all rheumatological conditions an accurate diagnosis is essential. The application of the general treatments of knee pain, such as knowledge of quadriceps exercises and other joint protection mechanisms, is essential. The association between obesity and knee pain is well recognized and weight management should be part of the overall programme. It is also important to examine and re-examine the knees regularly to look for the development of deformities and instability, such as a valgus or varus deformity, which may require the use of splints or earlier orthopaedic surgery. The types

of acupuncture used can be examined under the heading of acute pain, chronic pain or anterior knee pain; some suggested points and forms of stimulation are shown in Box 17.3.

There are two additional important factors to be remembered in treating knee pain. The first is that apparent primary knee pain may very frequently be referred pain from the hip. Careful examination of the hip joint is extremely important in all patients, even when difficulties in hip movement are denied by the patient. The second is that the synovial membrane is very superficial around the knee joint and therefore careful attention to asepsis is important.

Treatment of osteoarthritis of the knee by corticosteroid injections is time honoured and is of proven benefit. The question of whether to use acupuncture or corticosteroid injection as the prime treatment depends upon the preference and training of the practitioner and the patient's expressed wishes. It is not surprising that, with such a simply applied treatment, comparison between corticosteroid injections and acupuncture have been the subject of clinical trials for both the knee and hip joint (Christensen et al 1992, A Kirk, A Mickiewicz & A V Camp, unpublished work 1992, McIndoe, Young & Bone 1995). These studies seemed to indicate that acupuncture, although more time consuming and possibly more delayed in its effect than corticosteroid injections, is at least as effective. The side-effects profile for acupuncture is certainly better than that of corticosteroid injections. The theoretical

---

Box 17.3 Treatment of the knee joint
  • *Acute pain/stiffness*: SP-9, SP-10, BL-54, BL-57, ST-33, ST-36 'Eyes of the knee' Electrical or manual stimulation • *Chronic pain*: SP-9, XLI, BL-54, BL-57, LR-3, LR-9, ST-33, ST-36, SP-10 Tender and trigger points Ear points can be added 'Eye of the knee' points—penetrate synovium only • *Anterior knee pain*: Add—periosteal stimulation of patellar margins 'Fanned' stimulation of patellar attachment SP-6

danger of corticosteroid injections to joint cartilage has not been borne out in practice, but the possibility of systemic effects and a local effect from bruising, thinning of the skin and fat necrosis should be discussed with the patient.

The nerve suppy to the knee joint is extremely rich. It should be well known and can be used to aid treatment both in the correct application of electroacupuncture for knee pain and in considering the possibility of further points to add to the treatment, as well as in directing the search for tender points (Box 17.4). The same approach may be used in treatment of other joints—that is, examining the nerve supply in order to decide upon point selection and improve the efficacy of acupuncture treatment (Figs 17.4–17.7).

Other joint problems

There have been isolated reports of acupuncture treatment for the hip (Clinical Standards Advisory Group 1994), the elbow (Molsberger & Hills 1994) and the shoulder (Moore & Berk 1976). The paucity of trials, the variation of the results and the mixed nature of the patients treated mean that no conclusions can be made from these studies. Suggested treatment schedules are therefore anecdotal. Pain from these three joints, together with that from the knee, cause some of the commonest problems presenting in general practice in this country and lead to a great deal of disability in the older population. It is therefore well worth trying acupuncture, assuming that other treatments have been tried and found ineffective or are contraindicated. The points used should be a combination of local treatment of the individual joint, using classical acupuncture points where they relate to tender areas or the nerve supply of the joint, together with the treatment of related trigger spots in local muscles to try and aid mobility of the joint and peripheral points in the arms and legs such as LI-4 or LR-3. The hip joint is traditionally treated by the Gall Bladder meridian and the shoulder by Stomach meridian points in the legs. These can often lead to a successful outcome when combined with careful examination of the spine and other joints, where tender points may be identified and

---

Box 17.4   Nerve supply to the knee

- *Cutaneous*:
  Anterior—femoral nerve (L2, 3 and 4) → patellar plexus
  Medial—medial cutaneous nerve and saphenous nerve (L2, 3 and 4)
  Posterior—posterior cutaneous nerve (S1, 2 and 3)
  Lateral—lateral cutaneous nerve of thigh (L2 and 3)
- *Knee joint*:
  Anterior—femoral and saphenous nerve
  Lateral—anterior tibial nerve or lateral popliteal nerve (L4 and 5, S1 and 2)
  Posterolateral—lateral popliteal nerve
  Posteromedical (L4 and 5, S1, 2 and 3)

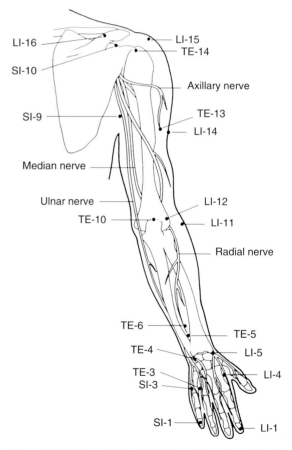

Figure 17.4   The relationship between the main points of the lateral aspect of the upper extremities and the nerves. Adapted from Ellis 1994, with permission.

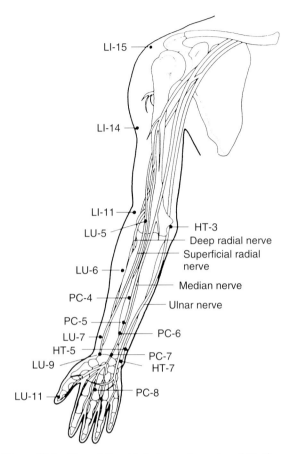

Figure 17.5 The relationship between the main points of the medial aspect of the upper extremities and the nerves. Adapted from Ellis 1994, with permission.

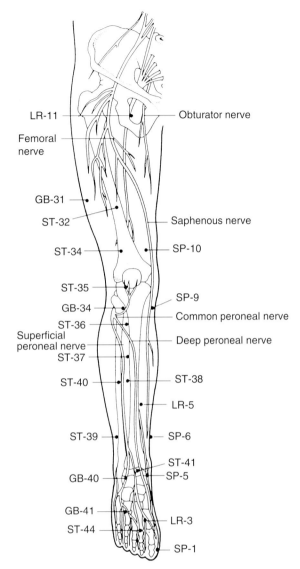

Figure 17.6 The relationship between the main points of the anterior aspect of the lower extremities and the nerves. Adapted from Ellis 1994, with permission.

treated, together with education of the patient and exercises to mobilize and strengthen the joint. Acupuncture for the hip joint can also be used in those with intractable pain on the waiting list for hip surgery and should certainly be tried for the elbow and shoulder pain associated with severe osteo- or rheumatoid arthritis, where joint arthroplasty is not yet universally available. Points suggested as of most use are LI-9 and LI-11 for the elbow, LU-2 and GB-21 for the shoulder and GB-30 and GB-34 for the hip.

Spinal pain

Spinal pain is common, disabling and inadequately treated by medical and surgical techniques. The origin of the pain is usually poorly understood and, even with modern imaging techniques such as MRI, a clear diagnosis of an individual problem is not made. Back pain is one of the commonest conditions managed in primary care and costs the country 50 million lost working days and 500 million pounds of NHS care each year (Clinical Standards Advisory Group 1994). Many studies of non-invasive treatment for back

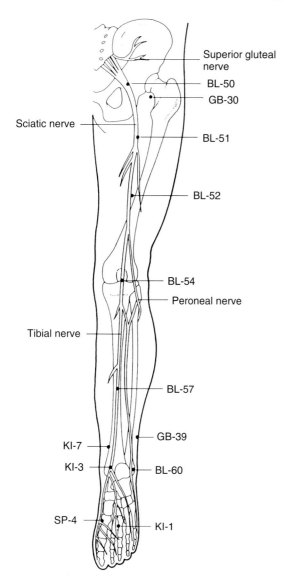

Superior gluteal nerve

BL-50

GB-30

Sciatic nerve

BL-51

BL-52

BL-54

Peroneal nerve

Tibial nerve

BL-57

GB-39

KI-7

KI-3

BL-60

SP-4

KI-1

Figure 17.7 The relationship between the main points of the posterior aspect of the lower extremities and the nerves. Adapted from Ellis 1994, with permission.

pain in recent years have shown the benefits of manipulative therapies (Koes et al 1991), and fitness and exercise programmes (Fass et al 1993) including those taking a psychological approach (Lindstrom et al 1992). Non-specific spinal pain, as with the majority of rheumatological conditions, is disabling but not life threatening. Treatments have moved away from the invasive and potentially dangerous treatments used in the earliest pain clinics to simpler and more patient-controlled methods (Melzack & Wall 1982).

Much distress is caused to both patients and therapists by the inability to control chronic pain. The use of acupuncture for back pain may offer a further treatment modality, although the success rate of 50 to 60% is lower than that for other conditions. There have been more published trials of acupuncture for spinal pain than for any other area of the body. Some of these have had negative results (Mendelson et al 1983, Petrie & Hazleman 1986). Although these have been criticized by others, they should not be ignored. Positive results have been recorded in studies on acute pain (Hackett, Seddon & Kaminski 1988), those using classical acupuncture (Coan, Wong & Coan 1980, Coan et al 1980, Lisenyuk & Yakupov 1992), electroacupuncture and TENS (Fargas-Babjak, Pomeranz & Rooney 1992, Lehmann et al 1986), superficial acupuncture (MacDonald et al 1983), and trigger point needling (Garvey, Marks & Wiesel 1989, Gunn et al 1980). There is a definite bias towards more positive studies and a recent careful series of trials from Scandinavia, using different methods of measuring response, such as sleep restoration (Carlssen & Sjölund, unpublished work, 1994), point a possible way forward for future trials of acupuncture in chronic back pain.

Acupuncture can be used as part of an overall back management programme. The programme must address patient attitudes, perceived disability, pain behaviour, lack of activity and conditioning, as well as the pain itself (Melzack & Wall 1982). Patients would certainly prefer to be cured of their back pain by outside means but this is seldom possible. Self-help programmes are as important in the management of back pain problems as in arthritis (Lorig et al 1989). In addition, knowledge of the presenting symptoms of serious primary and secondary pathology in the spine is vital. Serious neurological sequelae can result from ignoring key symptoms and signs accompanying back pain. A significant proportion of general practitioners have been shown to be at fault in this (Little et al 1996). The recommendations for the application of acupuncture and the treatment of spinal pain are:

- no one treatment will suffice
- patients require continuing support and a listening ear
- constant evaluation and examination for neurological signs are required
- secondary malignant disease can produce the same symptoms and signs as osteoarthritis or disc disease
- acute onset of back pain in middle age should be investigated
- saddle anaesthesia, incontinence and spasticity occurring de novo require urgent specialist assessment
- plain lumbar X-rays are seldom of diagnostic help
- minimal trauma fractures or loss of vertebral height should be investigated.

It should be noted that, provided a reasonably accurate diagnosis is made and even in the face of serious pathology, such as secondary malignancy or osteoporotic fracture, acupuncture can be very effective in relieving distressing symptoms and aiding disability for all types of spinal pathology (Box 17.5). Acupuncture is contraindicated if there is an unstable spine caused by trauma, malignancy or infection because it may remove protective spasm and, theoretically, lead to transection of the spinal cord.

It is important to carry out a careful and detailed examination of the whole patient before planning acupuncture treatment for spinal pain. This should include looking at the patient's gait for signs of abnormal pain behaviour, shortening

---

Box 17.5 Spinal problems potentially responsive to acupuncture

Non-specific acute and chronic pain
Discogenic disease
Postlaminectomy pain
Cervical headache
Occipital neuralgia
Nerve root pain of arm or leg
Fracture pain
Malignant pain
Arachnoiditis pain
Postherpetic and other neuralgias
Ankylosing spondylitis
Osteoarthritic symptoms

---

of one leg or previously undiagnosed neurological sequelae such as muscle wasting or weakness. In addition, spinal mobility should be examined and spinal deformity noted, both so that areas of muscle spasm can be identified and to ensure that pathologies such as osteoporosis or spondylolisthesis are not ignored. Standard examination of straight-leg raising, reflexes, sensation and muscle power will pick up neurological signs. This should be followed by detailed examination for trigger points, tender points in the spine and hyperaesthesia or temperature change of the skin. The patient should be asked to describe and draw the radiation of the pain, which may give a clue as to the best approach to the segmental application of acupuncture.

In general, pain above the waist arising from spinal problems responds better to acupuncture than does that below the waist. The pain of spinal osteoarthritis tends to be unresponsive to all forms of treatment but may be relieved for short periods by acupuncture. The approach to treatment with acupuncture is a combination of the needling of trigger or tender spots, some periosteal pecking, particularly around tender bony areas of the pelvis or the greater trochanter of the femur, and the use of peripheral points in the hands and feet. The areas of radiation of the pain (see Ch 4) will give an idea of the segmental approach to the pain areas. Knowledge of the nerve supply to the limbs and related acupuncture points, as in knee pain, can be very useful to arrive at extra points. Very frequently the course of the sciatic nerve in the leg is extremely tender, particularly over the classical acupuncture points on the Bladder meridian, and gentle needling of these is well worth while. A recent study of different modes of acupuncture for spinal pain indicated that low-frequency electroacupuncture may have a more prolonged effect in reducing pain than either manual stimulation of needles or high-frequency electroacupuncture (Thomas & Lundeberg 1994)

Autonomic symptoms are very common with spinal pain and include hyperaesthesia, coldness, bladder problems and abdominal pain. Such symptoms can be treated by acupuncture using sacral flats or an anatomical or classical

Chinese approach, but may sometimes be relieved only by deep needling of trigger points. The use of electroacupuncture may help neurological symptoms; when applied in the sacral area it can be particularly beneficial for the treatment of bladder symptoms and autonomic symptoms in the lower limbs. TENS machines can be used to supplement acupuncture treatments between courses. Unfortunately acupuncture for chronic spinal pain seldom lasts very long and the need for repeat courses must be expected.

Soft tissue rheumatism

The term 'soft tissue rheumatism' is now used as a generic description of a heterogenous collection of conditions, varying from traumatic lesions of tendons to fibromyalgia. The conditions encompassed are:

- trauma (rotator cuff tendinitis)
- inflammation (ankylosing spondylitis)
- degenerative (tennis elbow)
- myofascial syndrome
- fibromyalgia
- endocrine disorders (parathyroid disease)
- drug withdrawal (anxiolytics)
- repetitive strain injury.

The typical sites of pain are:

- **wrist**:–de Quervain's
- **elbow**:–epicondylitis
- **shoulder**:–rotator cuff, biceps
- **hip**:–greater trochanter
- **knee**:–patellar insertion
- **spine**:–interspinous ligaments.

Some are easily localized and diagnosed for instance lateral epicondylitis of the elbow.

Tendinitis

Acute or chronic tendinitis, confined to one or two areas and related to acute or repeated trauma, is traditionally treated by physiotherapy or injections. Acupuncture has been shown to help this condition, at least in the short term, and is well worth trying (Molsberger & Hills 1994). The tendon may be treated by direct needling with fanning of the needle from its insertion (see Fig. 17.1, p 345) or the area can be treated segmentally. Trigger points should be sought and treated in related muscle. A brief ergonomic history of the cause of the condition should be taken, to try and avoid repeated lesions. It should be remembered that soft tissue rheumatism may be the presenting symptom not only of metabolic diseases such as those of the thyroid and parathyroid glands, but also of the inflammatory arthritides, notably ankylosing spondylitis and psoriatic arthritis. A high index of suspicion for systemic disease should be kept where a patient presents more than twice with an acute tendonitis. Epicondylitis may also be an area of referred pain from pathology in the neck or part of early osteoarthritis. The success of acupuncture may be increased by examining and treating other parts of the upper limb or related areas of the spine.

Repetitive strain injury

Repetitive strain injury (RSI) is a condition, frequently occupational, that is characterized by pain arising in a particular area, usually the hand and the forearm, as a result of repetitive muscle activity. The pain responds initially to rest, but not to treatments such as injection, which are appropriate for tenosynovitis or ligamentous damage. RSI can be said to exist when pain no longer responds to out-of-work rest and starts to interfere with work and leisure. RSI is a poorly understood problem which is the subject of much litigation world-wide. It has a complex presentation where chronic pain, loss or work, compensation and immobility all combine and lead some patients to severe disability in everyday life (Fig. 17.8). It typifies the many conditions where pain has complex multifaceted causes interacting with one another to worsen the situation. No published studies of acupuncture have been found for this condition. Experience has shown that these patients have a heightened awareness of pain and frequently experience severe rebound pain after acupuncture. Treatment of RSI is time consuming and only a combination

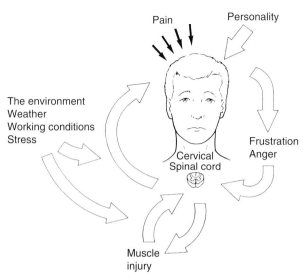

Pain   Personality

The environment
Weather
Working conditions
Stress

Frustration
Anger

Cervical
Spinal cord

Muscle
injury

Figure 17.8 The mechanism of RSI: The whole complex interaction of injury, reflex arcs, personality, anxiety and other changes resulting from pain are influenced by the environment, the weather, the condition of adjacent workers and working conditions including stress.
Reproduced with permission from Huskisson (1992).

of physiotherapy, counselling and graded functional exercises together with acupuncture can hope to achieve significant benefit (Box 17.6). The pain of RSI is very diffuse but in general follows a segmental pattern and spreads up the arms to the spine. Tension of nerves (adverse neural tension) is recognized by physiotherapists through special techniques. It can usually be picked up by stretching the worst-affected muscles and looking for the pattern of pain produced. This will indicate the segment to be treated by

---

Box 17.6 Treatment of RSI

Prevention is better than cure. Diagnosis is the first step:
- Rest from causative occupation.
- Correction of work ergonomics.
- Identification of stress.
- Counselling employer.
- Correction of upper arm use.
- Exercise—aerobic, whole body.
- Physiotherapy.
- Cognitive behavioural therapy.
- Sleep correction.
- Splints—early treatment only.
- Rehabilitation to and in the workplace.

---

acupuncture. Treatment should be graded in terms of strength, length and anatomical area used. In early cases, myofascial treatment can be applied. In later cases this will usually worsen pain so much that the patient refuses to continue acupuncture. Gentle treatment using only peripheral points to cause an endorphin response should be tried initially. Established RSI is an intractable and difficult condition to treat.

Fibromyalgia

The same difficulties apply to the treatment of fibromyalgia. This recently redescribed and fashionable condition is not universally accepted as a diagnosis. It is a chronic condition of widespread musculoskeletal pain, associated with multiple bony tender points, fatigue, morning stiffness and poor sleep pattern (Yunus et al 1981). Controlled studies have shown that patients may be helped by electroacupuncture (Deluze et al 1992), tricyclic antidepressants given at night, aerobic exercise and cognitive therapy. Such treatments are long winded and require a great deal of application from the patient. The wish for less hard work to achieve results can lead to trying acupuncture in a number of patients with limited success; these patients are hypersensitive to needles and therefore periosteal pecking of the bony areas or trigger point needling will be successful only in driving patients to other practitioners. Acupuncture should be gentle, with minimal stimulation and, at least initially, the use of no more than four needles. The points to be tried are:

- LI-4, LI-11
- ST-36
- SP-6
- KI-3.

If a change of sleep pattern can be obtained by an endorphin response, a great deal can be achieved. The time spent in giving acupuncture treatment can also be used to give lifestyle advice about stress, work, overtime, exercise and relaxation. If the patient proves to be hypersensitive to acupuncture (see Ch 5) then the use of needles on the contralateral side only can be tried. Treatment strength and a change to other forms of acupuncture can be added gradually as matters improve.

Chronic fatigue syndrome

The use of acupuncture for chronic fatigue syndrome presents the practitioner with even more difficulties. Pain is very frequent and widespread. It is mainly of non-specific distribution and associated with fatigue. The establishment of the diagnosis is often patient directed and unclear; the use by the patient of numerous different therapies simultaneously, such as exclusion diet, vitamins, herbal remedies and many others, means that evaluating the effects of acupuncture is extremely difficult. In addition most patients will attend a large number of practitioners at one and the same time and there are few true specialists in the treatment in the United Kingdom. Acupuncture is sought by many of these patients for its pain-relieving potential but is successful only in the long term. Its true contribution is very difficult to evaluate. Patients are hypersensitive to pain and the adverse effects of acupuncture. The approaches to treatment should be very much those for fibromyalgia.

CONCLUSIONS

Acupuncture can be extremely successful in the treatment of a number of musculoskeletal conditions and has proved very successful and popular with patients. It does not, however, prevent the deterioration of the overall condition, nor treat arthritis systemically. It should never be used as a sole treatment for any condition other than simple localized and reversible musculoskeletal pain. It is vitally important that all other treatments are explored, that overall response to acupuncture is assessed on each patient, that exercises are continued and that aids, appliances and daily living assessment are provided as required. It is also important where peripheral joints are being treated that the need for surgery is constantly evaluated. Initial treatment courses should be brief, perhaps consisting of four to six treatments over 6 weeks, and allowance should be made for a delayed response to acupuncture.

When acupuncture is successful in the treatment of such conditions, it is safe, relatively inexpensive and can be repeated with ease. Patients require some preparation for acupuncture, which should neither be a painful nor an uncomfortable type of technique. Acupuncture can change the dimensions of treatment that can be offered to rheumatology patients, but further critical appraisal through controlled trials is necessary before its true place will be found.

REFERENCES

Bhatt-Sanders D 1985 Acupuncture for rheumatoid arthritis, an analysis of the literature. Seminars in Arthritis and Rheumatism 14:225–231

British Medical Association 1993 Complementary medicine—new approaches to good practice. Oxford University Press, Oxford

Brooks P, Kirwan J R 1995 Evidence-based medical practice: the Cochrane Collaboration and osteoarthritis. British Journal of Rheumatology 34:403–404

Camp A V 1992 Acupuncture in the rheumatology department. Rheumatology Now 9:15–18

Camp A V 1995 The place of acupuncture in medicine. British Journal of Rheumatology 34:404–405

Chapman C R, Sato T, Martin R W, Tanaka A, Okazaki N, Colpitts Y M, Mayeno J K, Gagliardi G J 1982 Comparative effects of acupuncture in Japan and the US on dental pain

perception. Pain 12:319–328

Christensen B V, Iuhl I U, Vilbeck H, Bulow H H, Dreijer N C, Rasmussen H F 1992 Acupuncture treatment of severe knee osteoarthritis. A long term study. Acta Anaesthesiologica Scandinavica 36:519–525

Clinical Standards Advisory Group 1994 Management guidelines for back pain. HMSO, London

Coan R M, Wong G, Coan P L 1980 The acupuncture treatment of neck pain—a randomised controlled study. American Journal of Chinese Medicine 9:326–332

Coan R M, Wong G, Ku S L, Chan Y C, Wang L, Ozer F T, Coan P L 1980 The acupuncture treatment of low back pain: a randomised controlled study. American Journal of Chinese Medicine 8:181–189

Collier S, Philips D, Camp V, Kirk A 1995 The influence of attitudes to acupuncture on the outcome of treatment.

Acupuncture in Medicine 13:74–77

Deluze C, Bosia L, Ziebs A, Chantiaine D, Vescher T L 1992 Electroacupuncture in fibromyalgia: results of a controlled trial. British Medical Journal 305:1249–1252

Dowson D I, Lewith G T, Machin D 1985 The effects of acupuncture versus placebo in the treatment of headache. Pain 21:35–42

Ellis N 1994 Acupuncture in clinical practice: a guide for health professionals. Chapman and Hall, London

Ernst E 1995 Complementary therapies, the baby and the bath water. British Journal of Rheumatology 34:479–480

Fargas-Babjak A M, Pomeranz B, Rooney P J 1992 Acupuncture like stimulation with codetron for rehabilitation of patients with chronic pain syndrome and osteoarthritis. Acupuncture and Electrotherapeutics Research 17:95–105

Faas A, Havannes A, van Eijk J, Gubbels J 1993 A randomised placebo controlled trial of exercise therapy in patients with acute low back pain. Spine 18:1388–1395

Fitzpatrick R, Hopkins A 1976 Patients' satisfaction and reported acceptance of advice in general practice. Journal of the Royal College of General Practitioners 26:720–724

Garvey T A, Marks M R, Wiesel S W 1989 A prospective randomised double-blind evaluation of trigger point injection therapy for low back pain. Spine 14:962–964

Gunn C C, Milbrandt W E, Little A S, Mason K E 1980 Dry needling of muscle motor points for chronic low back pain: a randomised clinical trial with long term follow up. Spine 5:279–291

Hackett G I, Seddon D, Kaminski D 1988 Electroacupuncture compared with paracetamol for acute low back pain. Practitioner 232:163–164

Higham C, Ashcroft C, Jayson M I V 1983 Non-prescribed treatments in rheumatic diseases. Practitioner 227:1201–1205

Ho W K K, Wen H L 1989 Opioid-like activity in the cerebrospinal fluid of pain patients treated by electroacupuncture. Neuropharmacology 28:961–966

Huskisson E C 1992 Repetitive Strain Injury: the keyboard disease. Charterhouse Conference and Communications, London

James R, Fox M, Taheri G 1983 Who goes to a natural therapist? Why? Australian Family Physician 12:383–386

Kestin M, Miller L, Littlejohn G, Wahlqvist M 1985 The use of unproven remedies for rheumatoid arthritis in Australia. Medical Journal of Australia 143:516–518

Knox V, Handfield Jones C, Shum K 1979 Subject expectancy and the reduction of cold pressor pain with acupuncture and placebo acupuncture. Psychosomatic Medicine 41:477–486

Koes B, Assendelft W, van der Heijden G, Bouter L, Knipschild P 1991 Spinal manipulation and mobilisation for back and neck pain—a blinded review. British Medical Journal 303:1298–1303

Kreitler S, Kreitler H, Carasso R 1987 Cognitive orientation as a predictor of pain relief following acupuncture. Pain 28:323–341

Kronenfeld J J, Wasner C 1982 The use of unorthodox therapies and marginal practitioners. Social Science Medicine 16:1119–1125

Lehmann T R, Russell D W, Spratt K F et al 1986 Efficacy of electroacupuncture and TENS in the rehabilitation of chronic low back pain patients. Pain 26:277–290

Ley P, Whitworth M, Skilbeck C, Woodward R, Pinsent R,

Pike L 1976 Improving doctor–patient communications in general practice. Journal of the Royal College of General Practitioners 26:720–724

Lindstrom I, Ohlund C, Eek C et al 1992 The effect of graded activity on patients with sub-acute low back pain: a randomised prospective clinical study with an operant-conditioning behavioral approach. Physical Therapy 72:270–293

Lisenyuk V P, Yakupov R A 1992 Osteoelectroacupuncture in the management of vertebrogenic pain syndromes in the lumbar region and lower extremities. Acupuncture and Electrotherapeutics Research 17:21–28

Little P, Smith L, Cantrell T, Chapman J, Langridge J, Pickering R 1996 General practitioners management of acute back pain: a survey of reported practice compared with clinical guidelines. British Medical Journal 312:485–488

Liu X, Sun L, Xiao J, Yin S, Liu C, Li Q, Li H, Jin B 1993 Effect of acupuncture and point injection treatment on immunologic function in rheumatoid arthritis. Journal of Traditional Chinese Medicine 13:174–178

Lorig K, Cox T, Cuevas Y, Kraines R G, Britton M C 1984 Converging and diverging beliefs about arthritis; Caucasian patients, Spanish speaking patients and physicians. Journal of Rheumatology 11:76–79

Lorig K, Lubeck D, Kraines R G, Sleznick M, Holman H R 1989 Outcomes of self-help education for patients with arthritis. Arthritis and Rheumatism 32:91–95

MacDonald A J R, Macrae K D, Master B R, Rubin A P 1983 Superficial acupuncture in the relief of chronic low back pain. Annals of the Royal College of Surgeons of England 65:44–46

McIndoe A K, Young K, Bone M E 1995 A comparison of acupuncture with intra-articular steroid injection as analgesia for osteoarthritis of the hip. Acupuncture in Medicine 13:67–70

Man S C, Baragar F D 1974 Preliminary clinical study of acupuncture in rheumatoid arthritis. Journal of Rheumatology 1:126–129

Melzack R 1987 The short form McGill pain questionnaire. Pain 30:191–197

Melzack R, Wall P 1982 The challenge of pain. Penguin, Harmondsworth

Mendelson G, Selwood T S, Kranz H, Loh T S, Kidson M A, Scott D S 1983 Acupuncture treatment of chronic back pain: a double-blind placebo controlled trial. American Journal of Medicine 74:49–55

Molsberger A, Hille E 1994 The analgesic effect of acupuncture in chronic tennis elbow pain. British Journal of Rheumatology 33:1162–1165

Moore M E, Berk S N 1976 Acupuncture for chronic shoulder pain. Annals of Internal Medicine 84:381–384

Moore J, Phipps K, Marcer D, Lewith G 1985 Why do people seek treatment by alternative medicine? British Medical Journal 290:28–29

Norton G, Coszer L, Strub H, Man S 1984 The effects of belief on acupuncture analgesia. Canadian Journal of Behaviour Science 16:22–29

Petrie J P, Hazleman B L 1986 A controlled study of acupuncture in neck pain. British Journal of Rheumatology 25:271–275

Pruyn J, Rijckman R, vanBrunschot C, van den Borne H 1985 Cancer patients personality characteristics, physician–patient communication and adoption of the Moerman diet. Social Science Medicine 20:841–847

Puett D W, Griffin M R 1994 Published trials of non-medicinal and non-invasive therapies of hip and knee osteoarthritis. Annals of Internal Medicine 121:133–140

Struthers G R, Scott D L, Scott D G 1983 The use of alternative treatments by patients with rheumatoid arthritis. Rheumatology International 3:151–152

Thomas M, Lundeberg T 1994 Importance of modes of acupuncture in the treatment of chronic nociceptive low back pain. Acta Anaesthesiologica Scandinavica 38:63–69

Visser G J, Peters L, Rasker J J 1992 Rheumatologists and their patients who seek alternative care: an agreement to disagree. British Journal of Rheumatology 31:485–490

Weisenberg M, Kreindler M L, Schachat R, Werboff J 1975 Pain, anxiety and attitudes in black, white and Puerto Rican patients. Psychosomatic Medicine 37:123–135

Yunus M B, Masi A T, Calabro J J, Miller K A, Feigenbaum S L 1981 Primary fibromyalgia (fibrositis): a clinical study of 50 patients with matched normal controls. Seminars in Arthritis and Rheumatism 11:151–171

18

Acupuncture for the withdrawal of habituating substances

Paul Marcus

INTRODUCTION

Acupuncture, particularly when combined with electrical stimulation, has been widely used in the management of patients addicted or habituated to drugs, alcohol, cigarettes or over-eating. There is quite an extensive published literature on this subject, particularly in the case of opiates, although it is interesting that, in respect of the commonest drugs of habituation in the Western world, the benzodiazepines, there is very little published evidence. Acupuncture is used in the withdrawal of addictive substances in one of two general ways. Either it is utilized non-specifically to relieve neurotic symptoms such as anxiety or depression occurring during withdrawal, and here it may be adjunctive to other drugs or psychotherapy, or it may be used quite specifically to combat the manifestations of the withdrawal syndrome. It is the latter topic that will be dealt with here.

Acupuncture seems equally effective in all forms of habituation so far studied, and this is important evidence suggesting a mechanism of action (see below). The general method of application is to give treatment in parallel with abrupt or gradual withdrawal, and this may be done on an inpatient or outpatient basis. At one end of the scale, for instance, during a clinic visit an indwelling needle may be placed in the pinna of a person who then throws away their cigarettes and is not followed up again. At the other end, EA may be given at hourly intervals during a rapid methadone withdrawal programme to a heroin addict treated as an inpatient.

METHOD OF TREATMENT

From the literature, the most commonly used points for alleviating withdrawal symptoms are those on the pinna of the ear: Lung, Shenmen and Stomach (Fig. 18.1). The general technique will now be described, although modifications to the choice of points, frequency and duration of treatment, etc. will obviously be needed according to the condition being treated and general acupuncture principles.

As is usual in auriculotherapy, careful localization of the point is important. The anatomical area where the point is expected is probed for tenderness and then examined for sites of low electrical resistance. The ear is carefully cleaned with isopropyl alcohol (partly for reasons of sterilization and partly to ensure adherence of sticking plaster) and allowed to dry. An indwelling needle, such as a press needle or an ASP Sedatelec, may be inserted and secured with adhesive plaster.

An example of the use of these devices would be in patients wishing to lose weight or stop smoking. Here, together with a diet sheet or injunction to cease buying cigarettes, a press needle inserted into one or more of these points is left in situ for a week or so. It is stressed to the patient that self-control will be required but that the needle will help reduce the appetite or the desire for cigarettes, especially if it is manipulated between finger and thumb when the craving occurs.

As with all indwelling needles, an aseptic technique is most important as there is a higher chance of infection than with brief insertion of acupuncture needles. (For this reason some authorities recommend use of stainless steel 'magraine' balls instead of press needles.) Indwelling needles are contraindicated in rheumatic valvular disease, in diabetes and during treatment with immunosuppressants or with steroids. The patient must be instructed on the action to take if infection does occur: that they should remove the needle and clean the area with soapy water.

Withdrawal of more frankly addicting substances such as psychomimetic drugs and narcotics demands more vigorous treatment, probably using electroacupuncture applied to the same points. Such cases can be managed during clinic attendances, for instance during benzodiazepine dosage tapering off over a period of weeks, but opiate withdrawal, or the more rapid withdrawal of high intakes of alcohol or some other drugs, will require admission with continuous or frequently repeated treatment over a few days.

Manual stimulation with a standard fine acupuncture needle may be carried out, or alternatively a pulse stimulator may be connected across bilateral needles to give electrical stimulation for 20 to 30 minutes. A frequency of 100–125 Hz is used. Initially the amplitude is set so that the patient just feels the flow of current, and then it is adjusted after a period of a few minutes when adaptation has occurred. Unless a bipolar waveform is used, the polarity should be changed halfway through the treatment period.

It is important to control the depth of insertion carefully when treating ear points. The cartilage should not be needled, since infection introduced here can be difficult to treat and can lead to a poor cosmetic result. The usual contraindications to EA apply (Ch 10), particularly the use of a demand cardiac pacemaker. Patients

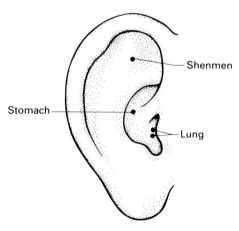

Figure 18.1 Ear points used for alleviating withdrawal symptoms.

should be treated lying down and a watch kept on their general condition since the ear has a rich innervation, with both somatic and autonomic fibres, and therefore strong stimulation may be expected to produce cardiovascular effects.

For specific withdrawal symptoms, other acupuncture points may be utilized sequentially or concomitantly such as: PC-6 for nausea and vomiting; LI-4, 11 and 20 for nasal congestion; GV-14 and LI-4 for anxiety; CV-12 for poor appetite; LU-7 for cough; LR-3 for headache; HT-7 for insomnia; tender (Ah Shi) points for muscle aching; and SP-6 for pain.

Drug therapy may be used adjunctively to EA in treating withdrawal. For instance, methadone may be substituted for heroin or morphine before withdrawal, while propranolol may be used to manage the somatic symptoms of anxiety; short courses of hypnotics may be given to treat insomnia and of anxiolytics to treat anxiety.

USE OF EA FOR WITHDRAWAL OF OPIATES

Most of the published data concerning treatment of addictions with acupuncture, and indeed the seminal paper discussed below, concern opiates.

Early studies

In the early 1970s Wen & Cheung, working at the neurosurgical unit at Kwong Wah Hospital, Hong Kong, discovered that EA used for inducing surgical analgesia modified withdrawal symptoms in patients suffering from addiction to opiates. In 1973 they described the use of electrical stimulation of acupuncture points on the ear to treat 30 opium and 10 heroin addicts (Wen & Cheung 1973). The addictive substance was stopped and EA was performed when withdrawal symptoms occurred. Needles were inserted subcutaneously into the Lung point of the concha on both sides. A 125 Hz alternating current was then passed through the needles from an electrical stimulator. The intensity was increased until the patient just felt

the flow of current. Stimulation was carried out for half an hour two or three times per day for 2–3 days, followed by one stimulation per day for the next 4–5 days. Wen & Cheung (1973) stated that, within 10–15 minutes the ear, nose and mouth became dry, aching, shivering or abdominal pain gradually disappeared and the patients felt well, warm and relaxed. They reported better appetite and appeared much less withdrawn. One patient dropped out of the study but all of the remainder were described as free from drug addiction afterwards. Although the inadequacies of this study have been pointed out (Whitehead 1978) this strongly optimistic report caused much interest, and over the next decade EA was used in several studies of addicts withdrawn from opiates. Sainsbury (1974) published a single case report in the Medical Journal of Australia, which was accompanied by an enthusiastic editorial (1974) talking of considerable financial savings.

Comparative and experimental studies

Wen & Teo (1975) compared 35 female heroin addicts treated with EA with another 35 given gradually reducing doses of methadone. The EA group was symptom free in 8 days compared with 14 for the methadone group, and 51% of the EA group compared with 29% of the methadone group were off drugs after one year. Ng et al (1975) reported experiments in rats implanted with morphine pellets and then administered naloxone in which EA reduced the resulting withdrawal symptoms, and these findings were later confirmed in mice by Choy et al (1978).

Shuaib (1976) used Wen & Cheung's (1973) technique to treat withdrawal symptoms in 19 opium addicts in the Military Hospital, Rawalpindi and confirmed the immediate response to treatment. All patients were symptom free and chemical free in 6–8 days. He stated also that if the siting of the needles was incorrect the effect was unsatisfactory. Tennant (1976) compared electro- and manual stimulation of skin staples with methadone detoxification in heroin addicts. A 7 Hz frequency was used, and the results were disappointing. Only a few acupuncture patients remained in the study after 5 days and only one became heroin free. However, all 18 felt that acupuncture provided partial temporary relief.

Work by Severson, Markoff & Chun-Hoon (1977) at the University of Hawaii, Institute of Psychiatry, on eight heroin addicts used high-frequency stimulation. It confirmed that the technique was feasible for this drug but suggested it was less effective in heavy users. Short-term follow-up showed that the incidence of reversion was comparable with other techniques and that a postdetoxification programme might be beneficial. Severson and colleagues presented useful criteria for the acceptability of the technique:

1. a minimum addiction pattern
2. absence of medical disease that would contraindicate other than very gradual drug withdrawal or would produce confusing symptoms
3. absence of severe psychiatric disease since effects of EA might be unpredictable
4. voluntary choice of EA.

Five out of the eight patients in this series were detoxified successfully and there was one dropout. Pointing out that the Lung point is innervated by the auricular branch of the vagus nerve, these workers suggested that central suppression of vagal activity might be the mechanism of action.

In the late 1970s and early 1980s there was further work. Leung (1977) carried out a double-blind comparison of real and sham EA using the Lung points and others including Shenmen and points on the body. Thirty-two patients were withdrawn from alcohol, narcotics and other drugs such as barbiturates and diazepam by the application of 125 Hz EA according to a variety of protocols. The numbers were too small for firm conclusions but the investigator felt the results were 'encouraging'. The combination of Lung and Shenmen points was felt to control anxiety, irritability and insomnia to some extent. Wen (1977) presented an extension of the previously reported technique, combining EA with administration of naloxone to speed up withdrawal in 50 heroin addicts. EA was applied continuously for half an hour before an i.v. injection of naloxone and then for the next 3–4 hours, during which time several further injections of naloxone were given. Forty-one patients were detoxified successfully with diminished symptoms of opiate withdrawal, but in nine cases a full-blown abstinence syndrome occurred and the treatment had to be stopped. This technique had the advantage that it could be accomplished in a single day, although the desire for heroin was not abolished in these patients and a long-term follow-up showed that 15 out of 41 patients had reverted to drug taking. Man & Chuang's study (1980) of 35 heroin addicts treated with EA at 100 Hz applied bilaterally to the 'Lung' and 'Stomach' ear points was confounded by the fact that 83% of their subjects used illicit drugs during the research period, but, in an uncontrolled study in Italian psychiatric hospitals, Lorini et al (1982) found benefit from manual acupuncture in combination with various psychomimetic drugs in detoxifying heroin addicts. Patterson, Firth & Gardiner (1984) published a review of experience in 186 patients treated with 'neuro-electric therapy': TENS comprising an asymmetric regular pulse (0.22 ms, 1–2000 Hz, 1.5–3.0 mA) passed through 1 cm diameter skin electrodes above the mastoid. Inpatients habituated to a variety of substances including alcohol and tobacco were treated in this way, lower frequencies being used for narcotics and higher ones for stimulants. Ten days' treatment was said to reduce rapidly both acute and chronic withdrawal symptoms of all chemical substances with no negative effects; 98% of patients were successfully detoxified and, in 50% who responded to follow-up, 78.5% of drug addicts were addiction free 1–8 years later. However, in a further study, TENS applied to the mastoid processes at frequencies between 70 and 400 Hz continuously for periods of days was felt to be of minimal assistance in withdrawing opiates (Gossop et al 1984). Newmeyer, Johnson & Klot (1984) gave daily high-frequency electroacupuncture to opiate addicts and reported both short- and long-term benefits, although there was less success in heavily dependent cases. There was also a higher rate of withdrawal from treatment in those patients who chose to be treated with electroacupuncture. This freedom of choice of treatment unfortunately introduced bias into the study. Kroening & Oleson (1985) reported that 12 out of 14 chronic pain patients habituated to methadone were successfully withdrawn with EA. Comparisons were drawn with historical controls. The technique used here was a modification of Wen's (Wen & Cheung 1973), utilizing naloxone with electrical stimulation of the 'Shenmen' point with a 'dense-dispersed' wave-form (alternating trains of 1–3 Hz and 600–1000 Hz impulses) to avoid adaptation of the body to stimulation. Electrical point detection was used in this case.

Recent studies

A National Acupuncture Detoxification Association (NADA) was set up in the United States in 1985 to support the use of acupuncture in the treatment of drug dependency, conducting training programmes for physicians both in America and overseas. In 1988 Smith (Chairman of the NADA) and Khan (representing the WHO) reported on 13 years' experience at the Lincoln Hospital, New York (a city-owned institution located in the South Bronx) in using acupuncture as the primary method of treatment for drug addicts (Smith & Khan 1988). Their programme saw 200 outpatients daily undergoing detoxification. Ear acupuncture with needles, without electrical stimulation, was used at the Sympathetic, Shenmen, Kidney, Lung and Liver points. The same points were utilized whatever the drug to which the person was addicted. They wrote that acupuncture relieved withdrawal symptoms, prevented craving and increased the rate of participation of patients in long-term treatment programmes. The treatment worked better in an open group setting and when integrated into counselling and other psychosocial services.

Recently White & Georgakis reported a lack of success with six daily treatments with electro-acupuncture at alternating 2 and 110 Hz frequencies applied to Shenmen and Lung points on the pinna, judged by subject and observer ratings of symptoms and signs during the first 14 days of withdrawal (A R White & A Georgakis, personal communication, 1995). Forty-four patients with heavy opiate dependence were randomly allocated to active EA, to a no-treatment control group or to a further control group treated by needling non-acupuncture auricular areas. No significant differences were found, although the active group was less likely to withdraw from post-withdrawal rehabilitation. The authors pointed out that EA had also been less successful in the heavily addicted group of Newmeyer, Johnson & Klot (1984). They also suggested a benzodiazepine used concomitantly might have interfered with the action of the acupuncture.

MECHANISM OF ACTION

Vagal versus adrenergic/cholinergic effects

In the late 1970s, two contradictory theories were advanced to explain the evident efficacy of EA in treating opiate withdrawal symptoms. As stated previously, Severson, Markoff & Chun-Hoon (1977) had felt that the efficacy of EA applied to the concha might be due to parasympathetic inhibition via the ear's vagal innervation. They pointed out that parasympathetically mediated symptoms such as lachrymation and rhinorrhoea, chills, sweating, intestinal cramps and bowel hyperactivity were the first to respond, with anxiety and heroin craving. Next came bone and joint pain, which were often incompletely relieved. However, Mendelsson (1978) took an opposite view, suggesting that the symptomatology of narcotic withdrawal is due to an imbalance of adrenergic and cholinergic neurotransmitter systems with a state of central adrenergic predomination, and that the effect of EA is one of parasympathetic stimulation. The efficacy of the central noradrenergic inhibitor clonidine in ameliorating cigarette, alcohol and opiate withdrawal suggests that noradrenergic activity is a common characteristic in the pathophysiology of withdrawal syndromes. These conditions have different final stages.

The delirium tremens and hallucinations of alcoholic withdrawal are different from the agitation, muscle cramps and retching of opiate withdrawal, or from the tension and irritability of cigarette withdrawal. Before these final manifestations, however, there is a common craving. Maintenance of opiate-taking behaviour depends on the very strong craving for the drug associated with the onset of withdrawal. Similarly an intense urge for a drink occurs early in alcohol withdrawal.

In smokers studied by Glassman et al (1984) craving occurred consistently as a feature of the withdrawal syndrome. Craving is thus a common denominator across these various habituations, and Glassman has suggested a special relationship between noradrenergic activity and craving. This may be why, as is commonly found, stress increases craving. Stress increases central noradrenergic activity and with it the urge to drink alcohol, smoke or overeat. Consuming alcohol, smoking and binge eating reduce tension and noradrenergic activity, and this may be the root cause of habituation, since the individual learns the behaviour that reduces their discomfort.

Centrally active cholinesterase inhibitors are effective in reducing opiate withdrawal symptoms due to augmentation of central cholinergic activity. Beta-adrenergic blockers such as propranolol diminish sympathetic activity and so, by implication, and involving the same nervous pathways that Severson referred to, the effect of EA may be one of parasympathetic activation. Mendelsson (1978) included as supporting evidence the blockade of acupuncture's effect by atropine, although no references were cited.

Endorphin and enkephalin levels

Physiological changes suggesting parasympathetic stimulation are not usually prominent during EA treatment but a further reason for its wide applicability is suggested by evidence from the field of pain relief. The Lung and Shenmen points utilized in the studies quoted above are also frequently used when EA is employed to induce analgesia for operative procedures. It has been known for some years that acupuncture carried out to treat acute or chronic pain causes the release of endogenous opioids and that the analgesic effects produced may be reversed with naloxone. Chen (1977) first suggested that the efficacy of EA in the withdrawal of exogenously administered opiates might be due to their being supplanted by endogenously produced substances resulting from the stimulation. Clement-Jones et al (1979) reported the results of biochemical analysis at St Bartholomew's Hospital, London of biological fluids from patients undergoing EA-assisted heroin withdrawal according to Wen & Cheung's protocol (1973) at Wen's clinic in Hong Kong (Fig. 18.2). In comparison with non-addicted controls, heroin addicts showing features of withdrawal had elevated β-endorphin levels in the blood and CSF, although these did not change with treatment. Met-enkephalin levels in the blood and CSF were elevated before treatment. Blood levels of met-enkephalin did not change with treatment, but EA was associated with a rise in CSF met-enkephalin levels in all six patients studied. In association with the rise in CSF met-enkephalin, relief of the withdrawal symptoms occurred in four patients. One of those who failed to show a clinical response had the highest pretreatment response to acupuncture. A subsequent study by the same workers (Clement-Jones et al 1980) of low-frequency EA for recurrent pain showed elevations in CSF β-endorphin but not met-enkephalin, and an editorial in the British Medical Journal (1981) suggested that, whereas low-frequency EA releases β-endorphin whose effects may be blocked, at least in part, by naloxone, high-frequency stimulation as in the technique used for opiate withdrawal releases met-enkephalin, whose effects are not blocked by conventional doses of naloxone. No doubt it is for this reason that the modified rapid detoxification technique using EA and naloxone is effective.

The mechanism by which exogenously administered opiates such as morphine produce drowsiness, euphoria, altered affective response to pain and tranquillity is unclear but un-

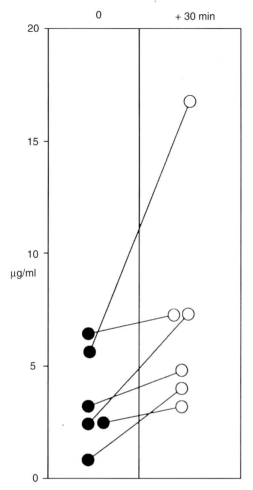

Figure 18.2   CSF immunoreactive met-enkephalin levels in heroin addicts before (●) and 30 minutes after (O) EA.

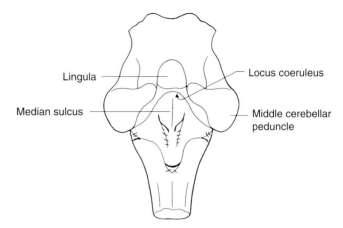

Figure 18.3   The rhomboid fossa—floor of the fourth ventricle

are both noradrenergic neurons and high concentrations of opioid receptors, and this structure is postulated to play a critical role in feelings of alarm, panic, fear and anxiety. The locus coeruleus contributes the main noradrenergic input to the brain (Copolov & Helme 1983) and this outflow is considerably increased by opiate withdrawal (Aghajanian 1978), probably contributing much to the concomitant subjective distress. Activity in the locus coeruleus is inhibited by α-adrenergic agonists such as clonidine and by both exogenous opiates and endogenous opiate-like peptides (Aghajanian 1978). EA might stimulate endogenous opioid release here, and perhaps at other relevant sites.

doubtedly in doing so they bind to the various opiate receptors, which are widely distributed in the brain. The activity of endogenous opioids is likely to be much more selective, in that they will be specifically released in different tissues in response to different stimuli, and since different members of this family have greater specificity for certain subtypes of receptor.

Locus coeruleus activity

In the locus coeruleus (Fig. 18.3; see also Ch 6), in the floor of the fourth ventricle on the posterior surface of the medulla oblongata, there

WITHDRAWAL OF BENZODIAZEPINES—THE CLINICAL PROBLEM

Benzodiazepines (BZs) are the most widely used psychotropic drugs in the Western world. In Britain about 1.5 million doses are consumed daily, and in one survey (Lloyd 1982) 26% of 287 consecutive patients seen at a psychiatric outpatient clinic had been taking BZs for a year or longer. Dependence after normal therapeutic doses has now emerged as a major problem in clinical practice. Withdrawal symptoms are reported to occur in 15–45% of long-term users, depending on the criteria used for definition, and they may last between 5 days and 2 months or even longer. Two groups of signs and symptoms may be experienced: those that mimic the anxiety originally treated and those that are distinct from this. The first group of symptoms include insomnia, restlessness, irritability, depersonalization and derealization, headache, tremor and palpitations. The second group include photophobia, hyperacusis, hyperaesthesia, hyperalgesia, paraesthesia, muscle twitching, a feeling of being in motion, difficulty in focusing, decreased perception of movement, a metallic taste in the mouth, facial pain and fitting.

A possible role for EA in BZ withdrawal?

We do not understand the full picture of the neurological and neurotransmitter response to acupuncture, but implication of so ubiquitous a group of neurohormones as the endogenous opioids, as well as the evidence we have so far from efficacy in other clinical addiction/ habituation syndromes, gives grounds for optimism that EA may be helpful in facilitating BZ withdrawal by shortening the withdrawal process and alleviating the unpleasant symptoms that many patients suffer. There is no reason to suppose that EA might have a direct effect on the BZ-receptor/GABA-receptor/ fluoride-channel axis but it seems entirely possible that the tranquillizing and euphoria-inducing effects of endogenous opioids produced by EA might offset the opposite manifestations caused by withdrawal of BZ from these receptors in habituated subjects. As stated previously, EA may counterbalance the excessive adrenergic activity characteristic of various forms of habituation. Additionally, certain neuropeptides such as vasopressin and CCK have been found to influence opioid analgesia, tolerance and dependence, perhaps acting as endogenous modulators of opioid receptor function, and EA has been shown to release at least one non-opioid neuropeptide: VIP.

The published evidence concerning acupuncture's utility in this situation has, so far, been slim.

Management of BZ withdrawal

Cases may be managed as outpatients or inpatients over periods of at least 4 or 2 weeks respectively, and the most critical factor is to avoid abrupt withdrawal. Gradual reduction is carried out at a rate adjusted for each patient but averaging 5 mg of diazepam (or the equivalent) per day. Manual or electroacupuncture, using the points previously listed, may be used to offset any withdrawal symptoms that do occur during this period.

Unless the patient can be admitted to hospital for more rapid withdrawal, it is best to convert the patient from whatever benzodiazepine they are taking to the equivalent dose of diazepam according to Table 18.1.

There are two reasons for this. First, diazepam, with its long half-life, is (paradoxically) easier to withdraw since there is no time during a 24-hour period when blood levels drop to very low values and symptoms are likely to be experienced. Secondly, a range of formulations exists that allows very fine reductions in the daily dose. Conversion to diazepam needs to be quite gradual. On successive days, or every other day, one of the daily doses of the other benzodiazepine is substituted with an equivalent dose of diazepam. Following conversion to diazepam slow, progressive withdrawal can ensue. Patients taking less than 20 mg daily can be given 1 mg a day less on successive weeks (so that the patient starting on a dose of 5 mg diazepam would take 15 weeks to withdraw completely). Patients receiving more than 20 mg daily will commence withdrawal with 2 mg o.d. decrements each week until they are receiving 20 mg daily, when withdrawal will slow to 1 mg weekly. The dosages and timings suggested are for guidance only, and variable individual needs can be catered for. Any withdrawal symptoms that emerge are then managed with EA sessions, given every few days or once per week.

Table 18.1 Benzodiazepines: approximate dosage equivalents*

Approved name	BNF[†]	Brand name	Half-life(h)[‡]	Dose (mg) equivalent to 10 mg diazepam
Chlordiazepoxide	a	Librium	5–30 (36–200)	25
Clobazam[§]	a	Frisium	12–60	20
Diazepam	a	Valium	2–100 (36–200)	10
Lorazepam	a	Ativan	10–20	1–2
Nitrazepam	h	Mogadon	15–38	10
Oxazepam	a	Serenid	4–15	20
Temazepam	h	Normison Euhypnos	8–22	20

* J Thompson and H Ashton, Personal Communication, 1986.
[†] BNF classification: a = anxiolytic; h = hypnotic.
[‡] Active metabolite shown in brackets.
[§] NHS prescription only for epilepsy.

Propranolol may be used to attenuate palpitations, tremor and muscle twitching, and non-BZ hypnotics can be used for insomnia. Acupuncture can also be used for symptomatic relief as for withdrawal of other substances. Antidepressants may be needed if depressive illness is unmasked or if depression arises from the withdrawal process. Some patients benefit from self-help groups and relaxation therapy. Most patients do withdraw satisfactorily but not without experiencing unpleasant symptoms and requiring considerable psychological support, and sometimes the course of withdrawal is protracted, with symptoms persisting for several months afterwards. The usual outcome of attempted withdrawal is that at 1 year about one-third of patients is problem-free, one-third has minor problems but has not restarted the use of BZs, and one-third has chronic anxiety and has restarted.

SMOKING

One of the most common uses of acupuncture in the field of habituation is as an adjunct to smoking cessation. Acupuncture is often combined with psychotherapy and counselling, distraction techniques and perhaps hypnotherapy or the use of nicotine gum or patches. There seems to be no evidence of a direct effect on the need for nicotine, and it is presumably the euphorigenic attributes of endogenous opioid release that are responsible for any benefit. Much of this treatment is carried out by lay practitioners, and outcome data are not available

for assessment but, with the growing evidence linking smoking with health risks, this is a subject of great medical interest and there have been two recent reviews, by Chockalingam & Schmidt (1992) and by Schwartz (1992), examining largely US data. Additionally a meta-analysis of 15 controlled trials by ter Riet, Kleijnen & Knipschild (1990) is available, covering European and North American studies of which three had a positive outcome and 12 a negative one. Chockalingam & Schmidt (1992) also used meta-analytic techniques summarizing across studies the success rate of various interventions and taking account of any significant statistical factors. They covered 23 different smoking cessation programmes evaluated in a total of 633 clinical studies. Of these, 19 studies were concerned with acupuncture (2292 patients). They calculated a 'mean quit rate' for each intervention based on the proportion of patients stopping smoking as a result. The range was from 7% for 'physicians advice' to 42% for programmes tailored for patients with cardiac disease. The initial 'quit rate' for acupuncture was 30% overall (compare smoking aversion 31%, hypnosis 36%, nicotine chewing gum 16%, group withdrawal clinic 30%); however, the success rates varied widely from one study to another (6–54%) as with other approaches.

Stopping smoking needs to be life long and Schwartz (1992) pointed out that, despite acupuncture's popularity in the US, there is only a handful of studies on its long-term efficacy. Most workers claiming high success rates base these on initial cessation or on very limited follow-up. Very few studies validate abstinence by biochemical measures.

ALCOHOL ABUSE

Like BZ habituation, alcohol dependence represents a very significant social and clinical problem in the UK. Most studies in the literature on the use of acupuncture to assist abstention from alcohol are open and uncontrolled.

Uncontrolled studies

Following brief mention of alcohol abuse in an overview of the use of electroacupuncture for substance withdrawal, which claimed the possibility of a 30–70% reduction of consumption shortly after treatment (Omura 1975), Smith et al (1982) reported clinical experiences at the Lincoln Hospital, South Bronx. Auricular therapy involving Lung, Shenmen and Sympathetic points plus LI-4 was used on each of 2–5 days on an in- or outpatient basis in combination with psycho-therapy and herbal treatments. About half of the patients were said to be abstinent for 6 months or longer as a result of this regimen. Olms (1984) then published a single case report utilizing bilateral auricular needling, and Lewenburg (1985) reported the results of 50 alcoholics treated with a combination of ear electroacupuncture and the antidepressant maprotiline. Patients were followed up at intervals for up to 6 months after treatment. Sixty-seven per cent of cases stopped drinking within 1 week of treatment and 38% remained abstinent for 6 months. None suffered withdrawal symptoms. The author called, as a consequence, for controlled studies to be carried out, but unfortunately there is a dearth of these. A further account of 310 patients treated in China was published (Shentian et al 1988). In this work points on the ear were treated with press needles or basil seeds retained for 3 days. This paper is somewhat difficult to interpret, but a success rate of 95.2% was stated for a subset of 250 patients who were cooperative and volunteered to give up drinking. The others were either unwilling to cooperate or were persuaded

to abstain from alcohol as part of a concurrent programme of medical treatment.

Controlled trials

One positive, placebo controlled study in recidivist alcoholics was reported (Bullock et al 1987) from the Hennepin County Hospital, Minnesota. In a paper in the Lancet, this group (Bullock, Culliton & Clander 1989) published data from a further 80 patients alternately treated with bilateral needling without electrical stimulation of the 'Shenmen', 'Lung' and 'Sympathetic' ear points and LI-4, or needling of adjacent non-specific points. Twenty-one of 40 patients in the treatment group completed the programme compared with one of 40 controls. Significant treatment effects persisted at the end of 6 months' follow-up: by comparison with treatment patients, more control patients expressed a need for alcohol and had more than twice the number of both drinking episodes and admissions to a detoxification centre. Unfortunately, as a later Lancet editorial (1990) pointed out, the controls may have been more severely affected cases since significantly more patients in the placebo group had been admitted to detoxification centres during the 2 years before entry into the study. None the less the study was carefully conducted and the results remain impressive.

In contrast a negative study was reported by Worner et al (1992) from the Long Island College Hospital, Brooklyn. Rampes & Pereira (1993) criticize this study for its lack of a primary outcome measure, lack of power calculation to justify sample size, the very large number of patients screened who refused entry or who did not fulfil the inclusion criteria, the lack of internationally recognized diagnostic criteria, the failure to exclude major psychiatric disorder and the lack of information about detoxification before study entry. Those who were enrolled were randomized either to body or auricular acupuncture three times a week for 3 months (LR-3, ST-36, TE-5, LI-4, GV-20, Shenmen and Lung points), to sham TENS, or to control. All three groups received counselling, education and group supportive activities. The patients were followed up for 3 months after the 3 months' treatment period. An analysis was carried out on the basis of the number of attendances at meetings of Alcoholics Anonymous. No significant difference between the groups was seen, but the relevance of this is uncertain. Nor were there significant differences between the numbers of detoxifications and relapses during treatment, but only a very small proportion of the patients completed the acupuncture or mock TENS treatment periods so conclusions are hard to draw, especially in view of the study's other deficiencies.

Mechanisms

Several studies have linked opioids and alcohol dependence, and Copolov & Helme (1983) have reviewed the data. Naloxone can reverse alcohol-induced coma in humans (although this may be due to a non-specific arousal effect) and it can inhibit ethanol-withdrawal convulsions in mice. If opioids are involved in alcohol dependence it is suggested that tetrahydroisoquinolines (TIQs), morphine-like alkaloids, are involved. These are formed from acetaldehyde, a metabolite of ethanol, and the neurotransmitter dopamine. TIQs bind to opiate receptors in the rat brain and lead to alcohol consumption after intraventricular injection in the rat. A receptor system for TIQs may mediate many phenomena of alcohol addiction. In the light of acupuncture's benefit in facilitating opiate withdrawal, an effect in alcoholism would not be surprising.

OBESITY

Vincent & Richardson (1987) reviewed the use of acupuncture for a number of common disorders, including ear stimulation for obesity. In this case they concluded that the three studies they assessed (Bin & Jiuzhi 1985, Giller 1975, Sacks 1975) had very significant design flaws that precluded valid conclusions despite the positive reports of the authors. Problems included absence of control groups, a lack of information about methodology and long and variable treatment periods.

Vincent & Richardson (1987) did not include the study by Mok et al (1976) mounted at Harbor Hospital UCLA specifically to avoid these difficulties. In this, 25 subjects, 3 to 25% overweight, were weighed five times once every 3 weeks. All subjects received no treatment during the first time period, and then at random either unilateral press needle application to the Mouth and Stomach points on the ear, bilateral applications to these points, or unilateral application to the Foot and Ankle points (not thought to be associated with appetite control). Appetite was assessed by questionnaire. The subjects manipulated their needles for a few minutes 30 minutes before eating. In parallel, a small animal study was carried out. Six guinea pigs were weighed weekly whilst being given free access to food pellets. Their weight increased steadily over a 2 month period, following which three animals selected at random received manual and electroacupuncture applied to the ear. There were no significant differences in the weights of humans or animals between the experimental groups, although in the humans a trend towards weight reduction occurred in the two active treatment groups (a loss of 0.9% ideal body weight) but not in the untreated or control groups. Results of the subjective assessments of the human subjects were very variable, although there was reportedly generally decreased hunger in the acupuncture-treated subjects. Power calculations were not provided in the paper, but numbers in both the human and animal arms of the study were obviously small. This was particularly so in the latter, and the authors admit that choice of the site on the guinea pig ear for stimulation was difficult.

So far, despite the suggestion that endogenous opioid release, which of course occurs in acupuncture therapy, modulates eating behaviour, (Thorens et al 1990) it must be said that the clinical efficacy of acupuncture in this situation is experimentally unproven.

META-ANALYSIS OF WITHDRAWAL STUDIES

A meta-analysis of 22 controlled clinical trials on

the efficacy of acupuncture in three fields of addiction: cigarette smoking (15 trials—three positive, and 12 negative), heroin (five trials—three positive, one negative and one neutral) and alcohol (two—both positive) was carried out by ter Riet, Kleijnen & Knipschild (1990). Like Vincent & Richardson (1987) 3 years earlier, these reviewers identified the poor quality of much clinical research into this subject, with inadequate numbers of patients, lack of biochemical validation of self-reported outcome, lack of randomization and of sham treatment, high dropout rates and imbalances in prognostic factors between index and reference groups at baseline. The researchers scored each study according to its methodology and showed that those in which a favourable outcome for acupuncture was claimed, in general scored lower than those in which investigators claimed no favourable effect. Put another way, this suggests that the better the study technique the less likely it is that acupuncture treatment surpasses the placebo effect. This is a disappointing result, as is the author's general conclusion in respect of heroin addiction: that the utility of acupuncture remains unproven. However, the number of studies reviewed in the case of opiate addiction was small, since the authors excluded uncontrolled work. While the lesser validity of uncontrolled trials is admitted, given the difficulty of setting up acupuncture controls this may be a little harsh, and uncontrolled trials can be at least indicative. Additionally, there is a new emphasis at present on the need for a 'content specialist' to participate in meta-analyses so that the most appropriate experimental features are given due weight. When an experienced acupuncturist reanalysed the data from ter Riet's sample of smoking studies according to his view of the excellence of each trial's design, the reverse result occurred, with the probability of a positive outcome correlating positively with good design. There was also a strong effect of return visits for treatment as against single sessions in studies comparing active acupuncture with sham (A R White, personal communication, 1995).

Perhaps the most important message here applies to all fields of acupuncture research: that there is no point in setting up poorly designed studies. Those that are open, not randomized and lack controls, even if strongly positive, will not convince the scientific community.

All in all, we should conclude that, despite much promise for acupuncture techniques in treating withdrawal, based on early studies in the field of opiate addiction together with a putative mechanism of action, there is not yet a sufficient body of valid evidence to confirm specific effects, particularly for alcohol, smoking and overeating. Certainly this is an exceedingly difficult area for research, not least because of the unreliability and lack of motivation of many of the subjects. It is also clear that a very wide range of other social and psychological factors, which it is very hard to control in any study, are massively important in deciding the outcome of treatment and whether relapse occurs. Acupuncture's role is merely to alleviate discomfort during the period of initial withdrawal. Then much depends on long-term follow-up and support, since the addict's personality and social circumstances are unlikely to change.

REFERENCES

Aghajanian G K 1978 Tolerance of locus ceruleus neurons to morphine and suppression of withdrawal response by clonidine. Nature 276:186–188

Bin X, Jiuzhi F 1985 Clinical observations of the weight-reducing effect of ear acupuncture in 350 cases of obesity. Journal of Traditional Chinese Medicine 5:87–88

Bullock M L, Umen A J, Culliton P D, Olander R T 1987 Acupuncture treatment of alcoholic recidivism: a pilot study, alcoholism. Clinical and Experimental Research 11(3):292–295

Bullock M L, Culliton P D, Olander R T 1989 Controlled trial of acupuncture for severe recidivist alcoholism. Lancet June 24:1435–1439

Chen G S 1977 Enkephalin drug addiction and acupuncture. American Journal of Chinese Medicine 5(1):25–30

Chockalingam V, Schmidt F L 1992 A meta-analysis comparison of the effectiveness of smoking cessation methods. Journal of Applied Psychology 77(4):554–561

Choy Y M, Tso W W, Fung K P et al 1978 Suppression of narcotic withdrawal and plasma ACTH by auricular electroacupuncture. Biochemical and Biophysical Research Communications 82:305–309

Clement-Jones V, McLoughlin L, Lowry P J, Besser G M, Rees L H, Wen H L 1979 Acupuncture in heroin addicts: changes in met-enkephalin and β-endorphin in blood and cerebrospinal fluid. Lancet August 25:380–382

Clement-Jones V, McLoughlin L, Tomlin S, Besser G M, Rees L H, Wen H L 1980 Increased β-endorphin but not met-enkephalin levels in human cerebrospinal fluid after acupuncture for recurrent pain. Lancet November 1:946–948

Copolov D L, Helme R D 1983 Enkephalins and endorphins—clinical, pharmacological and therapeutic implications. Drugs 26:503–519

Editorial 1974 Acupuncture in heroin withdrawal. Medical Journal of Australia 2:82

Editorial 1981 How does acupuncture work? British Medical Journal 283:746–747

Editorial 1990 Many points to needle. Lancet 335:20–21

Giller R M 1975 Auricular acupuncture and weight reduction. A controlled study. American Journal of Acupuncture 3:151

Glassman A H, Jackson W K, Walsh B T, Roose S P 1984 Cigarette craving, smoking withdrawal, and clonidine. Science 226:864–866

Gossop M, Bradley B, Strong J, Connell P 1984 The clinical effectiveness of electrostimulation vs oral methadone in managing opiate withdrawal. British Journal of Psychiatry 144:203–208

Kroening R J, Olesen T D 1985 Narcotic detoxification in chronic pain patients treated with auricular electroacupuncture and naloxone. International Journal of the Addictions 20(9):1347–1360

Leung A S 1977 Acupuncture treatment of withdrawal symptoms. American Journal of Acupuncture 5(1):43–50

Lewenburg A 1985 Electroacupuncture and antidepressant treatment of alcoholism in private practice. Clinical Therapy 7(5): 611–617

Lloyd G 1982 Is benzodiazepine dependence a cause for concern? Modern Medicine June:27–28

Lorini G, Fazio L, Fusari A, Cocchi R 1982 Soppressione della sindrome da astinenza da oppiacei con farmaci GABAergici psicofarmaci a basso dosaggio e agopunctura. Minerva Medica 73:707–710

Man P L, Chuang M Y 1980 Acupuncture in methadone withdrawal. International Journal of the Addictions 15(6):921–926

Mendelsson G 1978 Acupuncture and cholinergic suppression of withdrawal symptoms: a hypothesis. British Journal of Addiction 73:166–170

Mok M S, Parker L N, Voina S, Bray G A 1976 Treatment of obesity by acupuncture. American Journal of Clinical Nutrition 29:832–835

Newmeyer J A, Johnson G, Klot S 1984 Acupuncture as a detoxification modality. Journal of Psychoactive Drugs 16(3): 241–261

Ng L K Y, Douthitt T C, Thoa N B, Chalom A A 1975 Modification of morphine-withdrawal syndrome in rats following transauricular electrostimulation: an experimental paradigm for auricular electroacupuncture. Biological Psychiatry 10:575–579

Olms J S 1984 New: an effective alcohol abstinence acupuncture treatment. American Journal of Acupuncture 12:145–148

Omura Y 1975 Electroacupuncture for drug addiction withdrawal syndrome, particularly methadone and individualised acupuncture treatments for the withdrawal syndromes of drug addictions and compulsive habits of excessive eating, drinking alcohol and smoking. Acupuncture and Electro-therapeutics Research 1 (1,2,3):231

Patterson M A, Firth J, Gardiner R 1984 Treatment of drug, alcohol and nicotine addiction by neuroelectric therapy: analysis of results over 7 years. Journal of Bioelectricity 3(1,2):193–221

Rampes H, Pereira S 1993 Role of acupuncture in alcohol dependance abuse. Acupuncture in Medicine 11(2):80–84

Sacks L L 1975 Drug addiction, alcoholism, smoking, obesity treated by auricular staplepuncture. American Journal of Acupuncture 3:147

Sainsbury M J 1974 Acupuncture in heroin withdrawal. Medical Journal of Australia 2:102–105*h*

Schwartz J L 1992 Methods of smoking cessation. Medical Clinics of North America 76(2): 451–477

Severson L, Markoff R A, Chun-Hoon A 1977 Heroin detoxification with acupuncture and electrical stimulation. International Journal of the Addictions 12(7):911–922

Shentian S, Zhishun Y, Weibin G et al 1988 Clinical report of drinking intervention on 310 cases with auriculo-acupuncture. Journal of Traditional Chinese Medicine 8:123–124

Shuaib M 1976 Acupuncture treatment of drug dependence in Pakistan. American Journal of Chinese Medicine 4(4):403–407

Smith M O, Khan I 1988 An acupuncture programme for the treatment of drug addicted persons. Bulletin on Narcotics XL: 35–41

Smith M O, Squires R, Aponte J, Rabinowitz N, Bonilla-Rodriguez R 1982 Acupuncture treatment of drug addiction and alcohol abuse. American Journal of Acupuncture 10:161–163

Tennant F S 1976 Out-patient heroin detoxification with acupuncture and staplepuncture. Western Journal of Medicine 125:191–194

ter Riet G, Kleijnen J, Knipschild P 1990 A meta analysis of studies into the effect of acupuncture on addiction. British Journal of General Practice 40:379–382

Thorens P, Floras J S, Hoffmann P, Seals D 1990 Endorphins and exercise: physiological mechanisms and clinical implications. Medicine and Science in Sports and Exercise 22(4):417–428

Vincent A C, Richardson P H 1987 Acupuncture for some common disorders: a review of evaluative research. Journal of the Royal College of General Practitioners 37:77–81

Wen H L 1977 Fast detoxification of heroin addicts by acupuncture and electrical stimulation (AES) in combination with naloxone. Comparative Medicine East and West 5:257–263

Wen H L, Cheung S Y C 1973 Treatment of drug addiction by acupuncture and electrical stimulation. Asian Journal of Medicine 9: 138–141

Wen H L, Teo S W 1975 Experience in the treatment of drug addiction by electroacupuncture. Modern Medicine Asia 11(6): 23–24

Whitehead P C 1978 Acupuncture in the treatment of addiction: a review and analysis. International Journal of the Addictions 13(1):1–16

Worner T M, Zeller B, Schwarz H, Zwas F, Lyon D 1992 Acupuncture fails to improve treatment outcome in alcoholics. Drug and Alcohol Dependance 30:169–173

19

Adverse reactions to acupuncture

Hagen Rampes

In common with many of the complementary therapies, acupuncture is perceived as being natural and holistic. Because of these perceptions, there is a myth that acupuncture is completely safe. Practitioners are then considerably surprised to encounter their first serious adverse reaction and may be horrified to read the literature concerning adverse reactions including occasional deaths following acupuncture. There have been many reports of adverse reactions of acupuncture in the literature.

A recent literature survey (Rampes & James 1995) identified all reports of adverse reactions of acupuncture using the Complementary and alternative therapies database, Medline database (1966 to 1993) and by extensive cross-referencing. All English language articles identified were studied in detail. This comprehensive review concluded that there were over 216 reported instances of serious complications world-wide over a 20-year period. These figures suggest a low prevalence of adverse reactions, considering that 3% of the adult population of the United Kingdom alone consulted acupuncturists in 1984 (Fulder 1988). With wider availability of acupuncture in the National Health Service, however, there is a need for practitioners and patients to be aware of possible adverse reactions to acupuncture, the majority of which can be avoided with cautious and prudent use of this ancient therapy.

PAIN

Patients often expect pain during acupuncture.

Traditionally a strong needling sensation (De Qi) is obtained (Buck 1986). This is a characteristic sensation that arises when an acupuncture point is successfully stimulated. It is distinct from the simple pinprick sensation and is variously described as 'dull', 'numb', 'swelling', 'sore' or 'radiating along a limb' to nearby acupuncture points. It may be experienced as pain by some patients, especially if they have not been forewarned or if their pain threshold is low. Persistent pain following acupuncture has been reported (Lapeer & Monga 1988). A 42-year-old female received electroacupuncture for an acute attack of migraine. Needles were inserted bilaterally at LI-4 and a current of 60 mA at a frequency of 6 Hz (continuous waveform) was applied for 20 minutes. She developed tingling in both hands and her right arm following the treatment. This progressed to a severe pain in her forearm and paraesthesia in her right thumb. This pain lasted for several days and resolved following a course of diflunisal 500 mg for 10 days. The authors concluded that the pain may have been due to an irritation of either the superficial branch of the radial nerve and/or the digital branch of the median nerve. The authors discussed other possibilities such as carpal tunnel syndrome or radiculopathy but unfortunately the patient refused to have nerve conduction studies done. Another case report (Brougham 1988) concerned a 45-year-old man who had back pain and was found to have normal investigations. He received acupuncture treatment at a tender site in the lower thoracic spine and at distal points. He returned a few days later with a marked worsening of his back pain. Repeat investigations revealed a chest X-ray that had a suspicious lesion in the ninth thoracic vertebra. The patient died 5 weeks later from multiple secondaries. The author of the report remembered that she had been taught to 'beware the pain made worse by acupuncture'. One must remember that many successful treatments proceed with the patient feeling no sensation at all (Lewith 1982).

BLEEDING

A common adverse reaction is bleeding (Chung 1980) on withdrawal of the acupuncture needle. This is often minimal and easily dealt with but rarely can result in bruising at needle sites. In the case of facial acupuncture points, this can result in orbital ecchymosis (black eye) (Redfearn 1991, Tuke 1979). Petechiae (Butcha 1972) in a child have been reported. A 2-year-old child who was pyrexial and vomiting was seen in an accident and emergency department in the United States. On examination the child was noted to have multiple petechiae on her back, the clue to the aetiology of the lesions being their symmetrical nature and a history of acupuncture! Haematoma at the site of needle insertion has been reported (Chung 1980) and was possibly due to inadvertent arterial puncture; in this case, a hand was transfixed with one needle using the 'through needle method' to get to LI-4 from SI-3. This resulted in a golf-ball-sized haematoma. A pseudoaneursym (Fujiwara, Tanohata & Nagase 1994) was reported in a 58-year-old Japanese female who had acupuncture for shoulder stiffness. In a typical session she received 20 to 30 punctures with a thin needle around her shoulders, mostly along the spines of her scapulae. She experienced sharp pain in her left shoulder during her fourth session and noticed a nodule afterwards. Because the pain worsened she presented to hospital. A contrast-enhanced CAT scan showed a subcutaneous nodule with the same level of contrast as the cervical blood vessels. Arterial digital subtraction angiography of the left costicervical artery prior to surgery confirmed the diagnosis. The lesion was a thrombosed pseudoaneurysm.

SYNCOPE

A prospective cohort study of patients receiving acupuncture at the Centre for Traditional Medicine of Veterans General Hospital, Taipei in Taiwan reported that 0.19% (55 out of 28 285 acupuncture procedures) resulted in syncope (Chen et al 1990). Of those that had syncope, 35 were male and 17 female. Mean age was 45.2 (±16.7), with bimodal distribution of the young (20–29 years) and the elderly (60–69 years). Patients who experienced syncope or 'needle fainting' were all in a seated or upright posture when they received acupuncture. Occurrences of syncope were within 2 to 10 minutes of needle insertion. None of the patients developed complete loss of consciousness and all recovered without sequelae. The vasovagal fainting episodes usually occurred in young male and elderly patients in the early phase of the treatment. There have been case reports (Rajanna 1983, Verma & Khamesra 1989) of syncope following acupuncture. Two patients (Hayhoe & Pitt 1987) proceeded to have convulsions that were probably hypoxia induced.

DROWSINESS

Drowsiness is common during and after acupuncture; in fact, acupuncture can be soporific. There is thus a potential risk where patients driving home after treatment may be a danger to themselves and others. A study (Brattberg 1986) was conducted of 122 consecutive patients who received acupuncture at a pain clinic in Sandviken Hospital, Norway. Needles were inserted at the site of pain and manipulated (four to 20 needles) and 56% patients were deemed to be a significant traffic hazard had they driven a car home directly after the treatment. The authors were unable to predict which patient would become drowsy or when in the course of the treatment this drowsiness may appear. They recommended that a warning against driving a car while undergoing acupuncture treatment should therefore be issued to all patients. Excessive drowsiness with the risk of falling asleep was experienced by 36% of patients; 10% fell asleep after getting home; 25% were moderately drowsy even after their third acupuncture treatment; 23% were unaffected by the first three treatments and became drowsy only in subsequent treatments. The study made no mention of patients' concurrent medication, however, and whether such medication may have contributed to or enhanced acupuncture induced drowsiness. It is worth while noting that doctors are obliged to inform patients about medication that may impair a patient's ability to drive or operate machinery.

SKIN CONDITIONS

It is not uncommon to observe transient erythema at needle sites. This is most likely to be due to local histamine release from skin trauma. Patients with an atopic tendency are more likely to develop transient erythema at the needle site (Bodnar 1965, Dung 1987). There have been reports of contact dermatitis (Castelain, Castelain & Ricciardi 1987) to nickel (Fisher 1986, Romaguera & Grimalt 1979, 1981), chromium (Tanii et al 1991) and zinc (Koizumi et al 1989). All cases were reported in individuals who had a history of allergy and had positive patch tests for the respective metals. This reflects the diversity of the types of acupuncture needles employed: most are stainless steel, but some practitioners prefer silver and gold ones! Some workers have linked acupuncture with various dermatological oddities such as prurigo pigmentosa (Tanii et al 1991), blue macules of localized argyria (Tanita et al 1985), a case of multiple lymphocytoma cutis of the ears (Bork 1983) and even a case of skin carcinoma (Tsukerman 1970). The latter was one of the more speculative case reports and was published in Russian. Koebner phenomena at the needle insertion sites has been described in a patient suffering from psoriasis (Kirschbaum 1972). A case of abrasions of the shoulder (Carron, Epstein & Grand 1974) has been reported where a sharp instrument was used to abrade skin in addition to needle insertion. Localized lipoatrophy after acupuncture has been reported in two patients (Drago et al 1996). Both female patients developed symmetrical, symptomless depressions on the lateral aspect of their arms. These lesions developed 3 months after acupuncture treatment. Biopsy revealed characteristic histopathological changes seen in involutional lipoatrophy.

An interesting case (Chang 1974) of reactivation of cutaneous herpetic lesions following 12 hours after each acupuncture treatment has been reported. A 67-year-old female with cutaneous herpes had 15 recurrences after 20 acupuncture treatments over a 5-month period. The lesions occurred at the same site, which was distant from the needle site.

MOXIBUSTION

In China and the Far East, acupuncture has been combined with other therapeutic modalities such as herbs, massage and moxibustion. Moxa is the dried leaves of *Artemisia vulgaris* made into various forms: 'punk' is loose moxa, rather like green cotton wool, while 'moxa rolls' are like cigars. When lit, moxa smoulders constantly. The heat is usually applied gently by holding a glowing moxa roll about 2 cm from the point. Carelessness in the technique can result in accidental burns. However in the Far East 'cauterizing moxibustion' is often used, where cones of loose punk are burned intentionally on the skin until blisters form. Third-degree burns, eschars and scars (Carron, Epstein & Grand 1974) have been reported from the use of moxibustion. Hot-needle acupuncture, which entails inserting a heated needle, has also resulted in scarring (Hung & Mines 1991). Inhalations of moxa fumes during treatment resulted in a practitioner developing chest tightness, dyspnoea and mucus production (Umeh 1989). The practitioner had a tendency to asthma and bronchitis. Antihistamine prophylaxis minimized such attacks, confirming an allergic origin to the symptoms. The author recommended the cautious use of moxibustion in patients with asthmatic and allergic tendencies.

PNEUMOTHORAX

Pneumothorax is easily avoided by good anatomical knowledge and a high degree of caution in the needling of certain points. All practitioners have a responsibility to ensure that they have studied adequately the anatomy of all points at which they propose to insert needles. When needling points on the anterior, lateral or posterior surfaces of the thorax and in the anterior and posterior triangles of the neck, particular attention must be given to the depth and direction of needle insertion. There have been many reports (Lewis-Driver 1973, Goldberg 1973) of this serious adverse reaction world-wide. From an analysis of the reports, it is apparent that needle insertion on the thorax, particularly the intercostal spaces, paraspinal areas and supraclavicular

regions, resulted in the puncture of the pleura and the lung parenchyma, leading to unilateral or bilateral pneumothorax. A chest X-ray taken immediately failed to demonstrate the lesion in one case (Ritter & Tarala 1978). In such cases, it is important to repeat an X-ray of the patient 24 hours later. The diagnosis of pneumothorax was missed in one case even though it was evident on X-ray (Wright, Kupperman & Liebhaber 1991). All the cases reported were admitted and treated with chest drains leading to successful recovery. Haemothorax (Carron, Epstein & Grand 1974) has also been reported but is much rarer. Recent litigation has involved cases of acupuncture-induced pneumothorax (Evans 1989). One case was settled for 20 000 Australian dollars. Another case involved the failure of a practitioner to diagnose acupuncture-induced pneumothorax. A general practitioner gave acupuncture for frozen shoulder. Needles were inserted in both upper arms of the patient and at the midpoints of both scapulae. Ten minutes later the patient complained of pain and a burning sensation and became short of breath. It was 48 hours later that the condition was diagnosed by another doctor.

There is one case (Waldman 1974) of a male volunteering to have acupuncture demonstrated at a New Year's party by a man, who proceeded to insert needles in his anterior chest. The volunteer developed chest pain and whilst in hospital recalled that one needle inserted through his nipple had penetrated his chest much deeper than the other needles! This is clearly a case of malpractice, where the needle was inserted deeply resulting in pneumothorax and in any case the needle was inserted at a site forbidden in traditional acupuncture.

In a questionnaire sent to 1135 doctors and 197 acupuncturists in Norway (Norheim & Fonnebo 1995) enquiring about adverse reactions of acupuncture, 25 cases of pneumothorax were recalled by doctors. If extrapolated to the whole of the country, this would suggest that 250 cases may have occurred. Interestingly, the acupuncturists themselves recalled only eight cases. This may indicate that patients prefer to return to their family doctor for the diagnosis and treatment of potentially serious problems. Acupuncture practitioners may therefore be unaware of the adverse reactions they may have caused.

CARDIOVASCULAR TRAUMA

There has been a fatality due to self-acupuncture (Schiff 1965); the needle had penetrated the pericardium and caused cardiac tamponade. More fortunate victims of self-acupuncture have been operated upon and survived (Cheng 1991, Hasegawa et al 1991, Nieda et al 1973). In an acupuncturist-induced fatality in Norway (Halvorsen et al 1995), a 40-year-old woman died after treatment for fibromyalgia using CV-17, a midsternal point. The patient complained of chest pain and died about 2 hours after the insertion of the needle. Postmortem revealed the cause of death to be cardiac tamponade, following a puncture wound in the right ventricle. A congenital sternal foramen was present. The distance from the skin to the surface of the heart was estimated to be only 13–19 mm. This congenital abnormality is present in 9.6% of men and 4.3% of women, but does not show on plain chest X-ray. Most acupuncture textbooks give instructions that CV-17 should be needled obliquely, as parallel to the skin as possible.

A patient died of a myocardial infarction 5–6 hours after acupuncture for pains in the back and the left arm (Bostrom & Rossner 1990). One of the problems in most of the case reports referred to is the attribution of causality. It may well have been that this patient had referred pain from myocardial infarction and the practitioner missed the diagnosis and inappropriately treated with acupuncture.

A compartment syndrome has been reported (Smith, Walczyk & Campbell 1986) following acupuncture in an anticoagulated patient. A 68-year-old man who was on warfarin because he had a prosthetic heart valve had received acupuncture from a physician. One of the needles was inserted at ST-36. Almost immediately, the patient developed local pain that deteriorated. There was gradual swelling and discoloration over 4 days, resulting in hospital admission. An anterior compartment surgical decompression

fasciotomy was carried out. It is not clear whether the acupuncturist was aware of the patient's medical history and current medication. The authors caution that needle insertion for any reason in anticoagulated patients can result in soft tissue haemorrhage.

There have been two reports (Blanchard 1991, Ruchkin 1987) of deep venous thrombophlebitis following acupuncture. Another case (Gray 1996) mimicking a deep venous thrombosis was a 72-year-old female with rheumatoid arthritis, who had acupuncture around her right knee. One week later she returned with pain in the back of her knee and ankle swelling. Her practitioner arranged an urgent referral to the local hospital where she was commenced on anticoagulants. However, a venogram done later was normal and it was concluded that a Baker's cyst had burst.

TRAUMA TO SPINAL CORD

There have been a number of reports, mainly from Japan, of trauma to spinal cord and spinal nerve root during needle insertion (Isu et al 1985, Noumi et al 1976) or due to migration of cut or broken retained needles (Drake 1974). Trauma to the patient (e.g. a fall) can result in movement of a retained needle, leading to injury of vital structures. Patients present with focal neurological signs, and radiological examinations reveal the culprits, which then require surgical removal. There have been isolated reports of spinal arachnoiditis (Oka et al 1986) and subarachnoid haemorrhage (Keane, Ahmadi & Gruen 1993, Murata et al 1990). Nerve injury resulting in sympathetic dystrophy has been reported (Carron, Epstein & Grand 1974, Kataoka & Sakata 1958).

SEPTICAEMIA

There have been reports of septicaemia (Doutsu et al 1986, Izatt & Fairman 1977) due to *Staphylococcus aureus*. Two patients who had complex past medical histories and were debilitated died (Pierik 1982). Small indwelling press needles were used in both cases. In one case (Izatt & Fairman 1977) acupuncture around a knee joint resulted in septicaemia with fulminant disseminated intravascular coagulation.

ENDOCARDITIS

Bacterial endocarditis (Jefferys et al 1983, Lee & Mcilwain 1985, Scheel et al 1992) has been reported in three cases. Patients who had prosthetic heart valves underwent acupuncture that involved the use of press needles for a number of days. The reports of endocarditis raise important questions about patients' suitability for acupuncture. In the correspondence following the first report of endocarditis (Jefferys et al 1983), Cheng (1983) criticized prophylactic measures suggested by the authors of the report. It had been suggested that antibiotic prophylaxis be used in all patients with cardiac lesions undergoing acupuncture. However, acupuncture is not a single procedure but entails a course of treatment; therefore it would be impracticable and uneconomical to use antibiotics for each acupuncture session. The reported cases of endocarditis occurred with the use of press needles, retained in the skin for up to a week. It would be strongly advised for patients who have prosthetic or damaged heart valves not to have acupuncture involving press needles. When taking a history, practitioners should inquire whether patients have had cardiac surgery or rheumatic fever. Auscultation of the heart may well be important, yet is likely to be omitted where 'simple anti-smoking treatment' has been requested.

PERICHONDRITIS

Auricular acupuncture lends itself to the use of press needles (small needles for indwelling use in auricular therapy, which may be left in place for 1 week or longer to produce continued effect). The commonest use of press needles is for the treatment of smoking and obesity. These needles are inserted at known auricular acupuncture points or at any tender areas of the ear. Press needles were implicated in all the reports of perichondritis except one case where intradermal needles were inappropriately used (Allison & Kravitz 1975, Gilbert 1987). Perichondritis is a serious adverse reaction. The treatment may entail parenteral antibiotics and surgical intervention. Some of the patients were left with a cosmetically deformed ear following treatment. A recent litigation case (Evans 1989) involved a young female who received ear acupuncture for rheumatoid arthritis. The ear lobe was cleaned with a swab before the needle was inserted. The needle was left in situ for 6 days. The needle site became infected. She was prescribed fucidin and the ear was dressed. The infection progressed and developed into a perichondritis requiring three surgical operations. The patient was left with an unsightly cauliflower ear. Unfortunately none of the case reports of perichondritis had sufficient detail to scrutinize the method of acupuncture. For example, what aseptic technique (the adequate disinfection of the skin and avoidance of handling the sterile needles) if any was practised? Were patients instructed to stimulate the retained press needles? How long were the needles retained in the ear?

HEPATITIS

Doctors visiting China who have seen the practice of acupuncture in a rural setting have expressed concern (Alexander, Hamilton-Fairly & Smithers 1974) at the lack of aseptic technique. Some have speculated (Conn 1988, Li & Shiang 1980) about a link between the use of acupuncture and the high prevalence of hepatitis and hepatocellular carcinoma in China.

There have been definitive reports (Alexis, Lubin & Bichachi 1988, Slater et al 1988) of dissemination of hepatitis B. There was a recent report of three cases of hepatitis B between December 1990 and October 1992 from an acupuncture clinic in south-west London (Communicable Disease Report 1992). The first report in the United Kingdom (Boxall 1978, Communicable Diseases Surveillance Centre 1977) was influential because practitioners switched over to using sterile disposable needles and public health supervision improved. One practitioner was noted to have an appallingly poor hygienic technique; he was seen to handle the needle points before and after insertion. He infected 36 patients and himself became infected through a needlestick injury. His technique was also unusual in that he used hollow needles! Other well-documented hepatitis outbreaks occurred where standard solid acupuncture needles were used and the infections were all attributed to failure to adhere to strict aseptic technique. One practitioner dipped his used acupuncture needles into calendula ointment (Hussain 1974); another used a disinfectant (Stryker, Gunn & Francis 1986) to clean his needles. Neither technique is effective to sterilize the needles.

Transmission of hepatitis B and other blood-borne infections via acupuncture needles can be prevented by using sterile disposable needles. The need to autoclave reusable needles and the fact that these needles become blunt with repeated use are the main disadvantages of using such needles. It is far more convenient and relatively inexpensive to use sterile disposable stainless steel acupuncture needles. In fact the author's opinion is that the use of sterile disposable needles should be mandatory.

The British Blood Transfusion Service screening of potential blood donors inquires about acupuncture. If acupuncture has been performed by a registered medical practitioner, the donor is accepted. If acupuncture was administered by others then the donor is asked to wait 6 months (HMSO 1989).

ACQUIRED IMMUNE DEFICIENCY SYNDROME

There has been much publicity about acquired immune deficiency syndrome and speculation whether acupuncture can transmit human immunodeficiency virus. There have been no proven cases, although we have identified one reported case (Vittecoq et al 1989) suggesting that acupuncture was implicated. This was a 17-year-old French male who did not have any risk factors for acquired immune deficiency syndrome. He received acupuncture for tendinitis and subsequently developed the symptoms of acquired immune deficiency syndrome. In a study (Castro et al 1988) by the Centre for Diseases Control, USA, cases of acquired immune deficiency syndrome in patients who did not have any apparent risk factors were thoroughly investigated. Two of 2059 were found to have had acupuncture before symptoms developed.

The United Kingdom government produced acquired immune deficiency syndrome leaflets suggesting that acupuncture needles may transmit human immunodeficiency virus (DHSS 1986). However, there is no definite evidence that acupuncture needles have caused human immunodeficiency virus transmission. The risk to the practitioner from needlestick injury when treating a patient who has human immunodeficiency virus may be more important.

ELECTROACUPUNCTURE

This can impair the function of a demand type pacemaker (Fujiwara et al 1980). Low-frequency electroacupuncture employed for anaesthesia during a cervical operation deranged the proper function of a demand pacemaker. An applied voltage of about 20 V and a current of about 3 mA resulted in complete inhibition of the pacemaker. It would be prudent not to administer electroacupuncture to any patient with a pacemaker.

RETAINED NEEDLES

There have been reports of acupuncture needles in the abdominal cavity (Yin 1937), kidney parenchyma (Fukuda et al 1969, Yamaguchi, Kyakuno & Osafune 1989) and the urinary tract, leading to calculus formation (Aso, Murahashi & Yokoyama 1979, Keller, Parker & Garvin 1972, Yuzawa et al 1991). A man presented with haematuria and an X-ray revealed a metallic object in his pelvis. An acupuncture needle was retrieved by cystoscopy. He admitted inserting the needle into the urethral meatus to clear some glue that had become stuck to his penis (Roy 1974). Foreign body granuloma reaction to retained acupuncture needles has been noted (Asano 1969, Chun & Cho 1991). An accidentally broken needle has been surgically removed from the median nerve (Southworth & Hartwig 1990).

There have been reports (Behrstock & Petrakis 1974, Campbell 1982, Galuten & Austin 1988, Gerard, Wilck & Schiano 1993, Hollander, Dewitz & Bowers 1991, Imray & Hiramatsu 1975, Saenz, Lee & Mottram 1978) of fine linear metallic foreign bodies found incidentally on various X-rays. The differential diagnosis would include parasites, sutures, etc. The patients, usually of oriental origin, give a history of having had acupuncture by the okibari technique (a controversial technique peculiar to Japan, where gold needles are inserted into the skin permanently, the protruding part being cut off). The number of permanent subcutaneous needles varies widely; one patient had over 200 needles! A recent case (Chiu & Austin 1995) involved a 42-year-old Japanese male whose X-rays revealed many fine metallic opacities in the soft tissues of his back.

Needles do also occasionally break off accidentally (Rogers 1981) while in use. This is often because of muscle movement or spasm during treatment and is more likely to occur if old needles are being used. Patients should be advised not to move during treatment and the condition of the needles should be checked when they are removed. If breakage has occurred, the fragments must be removed immediately.

There are anecdotal cases of accidental retained needles following treatment. During the author's training in acupuncture, the author practised on a colleague and inserted many needles in him. The following morning, as the colleague woke up, he rubbed his hair to find a needle at GV-20! A needle had accidentally been left behind and he had slept with it protruding from his scalp. One way of remembering to remove all inserted needles is to keep a count, as is the practice for swabs used during surgical procedures.

MISCELLANEOUS

A 29-year-old man was found to have increased bone activity on bone scans (Kuno & Cerqueira 1995). He had a bone scan (scintigraphy with [^{99m}Tc]-methylene diphosphonate) for investigation of chronic back pain. Posterior and lateral images of the skull showed focal increased uptake in several regions of his skull. On further questioning, he related that he received acupuncture for his condition at the same regions as the increased uptake. The needle sites were confirmed by the patient's acupuncturist. The authors suggest that acupuncture be added as yet another cause for increased activity on bone scans! There have been isolated reports of spinal infection (Hadden & Swanson 1982) and a case of suspected osteomyelitis (Jones & Cross 1980). There has been one case (Carron, Epstein & Grand 1974) of an asthmatic who discontinued all his medication whilst undergoing acupuncture for his illness. He progressively deteriorated and developed status asthmaticus. This is not an adverse reaction of acupuncture, of course, but a consequence of inadvisedly discontinuing medication.

In a survey of Guardian newspaper readers, 386 people responded to an invitation to answer a questionnaire about their use of complementary therapies (Abbot, White & Ernst 1996). Interestingly 12.5% reported adverse reactions. A survey of general practitioners in Devon and Cornwall enquiring whether they had encountered patients experiencing adverse reactions due to complementary therapies elicited more serious adverse reactions than those reported by the users in the Guardian survey.

CONCLUSION

Ancient practitioners of acupuncture were aware of adverse reactions and the Nei Jing lists contraindications. For example, 'if the patient has come from far away, treatment should be given in a lying position after the patient has taken a good rest'. This is a sensible precaution. However, there are other more controversial recommendations such as 'needling is forbidden after sexual intercourse, and sexual intercourse should be avoided after needling'! (Luwen 1990).

The serious adverse reactions reported in the literature may easily be prevented by straightforward precautions, which are summarized in Box 19.1. Some of the adverse reactions were due to unusual or even controversial forms of acupuncture.

Box 19.1 Contraindications of acupuncture

Contraindication
- Anticoagulation
- Prosthetic and damaged cardiac valves (no press needles)
- Pacemaker (no electroacupuncture)

Caution
- Acupuncture points on thorax (practitioner must know anatomy of the pleura)
- Metal allergy
- Immunosuppression (note acupuncture may be valuable to people with lowered immunity; use scrupulous aseptic technique)
- Pregnancy (first trimester)

Precaution
- Use sterile disposable needles
- Use aseptic technique with press needles
- Lie down the patient during treatment
- Avoid driving after treatment
- Count needles in and out!
- Observe for bleeding

Clinical experience suggests that there are unexpected positive reactions due to acupuncture treatment. For example, the coincidental improvement of disorders that were not being treated by the acupuncturist (e.g. psoriasis). A randomized controlled trial investigating electroacupuncture for reduction of alcohol craving noted that one patient developed an aversion to smoking (Rampes et al 1996).

The majority of the case reports of adverse reactions of acupuncture did not have sufficient information to appraise them critically. One case report with an English abstract concerned a case of skin carcinoma following acupuncture (Tsukerman 1970) How much of this was speculation? Often it was not clear if the practitioner had any acupuncture training or whether they had a medical background or not. Future case reports of adverse reactions should give details about the type of acupuncture involved, who gave it, the timing of the adverse reaction, its reversibility and any confounding factors. All future clinical trials involving acupuncture should prospectively identify adverse reactions, a good example being the study by Kelleher et al (1994). Training and competence of the acupuncturist is an important issue and is an area that is given priority by the British Medical Acupuncture Society in their training programme.

Perhaps a national database for acupuncture adverse reactions similar to the Committee of Safety of Medicines system of reporting of drug adverse reactions should be set up to collect and evaluate reports of adverse reactions of acupuncture.

REFERENCES

Abbot N, White A R, Ernst E 1996 Complementary medicine. Nature 381:361

Alexander P, Hamilton-Fairly G, Smithers D W 1974 Repeated acupuncture and serum hepatitis. British Medical Journal 3:466

Alexis J, Lubin J, Bichachi A 1988 Acupuncture and non-A, non-B hepatitis. Southern Medical Journal 81:101

Allison G, Kravitz E 1975 Auricular chondritis secondary to acupuncture. New England Journal of Medicine 293:780

Asano K 1969 Foreign body granuloma caused by a broken sitren needle for acupuncture. Otolaryngology (Tokyo) 41:289–291

Aso Y, Murahashi I, Yokoyama M 1979 Foreign body stone of the ureter as a complication of acupuncture. European Urology 5(1):57–59

Behrstock B B, Petrakis N L 1974 Permanent subcutaneous gold acupuncture needles. Western Journal of Medicine 121:140–142

Blanchard B M 1991 Deep vein thrombophlebitis after acupuncture. Annals of Internal Medicine 115(9):748

Bodnar P N 1965 On the eosinopenic reaction to acupuncture in patients with bronchial asthma. Vrachebnoe Delo 9:147

Bork K 1983 Multiple lymphocytoma at the point of puncture as complication of acupuncture treatment. Traumatic origin of lymphocytoma. Hautarzt 34(10):496–499

Bostrom H, Rossner S 1990 Quality of alternative medicine—complications and avoidable deaths. Quality Assurance in Health Care 2(2):111–117

Boxall E H 1978 Acupuncture hepatitis in the West Midlands, 1977. Journal of Medical Virology 2:377–379

Brougham P A 1988 Case reports. An interesting acupuncture phenomenon. Acupuncture in Medicine 5:9

Brattberg G 1986 Acupuncture treatments: a traffic hazard? American Journal of Acupuncture 14(3):265–267

Buchta R M 1972 An unusual cause of petechiae. American Journal of Disease in Childhood 123:613

Buck C C 1986 Propagated needle sensation. Journal of

Chinese Medicine 22:15–16

Campbell A E R 1982 Hazards of acupuncture. British Journal of Radiology 55:875–877

Castelain M, Castelain P Y, Ricciardi R 1987 Contact dermatitis to acupuncture needles. Contact Dermatitis 16:44

Castro K G, Lifson A R, White C R et al 1988 Investigations of AIDS patients with no previously identified risk factors. Journal of the American Medical Association 259(9):1338–1342

Chang T W 1974 Activation of cutaneous herpes by acupuncture. New England Journal of Medicine 290:1310

Chen F, Hwang S, Lee H, Yang H, Chung C 1990 Clinical study of syncope during acupuncture treatment. Acupuncture and Electro-therapeutics Research 15:107–119

Cheng T O 1983 Acupuncture needles as a cause of bacterial endocarditis. British Medical Journal 287(6393):689

Cheng T O 1991 Pericardial effusion from self inserted needle in the heart. European Heart Journal 12(8):958

Chiu E S, Austin J H M 1995 Acupuncture needle fragments. New England Journal of Medicine 332:304

Chun S I, Cho S W 1991 Silica granuloma: scanning electron microscopy and energy dispersive X-ray microanalysis. Journal of Dermatology 18(2):92–96

Chung C 1980 Common errors and complications in acupuncture treatment. Acupuncture Research Quarterly 4:51–58

Communicable Diseases Surveillance Centre of the PHLS 1977 Acupuncture associated hepatitis in the West Midlands in 1977. British Medical Journal 2:1610

Communicable Disease Report 1992 Hepatitis B associated with an acupuncture clinic. 2(48) (27 November)

Conn H 1988 Acupuncture in epidemic HBV hepatitis: in China too? Hepatology 8(5):1176–1177

DHSS (Department of Health and Social Security) 1986 AIDS: don't die of ignorance. [leaflet] HMSO, London

Doutsu Y, Tao Y, Sasayama K et al 1986 A case of staphylococcus aureus septicemia after acupuncture therapy. Kansenshogaku Zasshi 60(8):911–916

Drago F, Rongioletti F, Battifoglio M L, Rebora A 1996 Localised lipoatrophy after acupuncture. Lancet: 347:1484

Drake T E 1974 Complication of acupuncture. Journal of the American Medical Association 229(10):1285–1286

Dung H C 1987 An immediate atopic erythroid reaction induced by acupuncture needles on the posterior thoracic wall. Alternative Medicine 2(3–4):209–214

Evans M 1989 Litigation and ethical issues affecting acupuncture. Acupuncture in Medicine 6(1):24–27

Fisher A A 1986 Allergic dermatitis from acupuncture needles. Cutis 38:226

Fujiwara H, Taniguchi K, Takeuchi J, Ikezono E 1980 The influence of low frequency acupuncture on a demand pacemaker. Chest 78(1):96–97

Fujiwara T, Tanohata K, Nagase M 1994 Pseudoaneurysm caused by acupuncture: a rare complication. American Journal of Roentgenology 162:731

Fukuda K, Kiriyama T, Kashawagi T et al 1969 Foreign bodies (acupuncture needles) in kidney combined with a stone. Acta Urologica Japonica (Kyoto) 15:233–236

Fulder S 1988 The handbook of complementary medicine. Oxford University Press, New York, Ch 2; p 28

Galuten A, Austin J H M 1988 Permanent subcutaneous acupuncture needles: radiographic manifestations. Journal of the Canadian Radiology Association 39:54–56

Gerard P S, Wilck E, Schiano T 1993 Imaging implications in the evaluation of permanent needle acupuncture. Clinical Imaging 17(1):36–40

Gilbert J G 1987 Auricular complications of acupuncture. New Zealand Medical Journal 100(819):141–142

Goldberg I 1973 Pneumothorax associated with acupuncture. Medical Journal of Australia 1:941–942

Gray P 1996 Baker's cyst burst after acupuncture. Acupuncture in Medicine 14(1):41–42

Hadden W A, Swanson A J G 1982 Spinal infection caused by acupuncture mimicking a prolapsed intervertebral disc. Journal of Bone and Joint Surgery 64A(4):624–626

Halvorsen T B, Anda S S, Naess A B, Levang O W 1995 Fatal cardiac tamponade after acupuncture through congenital sternal foramen. Lancet 345:1175

Hasegawa J, Noguchi N, Yamasaki J et al 1991 Delayed cardiac tamponade and hemothorax induced by an acupuncture needle. Cardiology 78:58–63

Hayhoe S, Pitt E 1987 Case reports. Complications of acupuncture. Acupuncture in Medicine 4(2):15

HMSO 1989 Guidelines for the blood transfusion services in the United Kingdom. Vol 1. HMSO, London, Chapter 5, p 22

Hollander J E, Dewitz A, Bowers S 1991 Permanently imbedded subcutaneous acupuncture needles: radiographic appearance. Annals of Emergency Medicine 20:1025–1026

Hung V C, Mines J S 1991 Eschars and scarring from hot needle acupuncture treatment. Journal of the American Academy of Dermatology 24(1):148–149

Imray T J, Hiramatsu Y 1975 Radiographic manifestations of Japanese acupuncture. Radiology 115:625–626

Isu T, Iwasaki Y, Sasaki H, Abe H 1985 Spinal cord and root injuries due to glass fragments and acupuncture needles. Surgical Neurology 23:255–260

Izatt E, Fairman M 1977 Staphylococcal septicaemia with DIC associated with acupuncture. Postgraduate Medical Journal 53(619):285–286

Jefferys D B, Smith S, Brennand-Roper D A, Curry P V L 1983 Acupuncture needles as a cause of bacterial endocarditis. British Medical Journal 287:326–327

Jones R O, Cross S J 1980 Suspected chronic osteomyelitis secondary to acupuncture treatment. Journal of the American Podiatry Association 70(3):149–151

Kataoka H, Sakata M 1958 Nerve injury due to an acupuncture treatment. Geka 20:578–582

Keane J R, Ahmadi J, Gruen P 1993 Spinal epidural hematoma with subarachnoid hemorrhage caused by acupuncture. American Journal of Neuroradiology 14(2):365–366

Kelleher C J, Filshie J, Burton G, Khullar V, Cardozo L D 1994 Acupuncture and the treatment of irritative bladder symptoms. Acupuncture in Medicine 12:9–12

Keller W J, Parker S G, Garvin J P 1972 Possible renal complications of acupuncture. Journal of the American Medical Association 222(12):1559

Kirschbaum J O 1972 Koebner phenomenon following acupuncture. Archives of Dermatology 106:767

Koizumi H, Tomoyori T, Kumakri M, Ohkawara A 1989 Acupuncture needle dermatitis. Contact Dermatitis 21:352

Kuno R C, Cerqueira M D 1995 Enhanced bone metabolism induced by acupuncture. Journal of Nuclear Medicine 36:2246–2247

Lapeer G, Monga T N 1988 Pain secondary to acupuncture

therapy. Cranio 6(2):188–190

Lee R J, Mcilwain J C 1985 Subacute bacterial endocarditis following ear acupuncture. International Journal of Cardiology 7(1):62–63

Lewis-Driver D J 1973 Pneumothorax associated with acupuncture. Medical Journal of Australia 2:296–297

Lewith G T 1982 Acupuncture: its place in Western Medical Science. Thorsons, Wellingborough, pp 34–35

Li F P, Shiang El 1980 Acupuncture and possible hepatitis B infection. Journal of the American Medical Association 243:1423

Luwen G 1990 Understanding the theory of acupuncture contra-indications according to the Nei Jing. Journal of Chinese Medicine 34(Sept):31–32

Maruoka N, Kinoshita K, Wakisaka S 1986 Cervical spinal cord injury caused by a broken acupuncture needle: a case report. No ShinKei Geka 14:785–787

Murata K, Nishio A, Nishikawa M, Ohinata Y, Sakaguchi M, Nishimura S 1990 Subarachnoid hemorrhage and spinal root injury caused by acupuncture needle. Neurologia Medico-Chirurgica (Tokyo) 30:956–959

Nieda S, Abe T, Kuribayashi R, Sato M, Abe S 1973 Cardiac trauma as complication of acupuncture treatment: a case report of cardiac tamponade resulting from a broken needle. Japan Journal of Thoracic Surgery 293:780

Norheim A J, Fonnebo V 1995 Adverse effects of acupuncture. Lancet 345:1576

Noumi T, Yamauchi Y, Kamimura K et al 1976 A broken acupuncture needle migrated into the spinal canal. Nippon Iji Shinpo 4:799–803

Oka N, Kanemaru K, Akiguchi I, Kameyama M, Koyama T 1986 Cervical adhesive arachnoiditis as a complication of acupuncture. Rinsho Shineigaku 26(8):847–850

Pierik M G 1982 Fatal staphylococcal septicemia following acupuncture: report of two cases. Royal Institute Medical Journal 65:251–253

Rajanna P 1983 Hypotension following stimulation of acupuncture point fengchi (GB 20). Journal of Royal College of General Practitioners (Sept) 33:606–607

Rampes H, James, R 1995 Complications of acupuncture. Acupuncture in Medicine 13:26–33

Rampes H, Pereira S, Mortimer A, Manoharan S, Knowles M 1996 Does electroacupuncture reduce craving for alcohol? A randomised controlled trial. Complementary Therapies in Medicine 5:19–26

Redfearn T 1991 Oh, what a surprise! Acupuncture in Medicine 9(1):2–3

Rogers P A M 1981 Serious complications of acupuncture: or acupuncture abuses? American Journal of Acupuncture 9(4):347–351

Romaguera C, Grimalt F 1979 Nickel dermatitis from acupuncture needles. Contact Dermatitis 5:195

Romaguera C, Grimalt F 1981 Contact dermatitis from a permanent acupuncture needle. Contact Dermatitis 7:156–157

Roy J B 1974 Acupuncture needle in bladder. Urology 4(5):584

Ruchkin J N 1987 Auriculo-electroacupuncture in rheumatoid arthritis (a double blind study). Teraperticheskii Arkhiv (Moskva) 59:26–30

Saenz L, Lee H, Mottram M 1978 Permanent acupuncture needles. Journal of the American Medical Association 240:1482–1483

Scheel O, Sundsfjord A, Lunde P, Andersen B M 1992 Endocarditis after acupuncture and injection treatment by a natural healer. Journal of the American Medical Association 267(1):56

Schiff A F 1965 A fatality due to acupuncture. Medical Times (London) 93(6):630–631

Slater P E, Ben-Ishai P, Leventhal A et al 1988 An acupuncture-associated outbreak of hepatitis B in Jerusalem. European Journal of Epidemiology 4(3):322–325

Smith D L, Walczyk M H, Campbell S 1986 Acupuncture needle induced compartment syndrome. Western Journal of Medicine 144(4):478–479

Southworth S R, Hartwig R H 1990 Foreign body in the median nerve: a complication of acupuncture. Journal of Hand Surgery (British) 15B:111–112

Tanii T, Kono T, Katoh J, Mizuno N, Fukuda M, Hamada T 1991 A case of prurigo pigmentosa considered to be contact allergy to chromium in an acupuncture needle. Acta Dermato-Venereologica (Stockh) 71:66–67

Tanita Y, Kato T, Hanada K, Tagami H 1985 Blue macules of localised argyria caused by implanted acupuncture needles. Archives of Dermatology 121:1550–1552

Tsukerman I M 1970 A rare case of carcinoma of the skin arising after acupuncture. Voprosy Onkologii 16:88

Tuke J 1979 Complication of acupuncture. British Medical Journal 2:1076

Umeh B 1989 Moxibustion: respiratory complications. Acupuncture in Medicine 6(2):61–62

Verma S K, Khamesra R 1989 Recurrent fainting—an unusual reaction to acupuncture. Journal of the Association of Physicians of India 37(9):600

Vittecoq D, Mettetal J F, Rouziova C, Bach J F, Bouchon J P 1989 Acute HIV infection after acupuncture treatments. New England Journal of Medicine 320(4):250–251

Yamaguchi S, Kyakuno M, Osafune M 1989 Foreign body in the kidney: a case report and a review of the Japanese literature. Hinyokika Kiyo 35(4):665–669

Yin Y C 1937 Wire needle in the abdominal cavity: an accident in acupuncture. Chinese Medical Journal 52:107–108

Yuzawa M, Hara Y, Kobayashi Y et al 1991 Foreign body stone of the ureter as a complication of acupuncture: report of a case. Hinyokika Kiyo 37(10):1323–1327

FURTHER READING

Baltimore R S, Moloy P J 1976 Perichondritis of the ear as a complication of acupuncture. Archives of Otolaryngology 102:572–573

Batisse C 1986 Acupuncture followed by hepatitis. Revue du Rhumatisme et Maladies Osteoartic 53(11):670

Bodner G, Topilsky M, Greif J 1983 Pneumothorax as a complication of acupuncture in the treatment of bronchial asthma. Annals of Allergy 51:401–403

Carette M F, Mayaud C, Houacine S, Milleron B, Toty L, Akoun G 1984 Acupuncture treatment of acute asthma:

probable role in the onset of pneumothorax with progression to a state of status asthmaticus. Revue de Pneumologie Clinique 40(1):69–70

Carron H, Epstein B S, Grand B 1974 Complications of acupuncture. Journal of the American Medical Association 228(12):1552–1554

Corbett M, Sinclair M 1974 Acu and pleuro-puncture. New England Journal of Medicine 290:167–168

Davis O, Powell W 1985 Auricular perichondritis secondary to acupuncture. Archives of Otolaryngology 111(11):770–771

De Galocsy C, Geubel A P, Gulbis A, Dive C 1982 Hepatite sur acupuncture: rapport de sept cas. Acta Gastroenterologica Belgica 45:224–230

Dominguez A, Milicua J M, Larraona J L, Barcena R, Fernandez-Rodriguez C M, Gil-Grande L A 1985 Viral hepatitis B transmitted by acupuncture: presentation of 5 cases. Medicina Clinica (Barcelona) 84(8):317–319

Fraser R M 1974 An unusual complication of acupuncture. Canadian Medical Association Journal 3:388–393

Garcia-Bengoechea M, Cabriada J, Arriola J A, Arenas J I 1985 Hepatitis B caused by acupuncture and the same acupuncturist. Medicina Clinica (Barcelona) 85(16):686

Gray R, Maharajh G S, Hyland R 1991 Pneumothorax resulting from acupuncture. Canadian Association of Radiologists Journal 42(2):139–140

Guerin J M, Tibourtine O, Lhote F, Segrestaa J M 1987 2 cases of pneumothorax following acupuncture. Revue de Medicine Interne 8(1):71

Hasegawa O, Shibuya K, Suzuki Y, Nagatomo H 1990 Acupuncture needles, straying in the central nervous system and presenting neurological signs and symptoms. Rinsho Shinkeigaku 30(10):1109–1113

Henneghien C, Bruart J, Remacle P 1984 A new iatrogenic pathology: pneumothorax after acupuncture. Revue de Pneumologie Clinique 40(3):197–199

Huet R, Renard E, Blotman M J, Jaffiol C 1990 Unrecognised pneumothorax after acupuncture in a female patient with anorexia nervosa. Presse Medicale 19(30):1415

Hussain K K 1974 Serum hepatitis associated with repeated acupuncture. British Medical Journal 3:41–42

Johansen M, Nielsen K O 1990 Perichondritis of the ear caused by acupuncture. Ugeskrift for Laeger (Copenhagen) 152(3):172–173

Kent G P, Brondum J, Keenlyside R A, Lafazia L M, Denman-Scott H 1988 A large outbreak of acupuncture associated hepatitis B. American Journal of Epidemiology 127:591–598

Kida Y, Naritomi H, Sawada T, Kuriyama Y, Ogawa M, Miyamoto S 1988 Cervical spinal cord injury caused by acupuncture. Archives of Neurology 45:831

Kishikawa K, Nakae Y, Fujiwara S, Namiki A, Mori T 1990 A spinal cord injury caused by acupuncture needles. Pain Clinic 3(3):179–184

Kiyosawa K, Gibo Y, Sodeyama T et al 1987 Possible infectious causes in 651 patients with acute viral hepatitis during a 10-year period (1976–1985). Liver 7(3):163–168

Kobler E, Schmuzigar P, Hartmann G 1979 Hepatitis nach Akupunktur. Schweize Medizinische Wochenschrift 109:1828–1829

Kojima Y, Ono K, Ogino H, Okada K, Kimura T 1985 Migration of the needle of acupuncture into the cervical spinal canal. Report of four cases. Chuba Nippon Seikeigeka Gakkai Zasshi 23:292–294

Kondo A, Koyama T, Ishikawa J, Yamasaki T 1979 Injury to the spinal cord produced by acupuncture needle. Surgical Neurology 11:155–156

Kropp R, Hassler R 1983 Accidental pneumothorax following injections and acupuncture in the thoracic region. Medizinische Welt 34(41):1143–1144

Kuiper J J 1974 Pneumothorax as complication of acupuncture. Journal of the American Medical Association 229(11):1422

Marchuk I K 1989 Pneumothorax developing as a result of acupuncture in the treatment of bronchial asthma. Vrachebnoe Delo 5:101–102

Matsui S, Matsuoka K, Nakagawa K, Kohno K, Sakaki S 1992 Cervical spinal cord injury caused by a broken acupuncture needle: a case report. No ShinKei Geka 20(4):499–503

Mazal D A, King T, Harvey J, Cohen J 1980 Bilateral pneumothorax after acupuncture. New England Journal of Medicine 302(24):1365–1366

Moro-Aguado J, De-la-Lama-Lopez-Areal J, Cortejoso-Gonzalo B 1985 Viral hepatitis B transmitted by acupuncture. Medicina Clinica (Barcelona) 85(8):344

Morrone N, Freire J A, Ferreira A K, Dourado A M 1990 Iatrogenic pneumothorax caused by acupuncture. Revue de Paulista de Medicine (Sao Paulo) 108(4):189–191

Negro F E, Bornoroni C, Bove G 1977 Complications in acupuncture: viral hepatitis. Minerva Medica 68(11):727–728

Ritter H G, Tarala R 1978 Pneumothorax after acupuncture. British Medical Journal 277(2):602–603

Sasaki H, Abe H, Iwasaki Y, Tsuru M, Itoh T 1984 Direct spinal cord and root injury caused by acupuncture. Report of 2 cases. No Shinkei Geka 12(10):1219–1223

Sato M, Yamane K, Ezima M, Sugishita Y, Nozaki H 1991 A case of transverse myelopathy caused by acupuncture. Rinsho Shinkeigaku 31(7):717–719

Savage-Jones H 1985 Auricular complications of acupuncture. Journal of Laryngology Otol 99:1143–1145

Schlenker G, Huegel A 1976 Complications of acupuncture. Deutsche Medizinische Wochenschrift 101:241–243

Schmid E, Hortling G, Kammuller H 1984 Inoculation hepatitis caused by acupuncture. Clinical cases studied over a 9 year period. Fortschritte der Medizin (München) 102(35):862–865

Schneider L B, Salzberg M R 1984 Bilateral pneumothorax following acupuncture. Annals of Emergency Medicine 13(8):643

Shiraishi S, Goto I, Kuroiwa Y, Nishio S, Kinoshita K 1979 Spinal cord injury as a complication of an acupuncture. Neurology 29:1188–1190

Smith P F, Rauscher C R 1974 Complication of acupuncture. Journal of the American Medical Association 229(10):1285–1286

Sorensen T 1990 Auricular perichondritis caused by acupuncture therapy. Ugeskrift for Laeger (Copenhagen) 152(11):752–753

Stack B H R 1975 Pneumothorax associated with acupuncture. British Medical Association 1:96

Stryker W S, Gunn R A, Francis D P 1986 Outbreak of hepatitis B associated with acupuncture. Journal of Family Practice 22(2):155–158

Takishima T 1983 Pneumothorax as a complication of acupuncture in the treatment of bronchial asthma. Annals of Allergy 51:401–403

Tomonaga I, Miyazaki M, Kondo T, Kono M, Ueno T 1984 Migration of the acupuncture needles into the cervical spinal cord. Orthopedic Traumatology (Fukuoka) 32:123–125

Trautermann H G, Trautermann H 1981 Perichondritis der Ohrmuschel nach Akupunktur. HNO (Berlin) 29:312–313

Waldman I 1974 Pneumothorax from acupuncture. New England Journal of Medicine 290:633

Warwick-Brown N P, Richards A E S 1986 Perichondritis of the ear following acupuncture. Journal of Laryngology and Otology 100:1177–1179

Willms D 1991 Possible complications of acupuncture. Western Journal of Medicine 154(6):736–737

Wright R S, Kupperman J L, Liebhaber M L 1991 Bilateral tension pneumothoraces after acupuncture. Western Journal of Medicine 154(1):102–103

Acupuncture past and future

20

Reinterpretation of traditional concepts in acupuncture

François Beyens

INTRODUCTION

The history of scientific acupuncture begins with the application of scientific methodology to explain, understand and evaluate acupuncture treatments, as well as their results, in the light of modern medicine. This history is relatively short, spreading over the past 30 years or so.

This scientific approach concerns a body of theories and methods that is much less coherent than would at first appear from the dozens of recent Chinese publications. A specific intention shows through these writings—that of providing a relatively united theoretical and practical front. However, publishing companies from Hong Kong and Taiwan often simply copy and publish treatises and manuals originating from mainland China. Moreover, in China itself, the same texts may appear under different authors or different publishing companies. This apparent duplication of works, owing to the lack of control of authorship rights in these three regions, adds to the partly false impression of coherence regarding the contents.

When using modern methods of analysis and investigation to look at the history of acupuncture, we need also to consider information collected through historical criticism, the sinological analysis of texts, and sociological and cultural studies. Such a rigorous and objective study will help to enrich the scientific approach and establish a fuller understanding of acupuncture, which in turn will allow for an expansion and development of the scientific approach.

In its restricted meaning, history is a chrono-logical sequence of facts, events, ideas and theories. We must take into account simultaneity or continuity in time, and the social, philosophical and epistemological background in which they appear. These issues apply also to acupuncture, the foundations for which were laid during the first millennium BC, at the heart of a civilization at the height of its development. To this day acupuncture has maintained its specificity and originality.

The ancientness of acupuncture does not justify a systematic acceptance of the Chinese vision of this particular technique. It does, however, oblige us to try to understand, not only how this therapy came into existence, but above all how it managed to establish the theoretical concepts that still underlie the tech-nique today.

Finally, we must not forget the constant pres-ence of TCM as a whole. This medical system has always tried to integrate and assimilate acu-puncture into its theoretical structures, giving the technique a dimension that extends far beyond the scope of a reflex therapy. As proof we have the Huang Di Nei Jing (or Nei Jing) (Husson 1973, Lu 1978, Sunu & Lee 1985, Van Nghi & Van Dong 1973, 1975, Veith 1972).

The Nei Jing

The Nei Jing, or the 'Classic (Jing) of internal (Nei) medicine of the Yellow Emperor (Huang Di)', the fundamental book of early acupuncture, takes a very prominent place in the history and making of TCM and, more importantly, of acupuncture. Here are some of the facts:

• Until recently it was the oldest text in our possession, although printed by Wang Bing in AD 762, that is, nearly 1000 years after it was supposed to have been assembled for the first time! It was certainly reshaped several times and some chapters were probably added by Wang Bing himself. Many contradictions can be found in the various chapters. It is however considered the 'Bible' of acupuncture and contains the essentials of the technique's theory.

• Text analysis dates some chapters to several centuries BC (not always the most interesting ones); others seem to have been written between the end of the second century and the beginning of the first century BC.

• The text was written in classical Chinese, which is concise, allusive, intellectual and some-times secretive. As a result there have been innumerable interpretations and commentaries.

• The few translations that have been pub-lished in Western languages (Husson 1973, Lu 1978, Sunu & Lee 1985, Van Nghi & Van Dong 1973, 1975, Veith 1972) must be approached with caution, not only because of the difficulties in understanding the text itself, but also because of the many terms related to physiological and patho-logical concepts of those times that don't always correspond with our modern knowledge. Actually we sometimes have no idea of what they are referring to!

• The work represents the starting point of a tradition of ideas. It is, indeed, the main reference for the many different schools of thought that have developed over the years and that have each applied their own meaning to the contents of this 'Bible'.

As far as TCM is concerned, in 1973 Chinese archaeologists unearthed from the tombs of Ma Wang Dui near Chang Sha (in the province of Hunan) fragments of texts dating from 168 BC (Unschuld 1986). These 'Prescriptions against 52 ailments' (Harper Donald 1982) contain many remedies based on spells, talismans and amulets, besides others that use herbal, animal or mineral extracts. This parallel existence of demonological and empirical therapies can still be found today. However, the most interesting part of this dis-covery is that the information about the more physiological aspects either confirm those found in the Nei Jing, or sometimes show different conceptual evolutions.

The Nei Jing is a compilation of various docu-ments originating at least in the first century BC. Its vision of acupuncture is coloured by the theories of the Chinese medical systems that were prominent at that time. It is therefore not easy to determine where the limits of acupuncture as an empirical technique end and where the process of phagocytosis and assimilation into a more general and complex system begins.

Astrology and other schools of thought, naturalism and social systems will thus each have coloured the way in which the Nei Jing was both observed and practised. The lack of objective rigour and of critical approach, very understandable for those times, allowed for the coexistence of contradictory theories, and for supposedly proven techniques to be combined together without exclusion. This process seems to us rather strange. However, different schools and publications abound throughout the centuries, as do ideas, theories and explanations.

THE NUCLEUS OF ACUPUNCTURE THEORY

This accumulation of different discourses gives little credibility to the history of acupuncture, at least in the early stages. However, if we look beyond this diversity we find a basic nucleus that gives a certain coherence to acupuncture practice. Directly based on observation and interpreted through a few fundamental concepts, it provides a relatively efficient therapeutic tool whose strength lies in a more or less conscious acceptance of its limitations.

One must try to understand the history before making a judgement about acupuncture, to understand the system before dismantling it, and to differentiate the useful from the fantastic and the efficient from the ornamental. To do this one must enter the structure of the system while keeping a critical mind and applying modern methods of thought. Take, for example, the following illustration. During the Shang dynasty (roughly the second part of the second millennium BC) diseases were attributed to the anger of ancestral spirits neglected by the living. Later on, during the next dynasty, the Zhou (roughly the first part of the first millennium BC), demons and devils became the cause of human sufferings. These evil spirits were supposed to enter the body and produce different torments. In order to get rid of them the shamans of those times used all kinds of talismans, amulets, magical decoctions

and ritual dances. Si Ma-Qian, a famous historian of the second century BC, describes the biography of a certain medical practitioner called Bian Que (Bridgman 1955, Ma 1992) who is supposed to have lived in the fifth century BC and performed many therapeutical 'miracles'. Another writer, Sun Si-Miao, a well-known doctor and acupuncturist living in the seventh century AD, mentions in his book Qian Jin Yao Fang (Prescriptions of a thousand pieces of gold, Despeux 1987) that Bian Que recommended the puncture of 13 points of the body corresponding to the presence of demons.

The presumed existence of Bian Que does not make it de facto a historical reality, although Si Ma-Qian had already developed an astonishing degree of critical skill. Could it be that these 13 'demon' points, which correspond to well-known acupuncture points, represent the beginning of modern acupuncture? It is certainly a possibility since most of the points still have precise indications today, although these have of course nothing to do with the presence of demons. The historical environment, however, is tainted by shamanistic practices and superstitions. To add to the problem, these 13 points have also been found in the Qian Jin Yao Fang as a treatment for psychiatric diseases and epilepsy!

Finally, it is also possible that Sun Si-Miao attributed these 13 points to Bian Que in order to enhance the importance of their use. The Chinese have a strong respect for the past and, because of this, discoveries and new concepts and ideas were often attributed to their ancestors. Indeed, this attitude still prevails in many fields.

What can we extract from this information? An unproven historical hypothesis was later adapted to vouch for a technique with little applicability. Take away the shamans and demons, however, and we are left with the empirical observation that links pain and its disappearance after the stimulation of a point. The first practitioners seemed to look for efficiency, albeit for reasons that are questionable today or that we would now consider unscientific. However, of striking importance is the relationship from cause to effect, which had been correctly observed and which represented without doubt the beginning of all scientific thought.

The theory of acupuncture soon found a structure, much more quickly than did herbal therapy, whose theories were constantly modified and improved over the course of the centuries to form the present-day profile. At the time of the Nei Jing (the contents of which show a reasonably organized trend of thought), medical prescriptions comprised long lists of medicinal formulae with no underlying theory. Moreover, superstition and misplaced pragmatism were often combined with the empirical logic of herbal, animal and mineral extracts. It is also true that, whilst simplistic in nature, the theory of acupuncture is complex and cannot withstand many modifications within the framework of traditional Chinese medical vision. Most of the basic information in acupuncture existed by the second century BC, as described in the Nei Jing, and this has undergone little change. The nucleus of this information concerns roughly two themes: the theory of meridians, points and related Organs or functions, and the philosophical and cultural concepts practically applied to explain health and disease in the living being.

Whether these explanations are scientific is of little importance here. What is important is the analysis and interpretation of phenomena taking place and observed in the human body in the light of a specific cultural environment. Why indeed should the scientific view have dominated the early days of acupuncture when science as we conceive it did not exist at that time? Does this mean then that Chinese medical thought was mistaken? And if so, up to what point? Does the archaic expression hide an error or just an anachronism?

We are confronted here with one of the major difficulties encountered by any twentieth century individual interested in acupuncture. The terminology used—established more than 2000 years ago, expressed in ideograms that possess a strong power of evocation, with many meanings depending on the context, and, more importantly, lacking equivalence with our modern terms—needs a semantic approach that only sinologists familiar with the field can provide. That is why the value of existing translations varies from one

to another. We must not assume, however, that the Chinese authors were protected from this weakness. As proof we have the numerous and different commentaries and annotations of the most important classical treatises, which make the work of translators all the more difficult. Paul Unschuld, a medical sinologist of international reputation, has grasped the problem very well. In his translation of the Nei Jing (The Classic of Difficulties) (Unschuld 1986), dating from the third century AD, he quotes the commentaries of more than 20 authors ranging from those times to the present day.

A long list of books, few of which are used, a long list of famous practitioners, and a few large and many small schools form the core of the history of acupuncture. Fortunately, a number of books have always been regarded more highly than others, for example the Zhen Jiu Jia Yi Jing (ABC of acupuncture), written by Huang Fu-mi in the third century, and translated in 1983 (Milkis 1986), or the Zhen Jiu Da Cheng (Compendium of acupuncture) of Yang J Z first published in AD 1701 (translated 1981), in which many practical and therapeutic suggestions can be found. The main ideas and theories, however, were already established during the era of the Nei Jing. So the evolution is poor and concerns only the following minor aspects:

1. the number of acupuncture points
2. the techniques of needle manipulation
3. the methods for choosing the points to be stimulated.

The official recognition of acupuncture and the control of its teaching and practice were seldom at the forefront of government thinking. Under the Tang and the Sung dynasties, representing the apogee of Chinese civilization, medical colleges were created to centralize the organization and teaching of medicine, of which acupuncture was naturally a part. Mostly, however, teaching and practice were left to private practitioners, the 'masters' who jealously kept their techniques and their 'secrets', and only ever passed them on to their disciples, seldom committing them to writing. This custom of master and disciple still exists today. The author of this chapter had to undergo, in 1970, a formal initiation by a master acupuncturist of his choice in Taiwan. This began with a harrowing bargaining session with an intermediary over tuition fees, and comprised a solemn and impressive ceremony before the ancestors' shrine, with bowing and the lighting of incense sticks and speeches, and ending superbly with an exquisite vegetarian banquet, and more speeches. In mainland China, from 1949 to the end of the Gang of Four, this practice disappeared, but as soon as a relative liberalization took place in medical practice it became once again part of the system.

We are fortunate that a number of famous acupuncturists have left fairly complete treatises giving details of theories and techniques. However, it was not until the second half of the twentieth century that complete and practical manuals were published.

The basic nucleus, common to acupuncturists of all times, all tendencies and all schools, is relatively easy to determine, although its limits are not very precise. It covers the knowledge of the following elements:

1. the pathways of the main and secondary meridians
2. the viscera or functions with which they have preferential relations
3. the acupuncture points, with their general functions and indications
4. the basic philosophical concepts, common to the medical system, which take here a concrete value
5. the instruments and the simplest techniques
6. the prescriptions of points, either for a general action or for a specific disease, including the necessary variations according to each individual case. Pain represents of course the field of preference, but one finds also quite a few functional syndromes.

Beyond this basic nucleus there is a whole world of theories and techniques, either specific to acupuncture or related to the Chinese medical system as a whole. Amongst other topics are the following:

1. Different categories of acupuncture points, representing particular systems of treatment; the balance between meridians, between different parts of the body, between meridians and viscera; the most important points according to a certain master or author; the symbolic points corresponding with a network of mutual influences such as the cycle of Five Elements; points following the hour and the date, or originating from a numerological relation; and hundreds of points located on meridian pathways, of which only a few belong to the basic nucleus.
2. The diagnostic procedure and its formulation. Here we are in the specific field of Chinese medicine in general.
3. The pathological patterns, the choice of points for a prescription, and how to justify this choice.
4. Numerous techniques of needle manipulation, each more complicated than the last.

It would seem from this account that acupuncturists have always treated every kind of disease with their techniques. Indeed, in the books one finds points and prescriptions for the treatment of tumours, tuberculosis, major bacterial infections, heart attacks and cerebrovascular accidents (CVAs). One could infer from this that Chinese acupuncturists lacked completely a reasonable sense of judgement by adhering to such an exaggerated extension of the powers of acupuncture. On the other hand it is necessary to remember the following issues:

1. Chinese acupuncturists usually have solid notions of TCM, and they know when medicinal prescriptions are more efficient than acupuncture.
2. In some cases, both methods are used together in the treatment of patients.
3. This apparent extension of acupuncture indications hides in fact a sound pragmatism. The practitioner knows what works best and what kind of treatment is most efficient, but why not use an extra technique, which might increase the chances of obtaining good results?

One gets the impression that scientific thought is a poor relation to the accumulated theories and techniques, coming mostly from abstract reasoning, numerological calculations and symbolic correlations, all of which bear little relation to reality.

Throughout the history of acupuncture the innovations, schools, theories and different reference systems are a constant proof of the trend against scientific thought. There are no barriers such as the ones raised by our modern methods of investigation, analysis and experimentation, or by leaning on critical arguments and using common sense.

Acupuncture then is often considered as a whole, whatever the approach, and sight is often lost of the basic nucleus, which is more consistent, more pragmatic, more constant and up to a point more reliable than the whole, and which has represented the strength of acupuncture over centuries. We must come back therefore to this nucleus, which is common to all treatises, all authors, all teachings and all practitioners.

THE MERIDIANS

Whether the concept of the meridians (Box 20.1) appeared before or after the concept of points is unknown, although the latter is more likely. Both are found in the Nei Jing, and the meridians are also mentioned in the 'Prescriptions against 52 ailments'. Meridians represent the preferential pathways of one of the categories of vital force, or 'energy', which are approximate translations of the Chinese term 'Qi'. Chinese medical thinkers were not very much interested in anatomy, and probably never tried to verify the macroscopic reality of these pathways. Their existence was

deduced from the many sensations, painful or abnormal, spontaneous or provoked, that an individual experienced even when in good health. These sensations appeared in an elongated or linear shape, like a strip. The earliest observations were concrete and correct, and were interpreted using the existing concepts of the times. However, there is no historical evidence covering the development of the meridian's pathways during the period from these earliest beginnings to their final description. It would indeed be fascinating to discover how this 'cartography' came about. As a matter of fact we find in the final circuitry of the meridians, zones and sections of different value as follows:

1. Some of these sections correspond with nervous pathways, though not especially the pathways of individualized nerves in the anatomical sense, but more the preferential pathway of a sensation when a nerve or a nervous trunk is stimulated. Here the correspondence is anatomical or neurophysiological.

2. Other pathways seem to be linked with the projection on the skin, or in the underlying structures, of groups of neighbouring cells within the spine, which would have a lower threshold for mutual influences. At the same time these groups of cells are related by other circuits to specific areas, tissues or organs. These probably correspond to particular levels of the spine.

3. Finally, some of these sections appear to have little anatomical or physiological justification, and shock our present-day common sense.

As far as the first two categories are concerned, one can imagine that they are the result of scrupulous and repeated observations of various sensations (pain, itching, burning, etc.), and even of the linear or strip manifestations of some dermatological diseases (herpes zoster, neuro-dermatitis). What, however, urged the medical practitioners to develop the third category, which probably represents an exaggerated extrapolation designed to complete those areas not covered by what we could call the justifiable categories? What was the cause of this overextension? Earlier texts than the Nei Jing could teach us a lot about the development and different evolutionary stages

---

Box 20.1 The 12 regular meridians

Yin meridians Interior, Zang (solid) Organs	Yang meridians Exterior, Fu (hollow) Organs
Lung (Hand Tai Yin)	Large Intestine (Hand Yang Ming)
Spleen (Foot Tai Yin)	Stomach (Foot Yang Ming)
Heart (Hand Shao Yin)	Small Intestine (Hand Tai Yang)
Kidney (Foot Shao Yin)	Bladder (Foot Tai Yang)
Pericardium (Hand Jue Yin)	Triple Energiser (Hand Shao Yang)
Liver (Foot Jue Yin)	Gall Bladder (Foot Shao Yang)

of this cartography. It is also worth noting that the boundaries between the concrete observations and the extrapolations are not always clear.

In Chinese medical thinking the meridians have a functional rather than anatomical base. Moreover, their physiology is based on the Chinese vision of Qi circulation and not on ours, which is expressed in terms of blood vessels or nerve pathways, of electric currents and neurotransmitters. The interpretation of the observations was developed according to the medical concepts of the era, expressed in terms of Qi and functions or Organs, and the relations between them. This leads us to examine the Qi and the Organs or functions.

THE QI

Of course Qi does not exist as a material substance in that it does not correspond to any kind of anatomical, nervous or hormonal entity. However, the concept of Qi in a medical sense is found in the pages of the Nei Jing:

1. In the beginning, the concept of Qi had nothing to do with medicine. It was at the centre of Chinese philosophical thinking, which was trying to define the relations between matter and change, substance and activity. Qi represented the energy that allowed change and activity, and was revealed in all the transformations and modifications observed in nature. Throughout the cultural and philosophical history of China, Qi was the subject of many thoughts and speculations, and was perceived in a wide variety of modalities.

2. Later, Qi became a popular concept and was even used in many vernacular expressions. For instance Sheng Qi, 'to produce Qi', means to be angry; Qi Ying, 'overflowing with Qi', means to be pleased with oneself; Yun Qi, the 'moving Qi', means chance; Qi Xing, the 'nature of Qi', means the character (of a person), etc.

3. Medical thought very quickly appropriated the concept of Qi. The body has a substance, it is made of matter and its existence shows in movements and changes: in the movements of the body and the mind; in the modifications of the

air inhaled and of ingested food; and in the modifications of the mind, feelings and behaviour caused by environmental information. So, very naturally, the concept of Qi found its place within the changing, internal relations of the body. It was considered to be a fundamental substance itself, although of a very subtle nature, whose function implied a potential for activity. So, for want of chemical and physical explanations, Qi was established as the source of all vital activities.

These activities are numerous and varied, even by the simplistic but at the same time complex standards of Chinese medical thought. Qi, this potential for activity, obviously had many different facets depending on the activities to which it was applied, and depending also on the components of the body. There were therefore many categories of Qi:

a. for the moving, fundamental substances such as the Blood, the Body Fluids and the Mind (considered also as an ethereal substance)

b. for each viscera or functional entity

c. for synthetic functions such as protection against the environment, nutrition, growth and development of the body, and circulation in the meridians.

In reading acupuncture treatises one falls under the impression that the Qi circulating in the meridians is the one and only manifestation of this concept in the body. This is partly true if one limits the pathological and therapeutic approach to disease to the meridian pathways. However, as soon as one increases the scope to include the many other functions of the organism such as respiration, digestion, thinking, etc., it becomes obvious that there are many different modalities of Qi.

In its cultural context, and taking into account the knowledge available at the time, this interpretation can be justified. It is true that the concept of Qi is an invention, and does not correspond with any specific physical or chemical reality. However, in some ways Qi has now moved from an abstract concept to a concrete notion by reflecting synthetically the potential hidden behind the activities of the organism. Qi became the reason for the very existence of these activities and the cause of organic movements, although its precise nature could not be determined. In this respect it leaves our scientific mind unsatisfied. However it does not pretend to be an objective reality; it is only the expression of an interpretation of phenomena. More importantly, it does not betray reality, because it does not claim to exist in the same way that an organ, a tissue or a function exists. It is rather the energetic motor that animates these organs, tissues and functions. It sheds light on vital activities. There is no scientific mistake as such; there is only the very intelligent use of a concept to explain the life of a body in all its manifestations. It does not even contradict our present knowledge; it is just a different way of expression, a different organization of data that we know to be of a chemical and physical order. It is a discrete but omnipresent concept.

Finally, the fact that TCM considered Qi to be a type of substance was irrelevant. More important were the different functions of Qi manifested in the many organic activities. In a way these activities were the very proof that something unseen existed.

THE ORGANS

The Organs belong mainly to the field of TCM, but we must examine a few aspects of the subject in relation to acupuncture for the following reasons:

1. The meridians are differentiated from each other by specific names that have nothing to do with the names of viscera. In classical texts they are mostly referred to by these specific names.

Each meridian is differentiated and named according to the following information:

a. whether it circulates through the upper limb, symbolized by the hand (Shou) or the lower limb symbolized by the foot (Zu).

b. which two ideograms represent the different categories of Yin and of Yang, in all six denominations: Tai Yang, Yang Ming, Shao Yang, Tai Yin, Shao Yin and Jue Yin.

Manuals would therefore describe the pathway of a meridian or indicate the use of points on that meridian by mentioning, for example, Shou Tai Yang, the Tai Yang meridian of the upper limb, or Zu Shao Yang, the Shao Yang of the lower limb.

2. At the same time, both the pathway of and the points along a particular meridian are supposed to be related in a physiological and therapeutic way with one particular Organ or function. So to the specific name of the meridian is added the name of the Organ or function.

Take, for example, the full name of a particular meridian: Shou Tai Yang Xiao Chang Jing. Shou is the hand (for the upper limb), Tai Yang is the specific name, in terms of modalities of Yin and Yang, that this meridian shares with another, Xiao Chang means literally Small Intestine, and Jing is the character for meridian.

The links between meridians and organs, even for the Chinese, are sometimes neither precise nor binding, and it does not automatically follow that to treat such and such an organ one has to use the points situated on the meridian related to it. The apparently systematic connection is due rather to the tendency to classify and organize in a logical way. The principle of the relation is stated, but when confronted with a practical application the choice will be more pragmatic.

A typical illustration is the following: the meridians supposedly related to the Large Intestine and to the Small Intestine both run on the upper limb to the face. However, the indications of these points only partly concern diseases of the intestines. They are mainly used for treating local or regional disturbances along their pathways. Moreover, in order to treat diseases or malfunctions of the intestines, practitioners will choose either points located on the skin projection of these organs on the back or on the abdomen, or points located on the lower limbs. These points have, from the reflex therapy point of view, more chance of being justified and effective than do points located on the upper limb.

The Chinese knew about anatomy, although not in any detail. The names given to the Organs or functions represent most of the large internal anatomical organs, from the heart to the large intestine, from the stomach to the bladder. Beyond the anatomical organ, however, the Chinese were much more interested in the concept of physiological functions. The functions that they attributed to each of the viscera had a wider range than those attributed to the named organ. Whilst these are not always in agreement with scientific knowledge, they are mostly in accordance with the Chinese way of organizing the results of observations. It must be noted, however, that the elaboration of the physiological functions of each of the Organs only began once the different concepts of acupuncture had already been fixed. It is only in the last few centuries that acupuncture has reached its present-day stage. Indeed, before our era acupuncture might well have enjoyed a more prominent role compared with the rest of TCM than it does today. At the same time, there might have existed different schools of thought and practice, running in parallel, and advocating the use of demonological medicine on the one hand, or herbal, mineral and animal prescriptions and the use of acupuncture on the other.

The first two categories of the meridians' pathway, as mentioned earlier, allow us to accept the hypothesis of reflex relations of different levels between meridians and the organs. This hypothesis, however, even in the eyes of the Chinese, did not represent an obligation of systematic relation. Some of the points on certain meridians will rarely be used for the treatment of organs after which the meridians are named. Pragmatism prevails over systematic organization.

To treat lung diseases the practitioner will use points located on the meridian that bears the name, as well as some points situated on the back or on the anterior part of the thorax in the projection zones on the skin corresponding to the lungs, and which belong to other meridians. On the other hand, the Bladder meridian, which is the longest of all and has 67 points from the fifth toe to the inner canthus of the eye, will seldom be used for treating bladder malfunctions. This is for two reasons. The first is obvious: the greater part of its pathway is in no way related to the bladder. The second is more subtle and belongs to the pathophysiological approach of TCM: most of the bladder problems will find their origin in malfunctions of other Organs such as the Kidneys or the Small Intestine.

The fondness of the first Chinese medical thinkers for classification, relations, numbers and balance is obvious. There are 12 meridians, 12 viscera or functions, divided into two groups of six Yin and six Yang, into two groups according to whether they circulate on the upper or the lower limbs, into two groups according to whether their beginning or their end is on the head or the trunk, and there are four groups of meridians that share these characteristics in an even way. In addition, the circulation of Qi in the meridians follows a set sequence, and reaches its peak in each meridian during 2 hours of the day or night (Fig. 20.1).

As in most of the systematic theories of TCM there is some truth in this, which must originate from correct observations. The circulation of Qi peaks in the Lung meridian between 3 and 5 a.m. and we know from experience that asthmatic crisis often occurs in the middle of the night. Qi peaks in the Large Intestine meridian between 5 and 7 a.m. and one of the first actions of the day is to empty one's bowels. After this comes the first meal of the day, which prompts the stomach into action. The Qi of the Stomach meridian is at

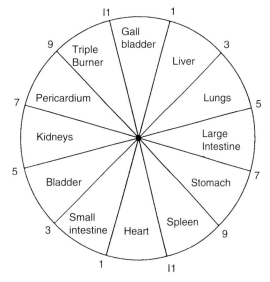

Figure 20.1 The 'midday–midnight law', showing the peak times of Qi in each of the meridians.

its peak between 7 and 9 a.m. These apparently logical correlations do not apply, however, to most of the meridians and correlated organs. The exaggerated extension of some logical relations into a whole system is a trend common to many theories of acupuncture and TCM.

The timings and distributions such as those mentioned above are very much favoured by the Chinese, satisfying their sense of rhythm, balance and harmony. It is difficult to ascertain, however, whether their concept of reality was different. Did they respect these classifications, as well as others that had the same arbitrary connotations, when confronted with a patient to be treated? Or did they rely more upon efficient empiricism? It seems that throughout history there have been partisans of each tendency. Even today there are traditional practitioners, though relatively few, who choose points in accordance with the hexagrams of the Yi Jing, the law of Five Elements, the hour and the date of treatment and other numerological systems.

A striking example is the theory called Zi Wu Liu Zhu. It is based on the use of the 66 Shu points related to the Five Elements, on the 10 Heavenly Stems and the 12 Earthly Branches, which, when combined, form the sexagenary cycle used to define the years. The 12 Earthly Branches also divide a day and a night into 12 hours. A system of relations was created by which, at each of the Chinese hours (corresponding to two of ours), there are one or two of the 66 Shu points which are 'open' and can therefore be stimulated in order to balance the Yin and the Yang of the body. This mathematical system has even been computerized for easy calculation of the points that are 'open' at each moment of the day. Although very elegant, this system is of course very questionable as far as therapeutic efficiency is concerned.

In the beginning there were six Yang viscera, five of them corresponding with anatomical organs and the sixth representing a kind of synthetic function, summarizing three groups of general functions, namely the cardiorespiratory, the digestive and the genitourinary. However, there were only five Yin viscera. In order to balance

the numbers, the Chinese created a sixth one, called the Pericardium. These Yin and Yang viscera were reflected in the names of the meridians. In practice, however, the points of the Pericardium meridian roughly duplicated those of the Heart meridian, and the points of the Triple Energizer meridian, the sixth Yang meridian, were mostly used for local or regional indications according to the areas covered by the meridian pathway. Once again the theoretical balance gave way to an efficient gesture.

The name of Triple Energizer (or Triple Warmer or Triple Burner) alludes to the heat generated by the body when one of its functions is predominant, symbolized by the work of a furnace transforming matter into energy that can be assimilated and used.

The same reasoning can be applied to all the point classification systems. Each meridian has a Yuan (Source) point, to be used in treating the related organ. Once again, in practice they are not all employed. The same applies to the Luo (Connecting or Collateral) points, the Xi (Accumulation or Cleft) points, those corresponding to the Five Elements, and those situated on the back, near to the spine, and corresponding each with one of the organs (Beijing College 1980, Cheng 1987).

It is essential to stress again that the names of anatomical organs linked with the 12 functions can be misleading. The physiological responsibilities of the Heart and of the Lungs correspond roughly with what we know scientifically. However, the functions of the Liver have very little to do with what science knows about the hepatic cells, and those of the Kidneys are a mixture of actions on water metabolism and actions related to the inherited trends of constitution, the potential activity acquired through nutrition and respiration, the growth and development of an organism and the sexual and reproductive capacities. The interesting thing is that practical treatment will aim at restoring the functions impaired and not especially at the well-being of an anatomical organ!

This is why the relations which exist between the meridians and the viscera are sometimes rather tenuous and fragile.

THE POINTS

In the Nei Jing 160 points are quoted, five centuries later their number has risen to 349, in the eleventh century Wang Wei-yi counts 354, and in the 'Acupuncture Compendium of Yang Ji-Zhou' (seventeenth century) there are 359. For our twentieth century mind several problems arise:

1. Their location. The Nei Jing does not give any location. The Jia Yi Jing of the third century gives insufficient details about how to locate the points, and later treatises don't fare any better. Why is this? Perhaps it is because this particular area was taught in a practical way with information passed on by word of mouth from master to disciple. The masters conferred importance upon the exact location of points. The disciples knew little, if anything, about anatomy and if the puncture of points was not precise there was the risk of piercing an organ, a large blood vessel or a nerve. The result is that throughout the centuries the teaching of acupuncture points has remained under the control of individual masters.

2. The precision of location. The precision of location depends very much on the methods used. These have multiplied over the years and, as they are no longer secret, are now published in modern manuals.

The various methods for locating points demonstrate the Chinese genius for scrupulous observation. Using sight, marks were registered on the surface of the body, for example bone reliefs, muscular bulges, body openings and skin creases. Using touch, the practitioner added palpable marks to the visual ones, for example the hollows between bones, muscle shapes or tendons. Some points, not apparent to sight or touch when the body was immobile, became visible or palpable in one or other positions of the body or limb. The practitioner also took into account the sensations experienced by the patient (some points being more sensitive than others), whether spontaneously or under the pressure of the finger.

This was not enough to locate all the points. The use of a precise measure of length was undermined by the variations in measurements from one person to another. So the Chinese developed a fairly original system: a unit of length particular to each individual, and therefore different for each person. Moreover, they divided the distances between some obvious body marks into a set number of units.

The collection of different methods produced a general technique for locating points. To this must be added the fact that the name given to each point was sometimes also an indication of its location.

Were these methods enough for the precise location of points to the exact millimetre? For some of them, yes. For many, however, they defined a particular area. The Chinese practitioners' awareness of this fact is reflected in the saying: 'What is important is to be on the meridian'. We certainly know that meridians were considered to be more like a band than a line.

Some modern authors (e.g. Mann 1992) tend to believe that acupuncture points do not exist, that there are only regions or areas. The truth lies probably somewhere between the two alternatives, as the different categories of points suggest.

3. The respective value of points. We must not believe that all points are equally significant. Many of them have only local and limited indications whilst others act upon neighbouring regions. A category of points is supposed to act from far away on another part of the body or on the functioning of an Organ. Some points are considered more important than others, and are regularly found in prescriptions, whereas numerous others are seldom mentioned.

To illustrate this let us look at the list of indications of a few points according to the Dictionary of Chinese Acupuncture published in 1985 simultaneously in Hong Kong and in China.

a. ST-1 (Chengqi), located just below the eye cavity: conjunctivitis, lacrimation, glaucoma, night blindness, blepharospasm, facial palsy. These are all local actions.

b. LI-15 (Jianyu), located at the tip of the shoulder: pain and stiffness in the shoulder, numbness of the upper limbs, spasms of the arm and hands, urticaria. Mostly local and regional actions, plus one indication of a general nature.

c. SP-6 (Sanyinjiao): located 3 'inches' above the inner malleolus: abdominal distension, due to insufficiency of the Spleen and Stomach, diarrhoea, irregularity of menses, abdominal masses, uterine haemorrhage, dysmenorrhoea, galactoschesis, spermatorrhoea, impotence, prospermia, enuresis, muscle atrophy at the lower extremities, insomnia, hysteria. A wide range of indications, digestive, gynaecological, sexual, two related to the psychological field, and one regional.

d. Houtinghui, an extrameridian point located behind the ear: tinnitus, deafness, mutism. Two local indications, and one that is often the consequence of a local condition.

The cartography of the acupuncture points is one thing. Their utilization is another. The value of each point is mainly dictated by its practical efficacy.

4. One unique point, general formulae or individual prescriptions? The policy of Chinese practitioners has always been to use as few points as possible. One of the reasons for this is that in the early days acupuncture needles were much thicker and longer than those used today and were therefore more aggressive and prone to create some damage, albeit minor. This 'economy' of needles and points reflected also the practitioner's mastering of the technique. Ma Dan-yang is said to have treated with only 12 points. Some practitioners limited themselves to using the points corresponding to the Five Elements. Others never stimulated more than two points at a time. But the dream of the unique point, vouching for the precision in diagnosis and in point prescription, remained in general what it is, a dream.

The other, much more frequent, tendency was to use formulae of points for each identified disease. These formulae were not completely rigid but represented a starting base to which other points were added according to the accompanying signs. Even though a disease might show itself differently from one patient to another, certain signs were constant. Here we see, although under another form, the idea of the basic nucleus applied to the formation of groups of preferential points for such and such an ailment.

What about the 'individual formula' advocated by the 'traditionalists'? This merely represents a variation of the above method. In 10 individual formulae for the same category of disease one will find the basic nucleus in each.

For more than 1000 years many manuals have given, for each point, a sometimes lengthy list of indications. However, the diseases or symptoms named do not automatically correspond with a modern category of identifiable disease (Kaptchuk 1983), and our critical minds must assess those indications that are credible and those that are not.

These manuals advise also, for various symptoms and diseases, the points to be stimulated. Only recently, however, have manuals been available that are both of practical use and demonstrate various methods for choosing points, which can be immediately applied.

5. The extrameridian points. These are points not located on meridian pathways. The Nei Jing and later treatises mentioned a few of these points, and their numbers grew rapidly thereafter. Today there are some 1500, including many 'new points', which are supposed to have been recently discovered. Each point has a name, a location and a few indications. More than 30 of these points are used frequently in practice; others correspond (like some meridian points) with trigger points. Most of these extrameridian points can, however, be criticized. Many are either very close together or very close to the meridian points, so it is difficult if not impossible to differentiate their location in practice. For example, in the small area between the angle of the lower jaw and the mastoid process one is supposed to locate about 20 acupuncture points belonging to all categories. How can we imagine that each of these points has a specific location and specific indications?

The same reservations discussed above with regard to meridian points apply to the extrameridian points. The accumulation of indications has not been subjected to a reasonable and pragmatic assessment. This does not mean, however, that we must retain only those actions that can be explained by our actual knowledge of reflex therapy. There still exists a field of neurophysiological relations that has to be explored, and might result in the justification of the use of this or that point for a symptom or a disease that at the present time seems illogical.

THE YIN–YANG

The Yin–Yang, symbolized by the symbol in Figure 20.2, is a splendid cultural concept, perhaps the most beautiful concept in Chinese civilization. It is also one of the major reasons for the constant condemnation and rejection of acupuncture. Perhaps this is because the concept is often misunderstood, oversimplified, and 'cliché'. It is true that if we believe that the Yin–Yang represents opposing aspects such as night and day, white and black, man and woman, etc. then we reduce the concept to a primitive and folkloric system of classifications with little purpose in scientific terms. Its scope is, however, much greater than this. Indeed, the very fact that it has taken root in the Chinese medical system at all levels demonstrates its very significant concrete value.

In the field of acupuncture this concept, as it is presented in the Nei Jing (Chs 5, 6 and 7 of the Su Wen), concentrates on the classification of meridians in different categories of Yin and Yang, as well as on the symptoms that appear when the Yin and Yang are disturbed. It is also linked with classifications of a spatial or structural order, assembling a certain number of opposing and complementary couples like upper and lower, Interior and Exterior, Heaven and Earth, clear and turbid, Cold and Heat, Blood and Qi, Water and Fire, etc. Disease is thought to be the exaggerated predominance of one aspect of the couples, breaking thereby the harmonious balance

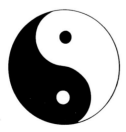

Figure 20.2 Yin and Yang Symbol of Taiji, the 'Great Unity'.

between them. The system remains, however, unsophisticated, and no matter how attentively one reads the Nei Jing, it is still difficult to find many practical elements within it.

Within the general framework of TCM, which as we know was constructed over many centuries, the concept of Yin–Yang became a key issue with much subtlety, which was adaptable to the complex reality of the human being. Yin–Yang became essential to the understanding of the phenomena observed, to the organization of symptoms, to the formulation of diagnoses, to the categories of pathological patterns, to the principles of treatment and to the practical applications. Its full dimension appeared mostly in the field of medicinal treatment. We find ourselves here, far from the sometimes disorderly observations and statements of the Nei Jing, which in fact represented the beginning of a prolonged way of thinking. Aspects that were partly naturalistic, partly abstract, progressively gave way to a system of classification that was much closer to organic reality. In this way the concept of Yin–Yang, with its mainly practical aims, established a central place in the Chinese medical system.

It became the pivot of the diagnostic procedure. Signs that were evident from patient examination were organized according to the general categories of Yin and Yang. These were then further categorized on the basis of three other couples: Interior and Exterior, Cold and Heat, Excess and Deficiency. This basic pattern had a mainly didactic objective, and Chinese practitioners recognized that reality was in fact much more complex. The variety of individual expressions of a disease, the interferences, the mutual influences and the evolutions formed a body of reasoning that moved as close as it could to organic reality, and as far as it could away from the earliest, simplistic classifications. The number and diversity of expressions of the Yin–Yang summarized, therefore, the individuality of each particular case.

Experience and the accumulation of symptoms therefore allowed signs to be attributed to a particular disorder: of the general state of the body; of a fundamental substance; of one of the viscera and functions; or of a mixture of two or more of these elements. The diagnosis was subsequently formulated in terms of Excess or Deficiency, Heat or Cold, and Yin and Yang was applied to a fundamental substance, a function or an Organ. This procedure is one of the most fascinating parts of TCM as different levels, categories and states are combined to define each individual case.

However, no part of Chinese medicine escapes criticism because it is, by definition, a closed and exaggerated system with false or misguided interpretations and unjustified extrapolations. What must be underlined here is the importance of the logical procedure that defined the countless facets of diseases and which presided over the development of Chinese medical thinking. It took a long time, however, for this logic to become sufficiently coherent in the domain of medical treatment.

Where is acupuncture positioned in this evolution? It has always followed two paths, at the same time parallel and intermingled. The first one is represented by the basic nucleus, applied practically to symptoms of pain and to some functional disorders. If one searches through 10 manuals and compares the points suggested for sciatic neuralgia, stiff neck, a sprained ankle, anxiety, irritability, facial palsy or insomnia, one finds a common group of points, and some others that vary according to the individual situation or to the differential diagnosis of a disease presenting similar symptoms. The basic nucleus, in dealing with pain patterns, refers mostly to abnormalities in the circulation of Qi along the meridians. So the acupuncture diagnosis is usually quite simple: obstruction in the circulation of Qi in one or several meridians, leading to pain, swelling and reduction of mobility. That is why, at this level, it is not really necessary to use the whole diagnostic procedure of TCM, and why it is quite possible to practise acupuncture within certain limits and without a deep knowledge of TCM!

The other path, much more ambitious, and also much more questionable, leads directly into the heart of the medical system. Acupuncture points find their indications according to the diagnostic procedure mentioned earlier, expressed in terms of Yin and Yang, or in one or other of the subcategories. So in theory any pathological pattern

could be therapeutically treated by acupuncture. In clinical practice, however, practitioners have progressively differentiated the respective fields of acupuncture, medicinal treatment, diet, massage and gymnastics.

Let us take the simple example of bronchopneumonia. The diagnosis in TCM would probably be something like: 'an attack of Wind-Heat in the Lungs with accumulation of Phlegm'. According to the theory of TCM, applied to acupuncture, there are points for dispelling the Wind, for reducing the Heat, for sustaining the Lungs and for eliminating the Phlegm. A formula of points could be created and an acupuncture treatment applied. What, however, happens in reality? Before the intrusion of Western medicine, Chinese practitioners would most certainly have chosen a medicinal prescription to reduce the Heat (antipyretic), to fluidify the Phlegm and help expectoration, to stimulate the respiratory function and help breathing, etc. Nowadays what do practitioners do? Prescribe antibiotics! Acupuncture or herbal treatment, or both, could eventually be of some help, but it would certainly not be as efficient as an antibiotic, at least statistically and in this example.

We are far from the original concept of Yin–Yang. We have, nevertheless, followed the impulse created by its evocative powers, its adaptability, versatility and subtlety, all of which have transformed the concept into an instrument of classification of the pathophysiological dynamics. Over time the concept moved closer to reality and, although expressed in archaic terms, this was based upon concrete observation and experience.

THE FIVE ELEMENTS

Even more than Qi and Yin–Yang, the concept of Five Elements and its regulating 'laws' have been the target of the modern disparagers of acupuncture. This is with some reason, because if Qi and Yin–Yang have been made to adapt as far as possible to the multiplicity of individual pathophysiological situations, the law of Five Elements, on the contrary, proposes an exaggerated simplification of the physiological and pathological relations by following the principles of symbolic correlations (or systematic correspondences). What exactly are these?

A school of thought in the fifth century BC (actually called the Yin–Yang school and headed by a certain Zou Yin) chose from the natural world five 'elements' that seemed to predominate: Fire, Earth, Metal, Water and Wood (Fig. 20.3). These elements were interrelated either in terms of production or in terms of domination and these two sets of relationships produced different sequences. The Yin–Yang school applied one set of these sequences to the succession of dynasties. Later, these rules of relationships were applied to all the categories to be found in nature, which were artificially divided by five: planets, grains, animals, cardinal points (to which a 'centre' had to be added), colours, climates, etc.

These correspondences and lists were not classified beyond their group of five, which showed the existence of relationships similar to those between the Five Elements. One can imagine the success of this vision for Chinese thinkers of all kinds and schools, who had so much affinity for order, balance, distribution and classification. From the second century BC

onwards this rule of relationships was found everywhere. It was, however, often criticized by rational thinkers, not because of its practical use, but because it encouraged infinite similarities in all fields, such as the Yin–Yang in its first stage of development and the distribution of couples. This was an abstract stage in the division of concrete aspects.

This rule of classification of macrocosmic phenomena was revived by the medical thinkers when it was applied to the microcosm, man and the organism. Viscera, sense organs and tissues were said to correspond to each of the Five Elements. However, the thinkers applied the system of mutual influences of production, domination and others only to the five Yin Organs, the Heart, Spleen, Lungs, Kidneys and Liver. As far as the other parts of the body were concerned, the system did not go further than the first stage of classification, without the notion of mutual influences. The physiological and pathological relationships existing between these five Yin Organs were dictated by the relations between the elements of nature. Moreover, it would be enough, on the therapeutic level, to favour this or that sequence of influence to obtain a result! No wonder people were fascinated by this elegant and synthetic method. We can imagine how arbitrary and artificial some of these reasonings might have been.

Acupuncture was also integrated into this system of relations. Each meridian had five special points, which corresponded with the Five Elements, and the use of these points was guided by the relationships existing between the Elements. The Nan Jing, in the second century AD, records a detailed account of the therapeutic potential of these points. We find this unacceptable since we can see only an abstract theory remotely related to organic reality, and not particularly useful in clinical practice.

The more Qi and Yin–Yang became part of the pathophysiological complexity of clinical practice, the more the rule of Five Elements appeared to apply external relations to an internal, unrelated field. How is it then that this 'law' enjoyed so much success, and that even nowadays treatises and practitioners vouch for it?

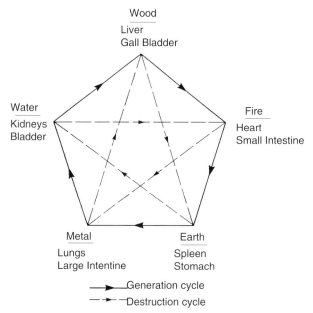

Figure 20.3 Law of the Five Elements.

The answer is simple: it is a question of perspective. The relationships between the Elements within the two sequences can be applied to all situations. Whether in the direction of production or domination, or away from it, each Organ is in contact with all the other Organs. There are therefore no physiological or pathological relationships that are not provided by the system. So, whatever the diagnosis, whatever the evolution, the relationships between the Organs are to be found in the sequences.

One can see the importance of this statement. The physiological relations between Organs, as well as their mutual pathological influences, follow the biological rules of the human body, and the therapeutic choices derive from clinical observation and experience. They can always be expressed in terms of Elements because the complete rule has covered all possibilities. Outwardly, diseases and treatments seem to follow this rule when in fact they are following the rules of the human organism, and are compared only with such and such a relationship between the elements. This parallel way of expression does not carry relationships of cause and effect. It is not because particular relations exist between Elements that these relations are going to be found between the Organs. The appearance of systematic correspondences, as much in classification as in pathophysiological dynamics, has not always been perceived in this way, and has often been confused with reality, as in so many treatises and schools.

The 'law' of Five Elements, condemned as an uncompromising model of dynamic relations within the body, is restored when it is considered as a method of systematic and organized expression of organic and clinical reality.

On the other hand, in the field of acupuncture, we find it difficult to accept the five Shu points and their therapeutic use according to the 'law' as a reflection of any kind of reality.

The Five Elements in Chinese medicine, even more than the five Shu points of acupuncture, are not part of the basic nucleus. It was necessary, however, to examine this concept in its proper and correct perspective.

Summary

The art and science of acupuncture has developed through a variety of routes and for a variety of reasons: practical, political, financial and cultural. Initially, the theory of acupuncture was firmly observation based, but the Chinese cultural love of symmetry and order caused the nucleus of practically based observation to be filled out and rounded off, so that it is now difficult to determine in the laws and theories that have been handed down to us by tradition where the scientific logic ends and the fantasy begins.

There has always been a spectrum in the way Chinese masters have interpreted the tradition of acupuncture, but throughout it there has run a strongly pragmatic approach to treatment; the theory is there to be used only in so far as it helps in the selection of an effective point prescription. In our modern use of acupuncture, we must take the same line.

It is well worth delving deeply into the traditional and cultural aspects of Chinese acupuncture. This is a fascinating intellectual exercise in itself, but far more importantly it enables us to distinguish what is of therapeutic value out of the beautifully constructed, but artificial, symmetry that is the traditional theory of acupuncture.

REFERENCES

Beijing College of Traditional Chinese Medicine, Shanghai College of Traditional Chinese Medicine, Nanjing College of Traditional Chinese Medicine, and the Acupuncture Institute of Traditional Medicine (1980) Essentials of Chinese acupuncture. Foreign Languages Press, Beijing
Bridgman R F 1955 La Médecine dans la Chine Antique. In: Mélanges Chinois et Bouddhiques, vol X. Institut Belge des Hautes Etudes Chinoises, Bruxelles, pp 17–24

Cheng Xin-nong (ed) 1987 Chinese acupuncture and moxibustion. Foreign Languages Press, Beijing
Despeux C (trans) 1987 Prescription d'acupuncture valant mille onces d'or: traité d'acupuncture de Sun Si-miao du 7 ème siècle. Guy Trédaniel, Paris
Harper Donald J 1982 Wu Shi Er Bing Fang: translation and prolegomena. University of California Press, Berkeley
Husson A (trans) 1973 Huang Di Nei Jing Su Wen.

Association Scientifique des Médecins Acupuncteurs de France, Paris

Kaptchuk T 1983 The web that has no weaver. Congdon and Weed, New York

Lu C H (trans) 1978 The Yellow Emperor's Classic of Internal Medicine and the Difficult Classic. Academy of Oriental Heritage, Vancouver

Ma K W 1992 The roots and development of Chinese acupuncture: from prehistory to early 20th century. Acupuncture in Medicine. 10(Suppl):92–99

Mann F 1992 Reinventing acupuncture: a new concept of ancient medicine. Butterworth Heinemann, London

Milkis C, Andrès G (trans) 1986 Zhen Jiu Jia Yi Jing. Revue de l'Association Française d'Acupuncture

The Canon of Acupuncture, Huangti Nei Ching Ling Shu 1985, compiled by Ki Sunu and Yunkyo Lee. Hong Sung Enterprises, Seoul

Unschuld P U (trans and annot) 1986 Nan Jing. University of California Press, Berkeley

Unschuld P 1982 Ma Wang-dui Materia Medica: a comparative analysis of early Chinese pharmaceutical knowledge. In: Zinbun Memoirs of the Research Institute for Humanistic Studies. Kyoto University Press

Van Nghi N, Van Dong M (trans from Vietnamese) 1973 Hoang Ti Nei King So Wen, Vol 1

Van Nghi N, Van Dong M (trans from Vietnamese) 1975 Hoang Ti Nei King So Wen, vol 2

Veith I 1972 The Yellow Emperor's classic of internal medicine. University of California Press, Berkeley

Yang J Z 1981 Zhen Jiu Da Cheng 1981 (French trans) in Editions Darras, Paris

Zhang R F, Wu X F, Wang N S 1985 The illustrated dictionary of Chinese acupuncture. Sheep's Publication Hong Kong; People's Medical Publishing House, Beijing

21

The future

Simon Hayhoe

A constant theme throughout this book is that, despite its long tradition and the enthusiasm of its practitioners, there is inadequate evidence for the efficacy of acupuncture, and more research is needed. There is no lack of publications, indeed there are many thousands of case reports, uncontrolled trials and even controlled trials with inadequate numbers to give a statistically meaningful result, but it is evident from the system reviews in this book that there are large areas with little or no evidence to support the substantial reliance placed on acupuncture in the East, or its popularity in the West. In view of the anecdotal benefit to so many for so long, it would be surprising if acupuncture did not prove efficacious for at least some of the traditional indications, so time spent on research is reasonably likely to bear fruit with positive results and is thus worthy of attention from experienced academic medical research workers.

This invites the question of why such an enormous volume of poor quality research is published, but so little that offers reliable clinical evidence. The causes are not difficult to find and most should be simple to rectify given goodwill in the right places.

CHINESE RESEARCH

The greatest volume of acupuncture publications comes from China, where a very different attitude to research exists. The Chinese 'know' that acupuncture works and therefore regard it as almost unethical to have a control group receiving a placebo or any other 'less effective' treatment. So the Western standard of the randomized, controlled trial is not even aspired to, being applied only by those few doctors who have had some training in the West. There is also a cultural tendency to overstatement, with an accepted exaggeration of benefits, so that any patient who feels better has had a 'miraculous cure' and anyone who has not actually got worse is included as a 'success'. Thus reported success rates of 100% are common and a recent review of journal articles found no success rate less than 87.5%. This is really a problem of translation since, where the lesser grades of benefit are excluded and only 'cure' or 'marked improvement' are accepted, a more reasonable success rate of around 70% emerges, showing that there is genuinely no intention to mislead, just a cultural difference in emphasis. Unfortunately this is not generally recognized in the West and Chinese reports are thus often needlessly rejected as simply unbelievable.

The majority of Chinese research is published in national journals and never becomes available in Western languages. Papers that are published in the West are usually translated by official translators rather than medical staff, so that often medical concepts are mistranslated and research techniques misunderstood; giving rise not only to the success rate problems, but to such unlikely diseases as 'gastroptosis' and 'wind stroke'.

Western authors normally refer to other literature on the same subject and discuss the relevance of their results to the findings of other experts. It is rare to find this in Chinese articles, and if there is discussion the references are usually given in Chinese characters—totally unavailable to Western assessment. With the difficulties involved in converting the philosophical and diagnostic basis of TCM into Western medical terms, it is not surprising that Chinese acupuncture research papers are viewed with suspicion.

How can these rather fundamental problems be resolved? Much of the difficulty arises from cultural differences that seem immutable, although no doubt as East–West trade and cooperation patterns become more comfortably established the differences will blur. What can be done is first to encourage proper research technique using adequately controlled trials—easy to say, but difficult to achieve: it is not until Western research papers are more widely read in China (and this is probably true of Eastern Europe as well) that they will have a peer model to follow. Perhaps I could set the ball rolling by sending my old medical journals to Chinese acupuncturists. But, more practically, a better means of translation must be provided, using medical linguists who are capable of translating concepts rather than mere words. The baffling nomenclature of TCM is a potent barrier to understanding what is essentially logical and, if explained in Western terms, surprisingly acceptable.

EXPERIENCE

The second major cause of low research quality is inexperienced researchers operating from general practice or small hospital units, with inadequate patient numbers, difficulty in finding suitable controls and no statistical advice.

Western acupuncture has tended to be practised by lone enthusiasts who are keen to promote the cause of acupuncture by lecturing, writing articles and research, but have little idea of how to go about it. In the first two cases their enthusiasm shows through to stir the listener or reader, and experience is soon gained; research, unfortunately, needs more than enthusiasm: it also needs expertise. There is nothing more frustrating than to find that a research project is rendered worthless after months or even years of work, by a minor point of design that could easily have been adjusted at the start. Not only is it a waste of time for the author, but it is ethically unfair on the patients involved. The following problems crop up regularly:

1. authors claim their patients come for acupuncture treatment, so a control group is unacceptable
2. patient and disease selection are inadequately defined, making the results difficult to interpret; for instance, a trial of facial pain has

included postherpetic neuralgia (notoriously resistant) and TMJ pain (highly responsive)

3. no statistical advice has been taken, so that inadequate numbers are entered into the trial to allow a statistically significant result

4. even if all these errors have been avoided, the final paper is often presented for publication in a format that invites instant rejection; the standard scientific layout of introduction, method, results and discussion is ignored so that important information such as needling technique is omitted, graphs and tables are unlabelled and seem to bear no relationship to the text, and the statistics are unconvincing with no standard deviation or other means of checking their accuracy.

University departments in teaching hospitals, which might have brought some measure of research expertise to the subject, have not generally shown much interest, an honourable exception being the anaesthetic unit at the Queens, Belfast, which has very effectively explored the use of PC-6 in nausea and vomiting. On the whole, if university staff do enter the field, not having had much training in acupuncture they make fresh errors, which could prove even more disastrous for medical acupuncture than those of the enthusiastic but inexperienced researchers.

The difficulty here is that the academics often have no feel for acupuncture, which is as much an art as a science at the moment, and tend to choose unsuitable points and methods of stimulation for the condition being investigated. Under the tutelage of non-medical acupuncturists, 'sham' controls have been selected that, although not using the traditional method of stimulation at the traditionally effective points, are none the less active, sometimes obviously so when viewed from a neurological standpoint as discussed in various chapters of this book. As a result, the trials show acupuncture to be no more effective than the control, which is erroneously thought of as an inactive placebo. Unfortunately, well-written-up trials of this sort, with excellent research design and perfect statistical handling, are readily published and then combined in meta-analyses to give

a probably erroneous impression of the efficacy of acupuncture in general.

A number of helpful changes could be made that ought to sort out these anomalies associated with research personnel. Here the question of cost appears at last. The late Professor Dundee once in conversation assessed the cost of his PC-6 research in Belfast at over £50 000, so the sums involved are not easily raised privately unless the cost of salaries can be avoided.

There is an urgent need for research grants to be made available to teaching hospital academic units for acupuncture research in a wide variety of specialties: dermatology, ENT, gastrointestinal, etc. But it is essential that practical advice on clinical technique and the suitability of placebo controls is given by an experienced medical acupuncturist, so that researchers avoid the mistake of assuming that any form of needling other than traditional Chinese acupuncture must be ineffective—there is still a touching belief in the magic of Chinese medical tradition, despite the down to earth evidence of modern neurophysiology as quoted widely in this book.

Money is not enough to provide the stimulus for research. There must be an interest in the subject and a reasonable expectation of a positive outcome. This can be induced only by our enthusiastic lecturer and writer of general acupuncture reviews: very often the general practitioner who is keen to do research, but lacks the expertise. If only that expertise were made available, what a rich source of enthusiasm could be channelled into research.

The simplest way to do this is for medical acupuncture associations to organize research committees, with a statistician, to give expert advice on the construction of trials, and for their journals to publish articles on research methodology, including a crash course in medical statistics and how to write a scientific paper, so that the enthusiastic amateur can produce work that shows the attention to detail and statistical sophistication of the academic researcher. Such a committee has been set up in Great Britain and already the standard of research articles being offered to the Society Journal (Acupuncture in Medicine) has noticeably improved. Other useful roles of the research committee are to coordinate multicentre trials, which are often the only way of accumulating sufficient numbers for statistical significance in general practice, particularly when investigating non-painful disease, and to assist in the planning of meta-analyses and systematic reviews, which have tended to suffer from either inappropriate analysis if performed by an academic, or unsystematic technique if by a medical acupuncturist.

THE JOURNALS

Finally, the Western journals that publish acupuncture papers, or in some cases don't publish them, are themselves an unexpected cause of the continuing lack of research articles. There are a few journals specifically for research and rather more devoted to TCM, but the majority of specialist acupuncture journals are in reality the magazines of national associations dedicated to publishing the news and views of members rather than encouraging research papers. This is a very necessary function, but has the disadvantage in a journal of giving the impression that there is no article of note within its covers. As a consequence, the medical database compilers will not list the journal, its readers do not take its contents seriously and have no good model to follow for their own research; so the standard of article never improves, and other medical readers conclude that acupuncture really isn't worthy of serious attention. Thus, when a reasonable article is submitted to a mainstream medical journal it is very difficult to persuade the peer reviewers that it is of sufficient importance to publish. Because little of worth is published, there is no stimulus to research. We have become firmly enclosed within this no-chicken-no-egg circle, with lots of interesting, but academically impoverished, journals circulating to a limited readership of society members.

It is unfair to expect more from this type of journal, which is really a superior newsletter, but I have several times noticed the same mediocre research articles reappearing in a selection of these journals, sometimes in different languages, over 2 or 3 years. Basic errors, such as percentage observations not adding up to 100%, have remained uncorrected throughout. There seems to be no peer review operating, nor do the editors

usually have the experience to challenge research technique themselves.

A lot needs sorting out here; none the less this should prove the cheapest route to more, available, quality research papers. It is surprisingly difficult to make the change from a magazine to a scientific journal, and in many ways I think a complete change could be counterproductive, as the news and views, photos and cartoons are needed to retain a readership and encourage the casual browser to move from the light material to serious articles and then, with luck, return for more. The difficulty really is in attracting research articles in the first place, since there are simply not enough to go round, leaving each journal with perhaps one per issue: insufficient to break that vicious circle and start generating new researchers.

My solution is to amalgamate the clinical and scientific content of all these society journals into a small number of carefully produced periodicals, perhaps a couple in English and one each in the other internationally used languages. With modern computer and design technology these can readily form the base around which each local society can wrap its own news and views magazine, enabling every acupuncture society to have an individualized journal. This has the advantage of gathering together all the research articles in a few publications and making them available to a really wide international readership, but without losing the attractiveness of the magazine approach. Readers are retained and treated to an improved diet of more and better research, the editors more rapidly gain experience in peer review and preparing research articles for publication, smaller societies that could not afford to produce their own journals are now able to buy in cheaply a ready-made issue, and the medical databases should be happy to accept the international journal provided the name and the page numbering of the scientific core remains the same for all national variants.

There is no doubt that a positive report of technically competent research breeds more work on similar topics. The protocol has already been worked out and success is likely, with probable quotation in future articles—what more could any author want? The perfect example is Dundee's investigation of nausea and vomiting using PC-6, which has led to a current total of 35 controlled trials on the same subject from 10 centres. Likewise, in our efforts to upgrade 'Acupuncture in Medicine', we have found that now randomized, controlled trials have started to feature regularly, we are being sent more trial reports from all over the world. Many are flawed, often by a failure to randomize or by inadequate blinding, so we are featuring a series of articles on research technique to help future authors. I know that other journals are working towards a similar goal. United we could have more control over quality, having sufficient material to reject the poorer papers, and thus achieve more rapidly the high standard needed to gain recognition of acupuncture's potential by the medical hierarchy.

EDUCATION

This brings me to the other major change that is to be looked for in the practice of acupuncture in future years: incorporation into the undergraduate curriculum, with consequent more widespread acceptance as part of standard medical practice.

There is already a fair degree of medical recognition by doctors, particularly the younger ones, that acupuncture benefits patients, but their understanding of the subject still relies on press and television reports that invariably have an orientation towards the bizarre. The average doctor, if asked how acupuncture is supposed to work, will mutter something about balancing the channels and restoring vital energy; those who have read this book will tell another, more scientific, story. So many patients now seek acupuncture treatment, often from non-medical therapists, that, whatever their attitude, doctors need to know the facts, and the ideal time to present the facts is at medical school. Several British universities now provide lectures on acupuncture to their medical students and one, Exeter, has a chair in Complementary Medicine (the first in the world). This is a start, but all medical students need to be exposed to clinical acupuncture as well as lectures, so medical schools will need to plan for this addition to their curriculum now. Since acupuncture has always been practised as

an integral part of medicine, it seems that a basic training in medical science should be a prerequisite for learning acupuncture.

The aim of this undergraduate teaching is partly to dispel the myths and enable future doctors to give knowledgeable advice on when acupuncture is an appropriate form of treatment, but more importantly to encourage them to learn more of the subject so that the pool of doctors capable of using acupuncture increases year by year. The stage must come when acupuncture is at last rightfully seen as an integral part of medical practice rather than an individual, alternative, therapy.

Medical acupuncturists at present regard their subject as a specialty in its own right, but it can very reasonably be argued that it should not be, any more than is the use of, say, local anaesthetic injections. Like local anaesthesia, there will similarly be those who are expert at the full range of techniques, but consultants in all hospital specialties should be capable of using the acupuncture methods applicable to their own subject; so that these can be considered along with any other suitable form of treatment for every patient, allowing the most appropriate to be chosen.

Likewise, although it is not necessary for every GP to be an effective acupuncturist, at least one in each group practice should be capable of basic acupuncture techniques, enough to treat musculoskeletal pain and a few other easy problems, and all GPs need the background knowledge to give advice and make appropriate referrals.

Once suspicion of the unknown and misunderstanding associated with the oriental tradition of acupuncture have been overcome, GPs ought to be confident to perform basic general treatments, while consultants should be able to give a specialized acupuncture service, keeping abreast of research and clinical advances in the same way as they do for all other methods of treatment in their field. There will then inevitably be an upsurge in the use of acupuncture in areas for which it has been proved effective, as such a simple, safe technique, that is already popular with the public, cannot fail to recommend itself to the medical profession in preference to more physically or pharmacologically aggressive treatments.

The wider use of acupuncture in hospital and general practice should not involve any additional costs, indeed it is likely that savings will be made on drugs, on referrals, and possibly on surgical time. Where new funding may be required is in the medical schools. If staff are expected to teach acupuncture to the students, they must themselves be taught. I would envisage the need for combined clinical, research and teaching posts, initially to train existing clinical staff, but ultimately to give the undergraduate lectures and organize their practical exposure to acupuncture, as well as providing an expert referral service for difficult cases and coordinating research projects within the hospital and in local general practice.

ACUPUNCTURE ASSOCIATIONS

In 1983 a group of medical acupuncture societies banded together to form the International Council of Medical Acupuncture and Related Techniques (ICMART). Their aim was to encourage a scientific approach to the investigation and use of acupuncture and thus to promote its medical acceptance worldwide. To this end, ICMART recommends a training programme that balances modern theory with traditional practice, and organizes regular congresses and seminars on the scientific theme. There are now over 40 national medical acupuncture societies as members, all aspiring to the scientific approach.

The West has recently assimilated a large number of societies from Eastern Europe that have a substantial and enthusiastic membership, but have been restricted in their scientific advance by lack of access to both Western and Chinese journals. It is important that these new national societies develop an understanding of modern acupuncture theory and that the enthusiasm of their members is guided into beneficial research.

Medical acupuncture societies throughout the world have been offering courses for doctors for many years now. That they have been successful in explaining the benefits of acupuncture to a doubting medical profession is witnessed by the number of course attenders who have joined their local society and become sufficiently enthusiastic to remain as long-term members; membership of the British Medical Acupuncture Society, for instance, has grown over the last 15 years from 80 to 1600.

Most courses were traditionally orientated at first, but now that so much more is understood of the basic science of acupuncture, doctors expect the subject to be presented to them in a Western, scientific manner, finding the ancient Chinese theories incompatible with modern knowledge. The points used remain essentially the same whichever approach is taught, but the number of hours in a Western course can be dramatically reduced for medical practitioners, as they have already learned sufficient in their medical training to give a firm base for the scientific theory and practice of acupuncture. None the less, the fund of accurate observation inherent in the Chinese tradition must not only be retained, but needs scientific investigation.

Just as Chinese herbal treatment is being analysed by drug companies in the search for new medicaments, so traditional acupuncture is likely to offer detail that will advance the understanding of modern physiology. In order to quell the medical sceptics, research has necessarily had to concentrate on demonstrating that the effects of acupuncture are more than placebo. This leaves the really important questions unasked: Which points, how to stimulate them and why? The answers could open the secret to medicine in the new millennium.

Appendices

APPENDICES CONTENTS

Appendix 1

Dermatome charts

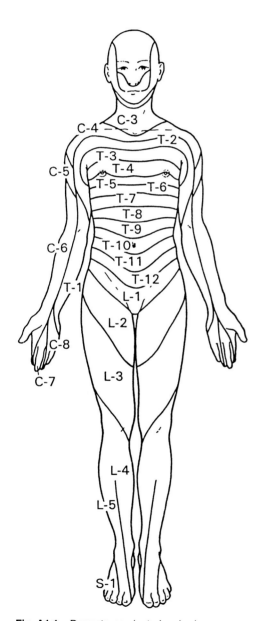

Fig. A1.1 Dermatomes (anterior view).

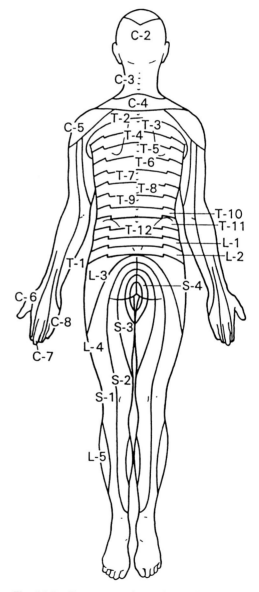

Fig. A1.2 Dermatomes (posterior view).

Meridian/channel charts

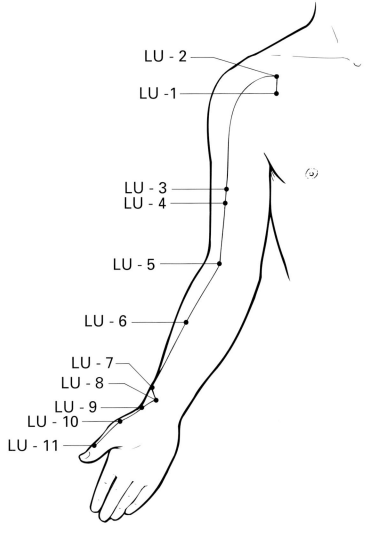

Fig. A2.1 The Lung channel.

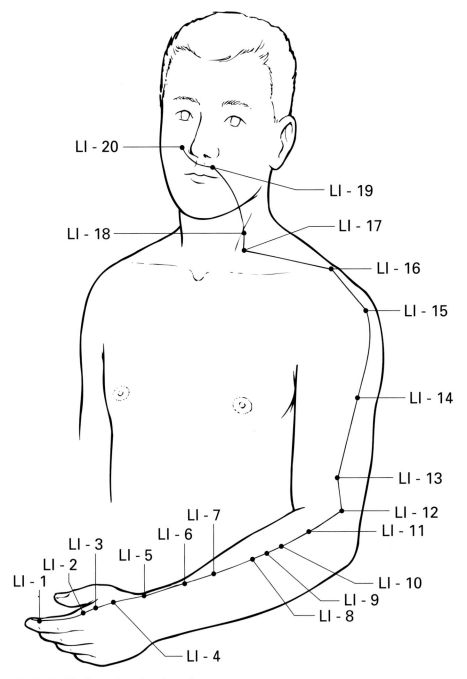

Fig. A2.2 The Large Intestine channel.

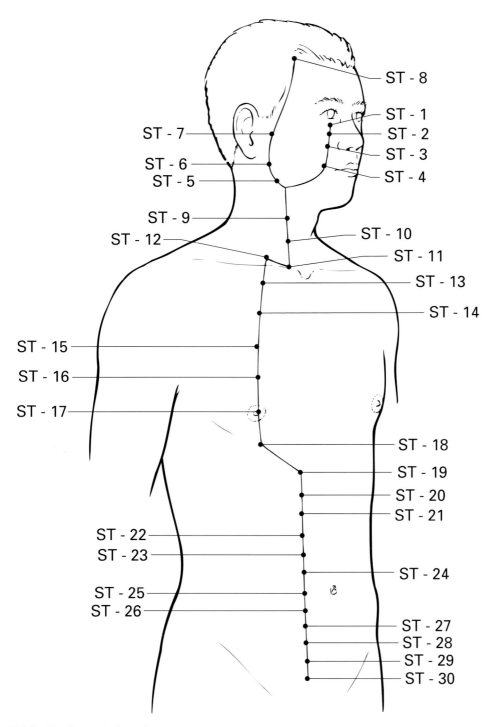

Fig. A2.3A   The Stomach channel.

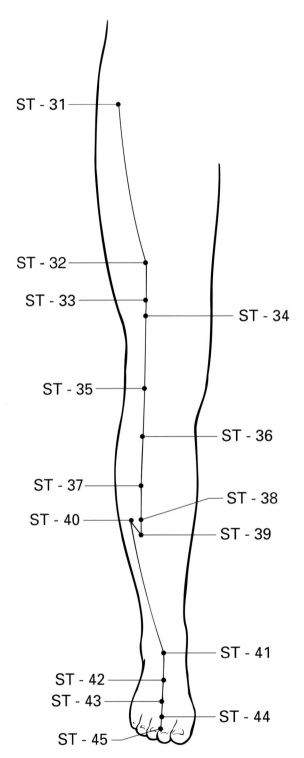

Fig. A2.3B The Stomach channel.

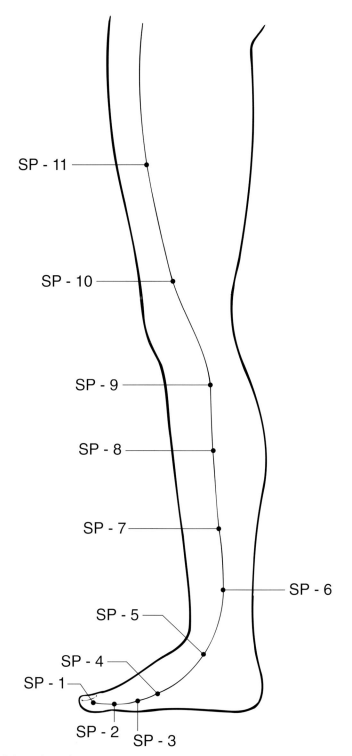

Fig. A2.4A   The Spleen channel.

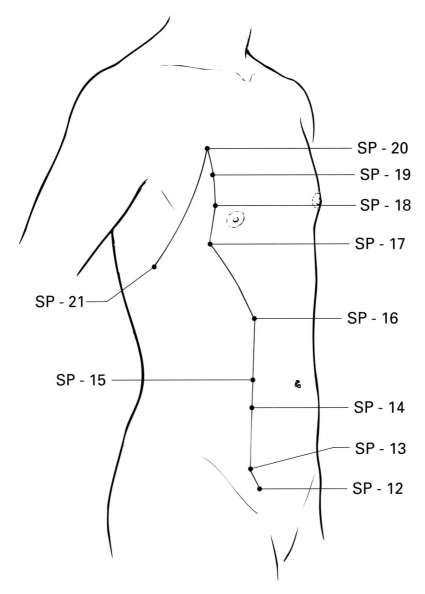

Fig. A2.4B The Spleen channel.

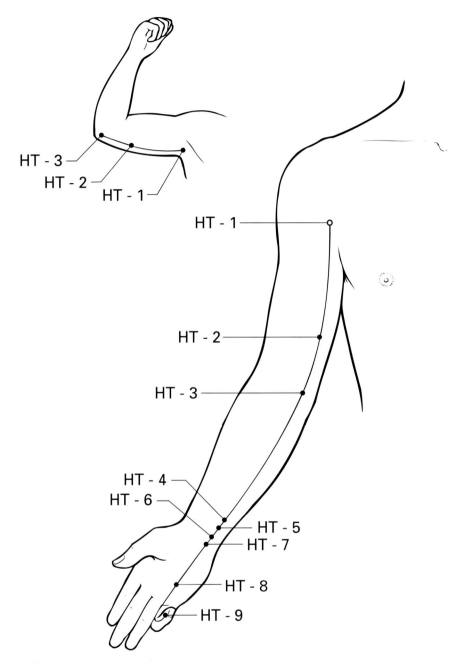

HT - 3

HT - 2

HT - 1

HT - 1

HT - 2

HT - 3

HT - 4

HT - 6

HT - 5

HT - 7

HT - 8

HT - 9

Fig. A2.5   The Heart channel.

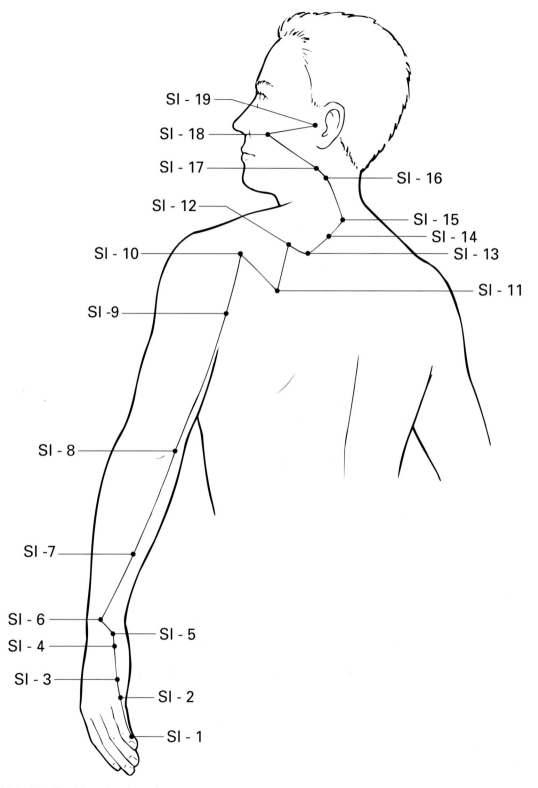

Fig. A2.6 The Small Intestine channel.

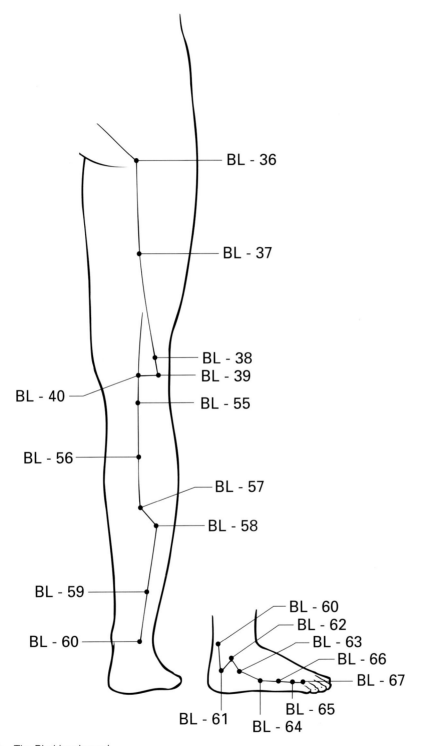

Fig. A2.7A The Bladder channel.

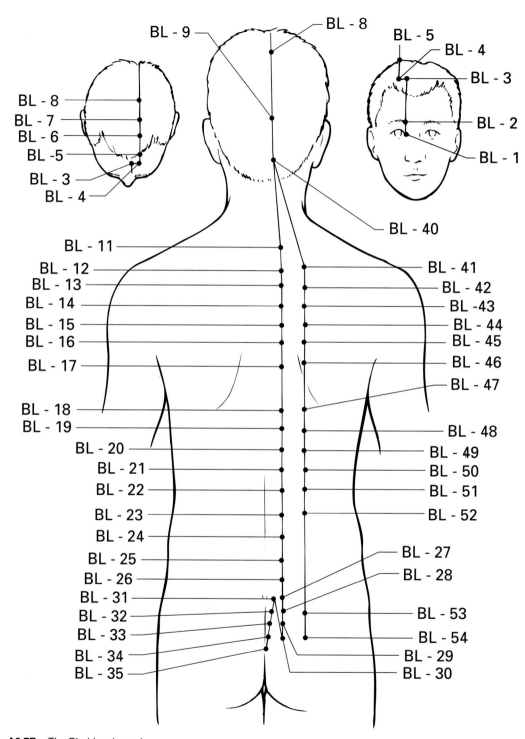

Fig. A2.7B The Bladder channel.

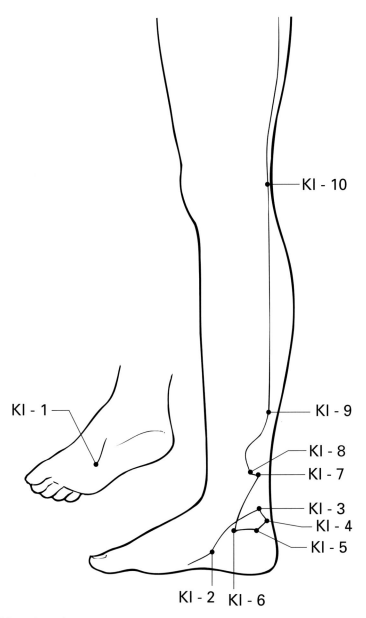

Fig. A2.8A The Kidney channel.

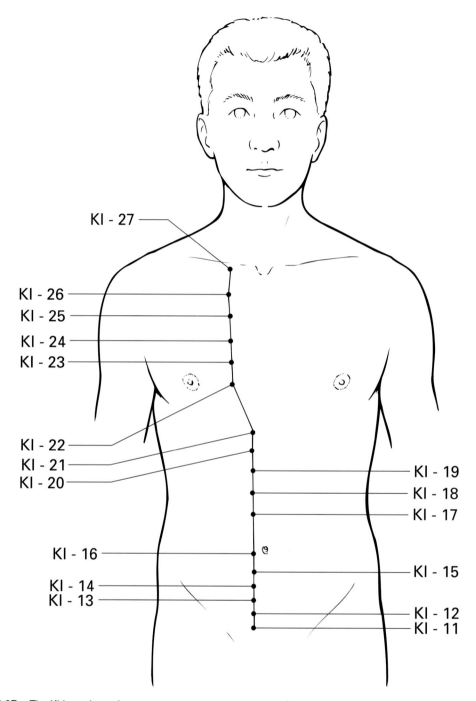

KI - 27
KI - 26
KI - 25
KI - 24
KI - 23
KI - 22
KI - 21
KI - 20
KI - 19
KI - 18
KI - 17
KI - 16
KI - 15
KI - 14
KI - 13
KI - 12
KI - 11

Fig. A2.8B The Kidney channel.

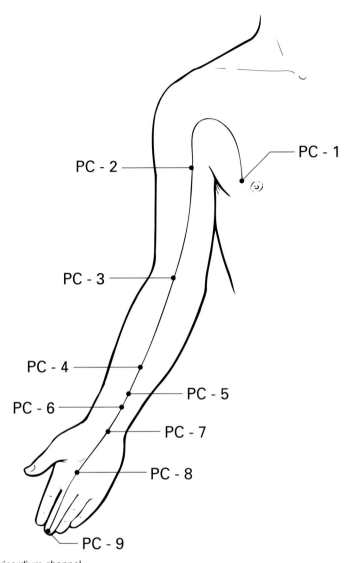

Fig. A2.9 The Pericardium channel.

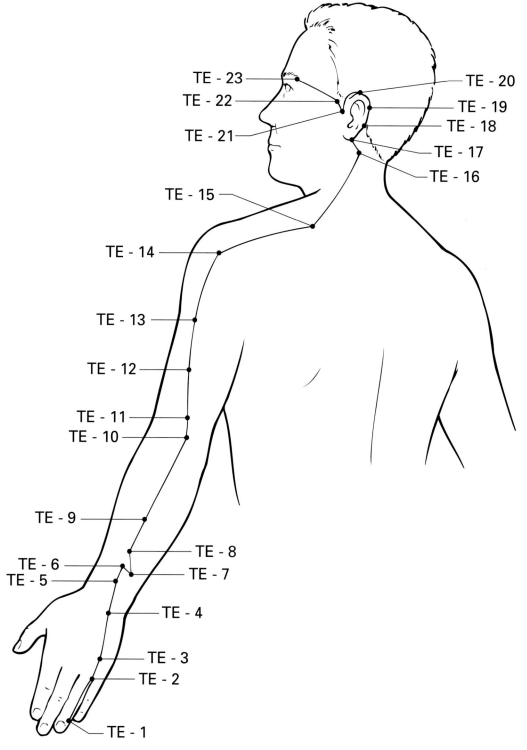

Fig. A2.10 The Triple Energizer channel.

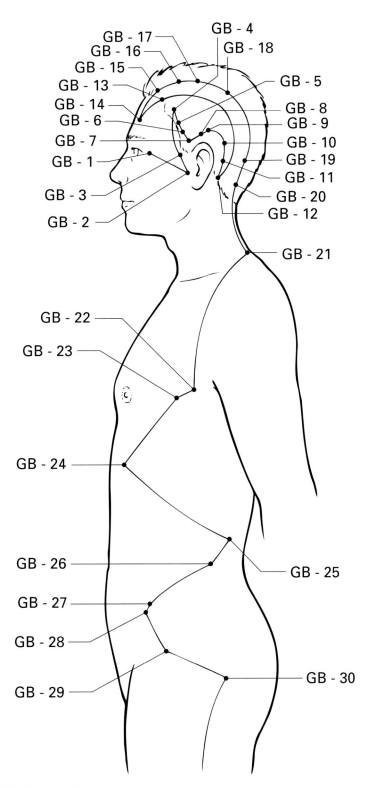

Fig. A2.11A   The Gall Bladder channel.

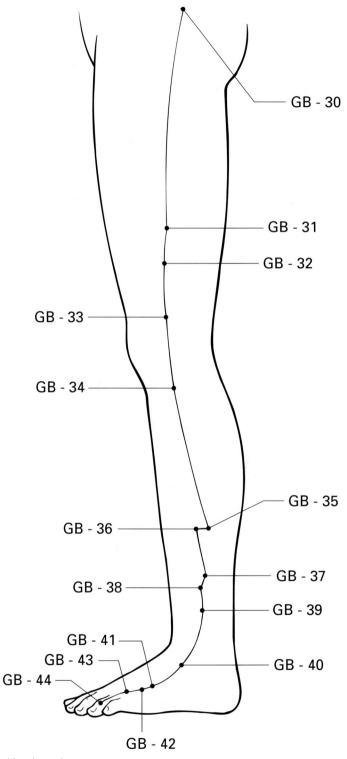

Fig. A2.11b The Gall Bladder channel.

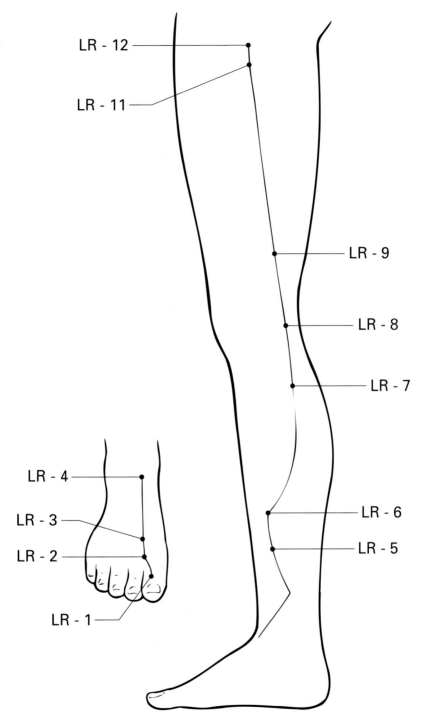

Fig. A2.12A   The Liver channel.

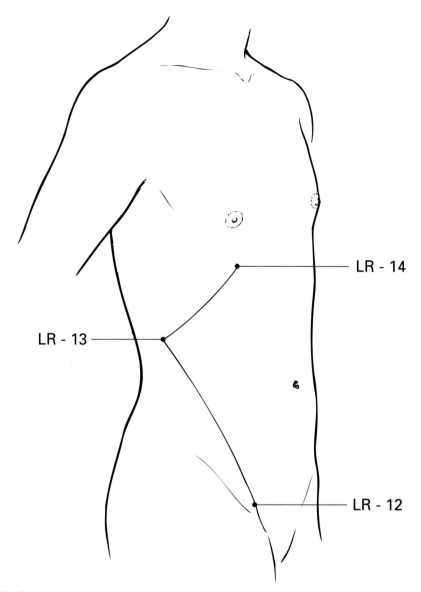

Fig. A2.12B The Liver channel

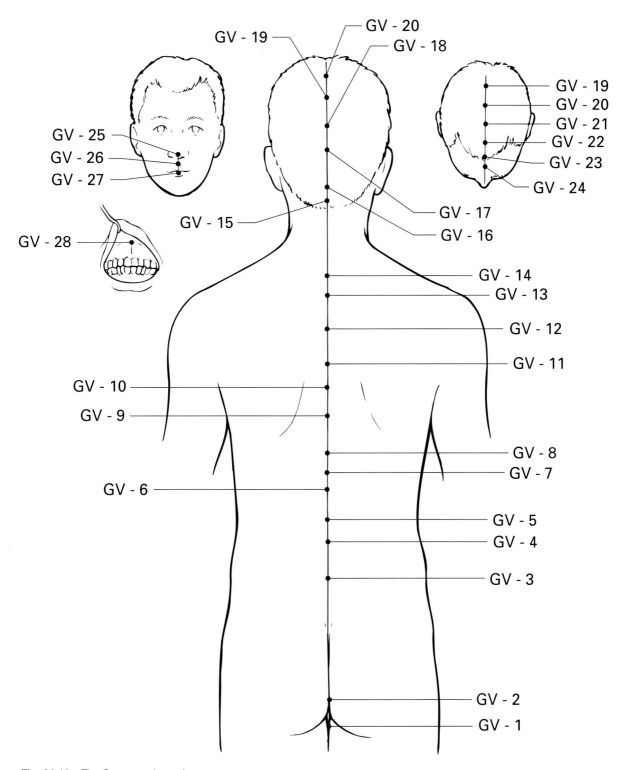

Fig. A2.13   The Governor channel.

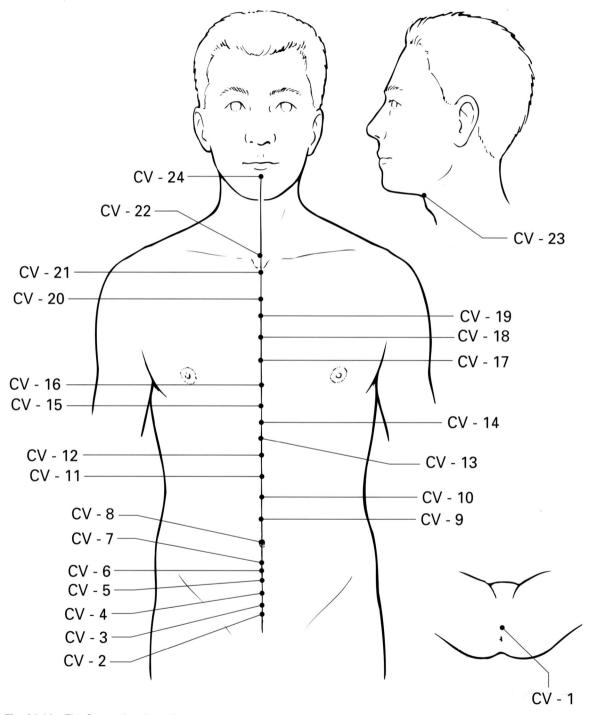

Fig. A2.14   The Conception channel.

Appendix 3

Standard international nomenclature for the 14 meridians

Name or meridian	Alphabetic code	
	Agreed	Former
Lung	LU	Lu, P
Large Intestine	LI	CO, Co, IC
Stomach	ST	S, St, E, M
Spleen	SP	Sp, LP
Heart	HT	H, C, Ht, He
Small Intestine	SI	Si, IT
Bladder	BL	B, Bi, UB
Kidney	KI	Ki, R, Rn
Pericardium	PC	P, Pe, HC
Triple Energizer	TE	T, TW, SJ 3H, TB
Gallbladder	GB	G, VB, VF
Liver	LR	Liv, LV, H
Governor Vessel	GV	Du, Du Go, Gv, TM
Conception Vessel	CV	Co, Cv, J, REN, Ren

Index